MEDICAL
DIAGNOSTICS

MEDICAL DIAGNOSTICS

Edited by

D. C. DUGDALE, M.D.

Assistant Professor of Medicine
University of Washington
Director, Internal Medicine Clinic
University of Washington Medical Center
Seattle, Washington

MICKEY S. EISENBERG, M.D., Ph.D.

Professor of Medicine
University of Washington
Director, Emergency Medicine Service
University of Washington Medical Center
Seattle, Washington

W.B. SAUNDERS COMPANY

Harcourt Brace Jovanovich, Inc.

Philadelphia, London, Toronto, Montreal, Sydney, Tokyo

W. B. SAUNDERS COMPANY
Harcourt Brace Jovanovich, Inc.

The Curtis Center
Independence Square West
Philadelphia, PA 19106

Library of Congress Cataloging-in-Publication Data

Medical diagnostics / editors, David C. Dugdale, Mickey
S. Eisenberg.
    p. cm.
    ISBN 0-7216-3499-0
    1. Diagnosis—Handbooks, manuals, etc.   I. Dugdale,
David C.
  II. Eisenberg, Mickey S.
    [DNLM: 1. Diagnosis. WB 141 M4888]
RC71.M453   1992
616.075—dc20
DNLM/DLC
for Library of Congress   91-37791
                                        CIP

Editor: John Dyson

MEDICAL DIAGNOSTICS   ISBN   0-7216-3499-0

Printed in the United States of America.

Last digit is the print
number: 9   8   7   6   5   4   3   2   1

To my parents, David and Barbara
Dugdale, and my wife, Colleen, and son,
Alex
D.C.D.

In memory of my father,
Louis Eisenberg
M.S.E.

CONTRIBUTORS

SAUNDRA N. AKER, R.D., C.D.

Clinical Instructor, Department of Physiological Nursing, University of Washington; Director, Clinical Nutrition Department, Fred Hutchinson Cancer Research Center, Seattle, Washington

Nutrition Assessment

RICHARD ALBERT, M.D.

Professor, Division of Pulmonary and Critical Care Medicine, Department of Medicine, University of Washington, Seattle, Washington

Tuberculosis

SCOTT BARNHART, M.D., M.P.H.

Associate Professor, Department of Medicine, University of Washington; Chief, Occupational Medicine Clinic, Harborview Medical Center, Seattle, Washington

Cough; Dyspnea; Hemoptysis; Pleural Effusions; Acute Respiratory Failure

DAVID BOLDT, M.D.

Professor and Chief, Division of Hematology, Department of Medicine, Health Science Center, University of Texas, San Antonio, Texas

Leukemia; Lymphoma

JAMES D. BOWEN, M.D.

Clinical Assistant Professor of Medicine; Chief, Division of Neurology, Pacific Medical Center, Seattle, Washington

Multiple Sclerosis; Neuropathy and Myopathy

EDWARD J. BOYKO, M.D., M.P.H.

Assistant Professor, Department of Medicine, University of Washington; Medical Service, Veterans Affairs Medical Center, Seattle, Washington

Principles of Diagnostic Testing

JAMES BRANAHL, M.D.

Clinical Associate Professor of Medicine, University of Washington; Director of Extended Care, Veterans Affairs Medical Center, Boise, Idaho

Urinary Incontinence

STUART L. BURSTEN, M.D.

Assistant Professor, Division of Nephrology, Department of Medicine, University of Washington; Research Associate Veterans Affairs Medical Center, Seattle, Washington

Electrolyte Disorders: Hyponatremia, Hypernatremia, Hypokalemia, and Hyperkalemia; Acute Renal Failure; Chronic Renal Failure

RICHARD C. CHERNY, M.D.

Senior Fellow, Division of Hematology, Department of Medicine, University of Washington, Seattle, Washington

Erythrocytosis

PETER COGGAN, M.D., M.S.Ed.

Associate Professor of Family and Community Medicine; Associate Dean for Medical Education, University of Nevada, Reno, Nevada

Alcoholism

CAROLYN COLLINS, M.D.

Assistant Professor, Division of Oncology, Department of Medicine, University of Washington, Seattle, Washington

Spinal Cord Compression; Localized Prostate Carcinoma

GEORGE J. COX, JR., M.D.

Clinical Instructor, Division of Gastroenterology, Department of Medicine, University of Washington, Seattle, Washington

Upper Gastrointestinal Disorders

MILES CRAMER, B.S., R.V.T.

Manager, Vascular Diagnostic Service, University of Washington Medical Center, Seattle, Washington

Acute Venous Thrombosis

JOSEPH J. CROWLEY, M.D.

Assistant Professor, Department of Medicine, University of Washington; Medical Service, Veterans Affairs Medical Center, Boise, Idaho

Pulmonary Embolism

RANDALL CULPEPPER, M.D., M.P.H.

Chief, Department of Occupational Health and Preventive Medicine, Naval Hospital, Great Lakes, Illinois

Lyme Disease

BARRY J. CUSACK, M.D., F.R.C.P.I.

Associate Professor, Department of Medicine, University of Washington; Chief, Geriatrics Section, Veterans Affairs Medical Center, Boise, Idaho

Dementia

ANDREW K. DIEHL, M.D., M.Sc.

Professor and Chief, Division of General Medicine, Department of Medicine, Health Science Center at San Antonio, University of Texas, San Antonio, Texas

Gallbladder Diseases

ROBERT DREISIN, M.D.

Clinical Associate Professor of Medicine, Oregon Health Sciences University; The Thoracic Clinic, Portland, Oregon

Chronic Interstitial Pneumonitis

DAVID C. DUGDALE, M.D.

Assistant Professor, Department of Medicine, University of Washington, Seattle, Washington

Fatigue; Acid-Base Disorders; Fever of Unknown Origin; Infectious Mononucleosis

CARIN E. DUGOWSON, M.D., M.P.H.

Assistant Professor of Medicine, University of Washington; Chief, Division of Rheumatology, Department of Medicine, Pacific Medical Center, Seattle, Washington

Polyarthritis; Osteoarthritis

MICKEY EISENBERG, M.D., Ph.D.

Professor, Department of Medicine, University of Washington; Director, Emergency Medicine Services, University of Washington Medical Center, Seattle, Washington

Diabetes Mellitus; Sexually Transmitted Diseases; Urinary Tract Infections

GEORGIANA ELLIS, M.D.

Acting Assistant Professor, Division of Oncology, Department of Medicine, University of Washington, Seattle, Washington

Cancer of Unknown Primary Site

RONALD H. FRIED, M.D.

Senior Fellow, Division of Gastroenterology, Department of Medicine, University of Washington, Seattle, Washington

Chronic Diarrhea

WILFRED Y. FUJIMOTO, M.D.

Professor, Division of Metabolism, Endocrinology & Nutrition, Department of Medicine, University of Washington, Seattle, Washington

Adrenal Gland Diseases

GREGORY C. GARDNER, M.D.

Assistant Professor, Division of Rheumatology, Department of Medicine, University of Washington, Seattle, Washington

Vasculitis

BRUCE GILLILAND, M.D.

Professor, Department of Medicine; Associate Dean for Clinical Affairs, University of Washington, Seattle, Washington

Spondyloarthropathies; Systemic Lupus Erythematosus; Systemic Sclerosis

JOHN HALSEY, M.D.

Senior Fellow, Division of Gastroenterology, Department of Medicine, University of Washington, Seattle, Washington

Abdominal Pain; Malabsorption; Pancreatitis; Hepatomegaly

JAN HILLSON, M.D.

Assistant Professor, Division of Rheumatology, Department of Medicine, University of Washington, Seattle, Washington

Arthralgias and Myalgias

DAVID HINDSON, M.D.

Clinical Professor of Medicine, University of Washington; Chief, Medical Service; Veterans Affairs Medical Center, Boise, Idaho

Hirsutism; Pheochromocytoma

MARY T. HO, M.D., M.P.H.

Assistant Professor, Department of Medicine, University of Washington, Seattle, Washington

Chest Pain and Angina

GEOFFREY JIRANEK, M.D.

Clinical Assistant Professor of Medicine, University of Washington; Department of Medicine, Virginia Mason Medical Center, Seattle, Washington

Gastrointestinal Bleeding; Colorectal Cancer

ELAINE C. JONG, M.D.

Associate Professor, Department of Medicine, University of Washington; Co-director, Travel Medicine Service, University of Washington Medical Center, Seattle, Washington

Malaria and the Febrile Patient from the Tropics

MITCHELL KARTON, M.D.

Seattle Medical Associates, Seattle, Washington

Amenorrhea; Thyroid Disease; Disorders of Serum Calcium Concentration

ARTHUR KELLERMAN, M.D., M.P.H.

Associate Professor and Chief, Division of Emergency Medicine, Department of Medicine, Center for Health Sciences, University of Tennessee, Memphis, Tennessee

Coma; Delirium

MICHAEL KIMMEY, M.D.

Assistant Professor, Division of Gastroenterology, Department of Medicine, University of Washington, Seattle, Washington

Abdominal Pain; Malabsorption; Pancreatitis; Hepatomegaly

THOMAS R. KLUMPP, M.D.

Assistant Professor of Medicine; Assistant Director, Bone Marrow Transplant Unit, Temple University Medical Center, Philadelphia, Pennsylvania

Anemia

THOMAS D. KOEPSELL, M.D., M.P.H.

Professor, Department of Epidemiology and Health Services; Adjunct Professor, Department of Medicine, University of Washington, Seattle, Washington

Polyarthritis; Osteoarthritis

JEFFREY B. KOPP, M.D.

Staff Fellow, National Institute of Dental Research, National Institute of Health, Bethesda, Maryland

Acute Glomerulonephritis and the Nephritic Syndrome

SHOBA KRISHNAMURTHY, M.D., M.B.B.S.

Clinical Associate Professor of Medicine, University of Washington; Division of Gastroenterology, Pacific Medical Center, Seattle, Washington

Constipation

PETER KUDENCHUK, M.D.

Assistant Professor, Division of Cardiology, Department of Medicine, University of Washington, Seattle, Washington

Palpitations and Cardiac Arrhythmias

DAVID K. LEE, M.D.

Clinical Associate Professor of Medicine, University of Washington; Associate Chief of Staff for Ambulatory Care, Veterans Affairs Medical Center, Boise, Idaho

Hyperlipidemia

JANE LEMAIRE, M.D., F.R.C.P.C.

Assistant Professor, Department of Medicine, University of Calgary, Calgary, Alberta, Canada

Hematuria

KEITH LEYDEN, M.D.

Acting Instructor, Department of Medicine, University of Washington, Seattle, Washington

Myocardial Infarction; Bronchitis and Pneumonia

RUSSELL MCMULLEN, M.D.

Assistant Professor, Department of Medicine, University of Washington; Co-director, Travel Medicine Service, University of Washington Medical Center, Seattle, Washington

Malaria and the Febrile Patient from the Tropics; Viral Hepatitis

CHRISTINA M. MARRA, M.D.

Acting Instructor, Division of Neurology, Department of Medicine, University of Washington, Seattle, Washington

Meningitis and Encephalitis

THOMAS R. MARTIN, M.D.

Associate Professor of Medicine, University of Washington, Division of Respiratory Disease, Veterans Affairs Medical Center, Seattle, Washington

Chronic Obstructive Pulmonary Disease

RICHARD MAUNDER, M.D.

Clinical Associate Professor of Medicine, University of Washington; Director, Pulmonary and Critical Care Services, Swedish Hospital Medical Center, Seattle, Washington

Adult Respiratory Distress Syndrome

TERRY J. MENGERT, M.D.

Assistant Professor, Department of Medicine, University of Washington, Seattle, Washington

Mediastinal Masses; Syncope

TIM OBERMILLER, M.D.

Senior Fellow, Division of Pulmonary and Critical Care Medicine, Department of Medicine, University of Washington, Seattle, Washington

Asthma; Sarcoidosis

DOUGLAS S. PAAUW, M.D.

Assistant Professor, Department of Medicine, University of Washington, Seattle, Washington

Otitis, Pharyngitis, and Sinusitis; Skin Infections; Infectious Diarrhea; Septic Arthritis and Osteomyelitis; Acquired Immunodeficiency Syndrome (AIDS); Chronic Hepatitis

BEVERLY M. PARKER, M.D.

Fellow in Geriatric Medicine, University of Washington; Medical Service, Veterans Affairs Medical Center, Boise, Idaho

Dementia

STEPHEN PETERSDORF, M.D.

Assistant Professor, Division of Oncology, Department of Medicine, University of Washington, Seattle, Washington

Hemostatic Disorders

JULIA PHISTER, M.D.

Clinical Assistant Professor of Medicine, University of Washington; Medical Service, Veterans Affairs Medical Center, Boise, Idaho

Multiple Myeloma

OLIVER W. PRESS, M.D., Ph.D.

Associate Professor, Division of Oncology, Department of Medicine, University of Washington, Seattle, Washington

Lymphadenopathy; Fever in the Immunocompromised Host

GANESH RAGHU, M.D.

Associate Professor, Division of Pulmonary and Critical Care Medicine, University of Washington, Seattle, Washington

Sarcoidosis

MERRIT T. RAITT, M.D.

Senior Fellow, Division of Cardiology, Department of Medicine, University of Washington, Seattle, Washington

Valvular Heart Disease

PAUL G. RAMSEY, M.D.

Professor and Acting Chairman, Department of Medicine, University of Washington, Seattle, Washington

Otitis, Pharyngitis, and Sinusitis; Skin Infections; Infectious Diarrhea; Septic Arthritis and Osteomyelitis

RAYMOND G. RAMUSACK, M.D.

Acting Instructor, Department of Medicine, University of Washington, Seattle, Washington

Urolithiasis

CARRIE A. REDLICH, M.D., M.P.H.

Assistant Professor of Medicine, Occupational and Environmental Medicine Program, Yale University, New Haven, Connecticut

Clinical Approach to Occupational Medicine

NORMAN R. ROSENTHAL, M.D.

Clinical Assistant Professor of Medicine, University of Washington; Section of Endocrinology and Diabetes, Virginia Mason Medical Center, Seattle, Washington

Metabolic Bone Disease

CURTIS SAUER, M.D.

Clinical Assistant Professor of Neurology, Hahnemann School of Medicine; Staff Neurologist, Veterans Affairs Medical Center, Wilkes-Barre, Pennsylvania

Coma; Delirium

ANTHONY SAWAY, M.D.

Rheumatology Associates, Birmingham, Alabama

Gout and Pseudogout; Polymyositis and Dermatomyositis

C. SCOTT SMITH, M.D.

Acting Instructor of Medicine, University of Washington; Medical Service, Veterans Affairs Medical Center, Boise, Idaho

Hypertension; Congestive Heart Failure; Infective Endocarditis

JEAN M. STERN, M.S., R.D., C.D.

Outpatient Nutrition Manager, Fred Hutchinson Cancer Research Center, Seattle, Washington

Nutrition Assessment

SUSAN STOVER-DALTON, M.D.

Hall Health Center, University of Washington, Seattle, Washington

Breast Nodules and Cancer

CHRISTINA M. SURAWICZ, M.D.

Associate Professor, Division of Gastroenterology, Department of Medicine, University of Washington, Seattle, Washington

Chronic Diarrhea; Idiopathic Inflammatory Bowel Disease

PHILLIP D. SWANSON, M.D., Ph.D.

Professor and Chief, Division of Neurology, Department of Medicine, University of Washington, Seattle Washington

Cerebrovascular Disease

JAMES TAYLOR, M.D.

Consultant in Pulmonary and Critical Care Medicine, Tacoma General Hospital, Tacoma, Washington

Solitary Pulmonary Nodule

HASI M. VENKATACHALAM, M.B., B.S., M.P.H.

Clinical Associate Professor, Division of General Medicine, Department of Medicine, Health Science Center at San Antonio, University of Texas, San Antonio, Texas

Headache

ALAN WATSON, M.D.

Associate Professor of Medicine, Division of Nephrology, The Johns Hopkins Hospital, Baltimore, Maryland

Nephrotic Syndrome

RICHARD A. WILLSON, M.D.

Associate Professor of Medicine, Division of Gastroenterology, Department of Medicine, University of Washington, Seattle, Washington

Jaundice

PREFACE

A good clinician has to be a good diagnostician. From the diagnosis all else flows. How do doctors reach this diagnosis? Clinical studies over many years suggest that good diagnosticians carefully follow a sequence of steps.

The first involves gathering clinical information (history, physical examination, laboratory results, imaging results, etc.). The second, which occurs simultaneously with the first, involves a consideration of possible diagnoses.

The physician begins to consider possible diagnoses upon entering the examining room and seeing the patient. Some diseases can be diagnosed almost at a glance, and the process can stop here. More likely, a third step is reached, in which diagnostic possibilities must be evaluated or refined. Further questions about the patient's history and additional laboratory tests or other studies allow this process to proceed. Clinicians use pattern-matching or feature-matching as a central strategy in this step. Features from the patient's history and laboratory data are matched against the doctor's mental picture of various possible diagnoses. Good clinicians can simultaneously weigh several diagnostic possibilities and "argue with themselves" for and against each one. Also factored in this "argument" are the probabilities of each diagnosis. The axiom that common diseases *are* common ("when hearing hoofbeats don't look for zebras") is true up to a point. Determining when that point is reached (i.e., when do less common diseases become serious contenders?) is part of the challenge of medical diagnosis.

The fourth step involves the selection of a tentative diagnosis. From the previous gathering of information, consideration of possible diagnoses, feature-matching, and factoring in probabilities, a diagnosis is reached. It should be stressed that these diagnostic steps are not a rigid sequence that must be slavishly adhered to. Rather, the process is a dynamic one, constantly flowing back and forth as new information is gathered and tentative diagnoses are considered.

Once a diagnosis is reached, the process does not end. As more information is obtained or as the physician learns more about a disease, the diagnosis may well be altered.

The dimension of time is another important ingredient in reaching a diagnosis. Time can be an ally, especially when the diagnosis is not immediately evident. A common failing among inexperienced clinicians is the urge to make a diagnosis when a reasonable diagnosis is not yet possible. Assuming a stable clinical situation, it is often useful to let the passage of time allow the problem either to declare itself or to resolve. It is OK to tell a patient that "it is not possible to reach a diagnosis this soon."

Despite all of the above, remember that the diagnostic process is not a straightforward, quantifiable sequence that can be easily taught or even programmed into a computer. Characterizing the steps of diagnosis is merely a way to organize a very complex and admittedly poorly understood phenomenon. The *science* of diagnosis must be combined with the *art* of diagnosis. Why are some physicians better than others at reaching correct diagnoses? Why, with the same information available, will two competent physicians reach two different diagnoses? Is the art of diagnosis related to experience, better ability to match diseases with symptoms, better knowledge about probabilities, different thresholds for reaching a decision with inadequate information, or just common sense?

Whatever the science and art of diagnosis may involve, we hope that this book will help physicians become better diagnosticians and thereby better clinicians. This book is intended as a handy companion that will provide a ready source of information. It should complement a manual of medical therapeutics.

We follow a time-honored approach and outline the most frequent signs, symptoms, and laboratory findings for various diseases. For each problem and diagnosis we have gathered, whenever possible, consensus statements of diagnostic criteria. Today many task forces, quality assurance committees, and consensus panels have attempted to define criteria for making selected diagnoses. Similarly, they often recommend specific laboratory and imaging studies. We have researched and presented these recommendations for as many problems and diseases as possible.

But we have attempted something more. We have supplied additional information to assist the clinician in the crucial third step of the diagnostic process: the evaluation of possible diagnoses. We have provided expected incidences and prevalences, quantitative differential diagnoses, and a critical appraisal of laboratory and imaging information.

The clinician must not only know the classic description of diseases and problems presented here, but must also consider competing explanations. This requires an understanding of possible diagnoses. Unfortunately, most books on differential diagnosis fail to supply information about the expected frequencies of the diseases contained within a differential diagnosis. Whenever possible, our contributors have supplied quantitative information about differential diagnoses. Often this takes the form of a simple statement of disease incidence, which is valuable information for diagnostic decision-making.

For every disease or condition we include a *recommended diagnostic approach*. Instead of including a simple list of recommended laboratory evaluations, we try to evaluate tests on the grounds of their reliability, accuracy, predictive values, sensitivity, and specificity. Unfortunately, many data for this task are not yet available. Perhaps this handbook will encourage others to perform needed evaluations of diagnostic technology.

We hope this book will assist physicians in problem-solving and help them to arrive at more discriminating diagnoses.

CONTENTS

SECTION I
GENERAL

1
PRINCIPLES OF DIAGNOSTIC TESTING   3
Edward J. Boyko

2
FATIGUE   9
David C. Dugdale

3
CONSTIPATION   14
Shoba Krishnamurthy

4
CHRONIC DIARRHEA   19
Ronald H. Fried and Christina M. Surawicz

5
COUGH   25
Scott Barnhart

6
URINARY INCONTINENCE   28
James Branahl

7
HYPERTENSION   32
C. Scott Smith

8
ELECTROLYTE DISORDERS: HYPONATREMIA, HYPERNATREMIA, HYPOKALEMIA, AND HYPERKALEMIA   39
Stuart L. Bursten

9
ACID-BASE DISORDERS   48
David C. Dugdale

SECTION II
CARDIOLOGY

10

CHEST PAIN AND ANGINA   59
Mary T. Ho

11

CONGESTIVE HEART FAILURE   77
C. Scott Smith

12

PALPITATIONS AND CARDIAC ARRHYTHMIAS   85
Peter Kudenchuk

13

MYOCARDIAL INFARCTION   116
Keith Leyden

14

VALVULAR HEART DISEASE   134
Merritt Raitt

SECTION III
PULMONARY

15

DYSPNEA   155
Scott Barnhart

16

HEMOPTYSIS   158
Scott Barnhart

17

PLEURAL EFFUSIONS   162
Scott Barnhart

18

ACUTE RESPIRATORY FAILURE   167
Scott Barnhart

19

SOLITARY PULMONARY NODULE   171
James Taylor

20

MEDIASTINAL MASSES   178
Terry J. Mengert

21

ASTHMA 184
Tim Obermiller

22

CHRONIC OBSTRUCTIVE PULMONARY DISEASE 189
Thomas R. Martin

23

PULMONARY EMBOLISM 193
Joseph J. Crowley

24

ACUTE VENOUS THROMBOSIS 198
Miles Cramer

25

ADULT RESPIRATORY DISTRESS SYNDROME 204
Richard Maunder

26

CHRONIC INTERSTITIAL PNEUMONITIS 208
Robert Dreisin

27

SARCOIDOSIS 217
Tim Obermiller and Ganesh Raghu

**SECTION IV
RENAL**

28

HEMATURIA 229
Jane Lemaire

29

ACUTE RENAL FAILURE 236
Stuart L. Bursten

30

CHRONIC RENAL FAILURE 245
Stuart L. Bursten

31

NEPHROTIC SYNDROME 251
Alan Watson

32

ACUTE GLOMERULONEPHRITIS AND THE
NEPHRITIC SYNDROME 257
Jeffrey B. Kopp

33

UROLITHIASIS 264
Raymond G. Ramusack

**SECTION V
GASTROINTESTINAL**

34

ABDOMINAL PAIN 279
John Halsey and Michael Kimmey

35

GASTROINTESTINAL BLEEDING 289
Geoffrey Jiranek

36

UPPER GASTROINTESTINAL DISORDERS 297
George J. Cox, Jr.

37

MALABSORPTION 306
John Halsey and Michael Kimmey

38

IDIOPATHIC INFLAMMATORY BOWEL DISEASE 323
Christina M. Surawicz

39

COLORECTAL CANCER 330
Geoffrey Jiranek

40

PANCREATITIS 337
John Halsey and Michael Kimmey

**SECTION VI
HEMATOLOGY**

41

ANEMIA 347
Thomas R. Klumpp

42

ERYTHROCYTOSIS 355
Richard C. Cherny

43

HEMOSTATIC DISORDERS 361
Stephen Petersdorf

44

LYMPHADENOPATHY 374
Oliver W. Press

45

LEUKEMIA 381
David Boldt

46

LYMPHOMAS 389
David Boldt

47

MULTIPLE MYELOMA 396
Julia Phister

SECTION VII
ONCOLOGY

48

SPINAL CORD COMPRESSION 405
Carolyn Collins

49

BREAST NODULES AND CANCER 411
Susan Stover-Dalton

50

LOCALIZED PROSTATE CARCINOMA 420
Carolyn Collins

51

CANCER OF UNKNOWN PRIMARY SITE 426
Georgiana Ellis

SECTION VIII
ENDOCRINOLOGY

52

HIRSUTISM 435
David Hindson

53

AMENORRHEA 443
Mitchell Karton

54

METABOLIC BONE DISEASE 453
Norman R. Rosenthal

55

THYROID DISEASE   461
Mitchell Karton

56

ADRENAL GLAND DISEASES   473
Wilfred Y. Fujimoto

57

PHEOCHROMOCYTOMA   485
David Hindson

58

DISORDERS OF SERUM CALCIUM CONCENTRATION 490
Mitchell Karton

59

DIABETES MELLITUS   498
Mickey Eisenberg

60

HYPERLIPIDEMIA   512
David K. Lee

SECTION IX
NUTRITION

61

NUTRITION ASSESSMENT   519
Jean M. Stern and Saundra N. Aker

SECTION X
INFECTIOUS DISEASES

62

FEVER OF UNKNOWN ORIGIN   533
David C. Dugdale

63

FEVER IN THE IMMUNOCOMPROMISED HOST   542
Oliver W. Press

64

OTITIS, PHARYNGITIS, AND SINUSITIS   552
Paul G. Ramsey and Douglas S. Paauw

65

BRONCHITIS AND PNEUMONIA   560
Keith Leyden

66

TUBERCULOSIS 574
Richard Albert

67

INFECTIVE ENDOCARDITIS 579
C. Scott Smith

68

SKIN INFECTIONS 590
Paul G. Ramsey and Douglas S. Paauw

69

SEXUALLY TRANSMITTED DISEASES 594
Mickey Eisenberg

70

URINARY TRACT INFECTIONS 610
Mickey Eisenberg

71

INFECTIOUS DIARRHEA 615
Paul G. Ramsey and Douglas S. Paauw

72

SEPTIC ARTHRITIS AND OSTEOMYELITIS 622
Paul G. Ramsey and Douglas S. Paauw

73

MENINGITIS AND ENCEPHALITIS 629
Christina M. Marra

74

ACQUIRED IMMUNODEFICIENCY SYNDROME 639
Douglas S. Paauw

75

MALARIA AND THE FEBRILE PATIENT FROM
THE TROPICS 653
Elaine C. Jong and Russell McMullen

76

LYME DISEASE 662
Randall Culpepper

77

INFECTIOUS MONONUCLEOSIS 668
David C. Dugdale

SECTION XI
RHEUMATOLOGY

78
ARTHRALGIAS AND MYALGIAS 675
Jan Hillson

79
POLYARTHRITIS 689
Carin E. Dugowson and Thomas D. Koepsell

80
OSTEOARTHRITIS 697
Carin E. Dugowson and Thomas D. Koepsell

81
GOUT AND PSEUDOGOUT 701
Anthony Saway

82
SPONDYLOARTHROPATHIES 709
Bruce Gilliland

83
SYSTEMIC LUPUS ERYTHEMATOSUS 718
Bruce Gilliland

84
POLYMYOSITIS AND DERMATOMYOSITIS 728
Anthony Saway

85
SYSTEMIC SCLEROSIS (SCLERODERMA) 733
Bruce Gilliland

86
VASCULITIS 738
Gregory C. Gardner

SECTION XII
NEUROLOGY

87
COMA 749
Arthur Kellerman and Curtis Sauer

88
SYNCOPE 761
Terry J. Mengert

89

DELIRIUM   769
Arthur Kellerman and Curtis Sauer

90

DEMENTIA   776
Beverly M. Parker and Barry J. Cusack

91

HEADACHE   784
Hasi M. Venkatachalam

92

CEREBROVASCULAR DISEASE   792
Phillip D. Swanson

93

MULTIPLE SCLEROSIS   799
James D. Bowen

94

NEUROPATHY AND MYOPATHY   804
James D. Bowen

95

ALCOHOLISM   812
Peter Coggan

**SECTION XIII
HEPATOLOGY**

96

JAUNDICE   821
Richard A. Willson

97

HEPATOMEGALY   827
John Halsey and Michael Kimmey

98

VIRAL HEPATITIS   833
Russell McMullen

99

CHRONIC HEPATITIS   852
Douglas S. Paauw

100

GALLBLADDER DISEASES   857
Andrew K. Diehl

SECTION XIV
OCCUPATIONAL MEDICINE

101

CLINICAL APPROACH TO OCCUPATIONAL
MEDICINE   865

Carrie A. Redlich

**APPENDIX: SELECTED NORMAL RANGES FOR
LABORATORY TESTS**   876

INDEX   883

SECTION I

GENERAL

PRINCIPLES OF DIAGNOSTIC TESTING

EDWARD J. BOYKO

The diagnosis of disease is often easy; often difficult, and often impossible.

PETER MERE LATHAM (1789–1875)

HOW DOES A PHYSICIAN MAKE A MEDICAL DIAGNOSIS?

A physician makes a medical diagnosis when the available information supports it.

When uncertain, a physician collects additional information to assist in the diagnostic process. In some cases, additional data are collected to help generate a hypothesis for the patient's problem. For example, a physician may order a complete blood count (CBC), chemistry panels, or a chest X-ray in a patient who presents with vague complaints such as fatigue or non–organ-specific findings such as unexplained weight loss. An abnormal finding on these "hypothesis-generating" panels of tests may lead eventually to the cause of the patient's problem.

However, this use of diagnostic testing can be overdone, particularly by physicians with little experience. An extensive hypothesis-generating diagnostic test protocol only rarely benefits the patient, and may in fact be responsible for much harm if dangerous diagnostic procedures are performed in response to results on tests that should not have been ordered in the first place. Thus it is important to know when to *stop* ordering diagnostic tests.

When expert internists (as judged by their peers) were compared to other internists, the diagnostic practice that distinguished the experts from the merely capable was their tendency to formulate, test, and reject hypotheses regarding the presence of a particular disease. For example, when evaluating the cause of chest pain in a 40-year-old man, the expert internist might postulate that myocardial ischemia is the root problem, and then go on to elicit the data necessary to test this hypothesis. This diagnostic method is called "hypothetico-deductive."

HOW IS DIAGNOSTIC TEST QUALITY EVALUATED?

If a diagnostic test were perfect, a positive test would mean that a disease is present (probability = 1), and a negative test would mean that a disease is absent (probability = 0). It is important to recognize that diagnostic tests rarely establish disease presence or absence beyond doubt, as seeking certainty in medical diagnosis is usually an exercise in frustration that may even harm patients. The level of certainty required varies by disease and depends on the costs and benefits of correctly treating the diseased and incorrectly treating the nondiseased.

For example, a physician evaluating a patient with chest pain may admit the patient to the coronary care unit for evaluation even if the probability of myocardial infarction (MI) is quite low (10%), because the potential harm due to missed treatment of this condition may far outweigh the costs in dollars and patient morbidity and mortality due to unnecessary admission for intensive monitoring. On the other hand, a physician who is trying to decide whether a patient with lymphadenopathy has lymphoma or a benign, self-limited cause of this condition may only begin treatment for lymphoma when the probability of malignancy has crossed a very high threshold (95%).

Few decision probability thresholds have been well described. They may differ from one disease to the next and also may differ depending on the opinion of the patient about the relative value of expected treatment benefits versus potential risks. Patient values regarding the outcome of treatments are important. For example, a patient may prefer a treatment of laryngeal cancer associated with a shorter life expectancy (radiation) but preservation of speech compared to surgical treatment leading to a longer life expectancy but inability to speak (laryngectomy).

MEASURES OF DIAGNOSTIC TEST QUALITY

The ability of a diagnostic test to determine the probability of disease presence if positive or negative depends on its sensitivity and specificity. *Sensitivity* is defined as the percentage of persons with the disease who test positive, while *specificity* is the percentage of nondiseased persons who test negative. Therefore, if a very specific test is positive, the presence of disease is highly likely, because few nondiseased subjects will test positive on a test of very high specificity. Also, when a very sensitive test is negative, the presence of disease is very unlikely, because almost all diseased subjects will test positive.

Diagnostic test sensitivity and specificity are related to the more clinically useful probabilities of whether a patient does or does not have disease. The positive predictive value (PPV) of a diagnostic test is the probability of disease given a positive test result, while the negative predictive value (NPV) is the probability of no disease given a negative test result.

An alternate concept to the PPV and NPV is the posttest disease likelihood, which is the probability of disease given a positive or negative test result. For example, the posttest likelihood of a positive test is the number of diseased with a positive test result divided by the number of diseased and

TABLE 1–1.

| TEST RESULT | DISEASE | |
	Present	Absent
Positive	a	b
Negative	c	d
Total	n	m

Test sensitivity = a/n
Test specificity = d/m
Pretest disease probability = n/(n + m)
Posttest disease probability, positive test = a/(a + b)
Posttest disease probability, negative test = c/(c + d)

nondiseased with a positive test result, while the posttest likelihood of a negative test result is the number of diseased with a negative test result divided by the number of diseased and nondiseased with a negative test result (see Table 1–1).

The patients in Table 1–2 have a disease probability ("pretest probability") of 0.5. When the results of the diagnostic test are known, a positive test result makes the presence of disease likely (0.78); a negative test result reduces the disease probability (0.27). If a disease probability of 0.78 exceeds the physician's threshold for further testing or treatment, then the diagnostic test has aided in the diagnostic process in this example. In addition, a disease probability of 0.27 may allow the physician to withhold further testing or treatment.

A disease probability of 0.27 *may* be *high* enough to justify treatment where the costs of not administering treatment outweigh the costs of unnecessary treatment (e.g., MI). In this situation, the diagnostic test should never have been performed, since the management decision would have been the same regardless of test outcome.

The pretest disease probability has a crucial effect on the interpretation of diagnostic test results (Table 1–3). In example A, the pretest probability of disease is low. When the diagnostic test is performed, the posttest disease probability, whether the test is positive or negative, is still very low, and possibly below the threshold for further action. In example B, the posttest probability is high even when the test is negative—possibly high enough to mandate further testing or treatment. In general, the probability of disease *after the test* depends greatly on the pretest probability.

HOW IS "NORMAL" DEFINED?

Test results are classified as "normal" or "abnormal" based on several different criteria. Most laboratory tests are defined as normal if the test result falls between 2 standard deviations from the mean value in either direction. This range encompasses 95% of subjects, and "normal" defined in this fashion causes 5% of subjects to be labeled as abnormal.

TABLE 1–2. Posttest Disease Probability

	DISEASE		
TEST RESULT	Present	Absent	
Positive	350	100	450
Negative	150	400	550
Total	500	500	1000

Sensitivity = 350/500 = 0.70
Specificity = 400/500 = 0.80
Positive predictive value = 350/450 = 0.78
Negative predictive values = 400/550 = 0.73
Posttest disease probability, positive test = 350/450 = 0.78
Posttest disease probability, negative test = 150/550 = 0.27
Overall (pretest) disease probability = 500/1000 = 0.50

When several laboratory tests with normal values, defined using these statistical criteria, are performed, the probability of obtaining an abnormal result *due to chance alone* increases with the number of tests ordered. If 5 such tests are ordered as a group, there is a 23% chance of obtaining 1 abnormal result. When 15 such tests are ordered, the probability of 1 abnormal result increases to 54%! Consequently, unexpected abnormal results obtained from a panel of multiple tests should be ap-

TABLE 1–3. Pretest Disease Probability and Diagnostic Test Results

	EXAMPLE A		
TEST RESULT	Present	Absent	Total
Positive	7	198	205
Negative	3	792	795
	10	990	1000

	EXAMPLE B		
	Present	Absent	Total
	665	10	675
	285	40	325
	950	50	1000

Sensitivity = 0.70 (for A and B)
Specificity = 0.80 (for A and B)
A, pretest disease probability = 10/1000 = 0.01
A, posttest disease probability, positive test = 7/205 = 0.03
A, posttest disease probability, negative
    test = 3/795 = 0.004
B, pretest disease probability = 950/1000 = 0.95
B, posttest disease probability, positive test = 665/
    675 = 0.99
B, posttest disease probability, negative test = 285/
    325 = 0.88

proached by repeating the test whose value was abnormal to exclude the possibility that the result was merely an artifact of multiple testing.

BIASES IN THE EVALUATION OF DIAGNOSTIC TESTS

Frequently research performed to evaluate the sensitivity and specificity of diagnostic tests applies only to limited populations or may even be biased. When diagnostic test performance is evaluated, the quality of the reference or "gold standard" test against which the diagnostic test is compared affects the apparent performance. A reference test that does not classify disease presence or absence accurately may lead to an erroneous judgment of the quality of the diagnostic test.

COMBINING THE RESULTS OF MULTIPLE DIAGNOSTIC TESTS

In many clinical situations multiple diagnostic tests are available for a particular disease. Certain general principles apply when the results of multiple diagnostic tests are combined.

If 2 independent tests, each with sensitivity and specificity equal to 0.7 and 0.8, respectively, are performed, and a positive result is defined as *both* tests being positive, the sensitivity of this dual test strategy (referred to as a serial testing strategy) decreases while the specificity increases. In this example, the sensitivity is $0.7 \times 0.7 = 0.49$, while specificity is $1 - (0.2 \times 0.2) = 0.96$ (note that $0.2 = 1 - 0.8$). The general principle illustrated is that tests performed in a serial strategy lead to a more specific result that is better suited to "ruling in" disease, if positive.

A different multiple testing strategy would define a positive result as *1 or more* positive results from 2 or more tests ordered (referred to as a parallel testing strategy). In this case, the sensitivity is $0.7 + 0.7 - (0.7 \times 0.7) = 0.91$, and the specificity is $1 - (0.2 + 0.2 - (0.2 \times 0.2)) = 0.64$. A parallel testing strategy, therefore, will lead to higher test sensitivity and would be better suited to ruling out disease if the test result is negative.

FOLLOW-UP AS A DIAGNOSTIC TEST

The most informative and widely used diagnostic test in medical practice today—clinical follow-up—requires no specialized instrumentation and no direct trauma to the patient. With the passage of time, additional symptoms or signs may become apparent that assist the diagnostic process, or difficult diagnostic problems may disappear, never to return again. The use of follow-up as a diagnostic test does not come naturally to many physicians in training, probably because the hospital-based nature of medical training puts pressure on housestaff to resolve problems before discharge. In the outpatient setting, however, one soon realizes how important follow-up is in resolving diagnostic dilemmas. The proper use of follow-up as a diagnostic tool is partly determined by disease severity. For example, a patient with chronic diarrhea so severe that dehydration and weight loss have become life-threatening problems requires rapid diagnostic evaluation rather than clinical follow-up.

SUMMARY

The following principles underlie the interpretation of all diagnostic tests:

1. Disease presence is usually ruled out by a negative result on the most sensitive test.

2. Disease presence is usually ruled in by a positive result on the most specific test.

3. Diagnostic tests are unlikely to be useful when the disease is either very likely or very unlikely. Diagnostic tests are often most useful when disease probability is "50-50."

4. Combinations of diagnostic tests may be more sensitive or more specific than single tests, depending on how a positive result is defined.

5. Determination of diagnostic test sensitivity and specificity may be biased by factors such as spectrum of disease tested, failure to blind observers to the results of other tests, or imperfect reference tests for the disease.

Bibliography

Boyko EJ, et al. Reference test errors bias the evaluation of diagnostic tests for ischemic heart disease. J Gen Intern Med 1988;3:476–481.

Kassirer JP. Our stubborn quest for diagnostic certainty. A cause of excessive testing. N Engl J Med 1989;320:1489–1491.

Pauker SG, Kassirer JP. The threshold approach to medical decision making. N Engl J Med 1980;302:1109–1117.

Ransohoff DF, Feinstein AR. Problems of spectrum and bias in the evaluation of diagnostic tests. N Engl J Med 1978;299:926–930.

Sackett DL, et al. Clinical Epidemiology: A Basic Science for Clinical Medicine. Boston, Little, Brown, and Co., 1985.

Weinstein MC, Fineberg HV. Clinical Decision Analysis. Philadelphia, W. B. Saunders Co., 1980.

FATIGUE

DAVID C. DUGDALE

> When Helen was quite old and with more energy left than strength, I asked her what her idea of heaven was. She replied, "Perpetual activity without fatigue."
>
> ANONYMOUS. Quoted in *Arch. Int. Med.* 114:557, 1964.

DEFINITION AND GENERAL COMMENTS

- Fatigue refers to an abnormally rapid onset or severe degree of global tiredness after activity. Careful questioning is necessary to determine that the complaint is true fatigue rather than localized pain or weakness, dyspnea, or lightheadedness.
- Abnormal fatigue is a loss of energy out of proportion to effort and/or tiredness not relieved by rest.
- Many patients have a short-term problem that resolves spontaneously or with appropriate treatment. Others develop the "chronic fatigue syndrome" (Table 2–1).

EPIDEMIOLOGY

Fatigue is the seventh most common symptom in primary care and is the reason for 3 to 4% of all office visits. The prevalence of fatigue in outpatients is approximately 20%.

DIFFERENTIAL DIAGNOSIS (Table 2–2)

- Many medical conditions may be associated with fatigue. The diagnostic process is guided by the age of the patient (serious disease is more likely in an older patient), epidemiologic (infectious or environmental illness may be suggested) and behavioral (possible psychiatric illness) factors, and the appearance of the patient ("appears sick" versus "appears well").
- Most organic illnesses causing fatigue have additional associated symptoms or signs.
- Most psychiatric illnesses associated with fatigue meet specific diagnostic criteria and are not diagnoses of exclusion. Up to two-thirds of fatigued patients have a psychiatric disorder that contributes to their complaint.
- Up to one-third of patients have no clear diagnosis.

TABLE 2–1. Working Definition of Chronic Fatigue Syndrome

A case of chronic fatigue syndrome must fulfill major criteria 1 and 2 and have the following minor criteria:

  1. Six or more of the 11 symptom criteria and 2 or more of the 3 physical criteria, *or*

  2. Eight or more of the 11 symptom criteria.

A. Major criteria

  1. New onset of persistent or relapsing, debilitating fatigue or easy fatigability in a person who has no previous history of similar symptoms, that does not resolve with bedrest, and that is severe enough to reduce or impair average daily activity below 50% of the patient's premorbid activity level for a period of at least 6 months.

  2. Exclusion of specific clinical syndromes associated with fatigue (see Table 2–2).

B. Minor criteria: To fulfill a symptom criterion, a symptom must have begun at or after the time of onset of increased fatigability and must have persisted over or recurred within a period of at least 6 months.

  1. Mild fever: oral temperature between 37.5 and 38.6° C (if measured by the patient) or chills

  2. Sore throat

  3. Painful lymphadenopathy in the anterior or posterior cervical or axillary distribution

  4. Unexplained generalized muscle weakness

  5. Muscle discomfort or myalgia

  6. Prolonged (24 hours or greater) generalized fatigue after levels of exercise that would have been easily tolerated in the patient's premorbid state

  7. Generalized headaches (different from headaches experienced in the premorbid state)

  8. Migratory arthralgia without joint swelling or redness

  9. Neuropsychologic complaints (photophobia, transient visual scotomata, forgetfulness, excessive irritability, confusion, difficulty thinking, inability to concentrate, depression).

  10. Sleep disturbance (hypersomnia or insomnia)

  11. Description of the main symptom complex as initially developing over a few hours to a few days

C. Physical criteria: These must be documented by a physician on at least 2 occasions, at least 1 month apart.

  1. Low-grade fever (oral temperature between 37.6 and 38.6° C, or rectal temperature between 37.8 and 38.8° C

  2. Nonexudative pharyngitis

  3. Palpable or tender anterior or posterior cervical or axillary lymph nodes

Source: Adapted from Holmes GP, et al. Chronic fatigue syndrome: A working case definition. Ann Intern Med 1988;108:387–389.

TABLE 2–2. Differential Diagnosis of Fatigue

A. Tumor
   1. Solid tumor: lung, breast, gastrointestinal, renal
   2. Hematologic malignancy: leukemia, lymphoma, myeloma
B. Infection
   1. Bacterial: subacute bacterial endocarditis, brucellosis, tuberculosis, localized infection (occult abscess)
   2. Fungal: histoplasmosis, blastomycosis, coccidioidomycosis
   3. Parasitic: toxoplasmosis, amebiasis, giardiasis, helminthic infestation
   4. Viral: hepatitis, human immunodeficiency virus, infectious mononucleosis
C. Toxin
   1. Medication use: sedatives, antidepressants, antipsychotics, analgesics, antihypertensives (beta blockers, central sympatholytics)
   2. Environmental: solvents, pesticides, heavy metals
   3. Substance abuse: alcohol, narcotics, sedatives
D. Inflammatory diseases: autoimmune diseases (e.g., systemic lupus erythematosus), sarcoidosis, Wegener's granulomatosis
E. Metabolic disorders: electrolyte abnormality, renal failure, diabetes mellitus, hypothyroidism, hyperthyroidism, hypoadrenalism, hyperadrenalism
F. Psychiatric: depression, personality disorder, psychosis, anxiety disorder, grief reaction
G. Neurologic: multiple sclerosis, myasthenia gravis, polyneuropathy
H. Miscellaneous
   1. Chronic cardiac disease (e.g., valvular heart disease, cardiomyopathy)
   2. Chronic pulmonary disease
   3. Anemia
   4. Fibrositis
   5. Chronic fatigue syndrome

Source: Adapted from Holmes GP, et al. Chronic fatigue syndrome: A working case definition. Ann Intern Med 1988;108:387–389.

CLINICAL FEATURES

- The general principles of the evaluation of fatigued patients are:
   1. Over 90% of diagnoses can be made from the history and physical examination.
   2. Psychosocial concerns must be addressed with an eye to specific psychiatric diagnoses. Treatable depression must be diagnosed.
   3. In a patient who appears healthy, extensive laboratory evaluation is of low yield. Clinical follow-up is appropriate for the majority of these patients.

- History
  1. The temporal pattern of fatigue may have diagnostic importance.
     a. Morning fatigue is common with depression or fibrositis.
     b. Purely exertional fatigue suggests cardiopulmonary disease.
     c. Specific factors in the onset of fatigue such as environment (e.g., toxin exposure), medication use, and relationship to substance use may be important.
  2. Localized fatigue syndromes suggest neuromuscular disease or a regional pain syndrome masquerading as fatigue.
  3. A history of unintentional weight loss (>10%) suggests the presence of underlying disease.
  4. The duration of the fatigue and associated symptoms may allow diagnosis of the chronic fatigue syndrome. Previous medical records should be obtained to save costly laboratory evaluation.
  5. Screening questions about mood and response to illness are important.
- Physical examination
  1. General: Fever (especially if above 38.6° C) suggests an infectious cause. Significant weight loss suggests a metabolic or malignant disease.
  2. Head and neck: Oral candidiasis or a goiter may be present.
  3. Lymph nodes larger than 2 cm usually require further evaluation for inflammatory and malignant disease.
  4. Cardiopulmonary examination may find evidence of chronic obstructive pulmonary disease, valvular heart disease, or congestive heart failure.
  5. The abdominal exam may find hepatosplenomegaly or masses.
  6. The breast, genitourinary, and rectal examinations are important for excluding malignancy.
  7. The skin may show evidence of endocrinologic (thyroid, adrenal) or infectious disease.
  8. The neurologic examination may show muscle abnormalities (wasting, fasciculations, localized weakness), or movement disorders. A formal mental status examination should be done.

LABORATORY FINDINGS

- Without a specific indication, laboratory testing is generally unrewarding. Appropriate screening tests include:
  1. A complete blood count.
  2. Serum electrolyte, glucose, urea nitrogen, creatinine, calcium, and transaminase levels.
  3. A free thyroxine index or thyroid-stimulating hormone level.
- Electrocardiogram: not indicated in the absence of a suggestive history.

- X-rays. A chest X-ray is indicated in a smoker, otherwise, this test should be limited to those with pulmonary symptoms.
- Tests for infectious diseases.
  1. An HIV test should be done, especially in a patient with a history of high-risk behavior.
  2. A heterophil antibody (e.g., Monospot) test may confirm a clinical diagnosis of infectious mononucleosis. Epstein-Barr virus serologies are not indicated in the evaluation of patients with chronic fatigue.
  3. Serologic tests for infections such as Lyme disease, brucellosis, and fungal diseases should be limited to those with suspicious clinical features.
  4. A tuberculin skin test should be done.
- Screening for malignancy: In the absence of clinical suspicion, this should be limited to stool test for occult blood, cervical cytology, and, depending on age, mammogram and sigmoidoscopy.

RECOMMENDED DIAGNOSTIC APPROACH

The importance of clinical guidance cannot be overemphasized. The diagnostic evaluation differs for patients with acute versus chronic fatigue, and those that "appear healthy" versus those that "appear sick." Older patients may require more laboratory evaluation.

Bibliography

Holmes GP, et al. Chronic fatigue syndrome: A working case definition. Ann Intern Med 1988;108:387–389.

Koo D. Chronic fatigue syndrome: A critical appraisal of the role of Epstein-Barr virus. West J Med 1989;150:590–596.

Kroenke K, et al. Chronic fatigue in primary care: Prevalence, patient characteristics, and outcome. JAMA 1988;260:929–934.

Kruesi MJP, et al. Psychiatric diagnoses in patients who have chronic fatigue syndrome. J Clin Psychiatry 1989;50(2):53–56.

Solberg LI. Lassitude. A primary care evaluation. JAMA 1984; 251:3272–3276.

3

CONSTIPATION

SHOBA KRISHNAMURTHY

Anyone who lives a sedentary life and does not exercise or he who postpones his excretions or he whose intestines are constipated, even if he eats good foods and takes care of himself according to (proper) medical principles—all his days will be painful ones and his strength will wane.

MOSES BEN MAIMON (MAIMONIDES) (1135–1204)

DEFINITION

- Stool weight, size, and consistency vary widely in normal people. Normal stool frequencies range from 3 stools per day to 3 per week.
- Constipation can be practically defined as the passage of less than 3 stools per week. It can be subjectively defined as small or hard stools or difficult passage of stools with abdominal discomfort and a feeling of incomplete evacuation.

EPIDEMIOLOGY

- National health surveys suggest that the prevalence of constipation is 1.2%, leading to 2.5 million physician visits per year.
- Constipation is more common in people over 65 years of age, is 3 times more common in women than men, and affects nonwhites more than whites.

DIFFERENTIAL DIAGNOSIS
(Tables 3–1 to 3–4)

A common cause of constipation in North America is an inadequate intake of dietary fiber. In addition, lack of exercise, voluntary suppression of the urge to defecate, and prolonged travel are often considered causes of constipation, though their frequency is not known.

HISTORY, SIGNS, AND SYMPTOMS

- Gastric and small bowel disorders. The diagnosis is indicated by predominant postprandial fullness and bloating, heartburn, nausea, vomiting, and upper abdominal distention associated with constipation.

14

TABLE 3-1. Drugs That Cause Constipation

Opiates
Antacids (Calcium and aluminum compounds)
Anticonvulsants
Antidepressants
Antihypertensives
Antiparkinsonian agents
Iron
Diuretics
Anticholinergics
Heavy metal poisoning

- Irritable bowel syndrome
  1. This is the most common GI disorder associated with constipation. Women sufferers outnumber men 2 : 1.
  2. The syndrome is characterized by disturbed motility and presents with abdominal pain, constipation, and/or diarrhea.
  3. Stress-induced symptoms are present in half of all cases. More than 50% of patients have abnormal psychologic features such as depression, anxiety, and panic-attack symptoms.
  4. Keys to diagnosis: a long history of symptoms beginning at a young age, with absence of weight loss (unless associated with depression), nocturnal abdominal pain, and hematochezia. There are no laboratory or radiologic abnormalities.
- Diverticular disease
  1. Diverticular disease is present in half of patients over 60 years old but symptomatic in only 20%.
  2. Symptoms are similar to those of irritable bowel syndrome. Diverticulitis and stricture formation are complications that can cause or worsen constipation.
- Colonic carcinoma
  1. This diagnosis must be considered in every patient over 40 with a recent history of constipation.

TABLE 3-2. Metabolic and Endocrine Disorders That Cause Constipation

Metabolic disorders
    Diabetes mellitus
    Porphyria
    Amyloidosis
    Uremia
    Hypokalemia
    Hypercalcemia
Endocrine disorders
    Panhypopituitarism
    Hypothyroidism
    Pheochromocytoma
    Glucagonoma
    Pregnancy

TABLE 3–3. Disorders of the GI Tract That Cause Constipation

Gastric-emptying disorders
   Gastric outlet obstruction (ulcer disease, tumor)
   Gastroparesis (postvagotomy, diabetes mellitus)
Small bowel obstruction
Colonic obstruction
   Extraluminal
     Tumors
     Chronic volvulus
     Hernias
   Luminal
     Tumors
     Strictures
       Infectious
       Ischemic
       Inflammatory
Abnormalities of colonic motor function
   Irritable bowel syndrome
   Diverticular disease
Pseudo-obstruction
   Disorders of intestinal muscle
     Scleroderma
     Hollow visceral myopathy
   Disorders of myenteric nerves
     Visceral neuropathy
     Paraneoplastic neuropathy
     Chagas' disease
     Neuronal intestinal dysplasia
     Hirschsprung's disease
Rectal disorders
   Rectocele
   Intussusception
   Prolapse
Anal disorders
   Stenosis
   Fissures

TABLE 3–4. Neurologic Disorders That Cause Constipation

Brain
   Parkinson's disease
   Tumors
   Cerebrovascular accidents
Other
   Trauma to nervi erigentes or lumbosacral nerve roots
   Cauda equina tumor
   Meningocele
   Autonomic insufficiency
   Tabes dorsalis
   Multiple sclerosis

2. Keys to diagnosis: recent onset, associated hematochezia, weight loss, or anorexia, or a past history of colonic polyps, ulcerative colitis, or family history of colonic cancer or polyposis.

- Hirschsprung's disease
  1. This is an uncommon (1 in 5000 live births) familial disorder that is caused by absence of ganglion cells in a segment of the distal colon. Spasticity of the affected aganglionic segment causes it to behave like an obstruction.
  2. Keys to diagnosis
     a. Symptoms have onset in childhood (infrequently in adult life) with abdominal distension and an empty rectal ampulla on examination.
     b. A barium enema may show rectal and distal colonic narrowing with a dilatation of the colon proximally (megacolon). Ganglion cells are absent on submucosal rectal biopsy.

- Neuromuscular disorders
  1. These affect either the colonic muscle (scleroderma or visceral myopathy) or the colonic myenteric plexus (paraneoplastic neuropathy or sporadic or familial visceral neuropathy).
  2. Keys to diagnosis include symptoms related to other viscera such as dysphagia, abdominal distention, nausea, vomiting, and urinary symptoms. The constipation responds poorly to laxatives.

- Metabolic and endocrine disorders
  1. Of the metabolic disorders, diabetes mellitus is the major cause of constipation. Thirty percent of diabetic patients without neuropathy and 80 to 90% with peripheral and autonomic neuropathy are constipated. Constipation is typically intermittent and alternates with diarrhea in 30% of cases.
  2. Among the endocrine disorders, hypothyroidism is the most common cause of constipation.

- Neurologic disorders
  1. Ten percent of patients with Parkinson's disease have megacolons, but a much higher number have constipation.
  2. Up to 43% of patients with multiple sclerosis complain of constipation.

RECOMMENDED DIAGNOSTIC APPROACH

- History
  1. Determine what the patient means by constipation. Many individuals who have normal bowel movements (3 to 5 times per week) think they are constipated.
  2. Include a detailed account of drug intake and symptoms of metabolic, endocrine, neurologic, and GI disease.
- Routine laboratory tests include complete blood count, stool test for occult blood, and serum tests of electrolytes,

calcium, fasting blood glucose, and renal and thyroid function.

- High-fiber diet: If routine laboratory findings are normal, the patient should be put on a diet with 20 g/day of fiber (1 cup of 100% bran cereal or 2 tablespoons of psyllium) for 30 days. If constipation persists, work-up should be continued.
- Sigmoidoscopy examines for anal fissures and rectosigmoid masses.
- Barium enema examines for intraluminal mass, stricture, or narrowed distal segment (Hirschsprung's disease).
- Rectal biopsy: Hirschsprung's disease and amyloidosis can be ruled out.
- Colonic transit time
  1. If the work-up described above reveals no abnormalities, the colonic transit time on a 20 g/day fiber diet should be measured by a radiopaque marker study. This test may be considered earlier if the patient's history is vague or inconsistent.
  2. The patient swallows 20 radiopaque marker pieces (cut a #12 French nasogastric tube into 5-mm bits) on day 0. Plain X-rays of the abdomen are obtained on days 5 and 7; 80% of the markers should pass by day 5, and 100% by day 7.
  3. The test should begin the day after the patient has had a stool, and the patient should avoid laxatives or enemas during the test. An abnormal test result is not specific for any disorder, but confirms delayed colonic transit.
- Other methods: If a neuromuscular disorder is suspected, consider:
  1. Esophageal manometry or upper GI and small bowel follow through X-ray
  2. An IV pyelogram to look for bladder dilatation or retention
  3. Anorectal manometry to rule out Hirschsprung's disease and study the expulsion pattern

Bibliography

Devroede G. Constipation. In: Sleisenger MH, Fordtran JS, eds. GI Disease: Pathophysiology, Diagnosis and Management. Philadelphia, W. B. Saunders Co., 1989, pp. 331–368.

Johanson JR, et al. Clinical epidemiology of chronic constipation. J Clin Gastroenterol 1989;11(5):525–536.

4

CHRONIC DIARRHEA

RONALD H. FRIED
and CHRISTINA M. SURAWICZ

A dirty cook gives diarrhoea quicker than rhubarb.

TUNG-SU PAI

DEFINITION AND INITIAL APPROACH

- Definition
  1. Subjectively, diarrhea is a change in stools: They are more frequent and more loose or watery.
  2. Diarrhea with a structural cause (see Table 4–1) occurs at night as well as during the day: "Functional" diarrhea (irritable bowel syndrome, "spastic colon") never wakes the patient up at night.
  3. Chronic diarrhea is one that lasts more than 4 weeks.
- Documentation of amount and type of chronic diarrhea. Because of the wide variation in patient definition of diarrhea, it should be documented by measuring stool weight. More than 200 g of stool in 24 hours is considered diarrhea. During the stool collection, the patient should continue a normal diet.
- Initial approach. The physician can classify the diarrhea as one of three types: fatty, watery, or bloody. Each type requires a different diagnostic approach.
  1. Stool fat. A negative Sudan stain in the presence of diarrhea excludes steatorrhea. A quantitative fat analysis should also be done. More than 5 g/24 hr indicates steatorrhea if the patient is eating an average diet.
  2. Gross or occult blood. Gross blood can be detected by visual inspection and occult blood by test cards (e.g., Hemoccult®).
  3. Fecal leukocytes. The presence of sheets of leukocytes suggests bacterial dysentery, which usually causes an acute diarrhea. However, fecal leukocytes are not always present, and they may also occur in inflammatory bowel disease.
  4. Stool culture and examination for ova and parasites (see Table 4–2).
     a. These tests are best done on fresh specimens.
     b. Protozoal cysts or trophozoites and the ova or larva of helminths may be seen.
     c. Routine stool culture tests for *Campylobacter, Salmonella,* and *Shigella* species should be used. Special media are required for organisms such as *Aeromonas* sp. and *Yersinia.*

TABLE 4–1. Causes of Chronic Diarrhea

A. Drugs
  1. Common
     Laxatives
     Lactulose
     Antacids
     Ethanol
     Coffee
     Digitalis
     Quinidine
     Colchicine
     Nonsteroidal anti-inflammatory agents
     Antibiotics
     Alpha-methyldopa
     Propranolol
     Chemotherapeutic agents
  2. Uncommon
     Excessive diuretics
     Excessive opiates
     Sorbitol (sugar-free chewing gum or candy)
     Eye drops (anticholinesterase, e.g., pilocarpine)
     Prostaglandins
B. Structural causes
  Inflammatory bowel disease
  Prior gastric intestinal surgery
  Celiac sprue
  Radiation enteritis
  Lactose intolerance
  Pancreatic insufficiency
  Gastrointestinal tumors (carcinoma, lymphoma, adenoma)
C. Motility disorders
  Irritable bowel syndrome
  Scleroderma
  Intestinal pseudo-obstruction
  Amyloidosis
D. Metabolic and endocrine disorders
  Zollinger-Ellison syndrome
  Carcinoid syndrome
  Pancreatic endocrine tumors (vasoactive intestinal peptideoma)
  Diabetes mellitus
  Hyperthyroidism
  Hypothyroidism
  Medullary carcinoma of the thyroid gland
  Addison's disease
  Amyloidosis

**TABLE 4–2. Infectious Causes
of Chronic Diarrhea**

A. Bacteria (usually cause acute, not chronic, diarrhea)
    Campylobacter
    Shigella
    Salmonella
    Yersinia
    Clostridium difficile
    E. coli
B. Parasites
    Amebiasis
    Giardiasis
    Coccidioidosis
    Cryptosporidiosis
    Helminthic infestation
    Trichuriasis (whipworm)
    Strongyloidiasis
    Capillariasis
    Hymenolepsis (dwarf tapeworm)
    Schistosomiasis (polyposis)
    Trichinosis (rare)
    Taenia sp.
C. In patients with acquired immunodeficiency syndrome
    (AIDS)
    Cryptosporidium
    Isospora belli
    Mycobacterium avium–intracellularis
    Cytomegalovirus
    Human immunodeficiency virus-enteropathy

    d. Cultures for *Clostridium difficile* and the assay for
       C. difficile toxin B should be done. This infection
       usually occurs in patients with recent antibiotic
       treatment or chemotherapy.

DIFFERENTIAL DIAGNOSIS

Fatty Diarrhea

There are two major causes of fatty diarrhea.

- Pancreatic insufficiency. Most often this is caused by recurrent episodes of pancreatitis. Keys to the diagnosis include a history of abdominal pain (often alcohol-related);
  marked steatorrhea (stool fat may be >40 g per day); an
  abdominal X-ray that shows pancreatic calcification; or
  a therapeutic response to oral pancreatic enzyme replacement.

- Small intestinal disease

  1. Celiac sprue is the most common in this category. This
     is a hereditary abnormality of small intestinal mucosa
     that causes sensitivity to gluten, a wheat protein. It
     may occur at any age. The key to diagnosis is a compat-

ible small bowel biopsy and improvement while on a gluten-free diet.
2. Small bowel bacterial overgrowth is seen after gastric operations and in intestinal pseudoobstruction. The diagnosis is made by jejunal aspiration and/or response to antibiotics.

Bloody Diarrhea

Blood in the stools is usually caused by colonic disease. It often requires sigmoidoscopy and air contrast barium enema (BE) or colonoscopy and may require upper gastrointestinal X-rays or endoscopy.

- Acute self-limited colitis (ASLC). ASLC is the most common cause of bloody diarrhea. The most common causative organisms are *E. coli, Campylobacter, Salmonella,* and *Shigella* (Table 4-2). Forty to sixty percent of patients are culture-negative. Keys to the diagnosis are abrupt onset, exposure or travel history, positive stool culture, and rapid (usually <2 weeks) spontaneous resolution.
- Idiopathic inflammatory bowel disease (IBD: ulcerative colitis and Crohn's disease; see Chapter 38). IBD is a primary bowel disease that may have systemic manifestations (in eye, skin, joint, or other areas). Rectal biopsies are often helpful in distinguishing between ASLC and IBD.
- Colon cancer. This condition occasionally presents with diarrhea. A change in bowel habits and weight loss are late clues to the diagnosis. Rectal examination, sigmoidoscopy, barium enema, and colonoscopy are necessary for diagnosis.
- Massive bleeding. In elderly patients this is usually caused by colonic diverticula or arteriovenous malformations. The key to diagnosis is painless bleeding. Colonoscopy and barium contrast studies are useful diagnostic tools.

Watery Diarrhea

The most common causes are medications, infections, lactose intolerance, prior bowel surgery, and irritable bowel syndrome. Rare causes include the Zollinger-Ellison syndrome and small bowel lymphomas.

RECOMMENDED DIAGNOSTIC APPROACH

The following is recommended for chronic diarrhea. This approach is not necessary for more acute, self-limited episodes.
- History
  1. Symptoms of night blindness, cramps (tetany), and easy bruisability result from the malabsorption of the fat-soluble vitamins A, D, and K.
  2. Medication use (especially antacids and antibiotics), prior bowel surgery, recent travel (especially foreign), and exposure to others who have diarrhea are important. Floating stools often indicate excess gas, not excess fat.

3. Patients who see fat globules in the toilet bowl water usually have pancreatic insufficiency (and severe fat malabsorption).

- Evaluation of stool. Subsequent evaluation of the patient who has chronic diarrhea depends on whether the diarrhea is fatty, bloody, or watery. Therefore, a 24-hour stool collection for fat and weight while taking a regular diet should be an early step.

    1. Chronic bloody diarrhea
        a. A stool culture should be obtained for *Campylobacter, Salmonella, Shigella, Clostridium difficile,* and *Yersinia.* Stool should be sent for *C. difficile* toxin determination if antibiotics or chemotherapeutic agents have been taken recently. A positive toxin determination diagnoses *C. difficile* (pseudomembranous) colitis. Positive stool cultures for *C. difficile* are not diagnostic in the absence of the toxin, although some patients respond to treatment with vancomycin or metronidazole.
        b. The physician should look for ova and parasites, especially *Entamoeba histolytica.* This diagnosis is excluded most definitely by paired amebic serologies 2 to 4 weeks apart.
        c. If cultures are nondiagnostic and symptoms persist, sigmoidoscopy and rectal biopsy should be performed. Colitis is best diagnosed by sigmoidoscopy. Prepared enemas or laxatives should not be used because they can damage the rectal mucosa and cause confusing artifacts. A tap-water enema can be used to cleanse the rectum.
        d. If the diagnosis is still unclear, an air contrast BE or colonoscopy, or both, should be done. Coloncosopy is more specific and sensitive, but its use in severe colitis is contraindicated because of the increased risk of perforation of the bowel.

    2. Chronic watery diarrhea. The evaluation often depends on clues in the history or physical examination (see above).
        a. The stool electrolytes and pH help determine whether the diarrhea is secretory or osmotic in origin. A low pH indicates carbohydrate malabsorption. The stool pH is elevated in patients taking antacids or milk of magnesia. The osmotic gap is the difference between the measured and the calculated stool osmolality—$([Na]_{stool} + [K]_{stool}) \times 2$. An osmotic gap >50 mOsm/L suggests osmotic diarrhea.
        b. Stool culture and examination for ova and parasites should be done to exclude infection. Amebic serologies should be considered.
        c. Sigmoidoscopy and BE may diagnose unsuspected IBD, polyps, or cancers.
        d. If results of these procedures are normal, an upper gastrointestinal X-ray with small bowel follow-through should be used to diagnose prior gastric surgery, fistulae, or small bowel mucosal disease.

e. If the radiograph appears normal, a lactose-tolerance test should be used to diagnose unsuspected lactose intolerance. This is best done by asking the patient to take 50 g of lactose in an 8-ounce glass of water on an empty stomach. This is equivalent to a quart of milk, but easier to take. Cramps, gas, or diarrhea over the next 4 hours suggest lactose intolerance.

f. A small bowel biopsy should be considered to look for mucosal small bowel disease or small bowel parasites such as *Giardia lamblia, Strongyloides,* or *Cryptosporidium.*

g. If the results of all of these procedures are normal, screening must be done for metabolic diseases such as carcinoid syndrome, Addison's disease, hyperthyroidism, and Zollinger-Ellison syndrome.

h. The last step in the evaluation of a patient with chronic watery diarrhea is to hospitalize the patient and give IV fluids for 36 hours. If the patient still has diarrhea with no oral intake, the diarrhea is secretory and may be due to laxative abuse or pancreatic cholera. If laxative abuse can be excluded, a serum VIP (vasoactive intestinal peptide) level and an abdominal CT scan should be obtained to diagnose endocrine tumors of the pancreas.

3. Chronic fatty diarrhea. A 24-hour stool fat content of greater than 5 g confirms fat malabsorption.

a. If the stool fat content is equivocal, the serum carotene should be measured. In fat malabsorption, the carotene is very low. A modest decrease in carotene may be caused by low dietary intake of vegetables even without malabsorption.

b. A small bowel biopsy should be considered to look for mucosal disease.

c. If pancreatic insufficiency is suspected, ultrasound or CT imaging of the pancreas should be performed to look for signs of chronic pancreatitis.

d. In theory, a D-xylose test separates luminal from mucosal disease. However, in practice the results are affected by many factors (e.g., gastric emptying, cardiac and renal function), so it is not a reliable test in the differential diagnosis of fat malabsorption.

Bibliography

Johnson DA, Cattau EL. Stool chemistries in patients with unexplained diarrhea. Am Fam Physician 1986;33:131.

Khouri MR, et al. Sudan Stain of fecal fat: New insight into an old test. Gastroenterology 1989;96:421.

Romano TJ, Dobbins, JW. Evaluation of the patient with suspected malabsorption. Clin Gastroenterol 1989;18:467.

Smith PD, Janoff EN. Infectious diarrhea in human immunodeficiency virus infection. Clin Gastroenterol 1988;17:587.

Surawicz CM. Diagnosing colitis. Gastroenterology 1987;92:538.

5

COUGH

SCOTT BARNHART

Cough and the world coughs with you. Fart and you stand alone.

TEVOR GRIFFITHS

GENERAL COMMENTS

- Cough is the sudden rapid expulsion of air through the glottis to expel mucus or other material. It results from the coordination of several actions, and it acts as one of the host's respiratory defense mechanisms.
- The neural control of the cough mechanism involves vagal afferents from receptors in the larynx, bronchi, and trachea, as well as trigeminal, glossopharyngeal, and phrenic afferents from receptors in the nose, sinuses, ear canals (vagal), pleura, stomach, pericardium, and diaphragm.
- Cough receptors respond to chemical and mechanical stimuli. They are most numerous in the larger airways and are not present beyond the respiratory bronchioles.

DIFFERENTIAL DIAGNOSIS (Table 5–1)

- The most common cause of an acute cough is a viral upper respiratory tract infection.
- For chronic or persisting cough, the most likely causes are postnasal drainage (29%), asthma (25%), and asthma with postnasal drainage (18%).

CLINICAL MANIFESTATIONS

- History
  1. Onset and duration
     a. Acute nonproductive coughs that later become productive and are associated with "flu"- or cold-like symptoms are likely due to an upper respiratory tract infection.
     b. A chronic productive cough in a smoker is most likely due to chronic bronchitis.
  2. Color of sputum
     a. Clear sputum is evidence against infection, and yellow or green sputum, especially if recently changed in color, suggests infection.

TABLE 5–1. Acute and Chronic Causes of Cough

1. Postnasal drainage
2. Asthma
3. Chronic bronchitis (12% of chronic cough cases)
4. Upper respiratory tract infection
5. Pneumonia
6. Foreign body
7. Hemoptysis
8. Pulmonary embolism
9. Aspiration
10. Gastroesophageal reflux (10% of chronic cough cases)
11. Left ventricular failure
12. Sarcoidosis
13. Neoplastic disease, including bronchogenic carcinoma or metastatic disease
14. Inhalation of allergens or irritant gases and fumes, including cigarette smoke
15. Irritation of receptors outside the lower respiratory tract, including ear canals, diaphragm, pleura, nose, and pharynx
16. Bronchiectasis
17. Psychogenic factors

     b. Bloody or blood-flecked sputum supports the diagnosis of hemoptysis and, while not infrequently due to bronchitis or bronchiectasis, should prompt consideration of malignancy.

   3. Amount of sputum

     a. Early viral infections, cough related to postnasal drainage, and psychogenic cough from irritation of receptors outside the lower respiratory tract are often nonproductive.

     b. Deep coughs productive of sputum suggest a source in the lower respiratory tract. Large quantities of sputum (up to a cup per day) may signify bronchiectasis.

   4. Associated symptoms

     a. Dyspnea or wheezing suggest asthma, pulmonary embolism, infiltrative disease, or pneumonia.

     b. Paroxysmal nocturnal dyspnea and orthopnea may suggest a cardiac origin.

     c. Patients with a history of allergies are at an increased risk of sinusitis or asthma.

     d. Hoarseness suggests a lesion that involves the vocal cords or the recurrent laryngeal nerve.

     e. Fever and chills suggest infection.

     f. Chest pain suggests esophageal reflux or ischemic heart disease causing pulmonary congestion.

• Physical examination. Pertinent findings may include:

   1. Vital signs including respiratory rate and temperature

   2. Sinus tenderness, which suggests sinusitis

   3. Discharge or inflammation of the nasopharynx

   4. Adenopathy suggesting infection or malignancy

5. Stridor, hoarseness, or visible lesion of the larynx on laryngoscopy
6. The lungs, for wheezes, rales, rhonchi, or decreased breath sounds
7. The cardiovascular system, for evidence of heart failure with elevated jugular venous pressure, gallops, or murmurs.

RECOMMENDED DIAGNOSTIC APPROACH

• A cough of acute onset and short duration associated with a history and examination suggestive of an upper respiratory infection does not require further evaluation.
• Chronic coughs usually require further evaluation with the following studies:
  1. Sputum examination
     a. This should include the general appearance, quantity, quality (specimens with >10 squamous epithelial cells per low power field have oropharyngeal contamination), Gram's stain, culture, and acid-fast smears and culture if indicated.
     b. If an allergic cause is suspected, a Wright's stain for eosinophils may be useful.
  2. Chest X-ray. If the chest X-ray is negative, the most likely cause is asthma, which can be diagnosed by spirometry or methacholine challenge, or both. Asthma is far more likely to cause cough than is an endobronchial tumor or foreign body.
• If these tests are negative, one of the other potential diagnoses should be pursued, with the evaluation often including sinus X-rays and/or an examination of the larynx and airways by bronchoscopy.

Bibliography

Bramman SS, et al. Cough: Differential diagnosis and treatment. Clin Chest Med 1987;92(3):529–530.

Irwin RS, et al. Chronic persistent cough in the adult: The spectrum and frequency of causes and successful outcome of specific therapy. Am Rev Respir Dis 1981;123:414–417.

Irwin RS, et al. Cough: A comprehensive review. Arch Intern Med 1977;137:1186.

Poe RH, et al. Chronic cough: Bronchoscopy or pulmonary function testing? Am Rev Respir Dis 1982;126:160–162.

6

URINARY INCONTINENCE

JAMES BRANAHL

As men draw near the common goal.
Can anything be sadder.
Than he who, master of his soul,
Is servant to his bladder?

ANONYMOUS

DEFINITION AND GENERAL COMMENTS

- Urinary incontinence is the involuntary passage of urine sufficiently severe to cause social or hygienic problems (see Table 6-1).
- Although individuals of any age group may develop this symptom, it is most frequent in the elderly, affecting over 15% of those living in the community and 50% of nursing home residents.
- The prevalence in females is twice that in males.
- Patients frequently underreport and physicians overlook urinary incontinence because of embarrassment or a sense of futility.

ACUTE VERSUS CHRONIC INCONTINENCE

1. Transient (acute) incontinence often occurs in hospitalized patients with acute medical or surgical problems and is usually reversible. Chronic or persistent incontinence requires a more detailed investigation.
2. The causes of acute incontinence have been organized by Resnick as follows ("DIAPERS"):

D: Delirium
I: Infection or inflammation of the bladder
A: Atrophic urethritis or vaginitis
P: Pharmaceuticals, psychological
E: Endocrine, e.g., glycosuria, hypercalcemia
R: Retention
S: Stool impaction

TABLE 6–1. Complications of Urinary Incontinence

Physical
  1. Skin rash
  2. Pressure sores
  3. Urinary tract infections
Psychosocial
  1. Depressive symptoms
  2. Social isolation
  3. Institutionalization

CLASSIFICATION OF CHRONIC URINARY INCONTINENCE

1. Urine loss occurs whenever intravesical pressure exceeds intraurethral pressure. Defining the pathophysiology is crucial to proper diagnosis and treatment.
2. Four basic types of incontinence are recognized in elderly patients (Table 6–2): stress, urge, overflow, and functional.
3. Although multiple mechanisms may interact in an individual, urge incontinence is the single most common type.

HISTORY

1. *Urinary symptoms:* frequency, urgency, nocturia, dysuria, force of stream, and characteristics of incontinence (amount, timing, precipitants). These symptoms are nonspecific except for the history of pure stress incontinence (urine loss only during sudden straining).
2. *Bladder record:* charting the timing of successful voiding and incontinent episodes during 24-hour periods may be both diagnostic and therapeutic.
3. *Other medical conditions:* dementia, delirium, neurologic disorders, diabetes, arthritis, congestive heart failure
4. *Past medical history:* childbirth, genitourinary surgery, urethral catheterization or dilation, pelvic irradiation
5. *Medications*
   a. Anticholinergic agents (including antidepressants, antihistamines, and neuroleptics), beta-adrenergic agonists, theophylline, calcium channel blockers, and narcotics may produce overflow by inhibition of bladder contractility.
   b. Alpha-adrenergic agonists increase sphincter tone, which promotes urine retention and overflow.
   c. Alpha-adrenergic blockers lead to stress incontinence by sphincter relaxation.
   d. Diuretics and alcohol induce polyuria and urgency.
   e. Any sedative may cause functional incontinence from confusion or excessive sedation.
6. *Functional/environmental:* Restraints, location of toilet, ability to walk, transfer onto toilet, manipulate clothing, and use bedpan or urinal.

TABLE 6–2. Mechanisms of Chronic Urinary Incontinence

TYPE	DEFINITION	COMMON CAUSES
Stress	Urine loss (small amount) with sudden increase in intraabdominal pressure, e.g., cough, laugh	Weakness of pelvic floor musculature Weakness or damage to urethral sphincter
Urge	Urine loss (moderate amount) due to uninhibited bladder contractions preceded by sensation of bladder fullness	Local bladder irritation (cystitis, stone, tumor) CNS disorder (mass lesion, stroke, dementia, parkinsonism, myelopathy)
Overflow	Urine loss (frequent small amounts) when pressure of urine in distended bladder exceeds urethral pressure	Obstructive (prostatic hypertrophy, stricture) Hypotonic bladder (peripheral neuropathy, cauda equina syndrome, medications) Detrusor-sphincter dyssynergy (CNS lesions, multiple sclerosis)
Functional	Urine loss caused by inability to reach toilet in time	Physical immobility Dementia

Source: Adapted from Ouslander JG. Commentary. Clin Geriatr Med 1986;2:711–713.

PHYSICAL EXAMINATION

1. Abdomen: mass, tenderness, bladder distention
2. Rectal: prostate, rectal mass, fecal impaction, perianal sensation, sphincter tone
3. Pelvic: mass, atrophic vaginitis, prolapse, stress-induced incontinence (patient strains with full bladder while standing)
4. Neurologic: mental status, signs of parkinsonism, stroke, neuropathy (especially perianal sensation), or myelopathy.
5. Functional: ability to ambulate, manipulate clothing, and use toilet.

LABORATORY STUDIES

1. Urinalysis (evidence of infection, stone, tumor).
2. Serum glucose, urea nitrogen, and creatinine.
3. Measurement of postvoid residual urine volume (PVR). A PVR volume greater than 100 ml suggests an overflow mechanism.

4. If the cause of incontinence remains unclear, simple cystometry may be performed at the bedside.

RECOMMENDED DIAGNOSTIC APPROACH

1. Elicit the symptom and duration of urinary incontinence.
2. Define the pathophysiologic mechanism (type) of persistent incontinence.
3. Provide appropriate therapy.
4. Refer to urologist or gynecologist if incontinence persists, mechanism is unclear, or if other referral criteria are met:
   a. Recent genitourinary or pelvic surgery
   b. Recent therapeutic pelvic irradiation
   c. Recurrent symptomatic urinary tract infections
   d. Stress incontinence unresponsive to medical management
   e. Marked pelvic prolapse
   f. Prostatic enlargement or nodule
   g. Palpable bladder, repeated elevation of the PVR, or severe hesitancy or straining
   h. Difficulty passing a urethral catheter
   i. Hematuria in the absence of infection

Bibliography

Consensus conference: Urinary incontinence in adults. JAMA 1989;261:2685–2690.

Ouslander JG. Commentary. Clin Geriatr Med 1986;2:711–713.

Ouslander JG. Diagnostic evaluation of geriatric urinary incontinence. Clin Geriatr Med 1986;2:715–730.

Ouslander JG, et al. Simplified tests of lower urinary tract function in the evaluation of geriatric urinary incontinence. J Am Geriatr Soc 1989;37:706–714.

Resnick NM, Yalla SV. Management of urinary incontinence in the elderly. N Engl J Med 1985;313:800–805.

7

HYPERTENSION

C. SCOTT SMITH

My fate cries out,
And makes each petty artery in this body
As hardy as the Newean Rion's nerve.

SHAKESPEARE (1564–1616) Hamlet, I, IV, 81

DEFINITION

The 1988 Joint National Committee on Detection, Evaluation and Treatment of High Blood Pressure (JNC) has defined hypertension in adults as 2 or more diastolic blood pressure (DBP) measurements on at least 2 occasions greater than or equal to 90 mmHg. Measurement is usually taken sitting, after a brief rest, with an appropriate-sized cuff (the rubber bladder should encircle at least 2/3 of the arm). No single elevated reading constitutes hypertension. Table 7–1 shows the definitions and follow-up recommendations as outlined by the JNC.

EPIDEMIOLOGY

Hypertension, as defined above, affects 10 to 20% of the adult U.S. population (nearly 60 million people). It is a powerful risk factor for cardiovascular disease. The prevalence of hypertension increases with age and is greater in blacks than in whites. Blacks also have more complications for any given blood pressure. The Framingham study has shown that the risk of cardiovascular complications increases steadily with increasing systolic or diastolic blood pressure without any clearly defined "at-risk" or "threshold" level.

Since the risk appears to continually increase with blood pressure level, the definitions of "high" and "normal" blood pressure are derived from evidence related to treatment. There have been 6 clinical trials comparing treatment to either placebo or no treatment which have shown that treating DBP in the mild range (>95 mmHg) improves mortality and morbidity from "hypertensive" complications (e.g., stroke, congestive heart failure, renal failure, left ventricular hypertrophy, or accelerated hypertension) but not from "atherosclerotic" complications (coronary artery disease).

DIFFERENTIAL DIAGNOSIS

The major item in the differential diagnosis for hypertension is "pseudohypertension," which is seen in the elderly. It is due

**TABLE 7–1. JNC Definitions
and Recommendations**

BLOOD PRESSURE (MM HG)	CATEGORY	FOLLOW-UP
Diastolic (mm Hg)		
<85	Normal	2 Years
85–89	High normal	1 Year
90–104	Mild HTN	2 Months
105–114	Moderate HTN	2 Weeks
≥115	Severe HTN	Immediate
Systolic (when DPB ≤ 90)		
<140	Normal	2 Years
140–159	Borderline systolic HTN	2 Months
>160	Isolated systolic HTN	—
>200	—	2 Weeks

to rigid, atherosclerotic blood vessels and the increased pressure needed in the sphygmomanometer cuff to compress them. Osler's maneuver screens for pseudohypertension: the radial artery is palpated as the sphygmomanometer is pumped up until Korotkoff's sounds disappear. If the radial artery is still felt, it is presumed due to the hardened walls of the artery and the patient most likely has some false elevation of blood pressure. If indicated, direct arterial cannulation can measure true intraluminal pressure.

CLASSIFICATION

Hypertension is usually described as primary (essential) or secondary, based on etiology (Table 7–2).

Aortic Coarctation

In adults a coarctation most often occurs below the left subclavian artery. The lesion may be congenital or caused by Takayasu's arteritis.

Renal Vascular Disease

1. Causes: There are two types of renovascular disease. Fibromuscular dysplasia (1/3 of cases) causes thickening of the media of the distal renal artery. It is most often seen in white women between the ages of 20 and 50. Atherosclerotic vascular disease (2/3 of cases) occurs in those prone to atherosclerotic disease anywhere, i.e., increased with age, male gender, smoking, diabetes, and hyperlipidemia. Renal artery stenosis is bilateral in approximately 20% of patients.
2. Clinical findings: Clues to renovascular disease as the cause of hypertension include accelerated or abrupt onset

TABLE 7–2. Frequency (%) of Various Forms of Hypertension in the General Population

Diagnosis	Percent
Essential hypertension	90–94
Renal hypertension	
Parenchymal	2–5
Renovascular	1–3
Adrenal hypertension	
Primary aldosteronism	0.1–0.5
Cushing's syndrome	0.1–0.2
Pheochromocytoma	0.1–0.2
Aortic coarctation	0.1–0.2
Oral contraceptives	2–4
Other	<2
Pregnancy	
Other medications (nonsteroidal anti-inflammatory drugs, estrogen, steroids)	
Endocrine (acromegaly, hyperthyroidism, hyperparathyroidism)	

hypertension, disease in young patients, new or refractory hypertension in the elderly, flank or abdominal bruits, disease refractory to two or more drugs, renal insufficiency after reasonable BP control with angiotensin converting enzyme inhibitors, hypokalemia, or relatively larger increases in blood ureanitrogen (BUN) than creatinine (a "prerenal" picture).

Cushing's Syndrome

This results in hypertension by four mechanisms: (1) the weak mineralocorticoid effects of excess glucocorticoids, (2) some increase in the secretion of true mineralocorticoids, (3) increased renin-angiotensin effects (due to stimulated production of renin substrate), and (4) increased activity of the sympathetic nervous system (due to enzyme induction by glucocorticoids).

Primary Aldosteronism

Increased levels of aldosterone are caused by benign adrenal adenomas (Conn's disease) or from bilateral adrenal hyperplasia (idiopathic hyperaldosteronism). This hormone acts to stimulate resorption (in exchange for other cations such as K^+ and H^+) at the distal tubule, and thus increases vascular volume.

Pheochromocytoma

These are tumors of chromaffin tissue that produce excess catecholamines. Catecholamines directly stimulate the heart to increase cardiac output and also directly cause blood vessel constriction and an increase in vascular resistance.

CLINICAL FEATURES

History

1. Family history of hypertension, renal disease, or endocrine disease
2. Patient's history of hypertension
   a. Age at onset
   b. Previous level of control
   c. Previous medications and side effects
3. History of weight gain, sodium intake, and alcohol intake
4. Current medications—prescription *and* nonprescription
5. History suggestive of secondary cause of hypertension
   a. Headache, sweating, palpitations: pheochromocytoma
   b. Muscle cramps, weakness, polyuria: hyperaldosteronism
   c. Changes in body fat, poor wound healing, easy bruising: Cushing's syndrome
   d. Cold feet, lower extremity claudication: aortic coarctation
6. History suggestive of end-organ damage
   a. Orthopnea
   b. Paroxysmal nocturnal dyspnea (PND)
   c. Angina
   d. Claudication
7. Co-morbid diseases that may affect choice of therapeutic agent
   a. Asthma: β blockers should be avoided, calcium channel blockers helpful
   b. Gout: diuretics aggravate the condition
   c. Migraine: β blockers are also efficacious for migraine
   d. Depression: aggravated by β blockers and central agents
   e. Sexual dysfunction: aggravated by β blockers, central agents, and diuretics

Physical Examination

1. Measurement of height and weight
2. Blood pressure readings lying, standing, and in both arms while sitting
3. Funduscopic exam
4. Neck exam for jugular venous distention, carotid bruit, and thyroid enlargement
5. Lung exam for rales
6. Cardiac exam for increased size, precordial heave, murmurs, arrhythmias, S_3 or S_4 gallop
7. Examination of the flank and abdomen for bruits, masses, and enlarged kidneys
8. Extremity examination for edema, pulses (including a check for radial-femoral pulse delay)
9. Neurologic exam

RECOMMENDED DIAGNOSTIC APPROACH

The goal of therapy is not to "normalize" a number, but rather to prevent end-organ disease. Therefore, there are 4 goals in the initial evaluation of hypertensive patients:

1. Assess other independent risk factors for cardiovascular disease that may also need modification: age, sex, total cholesterol, cigarette smoking, glucose intolerance, and ECG evidence of left ventricular hypertrophy.
2. Evaluate the extent of current end-organ disease (brain, heart, and kidneys).
3. Screen for secondary causes of hypertension.
4. Screen for any co-morbid disease that may affect your choice of treatment.

Initial Work-up (Table 7–3)

Most authors agree on a complete urinalysis and serum creatinine to assess renal function, a serum cholesterol and glucose to evaluate other risk factors, a serum potassium to screen for secondary causes, and an ECG to look for hypertrophy and check for lengthening of the PR interval (as this may preclude certain treatment options such as β blockers or calcium channel blockers). In addition, many authors recommend a chest X-ray (to evaluate heart size, look for evidence of CHF, and screen for coarctation), uric acid (a sensitive screen for early nephrosclerosis), or calcium as a screen for endocrine diseases.

Further Work-up

If the initial screening suggests secondary hypertension, the further diagnostic studies are as follows:

1. Aortic coarctation: If there is a radial-femoral pulse delay on exam, a chest X-ray should be obtained. If the chest X-ray is suspicious (aortic indentation, rib notching, etc.) then ultrasound duplex studies and/or aortography are performed.
2. Renal vascular disease: Screening tests should be restricted to those patients with suspected renovascular hypertension, as the positive predictive values (the probability that the patient has the disease if the test is positive) are unacceptably low when the tests are used on all

TABLE 7–3. Initial Laboratory Work-up of Hypertension

RECOMMENDED	OPTIONAL
Urinalysis	Uric acid
Creatinine	Chest X-ray
Cholesterol	Calcium
Glucose	
Potassium	
Electrocardiogram	

**TABLE 7–4. Sensitivities and Specificities
of Various Screening Tests for
Renovascular Disease**

Test	Specificity (%)	Sensitivity (%)
Hypertensive IVP	85–89	80–85
Renal scan	80	86
Peripheral renin	66	57
Captopril-stimulated renin	85	85
Ultrasound duplex scan*	92	94

* From the University of Washington Medical Center, Seattle, WA.

hypertensives (Table 7–4). If one studies only patients
with suggestive history, physical, or laboratory findings,
the increased sensitivity and specificity of newer tests
such as duplex studies yields a positive predictive value
of 70%.

If screening duplex is suspicious or unavailable and
aggressive therapy is contemplated, renal arteriography
and renal vein renin measurements should be performed.
A renin ratio of 1.5 to 1, affected to unaffected side, is an
excellent predictor of correctable disease. Renal arteriography alone is not sufficient to evaluate renal vascular

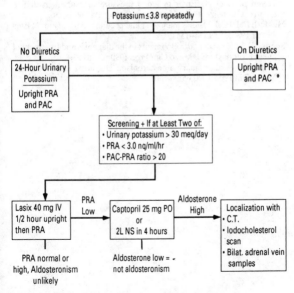

* PRA = plasma renin activity; PAC = plasma aldosterone concentration

Figure 7–1. Evaluation of Aldosteronism. (If possible, attempt to
stop diuretics for several days.)

disease because more than 30% of normals have some degree of stenosis on angiograms and would not benefit from surgical or angioplastic correction.

3. Cushing's syndrome: Screen with an overnight dexamethasone suppression test (1 mg p.o. at bedtime) or a 24-hour urine free cortisol.

4. Primary aldosteronism (Figure 7–1): Approximately 75% of these patients have a low serum potassium at the time of their initial presentation; 50% of untreated hypertensives presenting with a potassium <3.3 mEq/L have aldosteronism.

5. Pheochromocytoma (see Chapter 57): Screening is best done with a spot urine to check the metanephrine/creatinine ratio (≥1 μg metanephrine/mg creatinine is positive). This is both easier than obtaining 24-hour urines and more sensitive than total catecholamines or vanillylmandelic acid (VMA).

Bibliography

Alderman MH, et al. Treatment-induced blood pressure reduction and the risk of myocardial infarction. JAMA 1989;262:920–924.

Berglund G. Goals of antihypertensive therapy. Is there a point beyond which pressure reduction is dangerous? Am J Hypertens 1989; 2:586–593.

Joint National Committee on Detection, Evaluation, and Treatment of High Blood Pressure. 1988 report. Arch Int Med 1988;148(5):1023–1038.

Kannel WB. Some lessons in cardiovascular epidemiology from Framingham. Am J Cardiol 1976;37:269–282.

Maxwell MH, et al. Error in blood pressure measurement due to incorrect cuff size in obese patients. Lancet 1982;2:33–36.

Messerli FH, et al. Osler's maneuver and pseudohypertension. N Engl J Med 1985;312:1548–1551.

Sheps SG, et al. Recent developments in the diagnosis and treatment of pheochromocytoma. Mayo Clin Proc 1990;65:88–95.

Young WF, et al. Primary aldosteronism: Diagnosis and treatment. Mayo Clin Proc 1990;65:96–110.

8

ELECTROLYTE DISORDERS: HYPONATREMIA, HYPERNATREMIA, HYPOKALEMIA, AND HYPERKALEMIA

STUART L. BURSTEN

A grain of salt being added.

PLINY THE ELDER (23–79)

HYPONATREMIA

- General comments
  1. Hyponatremia indicates free water imbalance. In hyponatremia, water has diluted the serum sodium (Na) concentration.
  2. Hyponatremia may be hypotonic, isotonic, or hypertonic depending on the serum tonicity (osmolality). The normal serum osmolality is 280 to 295 mOsm/L.
  3. If total body sodium has changed significantly (i.e., with volume changes), the terms "hypervolemic" and "hypovolemic" are added.
- Isotonic hyponatremia
  1. Clinical occurrence. In this state, a true increase in total body water has not occurred. It occurs when the solid component of serum (the ash) is increased, such as in the dysproteinemic states of Waldenstrom's macroglobulinemia and multiple myeloma, and hyperlipidemias.
  2. Physiologic mechanism
     a. The normal solid component of serum (70 mL/L) is not sampled when serum is analyzed for sodium.
     b. If the ash content of the serum is doubled, as may occur in multiple myeloma, 140 ml of each liter is not available. The Na concentration is thus determined in 860 ml instead of 930 ml. The serum Na is falsely low at 129 (129/860 = 140/930).
     c. During infusions of isotonic solutions, such as mannitol or glucose, there is a transient dilutional hyponatremia due to proportional shift of water to serum.
- Hypertonic hyponatremia

1. This common finding is associated with hyperglycemia and infusions of hypertonic mannitol (for neurosurgical patients) or glucose (hyperalimentation). The hypertonicity due to glucose obligates water to cross into the extracellular space to dilute the serum Na, causing hyponatremia.

2. Correction factor

$$Sodium_{corrected} = Sodium_{measured}$$
$$+ \{[glucose \ (mg/dl) - 100]/100\} \times 1.8$$

3. For example, if the serum Na is 130, and the serum glucose is 750 mg/dl,

$$Na_{corrected} = 130 + \left(\frac{750 - 100}{100}\right) \times 1.8 = 141.7$$

- Hypotonic hyponatremia: hypovolemic type. In general, these states exist when salt is lost in greater amounts than water or when water is replaced in greater quantities than salt. Patients are placed in this category when signs of hypovolemia are present. Causes include:

1. Gastrointestinal disease: e.g., secretory diarrheas.
2. Lung: e.g., bronchorrhea as occurs with alveolar cell carcinoma.
3. Skin: e.g., sweating in a person not acclimated to a hot climate who still has a high–sodium-content sweat.
4. Adrenal insufficiency: e.g., renal salt-wasting.
5. Renal disease: e.g., diuretics, chronic renal failure with salt-wasting, and postobstruction diuresis.

- Hypotonic hyponatremia: isovolemic type. In this condition the volume status is normal, and there is no third spacing of fluid. Causes include:

1. Water intoxication. This is generally found in psychotic patients.
2. Potassium depletion. As potassium shifts out of cells in hypokalemic states, sodium shifts in, producing a dilutional hyponatremia. Potassium depletion also stimulates antidiuretic hormone (ADH) secretion.
3. Hypothyroidism and hypoadrenalism. These endocrinopathies decrease the ability to excrete a water load.
4. Syndrome of inappropriate antidiuretic hormone (SIADH) secretion. This can be caused by the following conditions:
   a. Ectopic ADH elaboration by tumors, particularly oat cell cancer of the lung.
   b. Inappropriate stimulation from pulmonary pathology (bacterial pneumonia, tuberculosis, lung abscesses, asthma).
   c. Medications: vincristine, cyclophosphamide, morphine, barbiturates, nicotine, oral hypoglycemic agents
   d. Uncontrolled secretion from any CNS problem (infections, trauma, vascular disease, neoplasms) or after stress such as trauma or surgery

- Hypervolemic hyponatremia
  1. This condition is associated with the late stage of processes that cause total body volume overload, such as end-stage congestive heart failure, cirrhosis, and nephrotic syndrome, and severe protein-losing enteropathies with edema.
  2. Pathophysiologic mechanisms include:
     a. Excessive stimulation of ADH by central hypoperfusion, poor right atrial return, and increased intrathoracic pressure
     b. Reduced renal blood flow and glomerular filtration rates
     c. Loss of diluting capacity as a result of diminished delivery of solutes to the renal tubules
     d. Increased activity of the renin-angiotensin-aldosterone system

Recommended Diagnostic Approach

- The serum osmolality and the patient's volume status determine the subsequent diagnostic pathway.
- Isotonic hyponatremia. When serum sodium determinations are consistently low and the serum osmolality is normal
  1. The total protein should be determined (this may be a clue to the diagnosis of multiple myeloma).
  2. The lipid fractions should be determined.
- Hypotonic hyponatremia: hypovolemic type
  1. Virtually all patients demonstrate postural changes in blood pressure and pulse if pulse is measured while standing for longer than 2 minutes, and a diminished skin turgor.
  2. Blood-urea nitrogen-creatinine (BUN/CREAT) ratio. This is usually >20 in this form of hyponatremia, although with renal failure it can be as low as 10.
  3. Urine sodium (U_{Na})
     a. With gastrointestinal, lung, and skin losses, U_{Na} is <20 mEq/L.
     b. With adrenal insufficiency and renal disease, the U_{Na} is >20 mEq/L.
  4. Urine osmolality (U_{osm}). The U_{osm} is usually greater than 400 mOsm/L except with renal failure when the urine is isosthenuric.
- Hypotonic hyponatremia: isovolemic type. To make the diagnosis of isovolemic hyponatremia, the patient must have no signs of congestive heart failure, hypovolemia, volume overload, or fluid "third spacing."
  1. Clinical and laboratory features of conditions 1–3 above should be sought.
  2. SIADH has the following laboratory findings:
     a. A U_{Na} that is initially elevated (>60 meq/L) and that subsequently falls to a level that reflects the daily sodium intake.

    b. The urine, which should be maximally dilute, has an inappropriately high U_{osm}. $U_{osm} > 100$ mOsm/L is too high in the face of a decreased serum osmolality.

    c. BUN and serum creatinine levels and the BUN/CREAT ratio may all be decreased.

    d. Serum ADH levels are normal to high.

- Hypervolemic hyponatremia
  1. The physician should examine for signs of volume overload, including peripheral and pulmonary edema, ascites, and hypertension.
  2. BUN/CREAT ratio. This ratio is greater than 20.
  3. U_{Na} is <20 mEq/L.

HYPERNATREMIA

- General comments
  1. Hypernatremia is caused by either loss of water in excess of loss of salt or by a gain of salt in excess of gain in water.
  2. The total body water deficit can be estimated as follows (desired sodium content is usually taken as 140 mEq/L):

$$[1 - (Na_{measured}/Na_{desired})] \times total\ body\ water$$

$$Total\ body\ water = 0.6 \times weight\ in\ kg$$

For example, if the serum sodium in a 70-kg person is 160, the total water deficit is:

$$\left(1 - \frac{160}{140}\right) \times (0.6 \times 70) = \frac{-20}{140} \times 42 = -6\ L$$

- Hypovolemic hypernatremia. This occurs when fluid loss is relatively salt-poor. It may also be caused iatrogenically when lost hypotonic fluid is replaced with hypertonic or isotonic fluid. Causes include:
  1. GI illness, including osmotic diarrhea and vomiting.
  2. Sweating after acclimation to hot climates (low-sodium sweat).
  3. Diuretic ingestion combined with increased salt intake and poor water intake.
  4. Partial urinary tract obstruction combined with administration of hypertonic fluids.
  5. Acute or chronic renal failure with loss of concentrating ability.
  6. Urea diuresis, particularly in catabolic patients.
  7. Glycosuria: Glucose spilling causes a urine that is 0.45% sodium chloride. Hypernatremia is common with hyperglycemia and sodium correction for hyperglycemia must be done.
- Euvolemic hypernatremia. This is characterized by selective loss of water and is caused almost exclusively by diabetes insipidus. Diabetes insipidus may be central or nephrogenic.

1. Central diabetes insipidus is characterized by diminished or absent production of ADH.
   a. Primary central diabetes insipidus accounts for 50% of cases.
   b. Secondary central diabetes insipidus is most often caused by cranial trauma or metastatic tumor, usually of lung or breast. Granulomatous diseases such as tuberculosis, sarcoidosis, and eosinophilic granuloma may be implicated.
2. Nephrogenic diabetes insipidus is characterized by diminished or absent renal response to ADH.
   a. Primary nephrogenic diabetes insipidus is rare, causing less than 1% of cases.
   b. Secondary nephrogenic diabetes insipidus is caused by electrolyte disorders such as hypokalemia and hypercalcemia and by renal disease such as acute tubular necrosis, obstruction, or myeloma and amyloid kidney.
   c. Up to 25% of nephrogenic diabetes insipidus is related to medications such as demeclocycline, methoxyflurane, and lithium carbonate. Half of patients taking lithium develop a concentrating disorder.
- Hypervolemic hypernatremia. This is almost always caused by iatrogenic administration of excess salt via hypertonic solutions. Other causes include primary hyperaldosteronism, Cushing's syndrome, and exogenous administration of corticosteroids. Iatrogenic hypernatremia may be suspected if there is inadequate replacement of cleared free water.

Recommended Diagnostic Approach

- BUN, serum creatinine, U_{Na}, and U_{osm} should be measured.
  1. Nonrenal causes of hypernatremia produce a BUN/CREAT ratio ≥ 20, a $U_{Na} < 20$ mEq/L, and a $U_{osm} > 400$ mOsm/L.
  2. Renal causes of hypernatremia usually produce a BUN/CREAT ratio of 10 because both BUN and CREAT levels are elevated. The U_{Na} is >20 mEq/L but less than the serum sodium content, and the urine is isothenuric.
- Twenty-four-hour urine output
  1. Central diabetes insipidus is characterized by large volumes of hypotonic urine (greater than 3 L/24 h); if there is complete absence of ADH the volume may be greater than 20 L/24 h.
  2. In nephrogenic diabetes insipidus there is a diminished output of isothenuric urine.
- Water deprivation test. In normal persons, water deprivation causes a fall in urine volume and an increased U_{osm} proportionate to the increasing serum osmolality.
  1. In central diabetes insipidus, patients have constant urine output and a rising serum osmolality, but little or

no rise in U_{osm}. The defect corrects with IM administration of ADH.

2. Nephrogenic diabetes insipidus responds in the same manner to water deprivation, but there is little or no response to ADH administration.

HYPOKALEMIA

- General comments. Hypokalemia is associated with cardiac arrhythmias and, when chronic, with renal tubular dysfunction and interstitial degeneration. It can be classified into one of three types, according to whether it is caused by:
    1. Redistribution of potassium
    2. Renal losses
    3. Nonrenal losses
- Redistributional hypokalemia. In these states the total body potassium content is normal. Causes include:
    1. Alkalosis. The depletion of protons with alkalosis causes an intracellular increase of negative charges. This obligates a potassium shift into cells and leads to hypokalemia (0.6 mEq/L of potassium decrease per 0.1 pH increase).
    2. Insulin administration. Insulin acts acutely to shift potassium into cells.
    3. Vitamin B_{12} therapy. As B_{12} stimulates myelopoiesis and rapid cell proliferation, there is a rapid sequestration of potassium in multiplying cells.
    4. Periodic paralysis. This is associated with thyrotoxicosis in Japanese persons and is an autosomal dominant genetic defect in whites.
    5. Beta$_2$ agonist administration. Stimulation of beta$_2$ receptors causes intracellular shifting of potassium.
- Hypokalemia from renal losses. By definition the 24-hour urine potassium content is greater than 20 mEq.
    1. Hypertensive states. Hypertensive states include:
        a. Conditions of elevated renin, such as renovascular and malignant hypertension.
        b. Conditions of low renin and elevated aldosterone, such as primary aldosteronism with bilateral adrenal hyperplasia.
        c. Conditions of low renin and low aldosterone, such as Cushing's syndrome and after intake of exogenous mineralocorticoids, licorice (glycyrrhizinic acid), chewing tobacco, and carbenoxolone.
    2. Normotensive states. Normotensive states include:
        a. Renal tubular acidosis, with serum bicarbonate concentration less than 23 mEq/L (types I and II).
        b. Alkalosis caused by vomiting, with urine chloride concentration less than 10 mEq/day.
        c. Alkalosis caused by diuretics, severe potassium depletion, or Bartter's syndrome.
        d. Drug-induced: carbenicillin and its derivatives, gentamicin, amphotericin B, cis-platinum, and beta$_2$ agonists (long-term use).

- Hypokalemia from nonrenal losses. These are uncommon, with the cause generally obvious from the history. The 24-hour urine potassium content is less than 20 mEq. Causes of fluid loss include:
  1. Skin losses, without acclimation.
  2. Biliary losses.
  3. Secretory diarrhea (e.g., villous adenomata) which is associated with bicarbonate loss and a corresponding acidosis.

Recommended Diagnostic Approach

- Clues to redistributional hypokalemia usually come from the patient's history. Measurement of the arterial pH can confirm alkalosis as a contributing factor.
- The 24-hour urine potassium excretion should be measured to distinguish renal and nonrenal losses.
- The serum electrolytes and patient's blood pressure may guide the diagnostic process. Cushing's syndrome and hyperaldosteronism should be excluded in hypertensive patients.

HYPERKALEMIA

- General comments. Hyperkalemia always represents a potential medical emergency. The electrocardiogram (ECG) should be examined for characteristic changes immediately. Early ECG changes are T-wave peaking, with progression to QRS widening. Imminent danger of ventricular fibrillation is signaled by merging of QRS–T complexes and formation of a poorly defined sine wave pattern.
- Pseudohyperkalemia (laboratory error)
  1. The serum potassium always exceeds plasma potassium by 0.1 to 0.3 mEq/L owing to release of potassium from white blood cells and platelets. To confirm this as the cause of the hyperkalemia, the plasma potassium should be compared with the serum potassium.
  2. The plasma-serum difference will be 0.5 to 2.0 mEq/L with:
     a. White blood cell count > 50,000/mm^3
     b. Platelet count > 750,000/mm^3
     c. Extensive hemolysis in the test tube
- Hyperkalemia from redistribution. This form of hyperkalemia occurs in the following conditions:
  1. Tissue necrosis: crush injuries, burns, rhabdomyolysis, and tumor lysis syndrome.
  2. Acidosis: The inverse of alkalosis occurs, with extracellular shifting of potassium. This may be acute after a generalized seizure.
  3. Insulin deficiency: This is exacerbated in diabetics who may also have simultaneous hypoaldosteronism.
  4. Medications
     a. Nonselective beta blockers with blockade of beta$_2$

receptors can cause extracellular leak of potassium.
b. Severe digitalis toxicity with inhibition of sodium-potassium ATPase may cause hyperkalemia.
c. Succinylcholine can produce rapid hyperkalemia, especially in trauma patients.

- Hyperkalemia from excessive intake or reduced excretion
  1. Hyperkalemia is not encountered in patients with chronic renal failure until their glomerular filtration rate is <8 to 10 ml/min.
  2. Causes of reduced potassium secretion in the distal tubules and collecting ducts include:
     a. Decreased extracellular fluid volume
     b. Interstitial nephritis
     c. Amyloid renal disease
     d. Urinary tract obstruction
     e. Use of potassium-retaining drugs, including triamterene, spironolactone, or amiloride
  3. Situations with excessive intake include:
     a. Potassium-penicillin administration
     b. Salt substitutes (often used as part of a low sodium diet)
     c. Transfusions

- Hyperkalemia from deficits in the renin-angiotensin-aldosterone system. Specific pathophysiologic categories include:
  1. Decreased renin
     a. Drugs, such as beta blockers, alpha-methyldopa, and prostaglandin inhibitors (nonsteroidal antiinflammatory drugs)
     b. Aging
     c. Interstitial nephritis (in addition to the secretory defects mentioned above)
     d. Diabetes mellitus
  2. Decreased angiotensin
     a. Glucocorticoid deficiency (Addison's disease)
     b. Hepatic failure
     c. Angiotensin converting enzyme inhibitors
  3. Decreased aldosterone
     a. Addison's disease
     b. Selective adrenal hemorrhage as with heparin administration
     c. Spironolactone
     d. Hydroxylase deficiencies

Recommended Diagnostic Approach

- Establish the diagnosis of true hyperkalemia. Identify diseases that may contribute to hyperkalemia.
- The decision to obtain serum renin, aldosterone, or angiotensin values may be guided by administration of 1.0 mg/day of fludrocortisone. If, after 3 to 5 days, there is kaliuresis and transition to normokalemia, the deficit is not renal, and measurement of renin, aldosterone, and angiotensin are appropriate.

Bibliography

Anderson RJ, et al. Hyponatremia. A prospective analysis of its epidemiology and the pathogenetic role of vasopressin. Ann Intern Med 1985;102:164.

Beck LH, ed. Body fluid and electrolyte disorders. Med Clin North Am 1981;65:251–448.

Gennari FJ. Serum osmolality: Uses and limitations. N Engl J Med 1984;310:102.

Narins RG, et al. Diagnostic strategies in disorders of fluid, electrolytes, and acid-base homeostasis. Am J Med 1982;72:496–520.

Ponce SP, et al. Drug induced hyperkalemia. Medicine 1985;64:357.

9

ACID-BASE DISORDERS

DAVID C. DUGDALE

In Physic, things of melancholic hue and quality are used against melancholy, sour against sour, salt to remove salt humours.

JOHN MILTON (1608–1674)

GENERAL COMMENTS AND DEFINITIONS

- Acid-base disorders are not a "diagnosis," but an indication for diagnostic evaluation. The approach to diagnosis of acid-base disorders has 3 facets:
  1. Recognition by clinical or laboratory features.
  2. Definition of the type(s) of disorder(s) present.
  3. Evaluation of the differential diagnosis of the acid-base disorder(s) present.

- Body functions produce acid continuously. The normal blood arterial pH is maintained by buffer systems and excretion of acid by the kidneys or lungs.
  1. Buffer systems maintain blood pH by rapidly absorbing acid that is produced. The major systems of the body include bicarbonate, phosphate species, and tissue proteins.
  2. Carbon dioxide (CO_2), produced from carbonic acid, is excreted by the lungs.
  3. The kidney regenerates bicarbonate (HCO_3) by sending hydrogen ions into the urine where they are buffered by ammonia and phosphate species.

- Analysis of acid-base disorders requires knowledge of the plasma pH, partial pressure of carbon dioxide ($PaCO_2$), and bicarbonate concentration (usually approximately 1 mEq/L less than the "measured" or "total" CO_2 of the serum electrolytes). When arterial blood gases are determined, only 2 (usually pH and $PaCO_2$) of the quantities are measured; the third is calculated using the Henderson-Hasselbalch equation:

$$pH = 6.1 + \log[HCO_3/(0.03 \times PaCO_2)]$$

  Normal arterial plasma pH: 7.35 − 7.45
  Normal $PaCO_2$: 35 − 45 mmHg
  Normal total CO_2: 24 − 30 mEq/L

- A pathologic process that affects the HCO_3 concentration is a metabolic disturbance (Table 9–1).

- A pathologic process that affects the $PaCO_2$ is a respiratory disturbance.

TABLE 9–1. Simple Acid-Base Disturbances

Disturbance	Primary Change	pH	Compensatory Change
Metabolic acidosis	Decreased HCO_3	Decreased	Decreased $PaCo_2$
Metabolic alkalosis	Increased HCO_3	Increased	Increased $PaCO_2$
Respiratory acidosis	Increased $PaCO_2$	Decreased	Increased HCO_3
Respiratory alkalosis	Decreased $PaCO_2$	Increased	Decreased HCO_3

- A *simple* acid-base disturbance has only one pathophysiologic process.
  1. The lung compensates rapidly by changing the minute ventilation. The kidney requires several hours to days to adjust its acid excretion.
  2. If over- or undercompensation occurs, a *mixed* acid-base disorder is present. The expected compensatory responses are summarized in Figure 9–1 and Table 9–2.
     a. In analyzing respiratory disturbances, many clinicians prefer to calculate the expected change in pH (Table 9–2) and compare it with the measured pH. A difference suggests the presence of a mixed disturbance.
        i. For example, if a patient has a $PaCO_2$ of 50 mmHg and the arterial pH is 7.32, a simple acute respiratory acidosis is present.
        ii. If the $PaCO_2$ is 50 mmHg but the pH is 7.40, a metabolic alkalosis is also present.
        iii. Clinical judgment must be used to determine whether to use the formula for acute or chronic disturbances with a specific patient.
     b. The expected $PaCO_2$ in a patient with a metabolic acidosis may be calculated with Winter's formula:

     $$\text{Expected } PaCO_2 = 1.5 \times (\text{plasma } HCO_3) + 8 \pm 2$$

     c. Respiratory compensation for a metabolic alkalosis may be estimated by the following, but compensatory elevation of the $PaCO_2$ above 50 mmHg is unusual:

     $$\text{Expected increase of } PaCO_2 = (0.25 - 1.00) \times \text{increase of } HCO_3$$

DIFFERENTIAL DIAGNOSIS

- A metabolic acidosis (Table 9–3) results from accumulation or administration of excess acid *or* loss of alkali.

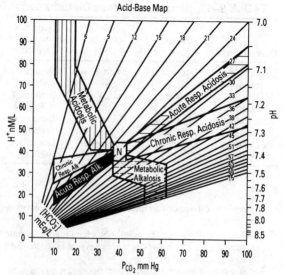

Figure 9–1. Graphic approach to acid-base disorders. The bands represent the 95% confidence interval for the compensatory response to a given primary disorder. The reader should work vertically from the $PaCO_2$ line. For example, consider a patient with a $PaCO_2$ of 70 mmHg, HCO_3 of 33 mEq/L, and pH of 7.30. The elevated HCO_3 could be caused by renal compensation for a chronic respiratory acidosis. The bands show that 95% of patients with $PaCO_2$ of 70 mmHg and chronic respiratory acidosis have a pH of 7.26 to 7.35 and HCO_3 of 32 to 39 mEq/L, which is the case for this patient, indicating appropriate compensation. However, if the HCO_3 were 30 mEq/L, which is outside the 95% confidence band for $PaCO_2$ of 70 mmHg, a mixed disorder would be suggested, such as an additional metabolic acidosis. (From Goldberg M, et al. Computer-based instruction and diagnosis of acid-base disorders. JAMA 1973;223:269–275.)

TABLE 9–2. Expected Changes in Acid-Base Disturbances

Expected change of plasma pH:

Acute respiratory disturbance:
$$\triangle pH = 0.008 \times (40 - PaCO_2)$$
Chronic respiratory disturbance:
$$\triangle pH = 0.003 \times (40 - PaCO_2)$$

$\triangle pH$ = change in pH

TABLE 9–3. Causes of Metabolic Acidosis

A. Normal anion gap
   1. Bicarbonate loss
      a. Proximal renal tubular acidosis
      b. Dilutional acidosis
      c. Carbonic anhydrase inhibitors (e.g., acetazolamide)
      d. Primary hyperparathyroidism
      e. Gastrointestinal loss (diarrhea, ureterosigmoidostomy)
   2. Failure of bicarbonate regeneration
      a. Distal renal tubular acidosis (including obstructive uropathy, interstitial nephritis)
      b. Hyporeninemic hypoaldosteronism
      c. Potassium sparing diuretics: triamterene, spironolactone, amiloride
      d. Medications: amphotericin B, cyclosporine
   3. Administration of acidifying salts
      a. Ammonium chloride
      b. Amino acid hydrochlorides (e.g., parenteral hyperalimentation)
B. Increased anion gap
   1. Reduced acid excretion
      a. Acute renal failure
      b. Chronic renal failure
   2. Accumulation of organic acids
      a. Lactic acidosis
      b. Ketoacidosis: alcoholic
                        diabetic
                        starvation
      c. Ingestion: salicylates
                    paraldehyde
                    methanol
                    ethylene glycol

Source: Adapted with permission from Andreoli TE. Disorders of fluid volume, electrolyte, and acid-base balance. In Wyngaarden JB and Smith LH, eds. Cecil Textbook of Medicine, 18th ed. Philadelphia, W. B. Saunders, 1988, p. 552.

Loss of anions with alkali equivalent (e.g., citrate in a patient with diarrhea) also causes metabolic acidosis.

1. The analysis of metabolic acidoses is aided by calculating the serum anion gap (AG) from the serum electrolyte concentration. The most common acute metabolic acidoses have an increased AG.

$$AG = Na - (Cl + CO_2)$$

   a. The normal range is 7 to 14 mEq/L, but variations in laboratory techniques may lower the reference range by up to 5 mEq/L.
   b. The AG is helpful in classifying metabolic acidosis and may provide a clue to the presence of a mixed disturbance (see Table 9–7).
   c. The AG is determined by the concentrations of

anions (other than Cl and CO_2) and cations (other than Na) that are required to maintain electroneutrality.

    i. A high AG usually indicates a metabolic acidosis with excess organic acids.

    ii. A low AG may result from excess cations (Li, Mg, Ca), excess cationic proteins (hyperglobulinemia), deficient anionic proteins (hypoalbuminemia), or bromide (which is counted as Cl by many colorimetric techniques).

2. Hyperchloremic metabolic acidosis due to bicarbonate loss or failure of HCO_3 regeneration is usually apparent from clinical clues. Patients who receive parenteral nutrition solutions without lactate or acetate (each of which has alkali equivalence) may receive excess acid.

3. Lactic acidosis occurs when there is inadequate tissue oxygenation; it may be induced by isoniazid toxicity or phenformin.

4. All types of ketoacidosis have accelerated lipolysis and ketogenesis due to relative insulin deficiency.

    a. In diabetic ketoacidosis (DKA), acetone, acetoacetate, and beta-hydroxybutyrate levels are elevated: the beta-hydroxybutyrate level is elevated to the greatest degree.

    b. Most "serum ketone" assays measure acetoacetate, and may thus underestimate the ketoacid concentrations.

        i. The relative proportions of the ketoacids is determined by the blood pH.

        ii. Coexistent lactic acidosis may depress acetoacetate production, also confounding assessment.

5. Alcoholic ketoacidosis often occurs in a poorly nourished patient following a recent alcohol binge (though 12 hours of abstinence is not unusual). Significant hyperglycemia is rare, and the serum glucose concentration is less than 50 mg/dl in 15% of patients.

6. Salicylate intoxication is suggested by a respiratory alkalosis accompanying the metabolic acidosis. Respiratory alkalosis is an early sign of salicylate intoxication.

7. Methanol ingestion leads to accumulation of formic acid and optic neuritis. Ethylene glycol ingestion causes glycolic and oxalic acid formation and oxaluria.

    a. Methanol or ethylene glycol ingestion may cause very high AGs, up to 50 mEq/L.

    b. An osmolal gap (between measured and calculated serum osmolality) is traditionally considered a marker of toxic alcohol ingestion, but it can occur in patients with alcoholic ketoacidosis or lactic acidosis.

- Metabolic alkalosis (Table 9–4) may be initiated by loss of acid, but maintenance of metabolic alkalosis requires an increase in the net rate of HCO_3 reabsorption by the proximal tubule of the nephron. Volume depletion and hypokalemia are the most common factors that maintain metabolic alkalosis.

TABLE 9–4. Causes of Metabolic Alkalosis

A. Low urinary chloride (usually less than 10 mEq/L)
1. Upper gastrointestinal loss (vomiting, gastric suction)
2. Chloride-losing diarrhea (e.g., villous adenoma of colon)
3. Diuretic administration
4. Decreased effective intravascular volume (with consequent increased mineralocorticoid activity, e.g., congestive heart failure, cirrhosis)
5. Carbenicillin therapy
B. High urinary chloride (usually greater than 20 mEq/L)
1. Primary hyperaldosteronism
2. Bartter's syndrome (secondary hyperaldosteronism)
3. Glucocorticoid excess
4. Licorice ingestion (glycyrrhizinic acid)
5. Severe hypokalemia
6. Severe hypomagnesemia
7. Occult diuretic abuse
8. After correction of chronic hypercarbia
9. After correction of organic acidosis (variably present)
C. Miscellaneous (urinary chloride variable)
1. Milk-alkali syndrome
2. Rapid blood transfusions (containing sodium citrate which is metabolized to bicarbonate)

---

1. Carbenicillin and other impermeant anions cause hydrogen ion secretion in the distal renal tubule, but since they are unmeasured anions, an elevated AG may be present.
2. Metabolic alkalosis due to excess consumption of alkali (e.g., antacids) is rare because the degree of consumption must be extreme.
3. The urinary chloride concentration is a useful quantity for distinguishing between metabolic alkalosis associated with volume depletion (urinary chloride concentration less than 10 mEq/L) and that associated with a primary increase in mineralocorticoid effect (urinary chloride greater than 20 mEq/L).

- Respiratory acidosis (Table 9–5). Patients with chronic respiratory acidosis have an increased serum HCO_3 level, but compensation requires 2 to 3 days. Therefore, increased HCO_3 in a patient with acute respiratory acidosis suggests a mixed disturbance.
- Respiratory alkalosis may be caused by a broad spectrum of clinical problems (Table 9–6). It may also occur transiently with anxiety due to obtaining the arterial blood gas specimen.
- Mixed acid-base disturbances (Table 9–7)
1. Two metabolic disturbances may be present simultaneously. Examples include:
a. DKA plus vomiting (AG acidosis + alkalosis)

TABLE 9–5. Causes of Respiratory Acidosis

A. Central nervous system depression
1. Medications (sedatives, anesthesia)
2. Respiratory center lesions (ischemia, trauma, tumor)
3. Infection (meningitis, encephalitis)
B. Neuromuscular disorders
1. Muscle disorders (muscular dystrophy, hypokalemia)
2. Nerve disorders (tetanus, poliomyelitis, Guillain-Barré syndrome, myasthenia gravis, amyotrophic lateral sclerosis)
3. Intoxication (botulism, pesticides)
4. Medications (curare, succinylcholine)
C. Lung motion impairment
1. Thoracic cage disease
   a. Kyphoscoliosis
   b. Thoracic injuries
   c. Ankylosing spondylitis
   d. Skin contractures (e.g., postburn)
   e. Obesity-hypoventilation syndrome
   f. Extreme abdominal distention
2. Intrathoracic disease
   a. Pneumothorax
   b. Pleural effusion or fibrosis
D. Lung disease
1. Mechanical obstruction
2. Obstructive lung disease (asthma, emphysema)
3. Severe intrinsic lung disease (e.g., pneumonia, pulmonary edema)

---

   b. Lactic acidosis plus diarrhea (AG acidosis + hyperchloremic acidosis)
   c. Vomiting plus obstructive uropathy (alkalosis + hyperchloremic acidosis)
2. Metabolic and respiratory disturbances may occur simultaneously:
   a. Salicylate toxicity (metabolic acidosis + respiratory alkalosis)
   b. Chronic obstructive pulmonary disease with diuretic therapy (respiratory acidosis + metabolic alkalosis)

CLINICAL FEATURES

- Changes in acid-base status may cause signs and symptoms. In many cases, they are overshadowed by those related to the underlying disorder.
- Metabolic acidosis may be associated with deep ("Kussmaul's") respirations, cardiac arrhythmias, hypotension, nausea, vomiting, lethargy, and coma.
- Metabolic alkalosis, when extreme, may cause cardiac arrhythmias and hypoventilation. The hypokalemia that

TABLE 9–6. Causes of Respiratory Alkalosis

A. Central nervous system disorders
1. Head trauma
2. Intracranial hemorrhage
3. Meningitis
4. Encephalitis
B. Metabolic disorders
1. Fever
2. Hypoxia
3. Marked anemia
4. Hyperthyroidism
5. Hepatic insufficiency
6. Sepsis
7. Drug effect: progesterone, salicylate toxicity
C. Pulmonary disorders
1. Pneumonia
2. Pulmonary edema
3. Asthma
4. Pulmonary embolism
D. Miscellaneous
1. Anxiety
2. Pregnancy
3. Mechanical hyperventilation
4. Pain

TABLE 9–7. Anion Patterns in Metabolic Acid-Base Disorders

CONDITION	SERUM ANION CONCENTRATION		
	HCO$_3$	Cl	Anion gap
Simple disorders			
Hyperchloremic acidosis	D	I	N
Anion gap acidosis	D	N	I
Metabolic alkalosis	I	D	N
Mixed disorders			
Metabolic alkalosis + anion gap acidosis	N, I, or D	D	I
Anion gap acidosis + hyperchloremic acidosis	D	I	I
Metabolic alkalosis + hyperchloremic acidosis	N	N	N

D = decreased; I = increased; N = normal.

Source: Reprinted with permission from Andreoli TE. Disorders of fluid volume, electrolyte, and acid-base balance. In Wyngaarden JB and Smith LH, eds. Cecil Textbook of Medicine, 18th ed. Philadelphia, W. B. Saunders, 1988, p. 556.

often accompanies metabolic alkalosis may cause muscular weakness or hyporeflexia.

- Respiratory acidosis is associated with dyspnea, tachypnea, headache, confusion, cardiac arrhythmias, lethargy, and coma. Accumulation of CO_2 may cause dilation of the blood vessels of the optic fundus or papilledema.

- Respiratory alkalosis, when acute, may be associated with paresthesia (extremities, circumoral), tetany, and light-headedness due to changes in the $PaCO_2$ and plasma ionized calcium concentration. Chronic respiratory alkalosis is usually asymptomatic.

RECOMMENDED DIAGNOSTIC APPROACH

- Measure the arterial blood gases and serum electrolyte levels. The pH indicates the primary disturbance unless there is acute respiratory alkalosis due to anxiety or a triple disturbance.

- For patients with a metabolic acidosis, calculate the anion gap. Other tests should be performed as indicated:
  1. Serum or urine ketone levels
  2. Serum lactate level
  3. Serum osmolality
  4. Serum levels of toxins, e.g., methanol, salicylate

- If the AG is normal in a patient with a metabolic acidosis, measure the urinary pH. A value greater than 5.5 during acidemia suggests a renal tubular acidosis.

- For metabolic alkalosis, measure the urinary chloride concentration (see Table 9–4).

Bibliography

Cogan MG, et al. Metabolic alkalosis. Med Clin North Am 1983; 67:901.

Emmett M, Narins RG. Clinical use of the anion gap. Medicine 1977;56:38–54.

Gabow PA. Disorders associated with an altered anion gap. Kidney Int 1985;27:472–483.

Gabow PA, et al. Organic acids in ethylene glycol intoxication. Ann Intern Med 1986;105:16–20.

Narins RG, Emmett M. Simple and mixed acid-base disorders: A practical approach. Medicine 1980;59:161–187.

Schelling JK, et al. Increased osmolal gap in alcoholic ketoacidosis and lactic acidosis. Ann Intern Med 1990;113:580–582.

Winter SD, et al. The fall of the serum anion gap. Arch Intern Med 1990;150:311–313.

Zunszein J, Baylor P. Diabetic ketoacidosis with alkalemia: A review. West J Med 1988;149:217–219.

SECTION II

CARDIOLOGY

10

CHEST PAIN AND ANGINA

MARY T. HO

The canker gnaw thy heart.

SHAKESPEARE (1564–1616)
Timon of Athens, IV, iii, 49.

EPIDEMIOLOGY

- Chest pain is the initial complaint of 4 to 7% of all patients seeking medical attention at emergency departments and walk-in clinics.
- Acute ischemic heart disease, including acute MI, unstable angina, and new onset angina, is the most common life-threatening cause of chest pain.
- Of patients hospitalized for suspected myocardial ischemia, only about one-third have acute ischemia (defined as unstable angina or acute MI) and need acute coronary care.

DIFFERENTIAL DIAGNOSIS (Table 10–1)

- In the outpatient setting, the most common diagnoses are chest wall pain and chest pain of unknown origin, presumably innocuous.
- Among patients with chest pain suggestive of ischemic heart disease who are referred for coronary arteriography, up to 30% have no detectable major vessel disease.
- Of patients with anginalike chest pain (but no evidence of coronary disease) who are referred for gastrointestinal evaluation, up to 50% have an esophageal etiology.

EVALUATION OF THE PATIENT WITH CHEST PAIN

There is urgency in rapidly identifying the subset of patients with chest pain who are having an acute myocardial infarction (AMI). Myocardial salvage (thrombolytic therapy or mechanical reperfusion) is now the goal in the management of AMI. Patients with chest pain may be categorized by their hemodynamic status. While the etiologies of the two categories overlap, the differential diagnosis for chest pain with abnormal hemodynamics is relatively limited (Table 10–2).

- Abnormal hemodynamics

TABLE 10–1. Causes of Chest Pain

Cardiovascular disorders
  Angina pectoris
  Myocardial infarction
  Tachyarrhythmia
  Bradyarrhythmia
  Aortic stenosis and insufficiency
  Mitral valve prolapse
  Mitral stenosis
  Hypertrophic cardiomyopathy (idiopathic hypertrophic
    subaortic stenosis)
  Pericarditis
  Postmyocardial infarction syndrome
  Aortic dissection
  Aortic aneurysm, leaking
  Superficial thrombophlebitis (Mondor's syndrome)
Pulmonary disorders
  Pneumothorax
  Pneumomediastinum
  Pleurisy and pleurodynia
  Pulmonary embolus or infarction
  Pulmonary hypertension
  Pneumonia
Gastrointestinal disorders
  Esophageal disorders (esophageal spasm, esophagitis,
    hiatal hernia)
  Perforated esophagus, stomach, or duodenum
  Peptic ulcer disease
  Pancreatitis
  Cholecystitis
  Splenic flexure syndrome
Musculoskeletal disorders
  Costochondrodynia
  Cervical and thoracic disc or joint disease
  Tietze's syndrome
  Thoracic outlet syndrome
  Muscle spasm and fibrositis
  Chest-wall tenderness (nonspecific)
Miscellaneous disorders
  Anxiety states (hyperventilation syndrome)
  Herpes zoster
  Intrathoracic neoplasm

1. Abnormal hemodynamics exist when either or both of the following conditions are present:
   a. Shock. Signs of shock include arterial hypotension, altered sensorium, oliguria or anuria, cool and clammy skin, and, frequently, rapid respiration. Milder degrees of shock may only be detected by postural blood pressure determinations.
   b. Central venous pressure elevation. This is manifested initially by distended, superficial neck veins and dyspnea and can progress to pulmonary edema with the appearance of rales and frothy

sputum. Peripheral edema, ascites, and hepato-megaly are usually absent when central venous engorgement is of acute onset. Pulmonary edema is usually not present in conditions causing pri-mary obstruction to venous return, such as pulmo-nary embolism and tension pneumothorax.

2. In addition to the conditions listed in Table 10–2, shock from any cause is a major stress that can precipitate myocardial ischemia or infarction, especially in the elderly and in patients with coronary vascular lesions that do not normally cause symptoms.

· Normal hemodynamics (Table 10–3). Initial evaluation should focus primarily on differentiating between causes that are potentially life-threatening from those that are more benign.

HISTORY

A carefully elicited, thorough history is the most useful step in diagnosing the cause of chest pain. Physical examination and routine laboratory tests are often nonspecific or useful mainly to confirm the diagnosis already suspected from the history.

· Quality of pain
1. The typical pain of ischemic heart disease is often described as squeezing, strangling, crushing, a tight-ness, pressure, heaviness, or more vaguely as a "funny feeling." The discomfort of angina or MI may not be perceived as pain by many patients.
2. A sharp, knifelike pain is not typical of myocardial ischemia but must be interpreted with caution, since patients may be referring to severity rather than the quality of pain.

· Location of pain
1. Discomfort related to myocardial ischemia is most commonly centered in the retrosternal region. The pain may radiate to the axilla, down the arms (more often the left), or to the back. Less commonly the pain may be confined to one of the areas in the usual path of radiation.
2. Pain of MI is also retrosternal, although up to 35% of patients may have pain located elsewhere, especially in the epigastric region. In patients with MI who have a history of angina, 94% experience the myocardial pain in the same location as the angina pain, even if the site of angina pain is atypical.
3. Esophageal dysfunction is the most common cause of central chest pain that is confused with myocardial ischemia. Fifty percent of patients with esophageal dysfunction have central chest pain, and one-third have "anginalike" chest pain.

· Duration of pain. Pain caused by angina usually lasts 2 to 10 minutes but can last up to 20 to 30 minutes or longer, especially when it is precipitated by emotional stress. Pain lasting a few seconds or less is not caused by myocardial ischemia.

Text continued on page 70

TABLE 10–2. Diagnostic Features of Conditions Causing Chest Pain with Abnormal Hemodynamics

HEMODYNAMIC STATE	DIAGNOSIS	SIGNS AND SYMPTOMS
Shock without central venous pressure elevation	Aortic dissection	Severe tearing chest pain, often radiating to back; history of hypertension or Marfan's syndrome; pulse deficits, especially if transient; widened mediastinum occasionally present on chest X-ray; angiogram or CT scan diagnostic.
	Leaking abdominal aneurysm	Abdominal or back pain also present; usually elderly with a history of hypertension; pulsatile abdominal mass; cross-table lateral or ultrasound (more sensitive diagnostic; surgical emergency.
	Myocardial infarction with excess vagal tone	Squeezing, retrosternal chest pain; nausea, vomiting, diaphoresis; bradycardia; EKG usually diagnostic.
	Gastrointestinal blood loss	Nausea, vomiting, abdominal pain; stigmata of liver disease or history of heavy ethanol use often present; hematemesis, melena, or maroon stools diagnostic; in early upper intestinal bleeding, stool guaiac may be negative and hematocrit normal; gastric lavage is diagnostic if positive.
Shock with central venous pressure elevation	Tension pneumothorax	Pleuritic chest pain; respiratory distress; deviated trachea with hyperresonant hemithorax and absent or decreased breath sounds; pulmonary edema absent; chest X-ray diagnostic.

Severe bradycardia or tachycardia	EKG shows ventricular rate <50 or >160 and ischemic pattern; pulmonary edema often present; usually necessary to rule out myocardial infarction
Cardiac tamponade	Dyspnea; faint heart sounds, narrow pulse pressure, elevated pulsus paradox; diffuse low voltage on EKG, electrical alternans; pulmonary edema often absent; globular heart on chest X-ray (absent if acute onset); echocardiogram diagnostic.
Cardiogenic shock (myocardial pump failure)	Severe dyspnea; marked pulmonary edema and often new murmur of mitral regurgitation or ventricular septal defect; bronchospasm due to cardiac asthma; EKG usually diagnostic of infarction.
Massive pulmonary embolus	Severe dyspnea with sharp pleuritic chest pain; predisposing conditions of peripheral venous disease, period of immobility or decreased activity, recent surgery, pregnancy, oral contraceptive use, malignancy, systemic infection; right heart strain on physical examination, EKG, or chest X-ray; pleural rub; chest X-ray with pleural effusion, consolidation, or truncated pulmonary vasculature; ventilation perfusion scan suggestive and pulmonary angiogram diagnostic.

TABLE 10–3. Diagnostic Clues to Causes of Chest Pain

Cause	HISTORY — Previous Attacks of Similar Pain	HISTORY — Pain: Location	HISTORY — Pain: Character	HISTORY — Pain: Onset	HISTORY — Duration	Common Associated Findings	Signs	Other Abnormalities	Other Comments
Angina	Usually	Retrosternal, radiating to left arm	Squeezing, oppressive	With stress or exercise	2–10 minutes up to 20–30 minutes	Occasionally dyspnea; dizziness and syncope rare	Often none; S$_4$ occasionally	EKG often normal between attacks.	Relieved by nitroglycerin.
Acute myocardial infarction	In some cases	Retrosternal, radiating to left arm, neck; rarely in back	Squeezing, oppressive, increases with time	No precipitating factor necessary	>20 minutes	Nausea and vomiting, diaphoresis, dyspnea	Heart failure, restlessness, shock; cardiac examination often normal	EKG may be diagnostic or normal.	Elevated CK, LDH, or CK MB isoenzymes. Normal isoenzyme levels on one determination do not exclude diagnosis.
Mitral valve prolapse	Usually	Variable	Variable	Variable	Variable; usually hours	Dyspnea, dizziness common; syncope in some	Midsystolic click or murmur in most cases	EKG may show inverted T waves on leads II, III, and aVF. Echocardio-	Arrhythmia or sudden death may occur. Usually seen in young women. High-

								gram is diagnostic.	arched palate or chest or spine deformities may be present. More common in older men.
Aortic stenosis	May have occurred	Like angina	Like angina	Like angina	Like angina	Syncope, dyspnea	Systolic ejection murmur transmitted to carotid arteries; delayed carotid pulse	EKG usually shows left ventricular hypertrophy. Echocardiography and angiocardiography are diagnostic.	
Aortic insufficiency	In some cases	Like angina	Like angina	Like angina	May be prolonged	Dyspnea	Diastolic murmur transmitted to carotid arteries; water-hammer and Quincke's pulse; wide arterial pulse pressure	EKG may be normal or may show left ventricular hypertrophy. Echocardiography and angiocardiography are diagnostic.	History of rheumatic heart disease, connective tissue disease, or syphilis.
Pericarditis	In some cases	Retrosternal	Variable; often pleuritic and relieved by sitting	Variable	Hours to days	Variable	Pericardial friction rub in many	EKG may be diagnostic, nonspecific, or normal.	Relieved by sitting. Perform echocardiography to detect fluid.

Table continued on following page

TABLE 10–3. Diagnostic Clues to Causes of Chest Pain *Continued*

	History								
			Pain						
Cause	Previous Attacks of Similar Pain	Location	*Character*	*Onset*	Duration	Common Associated Findings	Signs	Other Abnormalities	Other Comments
Aortic dissection	No	Retrosternal and back	Tearing, maximal at onset	Sudden	Variable	Myocardial infarction, stroke, limb ischemia, syncope	Stroke, absent pulses, hematuria, shock	Chest X-ray shows widened mediastinum. EKG may show acute myocardial infarction. Pulsatile abdominal mass.	Angiography or CT scan is definitive. Hypertension or connective tissue disease may be present.
Pleurisy	No	Variable, usually lateral thorax	Pleuritic	Usually sudden	Variable	Subjective dyspnea	Often none; occasionally friction rub, low-grade fever	Occasionally pleural effusion.	Negative lung scan or pulmonary angiogram.
Pneumothorax	In some cases	Variable	Variable; often pleuritic	Usually sudden	Variable	Dyspnea and cough; shock if tension pneumothorax is present	Tachycardia, lung collapse with or without mediastinal shift	Chest X-ray is diagnostic but needs careful examination.	

Pneumo-mediastinum	No	Retrosternal	Variable; often pleuritic	Usually sudden	Variable	Dyspnea	Mediastinal crunch	Chest X-ray is diagnostic.	Usually associated with pneumo-thorax.
Pulmonary hypertension	Usually	Retrosternal	Like angina	Like angina	Variable	Dyspnea, fatigue, exercise syncope	Loud P_2, right ventricular lift	EKG shows right heart strain. Chest X-ray shows signs of pulmonary hypertension.	
Pulmonary embolism	In some cases	Variable, usually lateral thorax	Usually strong pleuritic component	Usually sudden	Minutes to hours	Dyspnea, cough, and tachypnea; hemoptysis sometimes	Friction rub or splinting in some	Hypoxia and hypocapnia. Chest X-ray usually abnormal, but findings are not specific.	Abnormal lung scan or pulmonary angiogram.
Pneumonia	Rare	Over affected lobe	Pleuritic	Variable	Variable	Fever and chills, cough, dyspnea, sputum production	Fever, rales with or without consolidation, friction rub	Infiltrates on chest X-ray; purulent sputum.	
Esophagitis, esophageal	Usually	Retrosternal or epigastrium	Changes with eating	Usually gradual	Variable	Gastrointestinal symptoms;	None	Positive barium swallow	Relieved by antacids or

Table continued on following page

TABLE 10–3. Diagnostic Clues to Causes of Chest Pain *Continued*

| | | HISTORY | | | | | | |
| | Previous Attacks of Similar Pain | Pain | | | Common Associated Findings | Signs | Other Abnormalities | Other Comments |
Cause		Location	Character	Onset	Duration			
spasm, hiatal hernia						flushing, sweating		and Bernstein (acid perfusion) test. topical anesthesia.
Perforated duodenal ulcer	No, or milder pain of ulcer	Retrosternal to epigastrium	Severe	Variable	Variable	Variable	Epigastric pain	Free air in peritoneum; elevated amylase. Rare as cause of chest pain.
Pancreatitis	In some cases	Retrosternal to epigastrium	Variable	Variable	Hours to days	Vomiting, anorexia	Epigastric or upper quadrant tenderness	Markedly elevated urine or serum amylase. Rare as cause of chest pain.
Cholecystitis	Usually	Right upper quadrant; oc-	Variable	Usually sudden	Hours to days	Vomiting, anorexia	Epigastric or right upper	Abnormal liver function Rare as cause of chest pain.

| Musculo-skeletal disorder (Tietze's syndrome, stitch, etc.), rib fracture | Variable | Costochondral junctions; retrosternal and lateral | Pleuritic ache, "sticking" sensation | Gradual to sudden | Variable; fleeting for stitch | Splinting | Tender costosternal junctions, especially first and second ribs, or over affected ribs; rarely swelling over joints | None. | Relieved by lidocaine corticosteroid. |

Source: Reprinted with permission of the authors and publisher, from Mills J, Ho MT, Saunders CE, eds. Current Emergency Diagnosis and Treatment 2nd ed. San Mateo, Altos, Appleton & Lange. 1990, pp. 64–76.

69

- Provocation of pain
  1. Angina is often precipitated by exertion, emotional stress, or cold weather, food, or drink. Pain begins during the stress as opposed to after the event. Prinzmetal's or variant angina is caused by coronary artery spasm and usually occurs at rest, often at the same time each day.
  2. Pain of MI often occurs without any identifiable precipitating event and begins during rest or sleep in 20 to 40% of patients.
  3. Pain on swallowing, eating, or lying down is more frequently caused by esophageal dysfunction but may also occur with pericarditis or, less commonly, with angina.
  4. Pleuritic pain or pain with movement usually suggests pulmonary, musculoskeletal, or mediastinal involvement. Pain of pericarditis may be pleuritic.
- Relief of pain
  1. Pain caused by angina usually subsides within 1 to 15 minutes of the patient's cessation of the activity provoking the pain. Esophageal spasm, however, can be similarly relieved.
  2. Patients with pericarditis or esophageal dysfunction usually report improvement or relief of symptoms upon assuming the sitting position. Patients with dyspnea related to myocardial ischemia or pulmonary disease also feel better in a more upright position.
  3. Nitroglycerin usually relieves chest pain caused by angina within 5 to 10 minutes. Unfortunately, nitroglycerin is also very effective in relieving pain related to esophageal spasm within the same time period. Moreover, almost a fifth of patients with myocardial infarction also experience pain relief.
  4. Rapid relief with antacids is reported by only a quarter of patients with reflux esophagitis. Conversely, up to 4% of patients with myocardial ischemia may experience relief.
- Associated symptoms
  1. Complaints of nausea, vomiting, diaphoresis, or dyspnea are commonly associated with chest pain caused by myocardial ischemia but are nonspecific and occur frequently in patients with other conditions.
  2. Absence of associated symptoms does not exclude ischemic heart disease.
- Risk factors (see Table 10–4). The presence of risk factors does not in itself imply that an individual patient's chest pain is caused by ischemic heart disease; more importantly, the absence of risk factors does not exclude ischemic heart disease.

PHYSICAL EXAMINATION

Special attention should be paid to features of the physical examination that can rule in or exclude certain diagnoses. Occasionally, more than one disease process may be present.

TABLE 10–4. Risk Factors for Coronary Artery Disease

Gender (male > female)
Age
Family history of coronary artery disease
Cigarette smoking
Hypertension
Elevated serum cholesterol level (low high-density lipoprotein : low-density lipoprotein ratio)
Diabetes mellitus
Oral contraceptive drugs, estrogen, or menopause
Personality type (Type A)
Obesity
Elevated serum triglyceride level
Hyperuricemia or gout
Sedentary lifestyle
Excess alcohol consumption
Electrocardiographic evidence of left ventricular hypertrophy
Mediastinal radiation
Coffee (controversial)

For example, the stress of pneumonia may precipitate angina in a patient with aortic stenosis.

- Patients with angina, unstable angina, uncomplicated acute MI, esophageal disorders, pulmonary embolus, or psychogenic chest pain usually have no diagnostic abnormalities detectable by physical examination.
- Examine the fundus for diabetic or hypertensive changes and the pharynx for the high-arched palate often seen in patients with Marfan's syndrome and occasionally in mitral valve prolapse.
- Examine the chest wall carefully by inspection and palpation.
  1. The rash of herpes zoster (cluster of vesicles in a dermatome distribution) or Tietze's syndrome (erythematous nodules over the costochondral junction) are diagnostic.
  2. Pain on palpation of the chest wall may indicate musculoskeletal disorders such as costochondritis, rib fracture or contusion, thoracic outlet syndrome, or cervical or thoracic radicular syndrome.
     CAUTION: Care must be taken to ascertain that the pain elicited by palpation of the chest wall is identical to that of the patient's chief complaint.
- Percuss and auscultate over both the anterior and posterior lung fields and mediastinum, while listening for any abnormal sounds.
- Cardiovascular system
  1. Assess central venous pressure with the patient's upper body elevated 30°.
  2. Inspect and palpate for heaves, lifts, or thrills.

3. Auscultate for any abnormality in S_1 or S_2 and for any abnormal sounds such as S_3, S_4, click, murmur, or rub.
4. Determine the intensity and amplitude of carotid, femoral, and other peripheral pulses.
- Examine the abdomen carefully, looking especially for bruits, abnormal aortic pulse, or any evidence of intra-abdominal disease.
- Examine the patient's legs for evidence of thrombophlebitis such as swelling, redness, tenderness, increased warmth, and presence of cords.

LABORATORY STUDIES

Laboratory tests should be tailored to the individual situation. Limitations in the interpretation of test results must be recognized. In general, a positive test result is useful in a population with a high prevalence of a disease, and a negative test result is useful in a population with a low prevalence of disease. In the converse situations, some tests may increase the uncertainty of a diagnosis. (Table 10–5)

- Electrocardiographic (EKG) findings
  1. In angina, the characteristic EKG changes are transient ST-segment depressions or T-wave inversions while the patient is symptomatic. In Prinzmetal's angina, transient ST elevation is seen. A normal EKG, nonspecific changes, or transient bundle-branch blocks also can occur.
  2. Comparison to previous EKGs is most useful in determining presence and extent of changes.
  3. Absence of characteristic changes does not exclude acute ischemia as an etiology in patients presenting with chest pain.
  4. EKG changes consistent with acute myocardial infarction are new Q waves (in leads I, AVL, or in two diaphragmatic or precordial leads), ≥ 1-mm ST-segment elevation or depression in the same lead combinations, or new complete left-bundle-branch blocks.
- Cardiac enzyme analysis. Myocardial ischemia in the absence of infarction is by definition not associated with cardiac enzyme elevations. Thus, these tests are useful mainly to exclude the presence of acute infarction.
- Echocardiography
  1. Two-dimensional echocardiography can aid in differentiating acute ischemia from other causes of chest pain by detecting wall motion abnormalities and left ventricular dysfunction while the patient is symptomatic. This test should not be used as a criterion for whether or not a patient with chest pain is hospitalized.
  2. Detecting wall-motion abnormality by echocardiography may be a useful adjunct in identifying a subset of patients eligible for thrombolytic therapy but who have confounding EKGs with left-bundle-branch block or left ventricular hypertrophy.
  3. Echocardiography is most useful in identifying noncor-

TABLE 10–5. Pretest Likelihood of Coronary Artery Disease in Symptomatic Patients According to Age and Sex[a]

Age (yr)	Nonanginal Chest Pain		Atypical Angina		Typical Angina	
	Men	Women	Men	Women	Men	Women
30–39	5.2 ± 0.8	0.8 ± 0.3	21.8 ± 2.4	4.2 ± 1.3	69.7 ± 3.2	25.8 ± 6.5
40–49	14.1 ± 1.3	2.8 ± 0.7	46.1 ± 1.8	13.3 ± 2.9	87.3 ± 1.0	55.2 ± 6.5
50–59	21.5 ± 1.7	8.4 ± 1.2	58.9 ± 1.5	32.4 ± 3.0	92.0 ± 0.6	79.4 ± 2.4
60–69	28.1 ± 1.9	18.6 ± 1.9	67.1 ± 1.3	54.4 ± 2.4	94.3 ± 0.4	90.6 ± 1.0

[a] Each value represents the percent ± 1 standard error of the percent.
Source: Reprinted with permission of the author and publisher, from Diamond GA, Forrester JS. Analysis of probability as an aid in the clinical diagnosis of coronary artery disease. N Engl J Med 1979;300:1350–1358.

73

onary cardiac causes of chest pain. It should not be used as the sole test in the evaluation of patients suspected of having ischemic heart disease.

- Exercise electrocardiography
  1. Exercise testing is a useful initial screening test to determine the probability of significant (>75% occlusion) coronary artery disease in patients with chest pain atypical for ischemic heart disease. It should not be used in patients with rest angina or unstable angina.
  2. Criteria other than the degree of ST-segment depression must also be considered. For example, a drop in systolic blood pressure, attainment of a heart rate lower than expected, and shorter duration of exercise before developing ST-segment depression are all associated with a higher likelihood of significant coronary artery disease.
  3. In one study the false-positive test rate was 8% in men and 67% in women (average age 50 years). Conversely, the false-negative rate was 37% in men and 12% in women. Thus, a positive test result is useful to predict the presence of disease in men, and a negative test result is useful to exclude disease in women with low pretest probability of disease.

- Exercise thallium-201 imaging
  1. Sensitivity is 82%; specificity is 91%.
  2. Suboptimal exercise end-point and administration of beta-adrenergic blockers increase the false-negative rate.
  3. This is the initial test of choice in patients who have abnormal ST elevation or depression on the resting electrocardiogram that make interpretation of a simple exercise electrocardiogram difficult.

- Radionuclide angiocardiography
  1. Sensitivity is 82%; specificity is 84%.
  2. This test is useful mainly in patients with an indeterminate probability of having coronary artery disease after both exercise electrocardiography and exercise thallium imaging have already been performed and the patient is not a candidate for coronary angiography.

- Coronary angiography with ergot stimulation. This is currently the "gold standard" for the determination of the presence or absence of coronary artery disease. Coronary angiography is the initial test of choice in patients with anginalike chest pain at rest or in patients with an unstable chest pain pattern who are unresponsive to usual medical therapy.

- Laboratory tests for assessment of noncardiac causes of chest pain
  1. Ventilation perfusion scan. A perfusion scan alone is highly sensitive for detecting pulmonary embolism and are reliable in excluding disease when it is normal. However, specificity is low and pulmonary angiography may be required for definitive assessment.
  2. Gastrointestinal studies. Barium swallow, upper GI

series, upper tract endoscopy, esophageal manometry, and possibly Bernstein's test should be considered in patients with chest pain but no evidence of significant coronary artery disease. An esophageal disorder is the most common cause of chest pain in these patients.

RECOMMENDED DIAGNOSTIC APPROACH

- Rapid initial assessment should be followed by a thorough history and physical examination.
  1. Signs of shock or central venous distention should be sought.
  2. Examine the lungs, heart, and abdomen briefly for evidence of life-threatening conditions as listed in Table 10–2.
- Obtain an EKG as soon as ischemic heart disease is considered a possibility.
- At this point, the physician often has a probable or definite diagnostic opinion. Further laboratory evaluation may not be necessary or may be performed selectively, mainly for confirmation or documentation of the suspected diagnosis.
  1. The likelihood that acute ischemic heart disease is the cause of the patient's chest pain must be determined. Many guidelines have been proposed to aid the physician in this determination in order to improve the cost-effectiveness of the diagnostic process and to decrease the number of unnecessary coronary care unit admissions (see Chapter 13).
  2. If acute ischemic heart disease is a reasonable probability, the patient should be admitted to a coronary care unit and have the diagnosis confirmed or ruled out by serial electrocardiograms and cardiac enzyme measurements. Admission to an intermediate care unit can be considered for those patients with a lower likelihood of acute ischemic disease.
  3. If acute ischemic heart disease is ruled out by these tests or if the chest pain is not acute, other tests are necessary to establish a diagnosis.
     a. Exercise electrocardiography should be used as a screening test unless the patient has rest or unstable angina or an abnormal resting electrocardiogram.
     b. Exercise thallium imaging can be used to supplement a nondiagnostic simple exercise stress test. It is the first test of choice in patients with already abnormal ST segments on the resting EKG.
     c. Coronary angiography with ergot stimulation to detect coronary artery spasm is the definitive test to diagnose chest pain caused by coronary artery disease. It should be performed as the first test of choice in patients with atypical chest pain that is unstable or occurs at rest.
     d. In patients with anginalike chest pain and absence

of significant coronary artery disease as determined by these tests, gastrointestinal studies should be performed.

Bibliography

Chambers CE, Leaman DM. Management of acute chest pain. Crit Care Clin 1989;5:415–434.

Conti CR, Hill JA, Mayfield WR. Unstable angina pectoris: pathogenesis and management. Curr Probl Cardiol 1989;14:557–623.

Fesmire FM, Wears RL. The utility of the presence or absence of chest pain in patients with suspected acute myocardial infarction. Am J Emerg Med 1989;7:372–377.

Goldman L, et al. A computer protocol to predict myocardial infarction in emergency department patients with chest pain. N Engl J Med 1988;318:797–803.

Mills J, Ho MT. Chest pain. In Ho MT, Saunders CE, eds. Current Emergency Diagnosis and Treatment. San Mateo, CA, Appleton & Lange, 1990, pp. 64–76.

Pryor DB, et al. Estimating the likelihood of significant coronary artery disease. Am J Med 1983;75:771–780.

Rouan GW, et al. Clinical characteristics and outcome of acute myocardial infarction in patients with initially normal or nonspecific electrocardiograms (A report from the Multicenter Chest Pain Study). Am J Cardiol 1989;54:11087–11092.

Rusnak RA, et al. Litigation against the emergency physician: Common features in cases of missed myocardial infarction. Ann Emerg Med 1989;18:1029–1034.

Selker HP. Coronary care unit triage decision aids: How do we know when they work? Am J Med 1989;87:491–493.

11

CONGESTIVE HEART FAILURE

C. SCOTT SMITH

The heart is the root of life and causes the versatility of the spiritual faculties. The heart influences the face and fills the pulse with blood.

HUANG TI (The Yellow Emperor) (2697–2597 B.C.)

DEFINITION

- Heart failure is defined as the inability of the heart to deliver sufficient quantities of oxygenated blood to meet the needs of peripheral tissues. This syndrome is often accompanied by systemic or pulmonary vascular congestion, hence the term congestive heart failure (CHF).
- CHF is a descriptive term and does not imply a particular etiology. The most common etiology is dilated cardiomyopathy from ischemic heart disease or hypertension.

EPIDEMIOLOGY

- CHF affects more than 2 million Americans and is the leading cause of death among patients hospitalized with heart disease.
- Cumulative mortality is approximately 25% at 1 year and 55% at 5 years for the most common form, dilated cardiomyopathy. Of these deaths, 40% are due to disease progression, 40% to sudden death, and 20% due to other causes (e.g., pulmonary emboli, pneumonia, or unrelated).

DIFFERENTIAL DIAGNOSIS

- The main differential diagnosis is pulmonary disease. This includes lung diseases which present primarily with dyspnea, such as obstructive or restrictive lung disease, and diseases which present with pulmonary vascular congestion.
- Pulmonary function tests help assess the contribution of obstructive and restrictive diseases to symptoms. Obstructive lung disease is diagnosed by a decreased ratio of forced expiratory volume in one second to forced vital capacity (FEV_1/FVC). Restrictive lung disease is diagnosed by reduced lung volumes such as FVC or total lung capacity (TLC).

- Other diseases may cause pulmonary vascular congestion:
    1. Infectious pulmonary edema
    2. Smoke inhalation
    3. Salicylate intoxication
    4. Heroin overdose
    5. High altitude pulmonary edema (HAPE)
    6. Circulating or inhaled toxic lung disease
    7. Anaphylaxis
    8. Shock lung
- When the picture is confusing, measurement of pulmonary capillary wedge pressure (PCWP) and cardiac output will help to establish the pathologic abnormality.

ETIOLOGY (Table 11–1)

- The most common causes of CHF are hypertension and coronary artery disease. Excessive alcohol ingestion may cause up to 20% of the cases of CHF in Western society.

CLASSIFICATION

- Right-sided versus left-sided failure
    1. Division into right- and left-sided failure is useful in characterizing predominant symptoms. Left-sided failure results in increased left atrial filling pressure and pulmonary congestion. Right-sided failure causes passive liver congestion, peripheral edema, and prominent neck veins.
    2. Most processes contain an element of both right- and left-sided failure, and they are related in a complex fashion. For example, the most common cause of right-heart failure is left-heart failure.
    3. A predominance of right-heart failure should prompt the clinician to consider such etiologies as pulmonary emboli, cor pulmonale, restrictive cardiomyopathy, right ventricular infarct or constrictive pericarditis, which primarily affect the pulmonary circulation, or right ventricular compliance.
- Low-output versus high-output failure. Most heart failure is of the low-output variety. However, sustained increases in cardiac output can lead to failure as in thyrotoxicosis, pheochromocytoma, severe anemia, or pregnancy.
- Functional classification (New York Heart Association). This classification is useful in comparing groups of patients as well as the same patient at different times, and correlates well with survival (Table 11–2).

PATHOPHYSIOLOGY

- Systolic function is a complex interaction of myocardial preload, afterload, and contractility.
- In practice, preload is considered to be left ventricular end-diastolic pressure (LVEDP).

TABLE 11–1. Etiology of Congestive Heart Failure

A. Decreased myocardial contractility
 1. Coronary artery disease: ischemia or myocardial infarction (common)
 2. Pericardial tamponade
 3. Ventricular aneurysm
 4. Cardiomyopathy (alcohol common)
 5. Infiltrative diseases
  a. Myocarditis
  b. Amyloidosis
  c. Hemochromatosis
  d. Sarcoidosis
 6. Collagen vascular diseases
  a. Polymyositis
  b. Systemic lupus erythematosus
  c. Scleroderma
B. Excess myocardial workload
 1. Increased afterload
  a. Hypertension (common)
  b. Aortic or pulmonary stenosis
  c. Obstructive hypertrophic cardiomyopathy
  d. Cor pulmonale
 2. Increased preload
  a. Mitral or tricuspid valve insufficiency
  b. Aortic valve insufficiency
  c. Left to right shunting (congenital or acquired)
 3. Increased body demand
  a. Severe anemia
  b. Pregnancy
  c. Thyrotoxicosis
  d. Pheochromocytoma
  e. Paget's disease
  f. Arteriovenous fistulas
  g. Beriberi (vitamin B_1 deficiency)
  h. Erythroderma

- Afterload is the force resisting myofibril shortening throughout systole.
- Contractility is an assessment of the level of activity of actin-myosin crossbridge cycling during systole (i.e., "strength of squeeze").
- Compensatory mechanisms in dilated cardiomyopathy
 1. As contractility diminishes, the first compensation is increased LVEDP and dilation.
 2. Increasing LVEDP and ventricular size markedly increases wall stress. Therefore, the next compensatory change is hypertrophy.
 3. As the heart fails further, the body has several responses primarily aimed at volume repletion and maintenance of adequate perfusion pressure by vasoconstriction. Although they may initially augment perfusion, the net result is an increase in systemic vascular resistance and volume overload, leading to worsened failure.

TABLE 11-2. Functional Classification of CHF

1. Class I. No limitation: Ordinary physical activity does not cause undue fatigue, dyspnea, or palpitations.
2. Class II. Slight limitation of physical activity. Ordinary physical activity results in fatigue, palpitation, dyspnea, or angina.
3. Class III. Marked limitation of physical activity: Although patients are comfortable at rest, less than ordinary activity leads to symptoms.
4. Class IV. Inability to carry on any physical activity without discomfort: Symptoms are present even at rest. With any physical activity discomfort increases.

CLINICAL FEATURES

History/Symptoms

- Characterize clinical parameters (Table 11-3): Questioning may indicate whether the main problem is decreased output (fatigue, lethargy) or increased filling pressures (symptoms of congestion).
- History suggestive of underlying cause
    1. Angina, coronary artery disease, or MI
    2. Hypertension
    3. Valvular heart disease or rheumatic fever
    4. Alcohol intake
    5. Recent viral illness
    6. Any connective tissue disease
    7. Family history of CHF or sudden death (hypertrophic cardiomyopathy)
    8. Unusual exposures (anthracycline antineoplastic agents, antimony, cobalt, lead)
    9. Last menstrual period if fertile (pregnant?)
    10. Cocaine use (can lead to ischemic heart disease)
    11. HIV status or risk factors (HIV-related cardiomyopathy)
- Precipitating events. A detailed search for precipitating causes includes:
    1. Medication compliance
    2. Dietary sodium or alcohol excess
    3. Infection
    4. Iatrogenic (e.g., steroids, estrogens, nonsteroidal anti-inflammatories that cause fluid retention)

Physical Exam/Signs

- Vital signs: weight, blood pressure, pulse, respiratory rate
- Neck
    1. Check cartoid arteries for bruit and upstrokes: May reveal vascular disease or aortic stenosis.
    2. Jugular vein distention: indicates right-heart failure.

TABLE 11–3. Symptoms of CHF

1. Fatigue
2. Exercise intolerance
3. Cough
4. Right-upper-quadrant pain, anorexia: suggests right-heart failure and liver enlargement
5. Weight gain
6. Edema: suggests right-heart failure
7. Chest pain
8. Palpitations
9. Dyspnea on exertion or at rest: suggests left-heart failure
10. Orthopnea. This is not specific to CHF, and can be seen in restrictive lung disease, diaphragmatic dysfunction or massive ascites.
11. Paroxysmal nocturnal dyspnea (PND). PND may be considered an exaggerated episode of orthopnea and may be accompanied by wheezing.
12. Cheyne-Stokes respiration (alternating apnea and hyperventilation)

   3.   Hepatojugular reflux: indicates right-heart failure.

- Lungs
    1. Moist rales or rhonchi, or wheezes.
    2. Frothy or blood-tinged sputum in pulmonary edema (grossly bloody sputum is *not* a feature of CHF although "rusty" or blood tinged may be).
- Heart
    1. Precordial heave or thrill may occur.
    2. Laterally displaced point of maximal impulse (PMI): suggests dilated heart.
    3. Accentuated P_2: occurs with the development of left ventricular failure and increased pulmonary artery pressure.
    4. Third heart sound (S_3 gallop) occurs early in diastole and is a reliable sign of heart failure in middle-aged or elderly patients. An S_3 may be heard normally in children and young adults. Fourth heart sounds (S_4 gallop) represent ejection of atrial blood into a stiffened ventricle and can be seen in CHF, hypertension, and other disorders.
    5. Murmurs. Mitral and tricuspid regurgitation may occur as the ventricles enlarge and the annuli dilate. Murmurs of aortic stenosis or that associated with hypertrophic obstructive cardiomyopathy may suggest the cause of CHF.
- Abdomen: hepatomegaly, splenomegaly, or ascites may occur.
- Extremities: edema, cyanosis
- CNS: confusion, irritability

LABORATORY STUDIES

- Radiographic findings. The chest X-ray is the most important diagnostic tool after the history and physical exam. There may be a lag of 12 hours for X-ray changes to appear and delayed resolution of X-ray changes (for up to 4 days) after clinical improvement of CHF.

  1. Redistribution of flow and venous congestion. Blood flow to the lower lung field is reduced, and flow to the upper lung field is increased when the PCWP is elevated above 18 mmHg.

  2. Interstitial pulmonary edema. This may be seen as small lines found in the lower peripheral lung fields and extending to the pleural surfaces (''Kerley's B lines''). Fluid can also accumulate in the lobar septa and may be seen as lines extending into the lung parenchyma (''Kerley's A lines''). Pulmonary vessels may appear enlarged and, as interstitial fluid blurs their margins, indistinct. These findings suggest PCWPs of 20 to 25 mmHg.

  3. Alveolar edema. When PCWPs rise above 25 mmHg, fluid begins to accumulate in the alveolar spaces. The chest X-ray has bilateral hilar infiltrates in a butterfly pattern. Atypical chest X-ray patterns are not uncommon with preexisting lung disease (e.g., chronic obstructive pulmonary disease).

  4. Pleural effusions. Pleural effusions may occur at PCWPs greater than 20 mmHg and are transudates. They are usually bilateral; if unilateral, right-sided is more common.

  5. Enlarged cardiac silhouette. The cardiac silhouette is often enlarged (greater than half the transthoracic diameter) but may be normal in size.

- Electrocardiogram (ECG).

  1. Old myocardial infarction suggests coronary artery disease.

  2. Left ventricular hypertrophy suggests outflow obstruction (aortic stenosis, hypertrophic cardiomyopathy) or hypertension.

  3. Left atrial hypertrophy may be seen in the same conditions or in mitral valve disease

  4. Persistent ST-segment elevation suggests ventricular aneurysm.

  5. Recent-onset low limb lead voltages may indicate pericardial disease and/or effusion.

- Echocardiography. The echocardiogram is a powerful tool in assessing the causes and extent of CHF in a complicated patient. Characteristically a dilated left ventricle with poor wall motion is demonstrated. It may reveal ruptured papillary muscles, hypertrophic cardiomyopathy, aortic or mitral valvular abnormalities, or ventricular aneurysms as causes of CHF. It may suggest causes (as in the ''sparkling'' appearance of amyloid), and is the diagnostic modality of choice for pericardial effusions and myxomas.

- Laboratory. Laboratory abnormalities in CHF may be relatively minor.

1. Hyponatremia, a sign that vasopressin is stimulated, may suggest a poorer prognosis and guide treatment.
2. Evidence of renal dysfunction (usually BUN is elevated to a greater degree than creatinine) is common and is highly variable with heart function.
3. Liver enzymes may be elevated (usually a transaminitis) and albumin may be low.

- Hemodynamic monitoring may aid diagnosis, especially in confusing or unstable patients. The cardiac index is a guide to the forward pumping capabilities of the heart. Pulmonary capillary wedge pressure is a measure of the amount of congestion. If the cardiac index is particularly high, causes of high output cardiac failure should be addressed.

RECOMMENDED DIAGNOSTIC APPROACH (Figure 11–1)

The history, physical exam, chest X-ray, and electrocardiogram are the mainstay of the evaluation in the patient with

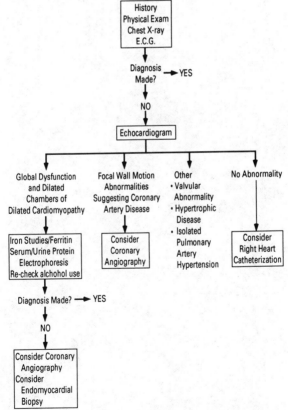

Figure 11–1. Recommended diagnostic approach to CHF.

CHF. The diagnostician should remember that CHF is a syndrome and not a diagnosis in and of itself. Therefore a cause for the CHF must always be sought.

Bibliography

Johnson RA, Palacios I. Dilated cardiomyopathies of the adult (parts one and two). N Engl J Med 1982;307(17):1051–1057; N Engl J Med 1982;307(18):1119–1126.

Packer M, et al. Role of neurohormonal mechanisms in determining survival in patients with severe chronic heart failure. Circulation 1986;73(2):257–267.

Rubin SA, et al. Accuracy of cardiac output, oxygen uptake, and arteriovenous therapy in patients with severe, chronic heart failure. Am J Cardiol 1982;50:973–978.

Weber KT, et al. Advances in the evaluation and management of chronic heart failure. Chest 1984;85:253–259.

12

PALPITATIONS AND CARDIAC ARRHYTHMIAS

PETER KUDENCHUK

I have tremor cordis on me, my heart dances.
THE WINTER'S TALE, I, II, 110.

DEFINITION OF PALPITATIONS

Palpitation refers to the patient's conscious perception of cardiac activity. It may be perceived as heavy or strong heart beats, or as skipped, early, or irregular beats. The preception of palpitations may not have any relationship to the actual presence of arrythmias.

CLASSIFICATION OF PALPITATIONS

1. Palpitations Caused by Diseases or Conditions Without Associated Arrythmias
   Examples include normal physical exertion and the following conditions:
   a. Fever
   b. Anemia
   c. Anxiety
   d. Thyrotoxicosis
   e. Pheochromocytoma
   f. Drugs (e.g., stimulants)
2. Palpitations Caused by Premature Beats
   a. Patients often use the term "skipped beats" or "fluttering sensation" to describe premature beats.
   b. Premature beats may occur in normal individuals; they may be associated with stimulant use or thyrotoxicosis.
   c. Ventricular premature beats (VPBs) are frequently benign, but must be interpreted by the company they keep. In digitalis toxicity, for example, VPBs should be considered serious.
   d. When supraventricular or ventricular premature beats group together (3 or more beats in succession), their significance is related to their rate and duration. Grouped beats at more rapid rates and of longer duration are more apt to cause symptoms or be dangerous.
3. Palpitations Caused by "Pauses" or Slowing of Heart Rhythm

CLASSIFICATION OF CARDIAC ARRHYTHMIAS

Arrhythmias can be classified according to *mechanism* (disorders of impulse formation, and disorders of impulse conduction), *anatomic location* (supraventricular or ventricular), and *rate* (normal, bradycardic, or tachycardic).

MECHANISM OF ARRHYTHMIAS

* Normal cardiac rhythm is the result of normal *impulse formation* and *impulse conduction*.
  1. An action potential is generated in the sinoatrial (SA) node (impulse formation). This action potential is then propagated (impulse conduction) over specialized conduction pathways to the atrioventricular (AV) node, and via the bundle of His, bundle branches, and Purkinje network to the ventricle.
  2. The rate of spontaneous depolarization normally slows along the conduction system from the SA node to the ventricle. Thus, if impulse formation in the SA node fails or is blocked enroute to the AV node, an "escape rhythm" will often be generated by depolarization in the AV node, usually at a slower rate than in the SA node.
* Automatic rhythms result from acceleration or slowing (change in automaticity) of *impulse formation*.
  1. Automatic rhythms are characterized by a gradual onset ("warm-up") and termination, similar to SA-node activity during and following exercise.
  2. Automatic rhythms can originate from any cardiac tissue (atrium, nodal, ventricle, or His-Purkinje system).
* Abnormal impulse conduction can cause both tachycardias and heart block.
  1. Tachycardia may occur when an impulse finds an abnormal conduction pathway within which it can "recirculate." The impulse repeatedly reenters its own path within this circular circuit, taking control of the heart rhythm and rate. Such tachycardias are described as *"reentrant"* or *"reciprocating,"* and usually have an abrupt onset and termination.
  2. Bradycardias occur due to impulse *conduction delay* or impulse blockade (*heart block*). When conduction block is persistent or prolonged, "escape beats" often result from a subsidiary pacemaker.

ANATOMIC LOCATION OF ARRHYTHMIAS

The AV node is the electrical "dividing line" between *supraventricular* (sinus, atrial, junctional) and *ventricular* rhythms.

RATE OF ARRHYTHMIAS

Rhythms may be bradycardic (<60 bpm), tachycardic (>100 bpm), or normal (60-100 bpm).

HELPFUL CLUES IN THE DIAGNOSIS OF ARRHYTHMIAS

1. Is it an arrhythmia? Frequently artifactual changes can mimic arrhythmias. The QRS complexes near the onset of the arrhythmia should be calipered and "marched through" the presumed arrhythmia. If sinus QRS complexes appear to coincide with the "arrhythmia," the most likely diagnosis is "artifact."

2. Is it a tachyarrhythmia or a bradyarrhythmia? Both atrial and ventricular rates should be measured to determine whether they are identical.

3. Is the arrhythmia precisely regular, regularly irregular (regular rhythm with a repeating pattern of irregularity) or irregularly irregular (beat-to-beat variability without any clear repeating pattern)?

   a. Irregularly irregular arrhythmias with uniform-appearing QRS complexes are usually due to atrial fibrillation or multifocal atrial tachycardia.

   b. Extremely irregular arrhythmias with wide variability in the configuration of QRS complexes are more likely to be ventricular (polymorphic ventricular tachycardia, torsades de pointes), but can also be seen in atrial fibrillation with variable antegrade conduction down an accessory pathway.

   c. A regular tachycardia at 150 bpm suggests atrial flutter with 2:1 AV block.

4. Is the QRS complex wide (>0.11 seconds) or narrow?

   a. A narrow complex QRS arrhythmias therefore suggests a supraventricular etiology.

   b. Wide complex QRS arrhythmias may be supraventricular with bundle-branch aberrancy, due to antegrade conduction down an accessory pathway, or be of ventricular origin (Table 12–1).

5. What is the relationship of P waves to QRS complexes?

   a. A P wave of different morphology than the usual sinus P wave implies an ectopic atrial rhythm focus.

   b. Arrhythmias which disrupt the normal 1:1 relationship of P wave preceding the QRS may be ventricular in origin or due to conduction block. In the various forms of conduction block, the atrial rate is characteristically faster than the ventricular rate. Conduction block may be "physiologic" at rapid atrial rates (e.g., atrial flutter with variable AV block), or "pathologic" at normal atrial rates (e.g., third-degree heart block).

   c. During ventricular tachycardia, there may be intermittent or constant "atrioventricular dissociation."

   d. Esophageal electrocardiography can be extremely

TABLE 12–1. Factors Suggesting a Ventricular Versus Supraventricular Etiology of a Wide Complex Tachycardia

FACTOR	VT	SVT
Ventricular rate precisely 150 bpm		X
Typical bundle-branch-block pattern		X
Presence of preexcitation on the ECG during normal sinus rhythm		X
Atypical bundle-branch conduction pattern	X	
QRS duration > 0.14 seconds	X	
"No-man's-land QRS axis" (−90 to −180)	X	
AV dissociation (regular P waves independent of QRS activity)	X	
Precordial concordance (all positive or all negative QRS complexes in chest leads)	X	
Fusion beats (beats of intermediate morphology between normal sinus and the wide complex tachycardia)	X	
R-on-T phenomenon (AV node refractory period is usually too long to allow conduction of a supraventricular beat so soon after a QRS complex)	X	
Variable first heart sound	X	
Irregular cannon "a" waves in jugular pulse	X	
History of myocardial infarction	X	

useful in identifying P waves. The lower half to one-third of the esophagus lies just posterior to the left atrium, and recording signals from this region results in amplification of P waves.

6. What is the response of the arrhythmia to carotid sinus massage? Carotid sinus stimulation decreases sympathetic and increases parasympathetic (vagal) tone to the heart. Vagal stimulation decreases the automaticity of the SA mode (slows impulse formation); and slows AV conduction. Usually, this has little or no impact on ventricular arrhythmias, but may slow or terminate supraventricular arrhythmias.

7. What is it about the patient that predisposes to arrhythmias?

SUPRAVENTRICULAR RHYTHMS AND ARRHYTHMIAS

- Sinus rhythms
   1. Normal sinus rhythm (Figure 12–1)
   Causes. normal

DIAGNOSTIC CRITERIA	PHYSICAL FINDINGS
Anatomic origin: SA node Mechanism: automatic Rhythm: regular	Jugular venous waves: normal

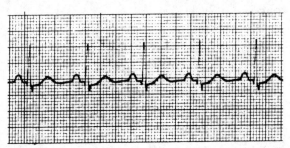

Figure 12–1. Normal sinus rhythm. (Reprinted with permission from Eisenberg MS, et al. Code Blue, Philadelphia, W.B. Saunders, 1987, p. 138.)

Rate: 60–100 bpm	Heart sounds: normal
P waves: upright in I, II, avF	Carotid massage: gradual slowing with return to normal rate upon termination
QRS: normal unless bundle-branch aberrancy is present	
P : QRS ratio: 1 : 1	

2. Sinus tachycardia

Causes. a physiologic response to the need for increased cardiac output, such as fever, exercise, anxiety, hypovolemia.

DIAGNOSTIC CRITERIA	PHYSICAL FINDINGS
Anatomic origin: SA node	Jugular venous waves: normal
Mechanism: automatic	
Rhythm: regular	Heart sounds: normal
Rate: >100 bpm, usually <160 bpm	Carotid massage: same as for normal sinus rhythm
P waves: upright in I, II, avF	
QRS: normal unless bundle-branch aberrancy is present	
P : QRS ratio: 1 : 1	

3. Sinus bradycardia

Causes. may be physiologic, as in a well-trained athlete, due to drugs (beta blockers), or SA-node disease.

DIAGNOSTIC CRITERIA	PHYSICAL FINDINGS
Anatomic origin: SA node	Jugular venous waves: normal
Mechanism: automatic	
Rhythm: regular	Heart sounds: normal
Rate: <60 bpm	Carotid massage: same as for normal sinus rhythm
P waves: upright in I, II, avF	

QRS: normal unless bundle-
branch aberrancy is
present
P : QRS ratio: 1 : 1

4. Irregular sinus rhythm (sinus arrhythmia, Figure 12–2)
Causes. physiologic response to respiration, with increased sympathetic tone during inspiration (resulting in
faster rate) and decreased sympathetic tone during expiration
(resulting in slowing of rate).

DIAGNOSTIC CRITERIA	PHYSICAL FINDINGS
Anatomic origin: SA node	Jugular venous waves: normal
Mechanism: variable automaticity	Heart sounds: normal
Rhythm: continuous variation of PP and resulting RR intervals	
Rate: 60–100 bpm associated with respiration. The rate speeds up during inspiration and slows during expiration. Breath holding eliminates the variability.	Carotid massage: same as normal sinus rhythm
P waves: upright in I, II, avF	
QRS: normal unless bundle-bunch aberrancy is present	
P : QRS ratio: 1 : 1	

5. Sinus block (also called SA block): classified as first-,
second-, or third-degree block (Figure 12–3) and is due
to a delay in conduction or block between the SA node
and atrium.
   a. First-degree SA block: There is a delay in conduction between SA node discharge and depolariza-

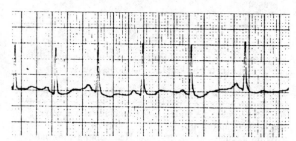

Figure 12–2. Sinus arrhythmia. (Reprinted with permission of author and publisher, from Huang SH, et al. Coronary Care Nursing, 2nd ed. Philadelphia, W. B. Saunders Company, 1989, p. 144.)

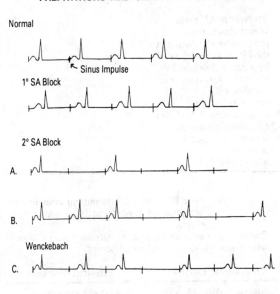

Figure 12–3. First-, second-, and third-degree SA node block. (Used with permission from Chou TC. Electrocardiography in Clinical Practice, 2nd ed. Orlando, Grune & Stratton, 1986, p. 358.)

tion of the atria. It is not recognizable on the routine ECG.

b. Second-degree SA block. Two varieties exist:

   i. Type I SA block (Sinus Wenckebach): There is a progressive slowing of conduction from SA node to atrium over a number of impulses, until a P wave is no longer generated. After the pause, cells surrounding the SA node recover, and conduction resumes.

Causes. increased vagal tone, coronary artery disease involving SA node, drugs (digoxin, quinidine, and other antiarrhythmic drugs, lithium). May be a normal phenomenon in athletes, children, and young adults.

DIAGNOSTIC CRITERIA	PHYSICAL FINDINGS
Anatomic origin: SA node	Jugular venous waves: normal
Mechanism: Conduction delay and block.	Heart sounds: normal
Rhythm: regularly irregular PP and resulting RR intervals; comparable to the progressive shortening of RR	Carotid massage: gradual slowing of sinus rate with return to normal; may worsen the degree of SA block observed

intervals in AV node Wenckebach, there is progressive shortening of the PP intervals followed by a pause. Longest PP interval is less than twice the shortest.
Rate: <60–100 bpm
P wave: upright in I, II, avF
QRS: normal unless bundle-branch aberrancy is present
P : QRS ratio: 1 : 1

ii. Type II SA block: intermittent complete interruption of conduction from SA node to atrium.

Causes. increases in vagal tone, coronary artery disease involving sinus node, antiarrhythmic drugs.

DIAGNOSTIC CRITERIA	PHYSICAL FINDINGS
Anatomic origin: SA node	Jugular venous waves: normal
Mechanism: conduction block	
Rhythm: regularly irregular PP and resulting RR intervals; pause between P waves is equal to an exact multiple of the PP cycle length (usually 2 : 1, but may be 3 : 1, 4 : 1, etc.)	Heart sounds: normal
	Carotid massage: gradual slowing of sinus rate with return to normal; may worsen the degree of SA block observed
Rate: <60–100 bpm	
P wave: upright in I, II, avF	
QRS: normal, unless bundle-branch aberrancy is present	
P : QRS ratio: 1 : 1	

iii. Third-degree SA block: total block of SA conduction to the atrium. Third-degree SA block cannot be distinguished from sinus arrest (in which an impulse fails to be generated altogether in the SA node) by surface ECG.

Causes. coronary artery disease involving SA node, increased vagal tone, inflammatory heart disease, antiarrhythmic drugs.

DIAGNOSTIC CRITERIA	PHYSICAL FINDINGS
Anatomic origin: SA node	Jugular venous waves: normal or absent
Mechanism: complete conduction block	Heart sounds: normal or absent
Rhythm: irregular PP and	

resulting RR intervals
owing to pause.

Rate: usually prolonged
asystolic period, unless
escape rhythm is present.

P wave: upright in I, II, avF

QRS: normal, unless bundle-
branch aberrancy is
present

P : QRS ratio: 1 : 1

Carotid massage:
contraindicated because
of potential worsening of
SA block, or slowing of
escape rhythm.

6. Sick sinus syndrome (bradycardia-tachycardia syndrome): This syndrome is defined by a wide variety of
interspersed rapid and slow supraventricular arrhythmias. The SA node is usually dysfunctional, and subsidiary escape pacemakers may also fail to adequately
sustain the heart rhythm.

Causes. coronary artery disease, inflammatory heart disease, fibrodegenerative conduction system disease, cardiomyopathy, hypertensive heart disease.

7. Sinus arrest: a failure of impulse formation in the SA
node. (Figure 12–4).

DIAGNOSTIC CRITERIA	PHYSICAL FINDINGS
Anatomic origin: SA node	Jugular venous pulse:
Mechanism: failure of	absent "a" waves, or
impulse formation	cannon "a" waves if
Rhythm: absent sinus	the escape rhythm
rhythm; usually regular	results in retrograde
escape rhythm from	atrial activation
subsidiary pacemaker	
Rate: variable ventricular	Heart sounds: normal or
rate, depending upon	absent
focus of escape rhythm.	Carotid massage: may
P wave: absent	prolong the duration of
QRS: configuration	the sinus arrest, or slow
dependent on location of	the rate of the escape
escape rhythm.	rhythm
P : QRS ratio: absent	

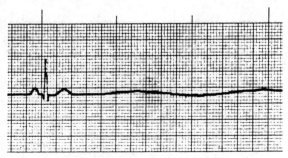

Figure 12–4. Sinus arrest.

- Supraventricular tachycardias (SVT): This term refers in general to tachycardias of atrial or AV nodal origin when these arrhythmias occur abruptly or in bursts with intervening normal sinus rhythm; they are referred to as paroxysmal SVT.

    1. Atrial premature beats (APBs) (Figure 12–5)
    Causes. normal variant, stimulants (caffeine, stress)

DIAGNOSTIC CRITERIA	PHYSICAL FINDINGS
Anatomic origin: atrium	Jugular venous waves: variable "a" waves with each APB
Mechanism: increased automaticity	Heart sounds: S_1 varies in intensity
Rhythm: regularly irregular atrial and ventricular rhythm	Carotid massage: no change in APBs
Rate: variable, depending upon frequency of APBs	
P wave: P wave of APB typically has different configuration and PR interval than sinus P wave	
QRS: Normal, unless bundle-branch aberrancy is present	
P : QRS ratio: usually 1 : 1, although P wave may be "buried" within a T wave, or a very premature P wave may fail to conduct to the ventricle and not be followed by a QRS ("blocked APB")	

   2. AV nodal reciprocating tachycardia (AVNRT): although frequently called "PAT" (paroxysmal atrial tachycardia), AVNRT (Figure 12–6) is due to a reen-

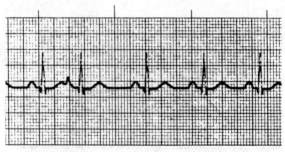

Figure 12–5. Atrial premature beats.

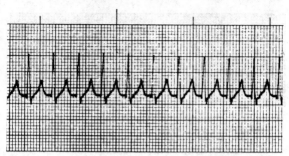

Figure 12–6. AVNRT. (Reprinted from Copass MK, et al. The paramedic Manual. Philadelphia, W. B. Saunders. 1987, p. 51.)

trant or reciprocating circuit within the AV node and is not an *atrial* arrhythmia per se.

Causes. most commonly seen in individuals with no evidence of heart disease; may be precipitated by sympathetic nervous system stimulation (emotion, fatigue, caffeine), or alcohol.

DIAGNOSTIC CRITERIA	PHYSICAL FINDINGS
Anatomic origin: AV node	Jugular venous waves:
Mechanism: reentry	constant cannon "a"
Rhythm: regular PP (if seen) and resulting RR intervals; usually starts and stops abruptly.	waves
Rate: 140–250 bpm	Heart sounds: normal
P wave: may not be evident. If evident, may be totally or partially superimposed on the QRS complex and inverted in II, III, and avF (retrograde P)	Carotid massage: abrupt termination or no effect
QRS: normal, unless bundle-branch aberrancy is present	
P : QRS ratio: 1 : 1 (if P waves can be identified)	

3. Wandering atrial pacemaker: The sinus node pacemaker is displaced by an atrial pacemaker (Figure 12–7), which spontaneously shifts its location, manifested by P waves which differ in rate and morphology from beat to beat.
Causes. normal variant, enhanced autonomic tone.

DIAGNOSTIC CRITERIA	PHYSICAL FINDINGS
Anatomic origin: atrium	Jugular venous waves: normal
Mechanism: increased automaticity of >1 atrial site	Heart sounds: S_1 may vary slightly in intensity
Rhythm: slightly irregular	Carotid massage: no effect

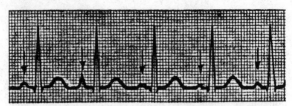

Figure 12–7. Wandering atrial pacemaker. Note the different contour of the P waves (*arrows*) with constant PR intervals. (Used with permission from Dunn MI, Lipman BS. Lipman-Massie Clinical Electrocardiography, Chicago, Year Book Medical Publishers, 1989, p. 350.)

atrial and ventricular rhythms	or increased AV node block
Rate: atrial rate <100 bpm	
P waves: variable (>1) distinct morphologies with variability in PR intervals	
QRS: normal, unless bundle-branch aberrancy is present	
P : QRS ratio: 1 : 1	

4. Ectopic atrial tachycardia (EAT): an atrial rhythm that originates at a site other than the sinus node. If abrupt in onset, EAT (Figure 12–8) may also be called "PAT" (paroxysmal atrial tachycardia).

Causes. organic heart disease, myocardial infarction, chronic obstructive pulmonary disease, alcohol, metabolic disturbances, stimulant drugs, digoxin.

DIAGNOSTIC CRITERIA	PHYSICAL FINDINGS
Anatomic origin: atrium	Jugular venous pulse: normal
Mechanism: increased atrial automaticity	Heart sounds: normal
Rhythm: atrial and ventricular rhythms are usually regular	

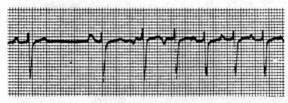

Figure 12–8. Ectopic atrial tachycardia (EAT). (Used with permission from Chou TC. Electrocardiography in Clinical Practice 2nd ed. Orlando, Grune & Stratton, 1986, p. 377.)

Rate: atrial rate 100–180 bpm	Carotid massage: may increase AV block, leading to slower ventricular rate
P wave: abnormal P axis	
QRS: normal, unless bundle-branch aberrancy is present	
P : QRS ratio: 1 : 1	

5. Paroxysmal atrial tachycardia (PAT) with block: This is an ectopic atrial tachycardia of abrupt onset, which is associated with block in the AV node.

Causes. most commonly seen in digitalis toxicity, coronary artery disease.

6. Multifocal atrial tachycardia (MAT) (chaotic atrial rhythm) (Figure 12–9)

Causes. chronic obstructive lung disease, coronary artery disease with congestive failure, alcohol, severe medical illness.

DIAGNOSTIC CRITERIA	**PHYSICAL FINDINGS**
Anatomic origin: atrium	Jugular venous waves: variable "a" waves.
Mechanism: increased automaticity of numerous (>3) atrial sites	Heart sounds: S_1 varies in intensity
Rhythm: irregularly irregular atrial and ventricular rhythms	Carotid massage: no effect or increased AV node block; gross irregularity remains
Rate: atrial rate usually >130 bpm; ventricular rate variable if AV node block is also present	
P waves: variable (>3) distinct morphologies with variable PR intervals, representing different foci of atrial rhythms	

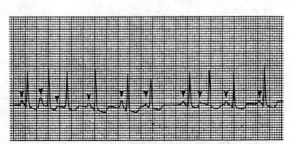

Figure 12–9. Multifocal atrial tachycardia. (Reprinted with permission from Dunn MI, Lipman BS. Lipman-Massie Clinical Electrocardiography. Chicago, Year Book Medical Publishers, 1989, p. 422.)

QRS: normal, unless
   bundle-branch aberrancy
   is present
P : QRS ratio: usually 1 : 1,
   with varying PR
   interval; AV block may
   occur with resulting
   variation in P : QRS ratio

7.   Atrial flutter (Figure 12–10)
Causes. coronary artery disease, mitral valve disease,
pulmonary embolism, hyperthyroidism.

DIAGNOSTIC CRITERIA	PHYSICAL FINDINGS
Anatomic origin: atrium Mechanism: reentry Rhythm: atrial rhythm is regular; ventricular rhythm may be regular or irregular depending on the degree of AV nodeblock. Rate: atrial 250–350 bpm (usually 300 bpm); ventricular rate variable, but 150 bpm is most common P wave: flutter waves, commonly described as saw-toothed pattern in which one P wave merges into the next without an intervening isoelectric line. QRS: normal unless bundle-branch aberrancy is present P : QRS ratio: usually 2 or more Ps (flutter waves) to each QRS, but may be variable.	Jugular venous waves: flutter "a" waves visible Heart sounds: S_1 may vary in intensity if AV block is changing; otherwise S_1 constant Carotid massage: may increase AV block and reveal flutter waves more clearly between QRS complexes

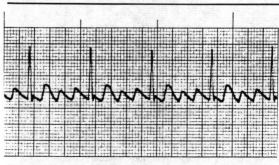

Figure 12–10. Atrial flutter. (Reprinted from Eisenberg MS, et al. Code Blue. Philadelphia, W. B. Saunders, 1987, p. 130.)

8. Atrial fibrillation (Figure 12–11)

Causes. congestive heart failure, hyperthyroidism, mitral stenosis, pulmonary embolism, recent cardiac surgery, coronary artery disease, cor pulmonale, pericarditis, alcohol, preexcitation (Wolff-Parkinson-White syndrome).

DIAGNOSTIC CRITERIA	PHYSICAL FINDINGS
Anatomic origin: atrium	Jugular venous waves: No "a" waves
Mechanism: reentry	
Rhythm: irregularly irregular atrial and ventricular rhythm.	Heart sounds: S_1 varies in intensity
Rate: atrial rate 350–600 bpm (fibrillation) with irregularly irregular ventricular rate due to AV node block, which ranges from 150 to 200 bpm if untreated.	Carotid massage: slowing of ventricular response due to increased AV node block; gross irregularity persists
P wave: no discernible P waves; usually there is irregular, undulating baseline between QRS complexes	
QRS: Normal, unless bundle-branch aberrancy is present	
P : QRS ratio: irregular ratio	

• Nonparoxysmal supraventricular arrhythmias: Unlike supraventricular *tachycardias,* these arrhythmias usually occur at rates similar to or slower than normal sinus rhythm. They do not usually manifest abrupt onset and termination.

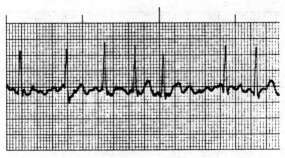

Figure 12–11. Atrial fibrillation.

Many of these rhythms are "escape beats" due to slowing or block in a rhythm focus higher in the conduction system; others result from increased automaticity in the AV node without any sinus-node abnormality.

1. Junctional premature beat (JPB) (Figure 12–12)
Causes. normal variant, digitalis excess, stimulants.

DIAGNOSTIC CRITERIA	PHYSICAL FINDINGS
Anatomic origin: AV node	Jugular venous waves: no "a" wave with JPB, unless atrium is captured retrogradely in which case cannon "a" is present
Mechanism: increased automaticity	
Rhythm: regularly irregular ventricular rhythm; atrial rhythm is frequently altered by JPB due to retrograde atrial activation	
Rate: variable ventricular rate depending upon JPB frequency	Heart sounds: S_1 constant if atrium is captured retrogradely; otherwise S_1 variable with JPB
P wave: when associated with JPB due to retrograde conduction, P wave is abnormal in configuration (inverted in II, III, avF) and may precede, coincide with, or follow QRS	Carotid massage: no effect upon JPB
QRS: normal, unless bundle-branch aberrancy is present	
P : QRS ratio: no association, unless retrograde P wave is caused by JPB	

2. Junctional rhythm (junctional escape, accelerated junctional rhythm) (Figure 12–13)

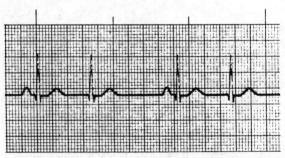

Figure 12–12. Junctional premature beat.

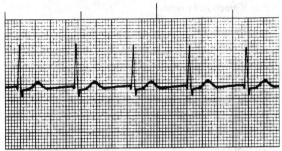

Figure 12–13. Junctional rhythm with retrograde P waves which follow each QRS complex.

Causes. suppression of SA-node activity due to excessive vagal tone, digitalis excess, carotid sinus disease, coronary artery disease, or inflammatory heart disease. An accelerated junctional rhythm is slightly faster than the normal junctional escape rate of 40–60 bpm, and is usually a benign phenomenon, due to increased automaticity in the AV node.

DIAGNOSTIC CRITERIA	PHYSICAL FINDINGS
Anatomic origin: AV node	Jugular venous waves: variables—without "z" waves, with intermittent "a" waves, or with cannon "a" waves if atria are captured retrogradely
Mechanism: escape or increased automaticity	
Rhythm: regular ventricular rhythm; atrial rhythm may or may not be evident, but if present will be at identical or slower rate than ventricular rate	
	Heart sounds: S_1 constant if atria are captured retrogradely
Rate: 40–60 bpm ventricular rate; accelerated junctional rhythm rate is 60–100 bpm	Carotid massage: no response, or slight slowing in ventricular rate
P wave: when seen, is abnormal in configuration, due to retrograde conduction from the AV node (inverted in II, III, avF). If junctional rhythm is due to AV nodal block, a slower but normally configured sinus P wave may be present.	
QRS: normal, unless bundle-branch aberrancy is present	
P : QRS ratio: if retrograde Ps are present, usually	

1:1; if junctional rhythm
is due to heart block,
P:QRS ratio is
inconsistent

· Ventricular arrhythmias

1. Ventricular premature beat (VPB) (Figure 12–14)

Causes. coronary artery disease, myocardial infarction, hypoxia, acidosis, hypokalemia, stimulants, normal variant. VPBs are common in elderly patients.

DIAGNOSTIC CRITERIA	PHYSICAL FINDINGS
Anatomic origin: ventricle	Jugular venous waves: intermittent cannon "a" waves
Mechanism: increased automaticity	
Rhythm: regularly irregular ventricular rhythm; atrial rhythm is usually unchanged	
Rate: variable ventricular rate depending upon frequency of VPB	Heart sounds: variable S_1; S_2 may be widely split
	Carotid massage: no effect upon VPB
P wave: usually sinus node P wave regularity is not disturbed by VPB; occasionally VPB may conduct retrograde to atrium to produce a retrograde P (inverted in II, III, avF) and disrupt the regularity of the sinus rate	
QRS: >0.11 sec. Morphology of QRS may be single (unifocal VPB) or multiple (multifocal VPBs)	
P:QRS ratio: usually no	

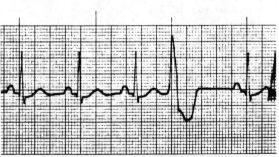

Figure 12–14. Ventricular premature beat.

relationship between P
wave and QRS of VPB

2. Idioventricular rhythm (IVR) (Figure 12–15)
Causes. myocardial infarction, hypoxia, acidosis. It frequently is an ''escape rhythm'' resulting from slowing or block higher in the conduction system.

DIAGNOSTIC CRITERIA	PHYSICAL FINDINGS
Anatomic origin: ventricle	Jugular venous waves: intermittent cannon ''a'' waves
Mechanism: escape or increased automaticity	
Rhythm: regular ventricular rhythm; regularity of atrial rhythm, if present, is not disturbed by ventricular rhythm.	Heart sounds: variable S_1
	Carotid massage: no response
Rate: 30–40 bpm	
P wave: usually not present; if present, cycle length is different from QRS, complex	
QRS: >0.11 sec	
P:QRS ratio: no association	

3. Accelerated idioventricular rhythm (AIVR)
Causes. myocardial infarction, escape focus due to slowing or block higher in the conduction system. This rhythm is identical to idioventricular rhythm except the rate is 60–100 bpm.
4. Ventricular tachycardia (VT)
    a. Three or more consecutive VPBs, usually at a rate > 100 bpm.
    b. Consecutive ventricular beats at rates slower than 100 bpm are called IVR or AIVR (see above).
    c. VT may have a single (monomorphic) (Figure 12–16) or multiple (polymorphic) (Figure 12–17) QRS configuration(s).

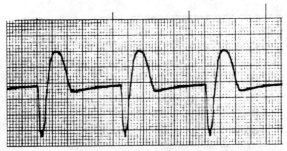

Figure 12–15. Idioventricular rhythm.

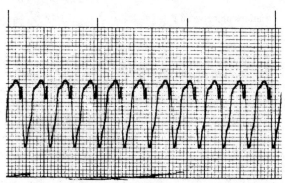

Figure 12–16. Monomorphic ventricular tachycardia. (Reprinted from Eisenberg MS, et al. Code Blue. Philadelphia, W. B. Saunders, 1987, p. 122.)

Causes. myocardial infarction or ischemia, hypoxia, acidosis, stimulants.

DIAGNOSTIC CRITERIA	PHYSICAL FINDINGS
Anatomic origin: ventricle	Jugular venous waves:
Mechanism: reentry;	cannon "a" waves
sometimes due to	present either constantly
increased automaticity	(with 1 : 1 retrograde
Rhythm: usually regular	atrial activation) or
ventricular rhythm,	intermittently (with
although polymorphic VT	intermittent or no
may be irregular; atrial	retrograde atrial
rhythm is usually regular	activation)
and not disturbed by VT	Heart sounds: variable S_1;
unless retrograde atrial	S_2 may be widely split
activation occurs	Carotid massage: no effect
Rate: >150–200 bpm, but	upon VT
occasionally slower (100–	
140 bpm)	
P wave: normal sinus P	
waves may be noted, but	

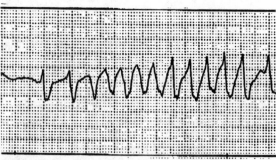

Figure 12–17. Polymorphic ventricular tachycardia.

SA activity is dissociated
from the VT
QRS: >0.11 sec
P : QRS ratio: no
relationship, unless
retrograde Ps are
produced by VT. If
retrograde Ps are
produced by VT, usually
there is some retrograde
AV block and not every
QRS is followed by a
retrograde P

5. Ventricular fibrillation (VF) (Figures 12–18 and 12–19)
Causes. same as for ventricular tachycardia.

DIAGNOSTIC CRITERIA	PHYSICAL FINDINGS
Anatomic origin: ventricle	Jugular venous waves: none
Mechanism: reentry	Heart sounds: none
Rhythm/rate: rhythm is completely disorganized, electrically	Carotid massage: no effect
P waves: not seen amid baseline undulations	
QRS: variable shapes and sizes	
P : QRS ratio: no association	

6. Torsades de pointes (Figure 12–20): a VT consisting of a prolonged QT interval on the baseline ECG and QRS complexes of changing amplitude that appear to turn around the isoelectric line of the ECG (''turning of the points'').
   There is a gradual change in QRS deflection over 5–20 beats to the opposite direction and back again.
Causes. congenitally prolonged QT syndrome or prolonged QT due to drugs, metabolic disturbances.

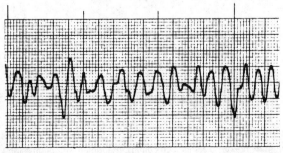

Figure 12–18. Coarse ventricular fibrillation. (Reprinted from Eisenberg MS, et al. Code Blue. Philadelphia, W. B. Saunders, 1987, p. 117.)

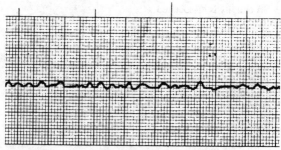

Figure 12–19. Fine ventricular fibrillation. (Reprinted from Eisenberg MS, et al. Code Blue. Philadelphia, W. B. Saunders, 1987, p. 117.)

DIAGNOSTIC CRITERIA	PHYSICAL FINDINGS
Anatomic origin: ventricle	Jugular venous waves: variable cannon "z" waves
Mechanism: probably, abnormal automaticity	Heart sounds: variable
Rhythm/rate: irregular and rapid (>200 bpm) ventricular rhythm and rate; atrial activity frequently not discernible	Carotid massage: no response
P waves: not discernible	
QRS: polymorphic with rotation of the QRS axis around the isoelectric line	
P : QRS ratio: no association	

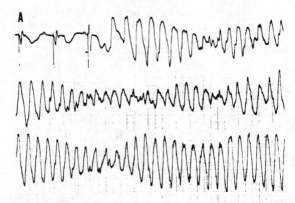

Figure 12–20. Torsades de pointes. (Reprinted with permission of publisher from Braunwald E. Heart Disease: A Textbook of Cardiovascular Medicine, 3rd ed. Philadelphia, WB Saunders, 1988, p. 699.)

- Preexcitation syndromes
    1. Preexcitation results from a pathway, in addition to the AV node and His bundle, through which an impulse can be conducted from atrium to the ventricle. It is usually congenital and often associated with mitral valve prolapse, cardiomyopathies, septal defects, or Ebstein's anomaly.
    2. Conduction along accessory pathways is more rapid than through the AV node. The ventricle is depolarized prematurely (preexcited) via the accessory pathway, reflected in an upward slur (delta wave) in the initial portion of the QRS complex and a shortening of the PR interval.
    3. The presence of an accessory pathway creates a circular "loop" between the atria and ventricles, with the accessory pathway serving as one limb and the AV node/His bundle as the other. When an impulse circulates within this loop, a "reciprocating" (reentry) tachycardia results.
    4. A *concealed* accessory pathway is one that only conducts from ventricle to atrium (retrograde only). Such a pathway can participate in SVTs, but does not produce delta waves during normal sinus rhythm or cause a short PR interval.
    5. A short PR interval (<0.12 seconds) with a normal QRS (no delta wave) implies either accelerated conduction through the AV node in the absence of any accessory pathway, or the presence of an accessory pathway which "bypasses" the AV node.
    6. A normal PR interval with a delta wave implies the presence of an accessory pathway which interconnects the distal conduction system with either a fascicle or ventricular muscle (Mahaim fiber).
    7. Arrhythmias associated with accessory pathways.
        a. Preexcitation syndromes are associated with reciprocating SVTs and atrial fibrillation.
        b. The constellation of preexcitation and supraventricular arrhythmias is referred to as Wolff-Parkinson-White syndrome.
        c. Atrial fibrillation can be particularly ominous with preexcitation. The accessory pathway, unlike the AV node, does not readily slow conduction of rapid atrial impulses to the ventricle. Rapid atrial fibrillation with preexcitation can precipitate ventricular fibrillation.
        d. Orthodromic reciprocating tachycardia (ORT) is a narrow complex SVT in which the reentry circuit consists of the atrium, AV node, ventricle and accessory pathway. Conduction is antegrade down the AV node to the ventricle, and retrograde up the accessory pathway to the atrium, which repetitively tracks along this "loop." Antegrade conduction down the normal conduction system results in a narrow QRS complex (not preexcited).
        e. Antidromic reciprocating tachycardia (ART): In this arrhythmia the reentry circuit consists of the atrium, accessory pathway, ventricle, and AV

node. Conduction is antegrade down the accessory pathway to the ventricle and retrograde up the AV node to the atrium, which repetitively tracks along this "loop." Because antegrade conduction is completely via the accessory pathway, the QRS complex is generally wide (totally preexcited).

f. Atrial fibrillation: Conduction from the atrium to the ventricle intermittently traverses the AV node, the accessory pathway, or both simultaneously. As a result, QRS complexes are variably preexcited and may manifest differing morphologies from beat to beat. If conduction down the accessory pathway is sufficiently rapid, the ventricular response may approach 300 bpm and produce ventricular fibrillation.

- Atrioventricular block
  1. First-degree AV block (Figure 12–21): The PR interval is prolonged but with consistent conduction of each P wave to the ventricle.

Causes. coronary artery disease, digoxin, antiarrhythmic drugs, rheumatic fever, congenital heart disease, endocarditis, increased vagal tone. May occur in healthy individuals.

DIAGNOSTIC CRITERIA	PHYSICAL FINDINGS
Anatomic origin: AV node	Jugular venous waves: normal
Mechanism: AV node conduction delay	Heart sounds: diminished S_1
Rhythm: regular atrial and ventricular rhythm	Carotid massage: gradual slowing of atrial and ventricular rate (identical to sinus rhythm)
Rate: atrial and ventricular rate 60–100 bpm	
P wave: normal	
QRS: normal, unless bundle-branch aberrancy is present	
P : QRS ratio: 1 : 1 with PR interval >0.20 sec	

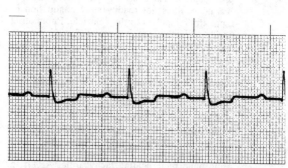

Figure 12–21. First-degree AV block. (Reprinted from Eisenberg MS et al. Code Blue. Philadelphia, W. B. Saunders, 1987, p. 135.)

2. Second-degree AV block, Mobitz type I (Wenckebach) (Figure 12–22): P waves are not consistently conducted to the ventricle. There is a gradual prolongation of the PR interval before a P wave is completely blocked.

Causes. myocardial infarction, rheumatic fever, endocarditis, digitalis, antiarrhythmic drugs, increased vagal tone. May occur in otherwise healthy individuals.

DIAGNOSTIC CRITERIA	PHYSICAL FINDINGS
Anatomic origin: AV node	Jugular venous waves: increasing a-c interval; "a" waves without "c" waves
Mechanism: AV nodal conduction delay and block	
Rhythm: sinus rhythm is regular; ventricular rhythm is irregular (grouped beats) when QRS complexes fail to be conducted	Heart sounds: S₁ cycles in intensity (correlates with PR interval)
Rate: overall SA node rate is faster than ventricular rate due to "blocked Ps"	Carotid massage: slowing of sinus rate with possible worsening of AV nodal block
P wave: normal; PP interval is constant.	
QRS: usually normal; the presence of bundle-branch aberrancy should raise concern over whether distal conduction system disease is also present	
P: QRS ratio: PR progressively prolongs until a P no longer produces a QRS. RR interval becomes progressively shorter until a QRS is "dropped"; PP interval remains constant. In order to distinguish	

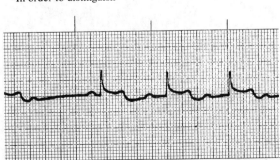

Figure 12–22. Mobitz type I (Wenckebach). (Reprinted from Eisenberg MS et al. Code Blue. Philadelphia, W. B. Saunders, 1987, p. 135.)

Mobitz I from Mobitz II
heart block, one *must*
observe at least 2
consecutively conducted P
waves before a blocked P
wave.

3. Second-degree AV block, Mobitz type II (Figure 12–23): Some P waves are not conducted to the ventricle. The failure of conduction is more abrupt and not heralded by prolongation of the PR interval. Mobitz II heart block implies conduction disease distal to the AV node.

Causes. myocardial infarction, distal conduction system disease, endocarditis.

DIAGNOSTIC CRITERIA	PHYSICAL FINDINGS
Anatomic origin: distal to AV node Mechanism: conduction block Rhythm: atrial rhythm is regular; ventricular rhythm is irregular Rate: atrial rate is usually normal; ventricular rate may be normal or slow P wave: normal with fixed PR interval on beats conducted to the ventricle QRS: usually >0.11 sec (implies distal conduction system disease) P : QRS ratio: ratio may vary over time (2 : 1, 3 : 1, 3 : 2, etc.) In order to distinguish Mobitz I from Mobitz II heart block, one *must* observe at least 2	Jugular venous wave: constant a-c waves, followed by "a" waves without "c" waves Heart sounds: S₁ variable in intensity Carotid massage: gradual slowing of sinus rate, usually no effect on Mobitz II block

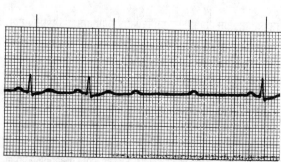

Figure 12–23. Mobitz type II. (Reprinted from Eisenberg MS et al. Code Blue. Philadelphia, W. B. Saunders, 1987, p. 136.)

consecutively conducted P
waves before a blocked P
wave.

4.   Third-degree AV block (complete heart block) (Figure
     12–24)

Causes.   coronary artery disease, myocardial infarction,
drug toxicity (digitalis, verapamil, antiarrhythmics).

DIAGNOSTIC CRITERIA	PHYSICAL FINDINGS
Anatomic origin: AV node or distal conduction system	Jugular venous waves: intermittent cannon "a" waves
Mechanism: conduction block	Heart sounds: variable S_1
Rhythm: atrial rhythm regular; ventricular rhythm precisely regular	Carotid massage: contraindicated in heart block (sinus and junctional escape rate may slow further)
Rate: normal atrial (SA node) rate which is faster than the ventricular rate; ventricular rate depends upon the focus of the escape rhythm (40–60 bpm with a junctional escape; 20–40 bpm with a ventricular escape)	
P wave: normal	
QRS: normal if junctional escape rhythm is present; >0.11 sec if ventricular escape rhythm is present	
P : QRS ratio: no relationship; atria and ventricles are independently contracting	

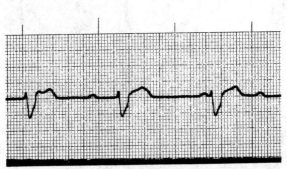

Figure 12–24.   Third-degree heart block. (Reprinted from Eisenberg MS et al. Code Blue. Philadelphia, W. B. Saunders, 1987, p. 136.)

- Intraventricular conduction defects (IVCD)
  When conduction of an impulse in the ventricle exits the normal conduction system, depolarization of the ventricle is less efficient, and occurs over a longer duration because of its reliance upon muscle-to-muscle conduction. The normal relationship of P waves to QRS complexes is not affected by the IVCD.

  1. Right-bundle-branch block (RBBB) (Figure 12–25)
  Causes. coronary artery disease, pulmonary embolus, right ventricular hypertrophy, cardiomyopathy, normal variant.

DIAGNOSTIC CRITERIA	PHYSICAL FINDINGS
Anatomic origin: right bundle branch	Jugular venous waves: normal
Mechanism: conduction block	Heart sounds: S_1 is constant, S_2 widely split

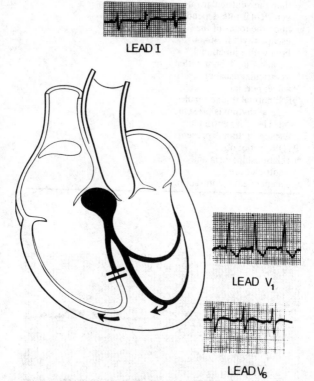

Figure 12–25. Right-bundle-branch block. (Reprinted with permission of publisher, from Phillips RE, Feeney MK. The Cardiac Rhythms, 2nd ed. Philadelphia, WB Saunders Company, 1980, p. 241.)

Rhythm/Rate: dependent upon underlying rhythm

P waves: normal

QRS: 0.12–0.16 sec duration with slurred R or R′ in V1-2, and wide S in I, V5, V6. If QRS = 0.11 sec, RBBB is incomplete

P : QRS ratio: 1 : 1, but depends upon underlying rhythm

Carotid massage: gradual slowing of sinus rate

---

2. Left-bundle-branch block (LBBB) (Figure 12–26)

Causes. reliable indicator of cardiac disease, including coronary artery disease, left ventricular hypertrophy, cardiomyopathy.

DIAGNOSTIC CRITERIA	PHYSICAL FINDINGS
Anatomic origin: left bundle branch	Jugular venous waves: normal
Mechanism: conduction block	Heart sounds: S_1 normal, S_2 paradoxically split
Rhythm/rate: usually normal, but depends upon underlying rhythm.	Carotid massage: gradual slowing of sinus rate
P wave: normal	
QRS: 0.12–0.16 sec duration with notched R	

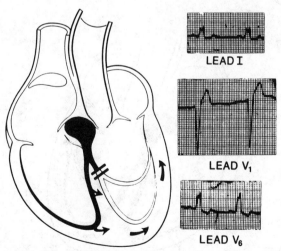

LEAD I

LEAD V_1

LEAD V_6

Figure 12–26. Left-bundle-branch block. (Reprinted with permission of publisher, from Phillips RE, Feeney MK. The Cardiac Rhythms, 2nd ed. Philadelphia, WB Saunders Company, 1980, p. 238.)

in I, avL, V6; rS or QS
in V1
P : QRS ratio: 1 : 1 but may
vary with arrhythmia
present

3. Left anterior fascicular block (LAFB) (Figure 12–27)
Causes. same as for LBBB.

DIAGNOSTIC CRITERIA	PHYSICAL FINDINGS
Anatomic origin: anterior fascicle of left bundle	Jugular venous waves: normal
Mechanism: conduction delay or block	Heart sounds: normal
Rhythm/rate: usually normal, but depends upon underlying rhythm	Carotid massage: same as for NSR
P wave: normal	
QRS: normal duration but with left axis deviation >−30 with small q in I and avL, and small r in II, III, avF	
P : QRS ratio: 1 : 1, but depends upon underlying rhythm	

4. Left posterior fascicular block (LPFB) (Figure 12–28)
Causes. same as for LBBB.

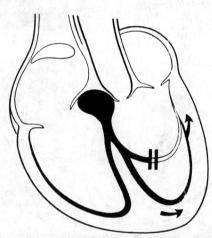

Figure 12–27. Left anterior hemiblock. (Reprinted with permission of publisher, from Phillips RE, Feeney MK. The Cardiac Rhythms, 2nd ed. Philadelphia, W. B. Saunders, 1980, p. 249.)

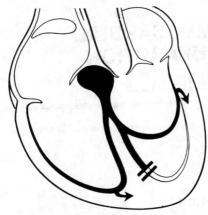

Figure 12–28. Left posterior hemiblock. (Reprinted with permission of publisher, from Phillips RE, Feeney MK. The Cardiac Rhythms, 2nd ed. Philadelphia, W. B. Saunders, 1980, p. 250.)

DIAGNOSTIC CRITERIA	PHYSICAL FINDINGS
Anatomic origin: posterior fascicle of left bundle	Jugular venous waves: normal
Mechanism: conduction delay or block	Heart sounds: normal
Rhythm/rate: usually normal, but depends upon underlying rhythm	Carotid massage: same as sinus rhythm
P wave: normal	
QRS: normal duration with right axis deviation >110 with small r in I, aVL and small q in II, III, avF	
P : QRS ratio: 1 : 1 unless underlying arrhythmia is also present	

5. Bifascicular block: RBBB coexists with either LAFB or LPFB.

Causes. coronary artery disease, acute myocardial infarction.

6. Trifascicular block: occurs when right-bundle-branch block alternates with left-bundle-branch block.

Causes. coronary artery disease, antiarrhythmic drugs.

7. Aberrant conduction (nonspecific IVCD): implies abnormal ventricular conduction of a supraventricular impulse. The QRS complex is wider than normal but the conduction abnormality is not characteristic of RBBB or LBBB.

Causes. coronary artery disease, cardiomyopathy, antiarrhythmic medications.

13

MYOCARDIAL INFARCTION

KEITH LEYDEN

As for me, except for an occasional heart attack, I feel as young as I ever did.

ROBERT BENCHLEY

DEFINITION

- Myocardial infarction (MI) is irreversible cellular injury and necrosis of cardiac muscle resulting from prolonged ischemia.
    1. Most MIs are due to atherosclerosis of the coronary arteries with superimposed thrombosis and possibly coronary artery spasm.
    2. Other less common mechanisms include coronary artery dissection, coronary artery embolism, coronary artery spasm (in the setting of normal arteries), coronary artery vasculitis, toxic injury (e.g., cocaine).
- The pathology of MI may be divided into:
    1. Transmural infarction. Myocardial necrosis involves the full thickness of the ventricular wall. The most common mechanism is complete coronary artery occlusion.
    2. Subendocardial infarction. Necrosis involves the subendocardium and/or intramural myocardium without extension to the epicardium. This frequently occurs in the setting of narrowed but still patent arteries.
    3. These processes have been clinically differentiated by the presence or absence of Q waves on the electrocardiogram (ECG). Autopsy studies have demonstrated a poor correlation between the presence of Q waves and transmural infarction, and the old terminology of transmural or subendocardial MI has been replaced by Q-wave or non–Q-wave MI. The natural history of patients distinguished by the presence or absence of Q waves is distinct (Table 13–1).

EPIDEMIOLOGY

- In the United States, approximately 1 million MIs occur annually. Nearly one-fourth of all U.S. deaths are due to MI.
- The risk factors for MI are identical to those of coronary

TABLE 13–1. Differences in Patients with Q-wave and Non–Q-wave Myocardial Infarction (MI)

CHARACTERISTIC	Q-WAVE MI	NON–Q-WAVE MI
Prevalence	60–70% of infarcts	30–40% of infarcts
Prior infarction	Rare	Frequent
Occluded infarct-related artery	80%	20%
Coronary collaterals	Less prominent	More prominent
ST-segment elevation	80%	40%
Peak creatine kinase	Higher	Lower
Time to peak creatine kinase	Longer	Shorter
Ejection fraction	Lower	Higher
Wall motion score	More dysfunction	Less dysfunction
Postinfarction ischemia	Less common	More common
Early reinfarction	8%	40%
In-hospital mortality	20%	8%

Source: Adapted from Taussig AS, et al. Misleading ECG's: Patterns of infarction. J Cardiovasc Med 1983; 9:1147.

artery disease in general and include male sex, age over 30, hypertension, smoking, hyperlipidemia, family history, systemic atherosclerosis, diabetes mellitus, and obesity. In a patient with chest pain, the absence of risk factors does not exclude ischemic heart disease.

DIFFERENTIAL DIAGNOSIS (Table 13–2)

CLINICAL FEATURES

The history and ECG remain the most useful tools in the diagnosis of MI and ischemia. There are no clinical features pathognomonic of acute ischemia.

TABLE 13–2. Differential Diagnosis of Acute Myocardial Infarction

Pericarditis and myopericarditis
Aortic dissection
Pulmonary embolism
Pneumothorax
Gallbladder disease
Peptic ulcer disease
Pancreatitis
Esophageal rupture
Acute cerebrovascular disease
Acute anxiety states
Spinal and chest wall diseases

Source: Lavie CJ, Gersh BJ. Acute myocardial infarction: Initial manifestations, management, and prognosis, Mayo Clin Proc 1990; 65:531–548.

- History
    1. Chest pain. Chest pain occurs in 80% of patients with MI. The character of the pain and the pattern of radiation are of most help diagnostically.
        a. Character. Ischemic pain is usually described as a pressure, heavy, cramping, burning and/or aching sensation not affected by respiration or movement. Sharp, stabbing, or positional chest pain is less likely to be due to ischemia.
        b. Location. Classically, the pain is substernal, but one-third of patients have epigastric discomfort. Shoulder, back, jaw, or arm pain is less frequent. Location does not help distinguish between patients with and without MI.
        c. Radiation. When substernal or precordial chest pain is accompanied by discomfort in the arms, neck, or jaw, the likelihood of MI increases three- to fourfold.
        d. Duration. Persistent pain >30 minutes in duration is characteristic of patients with MI.
        e. Relief. The use of nitroglycerin is of little value in differentiating acute ischemia from noncardiac chest pain. Only 20% of patients with MI have relief of pain with sublingual nitroglycerin.
    2. Non–Chest Pain Symptoms
        a. Dyspnea. Dyspnea is present in one-third of patients with acute MI. In 9% of patients with MI dyspnea is the only symptom.
        b. Diaphoresis. Diaphoresis occurs in 20 to 50% of patients with MI.
        c. Nausea and vomiting. Nausea and vomiting occur in almost 40% of patients with Q-wave MIs and in less than 5% of patients with unstable angina or non–Q-wave MIs. They are more likely to accompany inferior MIs.
    3. Silent MI and Atypical Presentation (Table 13–3)
        a. One-fourth of nonfatal MIs are unrecognized by the patient. Of these, one-half are truly silent. In one-quarter, the patients fail to seek medical attention, and the remaining patients have chief complaints other than chest pain.
        b. Silent MI occurs more frequently in elderly patients with diabetes or hypertension and in those

TABLE 13–3. Atypical Presentations of MI

Dyspnea/CHF
Syncope (secondary to arrhythmia)
Palpitation (secondary to arrhythmia)
Acute indigestion
Peripheral embolism
Apprehension and nervousness
Confusion (secondary to cerebral hypoperfusion, especially in elderly)
Stroke (embolism)

without antecedent angina. The comparative mortality in this group is 50% vs. 18% for patients with chest pain.

- Physical exam. The physical exam has limited utility in the diagnosis of acute ischemia. It is most helpful when it suggests a nonischemic etiology for a patient's complaints: abdominal tenderness, blood in the stool, or a very tender rib suggest noncardiac causes of chest pain.

  1. General appearance. Patients suffering from MI usually appear anxious and in considerable distress. Frequently, they massage their chests and describe their pain with a clenched fist held against the sternum (Levine's sign).
  2. Vital signs
     a. The most common rhythm is sinus tachycardia. Occasional premature ventricular contractions (PVCs) occur in 95% of patients with acute MI.
     b. The blood pressure usually is normal, although elevation or severe reduction may be present depending on the level of sympathetic or parasympathetic stimulation and degree of left ventricular dysfunction.
     c. Patients with MI develop fever as a nonspecific response to myocardial necrosis 24 to 48 hr after the onset of infarction.
  3. Chest. Tenderness to palpation over the chest is an important negative predictor of ischemia.
  4. Lungs. The lung examination usually is normal. In patients with left ventricular failure, rales or wheezes will be present (Table 13–4).
  5. Cardiac. The cardiac examination is often normal.
     a. A presystolic pulsation over the precordium indi-

TABLE 13–4. Killip Classification of Patients with Acute MI

	DEFINITION	PTS. WITH ACUTE MI IN CCU (%)	APPROX. MORTALITY (%)
Class I	Absence of rales over lung fields and absence of S$_3$	30–40	8
Class II	Rales over ≤50% of lung fields or presence of S$_3$	30–50	30
Class III	Rales over >50% of lung fields (frequently pulmonary edema)	5–10	44
Class IV	Shock	10	80–100

Source: Adapted from Killip T, Kimball JT. Treatment of myocardial infarction in a coronary care unit. A two-year experience with 250 patients. Am J Cardiol 1967; 20:457.

cates atrial contraction filling a ventricle with reduced compliance.

b. Auscultation may demonstrate the following:
   i. An S_4 reflects atrial contraction into a stiff ventricular chamber, but has little diagnostic utility.
   ii. An S_3 signifies extensive left ventricular dysfunction and is heard best at the apex.
   iii. New systolic murmurs in MI may result from papillary muscle dysfunction, mitral regurgitation as a result of ventricular dilatation, ventricular septal rupture, and acute severe mitral regurgitation due to papillary muscle rupture.
   iv. New diastolic murmurs in MI are rare. A new murmur of aortic regurgitation suggests aortic dissection.
   v. Pericardial friction rubs are audible in 7 to 20% of patients with MI.

6. Abdomen. The finding of occult blood in the stool can suggest a noncardiac etiology or, in the face of an obvious MI, help guide the use of thrombolytic therapy.

7. Extremities. The extremities may show evidence of peripheral vascular disease such as atrophic skin and hair loss, or pallor due to systemic emboli.

8. Neurologic exam. The neurologic exam is normal unless there is altered mental status from cerebral hypoperfusion or the patient has suffered a stroke secondary to hypoperfusion or an embolus from a ventricular thrombus. This complication occurs in 2% of all MIs.

• Thrombolytic therapy and clinical evaluation. The recent advent of thrombolytic therapy and its attendant risk of hemorrhage necessitate that additional historical and physical exam information be obtained when assessing a patient with suspected MI (Table 13–5).

TABLE 13–5. Contraindications to Thrombolytic Therapy

Absolute
   Major surgery within 1 month
   History of significant GI bleeding
   History of cerebrovascular disease
   History of intracranial neoplasm, aneurysm, or arteriovenous malformation
   Major bleeding diathesis
   Vigorous CPR
   Severe, uncontrolled hypertension (systolic BP > 180 or diastolic BP > 110)
   History of severe trauma within 6 weeks
Relative
   Advanced age (>75 years)
   History of peptic ulcer disease
   Agitation, confusion, or lethargy
   CPR

ELECTROCARDIOGRAPHY

- General comments. The ECG has definite limitations as a test for establishing or excluding acute MI or ischemia (Table 13–6).

  1. The initial ECG is consistent with ischemia or infarction in 64% of patients with acute infarction (sensitivity = 0.64). Thirty percent of patients with MI have only nonspecific changes, and 6% have normal ECGs. A completely normal ECG stratifies patients into a lower risk group.

  2. The ECG is a static representation of a dynamic process. A lag time of hours to days may exist before diagnostic changes become evident. Thus it is important to obtain serial ECGs to follow evolutional ECG patterns.

  3. The implications of ECG findings must be interpreted in their clinical context.

     a. In a patient likely to have coronary artery disease based upon presence of risk factors, when symptoms alone strongly suggest ischemia, a normal or minimally abnormal ECG will not substantially decrease the probability of ischemia.

     b. In patients who are unlikely to have ischemia based on a lack of risk factors and a history that is

TABLE 13–6. Conditions Simulating Infarction on ECG

Ventricular hypertrophy
  Right ventricular (cor pulmonale)
  Left ventricular
Conduction disturbances
  Left bundle branch block
  Left anterior fascicular block
Wolff-Parkinson-White syndrome
Primary myocardial disease
  Myocarditis
  Dilated cardiomyopathy
  Hypertrophic cardiomyopathy (obstructive and
    nonobstructive)
  Friedrich's ataxia
  Muscular dystrophy
Pneumothorax
Pulmonary embolus
Amyloid heart disease
Primary and metastatic tumors to the heart
Traumatic heart disease
Intracranial hemorrhage
Hyperkalemia
Pericarditis
Early repolarization
Sarcoidosis involving the heart

Source: Taussig AS, et al. Misleading ECG's: Patterns of infarction. J Cardiovasc Med 1983;9:1151.

atypical, an abnormal ECG, unless diagnostic for infarction, will only mildly increase the likelihood of infarction and certainly introduces diagnostic confusion.

4. The ECG is less definitive in non–Q-wave MIs.
5. ECG changes of acute MI may be obscured by competitive conditions (see following section).

- Electrocardiographic changes
  1. ST segment
     a. One of the earliest ECG findings of acute MI is ST elevations of 1 mm (0.1 mv of standard calibration) or greater.
     b. In patients with an appropriate history and ST elevations in two or more contiguous leads, MI will occur in 80 to 90%. For those without prior infarction, MI occurs in 99%.
     c. The ST segment can be elevated in many non-ischemic conditions:
        i. Early repolarization (Figure 13–1)
        ii. Pericarditis
        iii. Ventricular aneurysm
        iv. Left bundle branch block
        v. Left ventricular hypertrophy with strain
        vi. Hyperkalemia (rare)

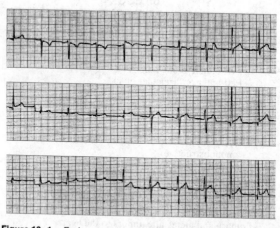

Figure 13–1. Early repolarization. Slight but definite ST-segment elevations are seen in leads I, II, aVF and V_2 through V_6. When the patient is young (under 30 years of age) and has neither cardiac signs or symptoms nor other electrocardiographic abnormalities, early repolarization (a benign variant of the normal ECG) is the likely explanation for relatively minor ST elevations. (From Scheidt S. Basic Electrocardiography. Summit, NJ, Ciba-Geigy, 1986, p. 117.)

d. ST-segment depression usually indicates "subendocardial" ischemia. Persistent and marked depression increase the likelihood of infarction. A true posterior infarction may be manifested initially by precordial (leads V_1, V_2, V_3) ST depression.

e. Nonischemic causes of ST depression include hyperventilation, digitalis, hypokalemia, and left ventricular hypertrophy with strain.

2. T wave

a. T-wave inversions may reflect acute ischemia. Of these patients, about 22% actually have infarction (Figure 13–2).

b. Other causes include previous (but not current) MI, left ventricular hypertrophy with strain, and subarachnoid hemorrhage and stroke.

c. Hyperacute T waves can be the earliest ECG finding of acute ischemia, but this is not always seen. Hyperkalemia is the other frequent cause of tall peaked T waves (Figure 13–3).

3. Q Wave

a. Abnormal Q waves develop early but are usually not seen within the first hours of MI. To be considered abnormal, a Q wave must be 0.04 sec in duration and greater than 25% of the R wave in depth, and should be present in more than one lead.

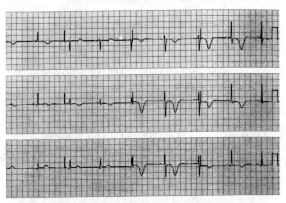

Figure 13–2. Subendocardial infarction. Widespread T-wave inversions without any significant Q waves. (From Scheidt S. Basic Electrocardiography. Summit, NJ, Ciba-Geigy, 1986, p. 117.)

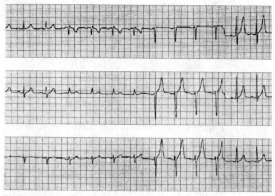

Figure 13–3. Tall, peaked T waves. (From Scheidt S. Basic Electrocardiography. Summit, NJ, Ciba-Geigy, 1986, p. 117.)

    b. Many Q waves are nonischemic or non–MI-related. In patients admitted with new inferior or anterior Q waves, MI is confirmed in only 51% and 77%, respectively. Q waves are rarely the sole manifestation of MI.

    c. Other causes of Q waves include transient Q wave associated with angina, normal young males (12% have inferior Q waves), chronic obstructive pulmonary disease, pulmonary embolism, spontaneous pneumothorax, left-bundle-branch block, and left ventricular hypertrophy.

  4. Reciprocal electrocardiographic changes

    a. These changes occur in leads facing the surface opposite the damaged myocardium and include ST-segment depression and upright T waves.

    b. In patients with inferior infarcts, ST depression in the precordial leads, particularly if persistent for more than 24 hr, is probably a reflection of posterior injury.

- Evolution of electrocardiographic changes (Figures 13–4 to 13–9)

- Location of infarction (Table 13–7). In patients with inferior infarction, an ECG with reversed precordial leads (i.e., right-sided) should be obtained to evaluate for right ventricular infarction. ST elevation of 1 mm or greater in V_4R is 100% sensitive for right ventricular infarction.

- Conduction disturbances and acute MI. An ECG diagnosis of acute anterior MI is obscured in the presence of left-bundle-branch block that either predates the infarction or results from it. The presence of right-bundle-branch block or fascicular blocks usually does not impede the diagnosis of acute MI.

INDICATIVE
CHANGES

RECIPROCAL
CHANGES

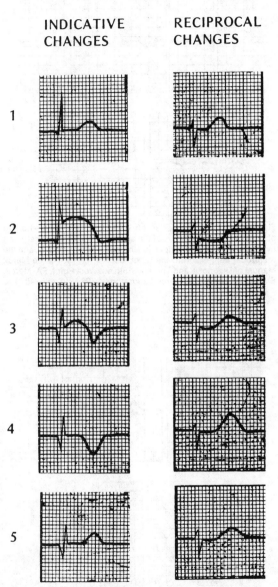

Figure 13–4. Evolutional ECG changes of myocardial infarction. 1. Normal tracing. 2. Hours after infarction. 3. A few days after infarction. 4. Many days to weeks later. 5. Months to years later. (From Huang SH, et al. Coronary Care Nursing, 2nd ed. Philadelphia, W. B. Saunders, 1989. p. 150.)

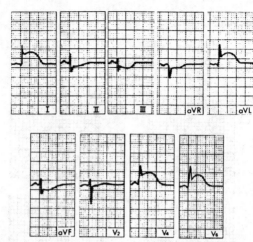

Figure 13–5. Acute anterior left ventricular infarction—tracing obtained within a few hours of the onset of illness. Note the striking hyperacute ST-segment elevation in leads I, aVL, V$_4$ and V$_6$, and the reciprocal depression in the other leads. (Berkow R. The Merck Manual of Diagnosis and Therapy, 15th ed. West Point, PA, Merck, Sharp, and Dohme Research Laboratories, 1987, pp. 486–487.)

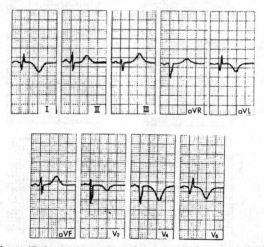

Figure 13–6. Acute anterior left ventricular infarction—several days later. Significant Q waves and the loss of the R-wave voltage persist. ST segments are now essentially isoelectric. The ECG will probably only change slowly over the next several months. (Berkow R. The Merck Manual of Diagnosis and Therapy, 15th ed. West Point, PA, Merck, Sharp, and Dohme Research Laboratories, 1987, pp. 486–487.)

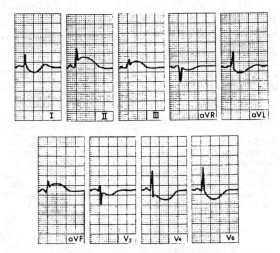

Figure 13–7. Acute inferior diaphragmatic left ventricular infarction—tracing obtained within a few hours of the onset of illness. Note the hyperacute ST-segment elevation in leads II, III, and aVF, and the reciprocal depression in the other leads. (Berkow R. The Merck Manual of Diagnosis and Therapy, 15th ed. West Point, PA, Merck, Sharp, and Dohme Research Laboratories, 1987, pp. 486–487.)

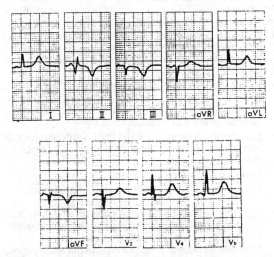

Figure 13–8. Acute inferior diaphragmetic left ventricular infarction—tracing obtained several days later. ST segments are isoelectric but abnormal Q saves are present in leads II, III, and aVF. Reprinted from Berkow R. The Merck Manual of Diagnosis and Therapy, 15th ed. West Point, PA, Merck, Sharp, and Dohme Research Laboratories, 1987, pp. 488–489.

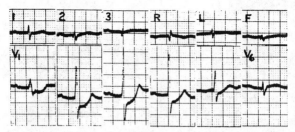

Figure 13–9. Probable acute true posterior infarction. Note prominent and wide R waves in V₁ and other right precordial leads accompanied by reciprocal ST-T changes in the same leads; these features in anterior leads suggest an acute infarction of the opposite, that is, posterior wall. (Reprinted with permission of author and publisher, from Marriott HJL: Practical Electrocardiography. 6th ed. Baltimore, Williams & Wilkins, 8th ed., 1988, p. 253.)

CARDIAC ENZYMES

Although the combination of history and electrocardiography is sensitive for detecting MI, an increase in the serum levels of cardiac enzymes (Figure 13–10) is more specific and can confirm the diagnosis. These levels must be measured serially, i.e., on admission and at 12 and 24 hr after admission. Initial enzyme determinations are only 40 to 50% sensitive for acute MI and are not useful to exclude acute ischemic heart disease in the emergency room setting.

- Creatine kinase (CK). Currently CK is the most sensitive laboratory test available for the diagnosis of MI. Its sensitivity is 96% when measured one day after MI, but its specificity is only 65%.
- Creatine kinase–MB isoenzyme (CK-MB). This isoenzyme of CK is the most specific laboratory test available (96 to 100%), although other cardiac and noncardiac conditions can cause it to increase (Table 13–8).
- Lactate dehydrogenase (LDH). LDH is 86% sensitive for MI but lacks specificity because it is elevated in a myriad of pathologic conditions.
- Lactate dehydrogenase isoenzymes
  1. A ratio of LDH1 : LDH2 > 1 is significantly more specific for MI than the LDH level alone.
  2. The LDH1 level can be elevated in conditions other than MI including hemolysis, megaloblastic anemias, renal infarction, and malignant solid tumors.
  3. LDH isoenzyme levels are most useful when patients seek medical attention 24 to 48 hr after their acute event.
- Aspartate aminotransferase (AST, previously known as SGOT). This enzyme is no longer routinely measured.

TABLE 13-7. Rapid Reference ECG Markers for Location of Infarct

MI LOCATION	LEADS	POSSIBLE ECGΔs	POTENTIAL CORONARY ARTERY INVOLVEMENT	RECIPROCAL LEAD	POSSIBLE ECGΔs
Inferior	II, III, aV_F	Q-wave, ST↑	RCA, LCx[a]	I, aV_L	ST↓
Anterior	V_1-V_4, aV_L	Q-wave, ST↑ R-wave[b]	LCA	II, III, aV_F	ST↓
Lateral	I, aV_L	Q-wave, ST↑	LCx	V_1, V_3	ST↓
Posterior	V_1, V_2	R[c]>S, ST↑	RCx	II, III, aV_F	—
Apical	V_3-V_6	Q-wave, ST↑ R-wave[b]	LAD, RCA	—	—
Anterolateral	I, aV_L, V_5, V_6	Q-wave, ST↑ T&R wave[b]	LAD, LCx	II, III, aV_F	ST↓
Anteroseptal	V_1-V_4	Q-wave, ST↑ R-wave[b]	LAD	—	—

[a] Less commonly occurring
[b] Loss of R-wave progression
[c] Followed in time by abnormally tall R-waves

129

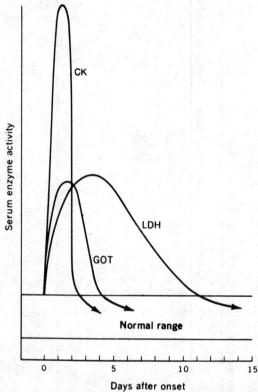

Figure 13–10. The time course of serum enzyme concentration changes following a typical MI. CK = creatine phosphokinase; LDH = lactate dehydrogenase; GOT = glutamic oxaloacetic transferase. (Reprinted from Braunwald E, et al. Harrison's Principles of Internal Medicine, 11th ed. New York, McGraw-Hill, 1987, p. 983.)

ECHOCARDIOGRAPHY

- Echocardiography readily detects regional wall motion abnormalities and identifies global systolic function of the left and right ventricles. Its limitations and cost prevent frequent use in the diagnosis of acute MI.

- Echocardiography is useful in detecting cardiac conditions which mimic MI including pericarditis, hypertrophic cardiomyopathy, and aortic dissection.

- Echocardiography is essential for diagnosing the complications of MI including septal or papillary muscle rupture, intracardiac thrombi, pericardial tamponade, and left ventricular aneurysm.

TABLE 13–8. Conditions Other Than Acute MI That Can Increase the CK-MB Isoenzyme Level

CARDIAC	NONCARDIAC
Cardioversion (>400 J)	Skeletal muscle trauma
Cardiac contusion	Skeletal muscle disease
Cardiac surgery	(e.g., myositis, muscular
Myopericarditis	dystrophy)
Percutaneous transluminal	Reye's syndrome
coronary angioplasty	Hypothyroidism
Prolonged supraventricular	Alcoholism
tachycardia	Peripartum period
	Acute cholecystitis
	Carcinoma (e.g., prostate,
	breast)
	Drugs (e.g., aspirin,
	tranquilizers)

Source: Lavie CJ, Gersh BJ. Acute myocardial infarction: Initial manifestations, management, and prognosis. Mayo Clin Proc 1990;65:535 with permission.

RADIONUCLIDE TECHNIQUES

*   Technetium-99m Pyrophosphate (TcPP)
    1. TcPP accumulates in an area of infarction as a "hot spot" on the nuclear scan. It has a sensitivity of 90% and a specificity of 86% in the diagnosis of acute MI. The sensitivity is somewhat higher in Q-wave than non–Q-wave MI.
    2. TcPP scanning is most likely to be positive 36 to 72 hr after the acute event and fades within 7 to 10 days. The test is most useful to document MI in patients who come to medical attention several days after the onset of their symptoms when ECG and enzyme changes are nondiagnostic.
*   Thallium-201. This isotope is distributed to the myocardium in proportion to blood flow. Ischemic or infarcted tissues appear as a "cold spot." This test is very sensitive for acute MI (100% if performed within 8 hr of symptoms), but its 20% false-positive rate (low specificity), inability to differentiate old from new MIs, and high cost preclude its routine clinical use in the diagnosis of acute MI.
*   Radionuclide ventriculography. This scan has no use in the diagnosis of acute MI. It aids in stratifying patients into prognostic groups by its ability to measure left ventricular ejection fraction.

RECOMMENDED DIAGNOSTIC APPROACH

*   Perform a rapid clinical evaluation in any patient presenting with chest pain or one of the atypical/silent symptoms discussed above. It is important to obtain the historical and

physical exam information, which helps to define the patient as high or low risk for ischemic heart disease.
- Obtain an ECG.
- Consider hospital admission for patients at risk for acute ischemia based upon positive clinical or ECG findings.
- On all admitted patients, obtain daily ECGs and cardiac enzymes at 0, 12, and 24 hr for definite detection of MI.
- In patients presenting several days after the onset of symptoms in whom ECG and enzyme analysis is nondiagnostic, consider TcPP scanning.

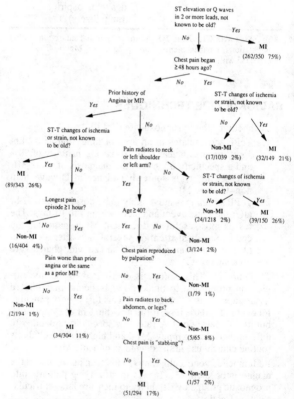

Figure 13–11. Computer-derived protocol for the evaluation of emergency department patients with chest pain. The likelihood of MI exceeds 7% for patients reaching an "MI endpoint" and is below 7% for those reaching a "non-MI endpoint". The numbers in parentheses are the number of study patients with MI divided by the number in that subgroup. (Reprinted from McCarthy BD, et al. Detecting acute cardiac ischemia in the emergency department. J Gen Intern Med 1990; 5:365–373.)

- Coronary care unit (CCU) utilization
  1. Given the number of acute interventions possible in patients with ischemic heart disease (i.e., thrombolytic therapy and arrhythmia detection and treatment) and the severe medico-legal consequences of missing the diagnosis of MI, physicians often overestimate the likelihood of ischemia in low risk patients and thus overutilize expensive CCU beds.
  2. Ninety-five to ninety-eight percent of patients with acute MI are admitted, however, only 30% of patients admitted to CCUs actually have acute MI, and only 50% have acute ischemia.
  3. Figure 13–11 is an example of a dignostic algorithm, which in small prospective testing equaled the sensitivity of physicians in predicting infarction and significantly improved upon their specificity (i.e., identified patients without ischemia.) A 30% decrease in CCU admissions was noted in patients without ischemia, while CCU admissions for those with acute ischemia did not change.

Bibliography

Bresler MJ, Gibler WB. Acute myocardial infarction: Subtleties of diagnosis in the emergency department. Monograph, Ann Emerg Med, February 1990.

Goldman L, et al. A computer protocol to predict myocardial infarction in emergency department patients with chest pain. N Engl J Med 1988;318:797–803.

Lavie CJ, Gersh BJ. Acute myocardial infarction. Initial manifestations, management, and prognosis. Mayo Clin Proc 1990;65:531–548.

McCarthy BD, et al. Detecting acute cardiac ischemia in the emergency department. J Gen Int Med 1990;5:365–373.

Pozen MW, et al. A predictive instrument to improve coronary care unit admission practices in acute ischemic heart disease: A prospective multicenter clinical trial. N Engl J Med 1984;310:1273–1278

14

VALVULAR HEART DISEASE

MERRITT RAITT

I am pained at my very heart; my heart maketh a noise in me.

OLD TESTAMENT. Jeremiah IV, 19

AORTIC STENOSIS

General Comments

- Aortic stenosis (AS) is the most common valve lesion in adults. In isolated AS deposits of calcium usually involve the valve cusps and their bases. This degenerative process is especially common in congenital bicuspid valves.
- Rheumatic AS is usually associated with mitral valve disease and results from valve thickening and fusion of the commisures. Unlike degenerative AS, rheumatic AS is frequently associated with significant aortic regurgitation (AR).
- AS produces a gradually increasing pressure gradient across the valve. Left ventricular (LV) output is maintained by compensatory LV hypertrophy resulting in a long asymptomatic period. Eventually, cardiac output cannot be increased with exercise, and symptoms of LV failure develop.

History

- The initial symptom of AS is dyspnea on exertion.
- Later, the cardinal symptoms of severe AS develop: angina, postexertional syncope, and congestive heart failure with average survival from onset of 5, 3, and 2 years, respectively.

Physical Examination (Table 14–1, 14–2)

- General. With progressive AS, pulse pressure narrows and systolic pressure drops, although it remains higher in the elderly and those with associated aortic regurgitation.
- Pulse. The rise of the carotid pulse is slow and sustained.
- Jugular veins. A prominent a wave is often present.
- Palpation
  1. The apical impulse is sustained, inferolaterally displaced, may precede the carotid pulsation, and is often

TABLE 14–1. Useful Maneuvers for Differentiating Similar Auscultatory Findings

PROBLEM	MANEUVERS	RESULTS
MS vs. TS	Respiration	Murmur of TS increases with inspiration; murmur of MS diminishes or does not change with inspiration.
S_2 and opening snap vs. widely split S_2	Position, respiration	S_2-opening snap interval widens with sudden standing, while split S_2 narrows; inspiration may widen S_2-opening snap into A_2-P_2– opening snap.
MR vs. TR	Respiration	Murmur of TR increases with inspiration; murmur of MR diminishes with inspiration.
MR vs. AS	Cycle length	Murmur of MR has no change with cycle length; murmur of AS increases after long cycle.
AS vs. MVP	Position	Murmur of AS increases with sudden squatting; murmur of MVP is diminished and delayed with sudden squatting.
AS vs. HC	Valsalva maneuver, position	Murmur of AS diminishes with the strain phase of the Valsalva maneuver and increases with sudden squatting; murmur of HC increases during strain phase of Valsalva's maneuver and diminishes with sudden squatting.
MVP vs. HC	Valsalva maneuver	Murmur of MVP begins earlier, lasts longer, and is diminished during strain phase of Valsalva maneuver; murmur of HC increases during strain phase of Valsalva maneuver.

double because of prominent presystolic filling with atrial contraction.
2. A thrill may be present at the second right intercostal space or along the carotid arteries.
- Heart tones. S_1 is normal or soft. A_2 (the aortic component of S_2) is often absent or delayed producing a single S_2 or a paradoxically split S_2. An ejection sound with opening of the valve may be heard just after S_1 if the leaflets are not rigid. An S_4 is frequently present. S_3 can be heard if there is end stage LV failure.
- Murmur
  1. The murmur is a low-pitched, harsh, rasping in character systolic crescendo-decrescendo sound beginning

TABLE 14–2. Auscultation of Valvular Heart Disease

Lesion	Murmur Diagram	Heard Best With	Point of Maximal Intensity	Characteristics and Radiation	Other Sounds
Mitral stenosis		Bell	Normal unless displaced by RV dilation	Low pitch, loudest at apex in left lateral decubitus position	Opening snap after S_2 at left lower sternal border
Mitral regurgitation Chronic		Diaphragm	Diffuse, hyperdynamic, displaced leftward	High pitch, holosystolic, loudest at apex, radiates to axilla	S_4 uncommon due to atrial fibrillation
Acute		Diaphragm	Hyperdynamic, displaced slightly leftward	Rough, early systolic, crescendo-decrescendo, loudest apex, may radiate to back, base, axilla	S_4 common
Mitral valve prolapse		Diaphragm	Normal	Murmur is mid- to late systolic, after the midsystolic click; loudest at apex	Midsystolic click more common than murmur

Aortic stenosis		Diaphragm	Sustained, displaced inferolaterally	Harsh crescendo-decrescendo murmur, loudest right 2nd intercostal space; radiates to neck, apex	Ejection click heard at left sternal border and S_4 common
Aortic regurgitation Chronic		Diaphragm: systolic and early diastolic murmurs; bell: Austin Flint murmur	Diffuse, hyperdynamic, displaced inferolaterally	Diastolic decrescendo murmur loudest at left sternal border; Austin Flint murmur loudest at apex; systolic ejection murmur loudest at base	Associated systolic ejection murmur and ejection click common
Acute		Diaphragm	Normal	Diastolic decrescendo murmur short and loudest at left sternal border	

Table continued on following page

137

TABLE 14–2. Auscultation of Valvular Heart Disease Continued

LESION	MURMUR DIAGRAM	HEARD BEST WITH	POINT OF MAXIMAL INTENSITY	CHARACTERISTICS AND RADIATION	OTHER SOUNDS
Tricuspid stenosis	S_2 ... S_1	Bell	Normal	Rumbling diastolic murmur loudest at lower left sternal border	Opening snap may be present; often accompanied by mitral stenosis
Tricuspid regurgitation	S_1 ... S_2	Diaphragm	RV heave at left sternal border common	High-pitched holosystolic murmur loudest at left sternal border, 4th intercostal space, and subxiphoid	Loud P_2 present if there is pulmonary hypertension; RV S_3 common (louder with inspiration)
Pulmonic stenosis	S_1 ... S_2	Diaphragm	RV heave at left sternal border common	Crescendo-decrescendo murmur loudest at left upper sternal border	Ejection click common
Pulmonic regurgitation	S_2 ... S_1	Diaphragm	Left parasternal heave frequently found	High-pitched diastolic decrescendo murmur, loudest along left sternal border in 2nd to 4th intercostal spaces	Right-sided S_3 and S_4 common

Source: Huang SH, et al. Coronary Care Nursing, 2nd ed. Philadelphia, WB Saunders Company, 1989, pp. 18–19.

after S_1 and ending before A_2. It is loudest at the second right intercostal space and radiates to the neck.
2. High-pitched components of the murmur can radiate to the apex, mimicking mitral regurgitation.
3. Significant obstruction usually produces a murmur of at least grade 3, though as the LV fails in end-stage AS, the murmur can soften.

- Dynamic auscultation. The intensity of the murmur increases with a prolonged diastole such as after a premature beat as well as with amyl nitrate, squatting, and lying down. It decreases with the strain of Valsalva's maneuver.

Laboratory Examination

- ECG. The rhythm is usually sinus. LV hypertrophy is present in 85% of patients with severe AS. An LV strain pattern and left atrial enlargement are also common.
- Chest X-ray. The heart shadow is usually near normal size, though it may have rounding of the left heart border and apex. Poststenotic dilatation of the aorta and valvular calcifications may be present.
- Echocardiography
  1. M mode and two-dimensional echocardiography (2D) can show a reduced range of valve opening, thickening and calcification of the valve, and LV hypertrophy diagnostic of AS but cannot quantify the gradient, valve area, or severity.
  2. Doppler allows reliable measurement of the peak instantaneous gradient across the valve and calculation of valve area.
  3. Critical AS is defined as a peak systolic gradient across the valve during normal cardiac output greater than 50 mmHg or a valve orifice area less then 0.75 cm².

AORTIC REGURGITATION

General Comments

- AR can be secondary to disease processes that primarily involve the aortic valve (2/3) or the aortic root (1/3).
- The causes of valvular AR include rheumatic fever, infective endocarditis, trauma, Marfan's syndrome, Ehlers-Danlos syndrome, and myxomatous degeneration of the valve.
- Diseases that can cause AR through aortic root dilatation include Marfan's syndrome, syphilitic aortitis, seronegative polyarthropathy, osteogenesis imperfecta, and systemic hypertension.

CHRONIC AORTIC REGURGITATION

- The diastolic return of blood through the aortic valve leads to compensatory LV dilatation and hypertrophy.
- Contractility and compliance increase and the ejection fraction becomes supranormal.

• As AR progresses, end diastolic pressure increases, end systolic volume increases, ejection fraction drops, and symptoms develop.

History

• AR has a very long latent period during which the only symptom may be a sensation of a forcefully contracting heart.
• Eventually symptoms of congestive heart failure develop, including dyspnea on exertion, orthopnea, and paroxysmal nocturnal dyspnea.

Physical Examination (Tables 14–1, 14–2)

• General
  1. Systolic blood pressure is usually elevated and diastolic blood pressure low.
  2. The Korotkoff sounds may persist down to a cuff pressure of zero, but the diastolic pressure correlates best with the pressure at which the sounds become muffled.
• Pulse. The wide pulse pressure leads to a bounding "water hammer" pulse that may be bisferiens at the carotid and is best palpated at the radial artery with the patient's arm raised. Classic signs of the wide pulse pressure include:
  1. Duroziez's sign: systolic and diastolic bruits heard over the femoral artery when it is compressed.
  2. Quincke's sign: capillary pulsations visible in the finger nail bed.
  3. Musset's sign: a head bob with each heartbeat.
• Jugular veins. No significant findings occur.
• Palpation
  1. The apical impulse is diffuse, hyperdynamic, inferolaterally displaced, and often with a prominent impulse of early diastolic filling.
  2. The increased stroke volume may cause a systolic thrill at the right upper sternal border and in the neck.
• Heart tones. S_1 and A_2 are soft, the pulmonic component of S_2 (P_2) may be obscured by the murmur. An ejection sound related to the increased stroke volume may occur after S_1. S_3 is frequently heard in severe AR.
• Murmur
  1. The murmur is a high-pitched blowing diastolic, decrescendo sound beginning immediately after A_2. It is loudest at the left sternal border and heard best with the diaphragm as the patient leans forward, breath-holding in end expiration.
  2. As AR becomes more severe, the murmur is louder and lasts through more of diastole.
  3. The Austin Flint murmur is a diastolic low-pitched rumbling, heard at the apex, and caused by displacement of the anterior leaflet of the mitral valve by the AR jet. It has no hemodynamic significance.
• Dynamic auscultation. The murmur of AR and the Austin

Flint murmur are made louder by squatting and isometric exercise.

Laboratory Examination

- ECG. LV hypertrophy including left axis deviation and strain pattern is a common finding in severe AR.
- Chest X-ray. Heart size increases as AR becomes more severe. Left atrial enlargement is rare in the absence of associated mitral valve disease. Depending on the etiology of the AR, a dilated ascending aorta may be present.
- Echocardiography
  1. M mode shows increased motion of the septum and posterior wall, increased end diastolic diameter, increased systolic shortening, and diastolic fluttering of the mitral valve.
  2. 2D provides clues to etiology by visualizing the valve cups and aortic root.
  3. Doppler is nearly 100% sensitive for the detection of AR. Color Doppler can map the dimension of the AR jet and provide information on the severity of regurgitation.

ACUTE AORTIC REGURGITATION

- Acute development of AR allows no time for compensation, and patients develop sudden severe cardiac collapse with rapid rise in LV end diastolic pressure and low forward output.
- The most common etiologies are infective endocarditis, aortic dissection, and trauma.

History

The patient complains of the sudden onset of severe weakness and dyspnea.

Physical Examination (Tables 14–1, 14–2)

- General. The patient is acutely ill, tachycardic, and hypotensive with near-normal pulse pressure.
- Pulse. None of the signs of chronic AR that result from wide pulse pressure are present.
- Jugular veins. Venous pressure may be elevated as a result of secondary right heart failure.
- Palpation. The apical impulse is near normal.
- Heart tones. S_1 is soft, absent, or heard in diastole. A_2 is soft or absent. P_2 is loud as a result of pulmonary hypertension. S_3 is usually heard. S_4 is absent.
- Murmur. The murmur is early diastolic low pitched and shorter in duration than chronic AR because of the rapid reduction in the pressure gradient across the valve. The Austin Flint murmur, if present, is brief.

Laboratory Examination

- ECG. Abnormalities are usually limited to nospecific ST-T changes.
- Chest X-ray. Slight cardiomegaly and pulmonary edema are the usual findings.
- Echocardiography
  1. M Mode and 2D show reduced opening of the mitral valve and early closure and near-normal diastolic volume and percent shortening. They may identify the etiology.
  2. Doppler is very sensitive to the presence of AR.

MITRAL STENOSIS

General Comments

- Rheumatic heart disease is by far the most common cause of mitral stenosis (MS). The inflammatory process involves the cusps, commisures, and chordae leading to obstruction to flow across the valve by thickening and, eventually, fusion of the cusps.
- The gradient across the valve depends on the valve area (normal: 4 to 6 cm^2, critical MS < 1 cm^2) and the square of the blood flow rate. As the gradient increases, pulmonary venous pressure rises and cardiac output is limited leading to the early development of symptoms.

History

- Two-thirds of patients are women with symptoms usually developing 10 to 20 years after the initial episode of rheumatic fever.
- The cardinal symptom is dyspnea. Initially, it occurs during periods of increased flow across the valve or decreased filling time due to tachycardia as in exercise, fever, stress, pregnancy, thyrotoxicosis, and rapid atrial fibrillation.
- Other symptoms include hemoptysis, chest pain, embolic phenomenon, and chronic or episodic atrial fibrillation. With progression, patients develop orthopnea, dyspnea at rest, and symptoms of right heart failure including ascites and edema.

Physical Examination (Tables 14–1, 14–2)

- Jugular veins. In the absence of atrial fibrillation there is often a prominent a wave.
- Palpation
  1. The apical impulse is normal unless displaced by right ventricular (RV) dilatation.
  2. In the presence of pulmonary hypertension, an RV heave may be present along the left sternal border. P_2 may be palpable in the second left intercostal space.
- Heart tones
  1. S_1 is loud when the valve is still mobile. P_2 is loud and

delayed in the presence of pulmonary hypertension causing a single loud S_2.

2. An opening snap (OS) depends on a mobile mitral valve, occurs after S_2, is heard at the apex with the diaphragm, and moves closer to S_2 as the degree of obstruction increases.

- Murmur
  1. The murmur of MS is low pitched, diastolic, and rumbling, heard best at the apex with the bell while the patient is in the left lateral decubitus position.
  2. The volume of the murmur does not predict severity, though murmurs of longer duration indicate more severe obstruction.
- Dynamic auscultation. The murmur is louder with exhalation, amyl nitrate, exercise, squatting, and hand grip. The S_2-OS interval widens with standing (unlike a split S_2, which narrows).

Laboratory Examination

- ECG. Left atrial enlargement, with broad notched P waves seen in lead II, appears in 90% of patients with moderate to severe MS. Atrial fibrillation with fibrillatory waves of greater than 1 millivolt in V_1 is common.
- Chest X-ray. Chest film shows straightening of the left heart border due to enlargement of the left atrium. In the presence of pulmonary hypertension there is enlargement of the pulmonary arteries, RV, and right atrium.
- Echocardiography
  1. M mode can confirm the diagnosis by documenting left atrial enlargement, thickening and limited motion of the mitral leaflets, and delayed rate of closure of the valve.
  2. 2D is no more sensitive than M mode for the diagnosis of MS but can measure the size of the mitral valve orifice.
  3. Doppler can accurately measure the pressure gradient across the valve and can be used to calculate the valve area.

MITRAL REGURGITATION

General Comments

Disease or dysfunction of the mitral valve leaflets, annulus, chordae, or papillary muscles can lead to acute or chronic regurgitation.

CHRONIC MITRAL REGURGITATION

The gradual progressive development of mitral regurgitation (MR) is usually caused by mitral valve prolapse or rheumatic heart disease. LV dilatation is another common cause, though the MR is not usually severe.

History

Symptoms occur late in the course of chronic MR because increased atrial compliance and LV contractility prevent significant elevations in left atrial pressure or a drop in effective cardiac output. Only when the LV begins to fail do symptoms of poor forward output such as fatigue and exertional dyspnea occur.

Physical Examination (Tables 14–1, 14–2)

- General. Atrial fibrillation is common.
- Pulse. The carotid pulse is rapid in upstroke and short in duration.
- Palpation. The apical impulse is diffuse, displaced to the left, and hyperdynamic.
- Heart tones. S_1 is soft, especially with valve leaflet disease. A widely split S_2 is produced by reduced LV ejection time. S_3 is common.
- Murmur. The murmur is a blowing high-pitched holosystolic sound that begins after S_1 and continues through A_2. It is loudest at the apex and radiates into the axilla. The intensity of the murmur does not correlate with severity.
- Dynamic auscultation. The murmur's intensity increases with exhalation, squatting, isometric exercise, and transient arterial occlusion. It decreases in intensity with inhalation, amyl nitrate, and the strain of Valsalva. There is no change in intensity of the murmur with variable diastolic intervals such as after a premature beat or in atrial fibrillation.

Laboratory Examination

- ECG. Atrial fibrillation and left atrial enlargement are common. LV hypertrophy is seen in one-third of patients.
- Chest X-ray. LV and left atrial enlargement are prominent.
- Echocardiography
  1. M mode and 2D are useful in determining the etiology of the valvular dysfunction.
  2. Doppler, both color and pulse, can assess the presence and severity of MR by determining the depth of the regurgitant jet in the left atrium relative to the size of the chamber.

ACUTE MITRAL REGURGITATION

Acute MR can result from infective endocarditis, trauma, prosthetic valve dysfunction, myxomatous degeneration, and papillary muscle rupture or dysfunction from acute myocardial infarction or ischemia.

History

With sudden valve dysfunction, left atrial compliance is low and the patient develops sudden pulmonary edema and/or hypotension.

Physical Examination (Tables 14–1, 14–2)

- General. Findings may include hypotension, sinus rhythm, pulmonary edema, and stigmata of infective endocarditis.
- Pulse. There is decreased volume and rapid upstroke.
- Jugular veins. Venous pressure is elevated and a waves are prominent.
- Palpation. The apical impulse is slightly laterally displaced and hyperdynamic. The impulse of LV filling with atrial contraction, an RV impulse, and an apical systolic thrill are all often detectable.
- Heart tones. Unlike in chronic MR, S_1 is normal in intensity. S_2 is widely split with a loud P_2. Both S_3 and S_4 are often present.
- Murmur
  1. The murmur is a loud rough early systolic crescendo-decrescendo sound beginning after S_1 and ending before S_2. The murmur can radiate to the base, back, or axilla.
  2. In some cases there is no murmur because extreme left atrial hypertension prevents significant retrograde flow.
- Dynamic auscultation. The murmur responds to maneuvers in the same way as chronic MR.

Laboratory Examination

- ECG. The rhythm is sinus, P wave duration is usually longer than 0.12 sec, and LV hypertrophy is seen in 25% of patients.
- Chest X-ray. In the absence of other underlying cardiac disease, the heart is normal size and the lung fields show pulmonary edema.
- Echocardiography
  1. M mode and 2D can show the etiology of the valve lesion and distinguish acute from chronic MR by the absence of enlarged left-sided chambers.
  2. Doppler is highly sensitive in detecting the presence of MR and is accurate in determining severity.

MITRAL VALVE PROLAPSE

General Comments

- Mitral valve prolapse (MVP) refers to displacement during systole of the valve leaflets into the left atrium. It is usually caused by disproportion between the connective tissue elements of the valve (cusps, annulus, chordae) and their muscular supports (papillary muscle, ventricle).
- MVP is frequently genetically determined and can be related to recognized connective tissue syndromes such as Marfan's and Ehlers-Danlos syndromes. Most often, however, it is inherited as an isolated finding.

History

- MVP is usually asymptomatic but in rare instances can be associated with syncope, endocarditis, palpitations, atrial arrhythmias, embolic phenomenon, autonomic instability, symptomatic mitral regurgitation, and chest pain.
- Though in the past MVP was felt to be related to dyspnea, panic attacks, and high levels of anxiety, these associations are no longer felt to be real.

Physical Examination (Tables 14–1, 14–2)

- Pulse, jugular veins, and palpation. No specific findings.
- Heart tones. S_1 and S_2 are normal. The classic MVP click is heard at least 0.14 sec after S_1 and after the initiation of the rise of the carotid pulse.
- Murmur. The murmur is less common than the click. It is mid- to late systolic beginning after the click at the apex.
- Dynamic auscultation
  1. The click and murmur of MVP may be intermittent in an individual.
  2. When present, the click and/or murmur occur earlier in systole with maneuvers that reduce LV size (standing, Valsalva strain, and amyl nitrate). Actions that increase chamber size (squatting, leg raise, isometric exercise, and release of Valsalva) move the click and murmur later in systole.

Laboratory Examination

- ECG and chest X-ray. No specific findings.
- Echocardiography
  1. M mode is the most sensitive, demonstrating posterior systolic motion of the mitral leaflet interface 2 mm behind the line connecting the opening and closing points.
  2. On 2D echo the systolic billowing of the mitral leaflets into the left atrium on a parasternal or apical four chamber view is diagnostic.
  3. Doppler can demonstrate the presence and magnitude of associated MR.

TRICUSPID STENOSIS

General Comments

In adults, tricuspid stenosis (TS) is rare, usually rheumatic in origin, and associated with mitral and aortic valve involvement. Like rheumatic MS, TS is often associated with tricuspid regurgitation (TR).

History

The symptoms of TS are secondary-to-low cardiac output and venous congestion including fatigue, edema, ascites, and hepatic congestion. As TS progresses, blood return to the left heart drops and the pulmonary congestion symptoms due to associated MS diminish.

Physical Examination (Tables 14–1, 14–2)

- General. Severe TS can result in edema, jaundice, hepatomegaly, and ascites.
- Jugular veins. The jugular pressure is increased with a prominent a wave and a slow Y descent.
- Palpation. TS is suggested by the absence of signs of pulmonary hypertension (i.e., RV heave) despite mitral stenosis and signs of RV failure. A diastolic thrill augmented by inspiration may be palpated at the left lower sternal border.
- Heart tones. S_1 and S_2 are usually consistent with lesions in other valves. A tricuspid opening snap may be heard at the left lower sternal border after the S_2 and mitral OS.
- Murmur. When audible, it is low-pitched, rumbling, diastolic sound with presystolic accentuation, heard best at the left lower sternal border.
- Dynamic auscultation. The murmur is louder with inspiration, leg raising, amyl nitrate, squatting, and exercise. It is reduced with exhalation and Valsalva strain.

Laboratory Examination

- ECG. Prominent right atrial enlargement without evidence of RV hypertrophy suggests TS.
- Chest X-ray. Cardiomegaly, prominent right atrial enlargement, and minimal pulmonary congestion are common.
- Echocardiography
  1. M mode and 2D echocardiography can document right atrial enlargement, thickening and limited motion of the valve leaflets, and delayed valve closure.
  2. Doppler can measure the pressure gradient across the valve, which can be used to calculate valve area.

TRICUSPID REGURGITATION

General Comments

- The most common cause of clinically important TR is dilatation of the valve annulus due to pulmonary hypertension or RV infarct.
- Other causes include endocarditis, Marfan's syndrome, rheumatic heart disease, Ebstein's anomaly, papillary muscle necrosis, trauma, and carcinoid syndrome.

History

TR is usually well tolerated unless it is associated with significant pulmonary hypertension. In that case, symptoms of poor forward cardiac output and venous congestion are prominent.

Physical Examination

- General. As TR becomes severe, findings on general exam include jaundice, cachexia, edema, ascites, and an enlarged, pulsatile liver.
- Jugular veins. Venous pressure is elevated with prominent v waves and a fast Y descent. Hepatojugular reflux with prolonged elevation of jugular pressure on hepatic compression is common.
- Palpation. An RV heave may be felt along the left sternal border.
- Heart tones. S_1 is normal. S_2 may contain a loud P_2 component if pulmonary hypertension is present. An RV S_3 is often heard especially on inspiration.
- Murmur. The murmur is high-pitched, holosystolic, and loudest in the left lower parasternal or subxiphoid regions.
- Dynamic auscultation. The murmur of TR is louder with maneuvers that increase return of blood to the right side of the heart, including inspiration, exercise, leg raise, hepatic compression, prolonged diastole, and release of the Valsalva's maneuver.

Laboratory Examination (Tables 14–1, 14–2)

- ECG. The rhythm is often atrial fibrillation. EKG may show evidence of right atrial enlargement, RV hypertrophy, or incomplete right-bundle-branch block.
- Chest X-ray. RV and right atrial enlargement are often present.
- Echocardiography
  1. 2D and M mode are useful in determining the etiology of TR.
  2. Doppler echo can, with high sensitivity, detect the presence of TR and quantify its magnitude using pulse or color mode by mapping the depth of the regurgitant jet in the right atrium.

PULMONARY STENOSIS

General Comments

Obstruction at the pulmonic valve is nearly always congenital and seldom increases in severity once adulthood is reached.

History

Most patients are asymptomatic. In severe pulmonary stenosis (PS), symptoms of limited cardiac output (exertional dyspnea and fatigue) are present with eventual development of TR and right-sided heart failure.

Physical Examination

- General. In severe PS there may be evidence of right-sided heart failure.

- Jugular veins. A prominent a wave may be seen.
- Palpation. An RV heave may be felt at the left sternal border with a systolic thrill at the left upper sternal border.
- Heart tones. S_1 is normal, P_2 may be delayed, and an ejection click may be heard.
- Murmur. The murmur is crescendo-decrescendo and loudest at the left upper sternal border.

Laboratory Examination

- ECG. As PS becomes more severe, right axis deviation, RV hypertrophy, and right atrial enlargement develop.
- Chest X-ray. Poststenotic dilatation of the main and left pulmonary arteries is common. Right atrial and RV enlargement is common in more severe cases.
- Echocardiography
  1. M mode and 2D can demonstrate PS and identify any associated congenital abnormalities.
  2. Doppler can reliably measure the gradient across the valve.

PULMONIC REGURGITATION

General Comments

Diastolic regurgitation of blood across the pulmonic valve is nearly always due to pulmonary hypertension. It seldom has any hemodynamic significance of its own.

History

Symptoms are due to pulmonary hypertension or its underlying cause and not the pulmonary regurgitation (PR) itself.

Physical Examination (Tables 14–1, 14–2)

- Palpation. A left parasternal heave and a diastolic thrill at the left upper sternal border may be present.
- Heart tones. S_1 is normal. S_2 is widely split with a loud P_2. Right-sided S_3 and S_4 may be present.
- Murmur. The murmur is a diastolic decrescendo high-pitched sound heard along the left sternal border.

Laboratory Examination

- ECG. RV hypertrophy may be present.
- Chest X-ray. The pulmonary artery and RV are usually enlarged.
- Echocardiography. M mode and 2D can demonstrate PR while Doppler can estimate severity.

THE DIFFERENTIAL DIAGNOSIS OF SYSTOLIC MURMURS

- Systolic murmurs may occur as a result of AS, MR, TR, ventricular septal defects (VSD), PS, hypertrophic cardiomyopathy (HC), and without associated pathology (benign).
- The first differential point is to distinguish right- and left-sided murmurs. Augmentation of the murmur on inspiration (when venous pressure is high, this maneuver should be done with patient sitting up) is sensitive and specific for the detection of right-sided murmurs (TR, PS).
- Right-sided murmurs
  1. TR can be differentiated from PS by its left lower sternal border location, holosystolic blowing quality, prominent jugular V waves, right-sided S_3, and association with atrial fibrillation.
  2. PS is loudest at the base, crescendo-decrescendo in quality, and produces a right-sided S_4.
- Left-sided murmurs
  1. Only the murmur due to HC, a harsh crescendo-decrescendo midsystolic murmur radiating to the base and axilla, becomes louder with Valsalva strain or standing from squatting and softer with squatting, passive leg elevation, or hand grip.
  2. MR and VSD can be identified by augmentation with hand grip. MR and VSD can be distinguished from AS by their association with atrial fibrillation, S_3, left atrial enlargement on chest X-ray, and the lack of change in murmur intensity after a prolonged diastole.
  3. To distinguish VSD from MR note that:
     a. MR is a blowing high-pitched holosystolic murmur loudest at the apex and radiating to the axilla.
     b. VSD is high-pitched pansystolic, crescendo-decrescendo, and heard best at the left midsternal border.
  4. No maneuvers are specific for AS, but it can be identified by exclusion of HC, MR, VSD and the presence of an S_4, slow delayed carotid upstroke, augmentation with prolonged diastole, and radiation of a low-pitched harsh crescendo-decrescendo murmur into the neck. AS commonly radiates to the apex, making differentiation from MR on the basis of location alone difficult.
- Benign murmurs are asymptomatic, brief, soft, medium pitched, and associated with normal heart tones. Although they can be heard anywhere in the chest, they are usually loudest along the left sternal border.

THE DIFFERENTIAL DIAGNOSIS OF DIASTOLIC MURMURS

- Diastolic murmurs may occur as a result of AR, MS, PR, TS, and the Austin Flint murmur.
  1. AR and PR are high-pitched, decrescendo, and heard best along the upper left sternal border.

2. MS, TS, and the Austin Flint murmur are low-pitched, rumbling, and heard best at the apex or lower sternal border.
- Regurgitant murmurs. AR is associated with a wide pulse pressure. PR is nearly always associated with findings of pulmonary hypertension.
- Stenotic murmurs
    1. TS is rare. MS is often present and predates significant TS. TS is heard more medially than MS, increases with inspiration unlike MS, and is associated with more significant findings of elevated venous pressure (edema, ascites, hepatic congestion).
    2. The Austin Flint murmur is produced by the anterior mitral leaflet as it is hit by the jet of AR. MS can be distinguished from the Austin Flint murmur by the presence of a loud S_1 and an opening snap in many cases of MS but not with the Austin Flint murmur.

Bibliography

Depace NL, et al. Acute severe mitral regurgitation. Am J Med 1985;78:293–306.

Devereux RBH, et al. Mitral valve prolapse: causes, clinical manifestations and management. Ann Int Med 1989;111:305–317.

Grewe K, et al. Differentiation of cardiac murmurs by dynamic auscultation. Curr Probl Cardiol 1988;13:669–721.

Lee RT, et al. Assessment of valvular heart disease with Doppler echocardiography. JAMA 1989;262:2131–2135.

Lembs NJ, et al. Bedside diagnosis of systolic murmurs. N Engl J Med 1988;318:1572–1578.

Morganroth J, et al. Acute severe aortic regurgitation. Ann Int Med 1977;87:223–232.

SECTION III

PULMONARY

15

DYSPNEA

SCOTT BARNHART

Give me some little breath, some little pause.
SHAKESPEARE (1564–1616) RICHARD III

GENERAL COMMENTS

- Dyspnea is a distressing sensation associated with labored breathing or breathlessness. A patient's assessment of dyspnea is subjective and cannot be directly measured.
- The sensation of dyspnea is directly related to the control of ventilation. Ventilation depends on the integration of afferent signals from mechanical and chemical receptors in the small airways, skeletal muscle, pulmonary vasculature, peripheral chemoreceptors, central chemoreceptors, cortical input, and a central pacemaker.

DIFFERENTIAL DIAGNOSIS

- Decreased oxygen delivery
  1. Nonpulmonary
     a. Decreased inspired oxygen tension
     b. Anemia
     c. Carboxyhemoglobinemia
     d. Hemoglobinopathy
     e. Decreased cardiac output
  2. Pulmonary: airways or pulmonary parenchyma
     a. Airflow obstruction
     b. Neoplasm
     c. Pneumonia
     d. Interstitial pneumonitis
     e. Emphysema
     f. Pleural effusion
  3. Pulmonary: vascular
     a. Pulmonary embolism
     b. Vasculitis
- Increased oxygen demands
  1. Exercise
  2. Infection
  3. Thyrotoxicosis
- Increased work of breathing
  1. Airflow obstruction
  2. Decreased lung compliance (e.g., diffuse infiltrative diseases)
  3. Increased carbon dioxide production (e.g., infection, increased metabolism)

- Miscellaneous
  1. Muscle weakness
  2. CNS stimulation
  3. Psychogenic factors
  4. Acidosis

CLINICAL MANIFESTATIONS

- History
  1. Onset
     a. Acute onset suggests pulmonary embolism, pneumothorax, or heart failure.
     b. Chronic dyspnea is much more likely to be the result of chronic left ventricular failure, chronic obstructive pulmonary disease, or interstitial fibrosis.
  2. Associated symptoms
     a. Chest pain may suggest MI or pulmonary embolism.
     b. Wheezing is often associated with asthma or chronic obstructive pulmonary disease (COPD).
     c. Cough, fever, and chills suggest an inflammatory process.
- Physical examination
  1. General appearance. The examination may detect the use of accessory muscles.
  2. Vital signs including the respiratory rate.
  3. Chest
     a. Appearance. Rate and depth of respirations, splinting, paradoxical chest wall and abdominal motion, and flail chest may be seen.
     b. Percussion. Dullness may suggest an effusion, and hyperresonance may support air trapping from airflow obstruction or pneumothorax.
     c. Auscultation. Wheezing, rales, and decreased or absent breath sounds may all point to the diagnosis.
     d. Cardiovascular examination. Elevated jugular venous pressure, cardiac enlargement, gallops, or murmurs may suggest a cardiac cause.

LABORATORY EXAMINATION

The choice of laboratory examinations is guided by the history and physical examination.

- Chest X-ray may detect abnormalities of the chest wall, pulmonary vasculature and parenchyma, and heart size.
- Spirometry
  1. Screening spirometry may indicate a low vital capacity or airflow obstruction.
  2. The diffusion capacity (DL_{CO}) may suggest or help quantify interstitial lung diseases.
  3. When dyspnea is out of proportion to the level of pul-

monary function test abnormality, exercise tests help quantify the limitations and assess cardiac derangement.

- Complete blood count. Anemia causing decreased ability to deliver oxygen must be ruled out. An elevated hematocrit may support chronic hypoxemia.
- Arterial blood gas
  1. The pH and $PaCO_2$ (arterial partial pressure of carbon dioxide) indicate the patient's acid-base status, the acuteness of the derangement (e.g., acute respiratory acidosis), and the patient's ability to maintain adequate ventilation.
  2. The PaO_2 (arterial partial pressure of oxygen) indicates whether hypoxemia is present and whether there is a widened arterial to alveolar O_2 gradient.
- Electrocardiography may suggest new or old ischemic cardiac disease or left ventricular hypertrophy.
- Additional studies to investigate cardiac or pulmonary disease may include exercise testing, ventilation-perfusion scans, or right- or left-heart catheterization.

RECOMMENDED DIAGNOSTIC APPROACH

- Initial evaluation
  1. Assessment of degree of distress
     a. Acute distress. Emergency evaluation and support may be required.
     b. Moderate distress or chronic problem. A full history and physical examination are indicated followed by the selected laboratory studies.
- Laboratory studies
  1. Pulmonary studies
     a. Chest X-ray
     b. Arterial blood gas
     c. Pulmonary function testing
        i. Spirometry
        ii. Diffusing capacity
     d. Exercise testing
  2. Cardiac studies
     a. EKG
     b. Exercise test
     c. Echocardiogram
     d. Right- and/or left-heart catheterization

Bibliography

Burki NK. Dyspnea. Clin Chest Med 1980;1:47.

Mahler DA. Dyspnea: Diagnosis and management. Clin Chest Med 1987;8(2):215–230.

Tobin MJ. Dyspnea. Arch Intern Med 1990;150:1604–1613.

Wasserman K, et al. Dyspnea: Physiological and pathophysiological mechanics. Ann Rev Med 1988;39:503–515.

16

HEMOPTYSIS

SCOTT BARNHART

Miniver coughed and called it fate, and kept on drinking.

EDWIN ARLINGTON ROBINSON (1869–1935)

DEFINITIONS AND GENERAL COMMENTS

- Hemoptysis is the coughing of blood from below the larynx. It must be carefully differentiated from the coughing of blood from the nasopharynx or the upper GI tract.
- Massive hemoptysis is defined as hemoptysis of 200 to 600 cm^3 over 24 or 48 hours.
- Hemoptysis may arise from sources fed by systemic or pulmonary arteries. Factors that contribute to hemoptysis include:
  1. Disruption of bronchial epithelium and capillaries by tracheobronchitis
  2. Injury to pulmonary parenchyma by infarction or necrotizing processes
  3. Pulmonary venous hypertension, as from mitral stenosis

DIFFERENTIAL DIAGNOSIS (Tables 16–1 and 16–2)

The most common cause of hemoptysis is bronchitis. Other common causes of hemoptysis include chronic suppurative processes, tuberculosis, pneumonia, neoplasms, and pulmonary embolism.

CLINICAL MANIFESTATIONS

- History
  1. The history should differentiate between true hemoptysis and blood arising from the GI tract or nasopharynx.
  2. Blood from the GI tract is frequently vomited, dark, acidic, never frothy, and may contain food particles.
  3. Important elements in the history include:
     a. The patient's age
     b. Onset, duration, and amount of blood
     c. The character of the hemoptysis, that is, bright red frothy blood or small flecks mixed in with purulent sputum
     d. Smoking, respiratory, and cardiac history

TABLE 16–1. Causes of Hemoptysis[a]

Bronchogenic carcinoma (56)
Lung abscess (49)
Pulmonary infarct (44)
Bronchiectasis (43)
Tuberculosis (36)
Congenital cyst (25)
Empyema (24)
Metastatic disease
Arteriovenous fistula
Bronchitis
Bronchoaortic fistula
Broncholithiasis
Foreign body
Goodpasture's syndrome
Idiopathic pulmonary hemosiderosis
Mycetoma
Parasitic infection
Left ventricular failure
Trauma
Wegener's granulomatosis

[a] Frequency (percentage) with which hemoptysis is associated with a condition is indicated by numbers in parentheses.

- Physical examination. Note the following:
  1. Gross examination of the sputum
  2. Vital signs, including respiratory rate and temperature
  3. Examination of the nasopharynx for a source of the bleeding
  4. Adenopathy
  5. The lungs, for wheezes or rhonchi suggesting chronic obstructive pulmonary disease, or rales suggesting pneumonia
  6. The heart, for evidence of left ventricular failure or mitral stenosis
  7. If the hemoptysis is massive, immediate attention must be directed to the patient's ability to maintain a patent airway as well as oxygenation and ventilation.

TABLE 16–2. Common Causes of Massive Hemoptysis[a]

Tuberculosis (49%)
Bronchiectasis (22%)
Lung abscess (12%)
Carcinoma (3%)

[a] Figures in parentheses indicate percentage of cases of massive hemoptysis caused by listed condition.

LABORATORY EXAMINATIONS

The following should be considered in every case of hemoptysis:

1. Chest X-ray
2. Sputum examination with Gram's stain, culture, and acid-fast smear and culture
3. Purified protein derivative skin test
4. Complete blood count, including platelet count
5. Prothrombin time
6. Sputum cytology
7. Arterial blood gas
8. Laryngoscopy
9. Bronchoscopy

RECOMMENDED DIAGNOSTIC APPROACH

- Almost all cases should be evaluated with a chest X-ray and sputum examination and should have evaluation for tuberculosis.
- The next step is dictated by the history, examination, and the results of the above mentioned studies.

  1. If bronchitis is the likely diagnosis, the patient should be observed and further evaluated with bronchoscopy only if
     a. The hemoptysis persists for 2 weeks
     b. The hemoptysis is recurrent
     c. Malignancy is suspected for other reasons, such as weight loss
     d. There is a possibility of undiagnosed infections such as tuberculosis
  2. If the chest X-ray suggests bronchiectasis or pneumonia, close observation is warranted.

- Clinical or radiographic evidence of malignancy should be evaluated promptly with bronchoscopy. Other appropriate studies may include:

  1. Chest CT
  2. Ventilation-perfusion scans
  3. Angiography
  4. Sputum examination for cytology or fungal or parasitic infection

- In the case of massive hemoptysis, immediate attention is directed to:

  1. The assessment of airway and respiratory reserve
  2. Identification of the site of bleeding, usually by rigid bronchoscopy followed by bronchial or pulmonary artery angiography as indicated
  3. Candidacy for surgery or arterial embolization

Bibliography

Garzon AA, Gourin A. Surgical management of massive hemoptysis. Ann Surg 1974;187:267.

Poe RH, et al. Utility of fiberoptic bronchoscopy in patients with hemoptysis and nonlocalizing chest roentgenographs. Chest 1988;93(1):70–75.

Santiago SM, et al. Bronchoscopy in patients with hemoptysis and normal chest roentgenographs. Br J Dis Chest 1987;81(20):186–188.

Wolfe JD, Simmons DH. Hemoptysis: Diagnosis and management. West J Med 1970;127:383–390.

17

PLEURAL EFFUSIONS

SCOTT BARNHART

A medical chest specialist is long-winded about the short-winded.

KENNETH T. BIRD (1917–   )

DEFINITIONS AND GENERAL COMMENTS

- Accumulation of more than 10 to 20 cm³ of pleural fluid in the pleural space.
- Pathophysiology
  1. Up to 2 to 3 L of fluid cross the pleural space each day. The passage of fluid through the pleural space is governed by opposing hydrostatic and oncotic pressures.
  2. The net effect is the passage of fluid from the parietal pleura into the pleural space, followed by the absorption by the visceral pleura and the lymphatics.
  3. The normal pleural space has a net negative pressure, which prevents the accumulation of fluid. Any process that upsets this balance leads to the development of an effusion.
- Pleural effusions are classified as either "exudates" or "transudates."
  1. Exudates generally result from diseases that directly involve the pleura. An exudate has fluid with one or more of the following criteria:
     a. Protein concentration greater than 3 g/dl.
     b. Pleural fluid lactate dehydrogenase (LDH) to serum LDH ratio greater than 0.6.
     c. Pleural fluid protein to serum protein ratio greater than 0.5.
  2. Transudates result from processes that do not directly involve the pleura. Further investigations of transudates are unnecessary other than to establish the primary process.

DIFFERENTIAL DIAGNOSIS (Table 17–1)

- Transudates. Two types of processes cause transudative pleural effusions:
  1. Diseases associated with hypoalbuminemia.
  2. Diseases associated with elevated venous pressure, primarily congestive heart failure.
- Exudative pleural effusions. These are most likely caused by:

TABLE 17–1.   Causes of Pleural Effusions[a]

Transudative Pleural Effusions
  Congestive heart failure (common)
  Cirrhosis
  Nephrotic syndrome
  Myxedema
  Hypoalbuminemia
  Meigs' syndrome
  Sarcoidosis
Exudative Pleural Effusions
  Infectious causes
    1. Bacterial infections
      a. *Staphylococcus aureus* (50%)
      b. *Streptococcus pneumoniae* (11%)
    2. Tuberculosis (38%)
    3. *Mycoplasma pneumoniae* (<20%)
    4. Viral (<20%)
    5. Fungal (common with *Nocardia* and *Actinomyces*)
    6. Parasites (frequent with *Entamoeba histolytica,* rare
      with *Pneumocystis carinii* and *Echinococcus*
      granulosus)
  Neoplasms
  Collagen vascular disease
    1. Rheumatoid arthritis (rare)
    2. Systemic lupus erythematosus (20 to 70%)
  Pulmonary embolus
  Gastrointestinal disease
    1. Pancreatitis (40%)
    2. Esophageal rupture (common)
    3. Subphrenic abscess
  Trauma
  Postoperative (50% after abdominal surgery)

  [a] Figures in parentheses indicate the percentage of a given cause that has associated effusions.

1. Inflammation of the pleura due to infection, as with a parapneumonic effusion or an empyema
2. Malignancy
3. Autoimmune disease
4. Pulmonary thromboemboli (effusions from which are exudative 3/4 of the time and transudative 1/4 of the time)
5. Pancreatitis

HISTORY AND PHYSICAL EXAMINATION

- History
  1. Dyspnea is the most common finding. Small pleural effusions are often clinically silent.
  2. Other prominent symptoms include pleuritic pain and cough or symptoms associated with the underlying disease.

- Signs
  1. Pleural effusions smaller than 200 to 300 cm³ are difficult to detect by physical examination or chest radiographs.
  2. If effusions of greater than 200 cm³ are present, the patient may have dullness to percussion, decreased breath sounds at the bases, and egophony just above the level of decreased breath sounds.

RECOMMENDED DIAGNOSTIC APPROACH

- The pleural effusion must be confirmed radiographically.
  1. 200 cm³ of fluid must accumulate in the pleural space before it becomes evident on a posteroanterior chest X-ray. Ultrasound examination may detect smaller effusions.
  2. The absence of free-flowing fluid on a lateral decubitus X-ray does not rule out a pleural effusion because the fluid may become loculated.
- Perform a thoracentesis.
  1. This leads to a diagnosis for 90% of pleural effusions.
  2. A thoracentesis is omitted for patients in whom the risk of a pneumothorax from the thoracentesis is greater than the benefits of a specific diagnosis.
- Analyze the pleural fluid. The fluid is classified as a transudate or an exudate by measurement of protein and LDH (see Table 17–2).
  1. Appearance. Clear straw-colored fluid can be either an exudate or transudate. Turbid fluid suggests an exudate with increased leukocytes, protein, or lipids. Frank pus is obvious, and a foul odor suggests an anaerobic empyema.
  2. Bloody effusion
     a. Bloody effusions are difficult to interpret, since it takes little blood (1 cm³) to produce a pink tinge, and the fluid often becomes contaminated with blood from the thoracentesis.
     b. Exudative pleural effusions that are genuinely bloody suggest tuberculosis, malignancy, trauma, and pulmonary emboli.
  3. White cell and differential count
     a. More than 1000 WBC/mm³ suggest an exudate, and over 25,000 WBC/mm³ suggest an empyema.
     b. A predominance of polymorphonuclear cells is consistent with an early inflammatory condition such as an empyema, parapneumonic effusion, or pulmonary embolus.
     c. Mononuclear cells are more common in chronic inflammatory processes or in transudates.
     d. Eosinophils suggest a pneumothorax, hemothorax, asbestosis, drug reaction, sarcoidosis, or parasitic fungal or autoimmune pleural disease.
  4. Gram's stain and culture
     a. Gram's stain and culture should be done immedi-

TABLE 17–2. Laboratory Findings in Pleural Effusions

DISEASE	APPEARANCE	WBC/MM^3	PREDOMINANT CELL TYPE	GRAM'S STAIN	GLUCOSE	OTHER
Transudate	Serous	<1000	Mononuclear	Negative	Equal to serum	
Exudate						
Parapneumonic	Serous	5000–25,000	Neutrophil	Negative	May be low	
Empyema	Cloudy to cloudy	Innumerable	Neutrophil	May be positive	Low	
Tuberculosis	Serosanguinous	>1000	Mononuclear	Acid-fast bacilli	Low	
Malignancy	Serosanguinous	<1000	Mononuclear	Negative	Normal	Cytology positive in 40%
Pulmonary embolism	Serosanguinous or serous	1000–100,000	Red blood cell	Negative	Normal	
Rheumatoid arthritis	Cloudy to serous	1000–2000	Mononuclear	Negative	Very low	
Pancreatitis	Cloudy	5000–20,000	None	Negative	Normal	Amylase may be high

ately on all exudates to rule out an empyema. Careful bacteriologic techniques should be used when an anaerobic infection is suspected.

b. Acid-fast smears and cultures should be obtained whenever tuberculosis is suspected.

5. Glucose. Low glucose levels are associated with pleural disease caused by rheumatoid arthritis, empyema, tuberculosis, and esophageal rupture.

6. Amylase. Elevated pleural fluid amylase levels suggest either pancreatic disease or esophageal rupture.

7. Cytology

a. Cytology can establish that a neoplasm is the source of a pleural effusion. With neoplastic involvement of the pleura, the yield is approximately 50%.

b. Malignancies that most commonly produce a pleural effusion are lung, breast, ovary, and stomach.

8. pH. A pH lower than 7.30 suggests an exudate, especially one caused by empyema or rheumatoid disease. A pH lower than 7.0 suggests empyema.

9. Other studies

a. Sudan stains for lipids can determine whether the thoracic duct has been ruptured.

b. Examination for antinuclear antibodies, immune complexes, and complement can help determine whether there is an autoimmune process.

- Other diagnostic procedures

1. The indication for a pleural biopsy is an unexplained exudative effusion. The biopsy is most useful to diagnose tuberculosis (70% sensitivity) or carcinomatous involvement (60 to 90% sensitivity) of the pleura.

2. Pleuroscopy may be useful when closed needle biopsies have been negative. In an undiagnosed effusion, it may increase the diagnostic yield approximately 20%.

Bibliography

Branch WT, McNeil BJ. Analysis of the differential diagnosis and assessment of pleuritic chest pain in young adults. Am J Med 1983;75:671.

Collins TR, et al. Thoracentesis: Clinical values, complications, technical problems and patient experience. Chest 1987;91:817–822.

Sahn SA. The differential diagnosis of pleural effusions. West J Med 1982;137:99–108.

18

ACUTE RESPIRATORY FAILURE

SCOTT BARNHART

Among the Haida Indians of the Pacific Northwest, the verb for making poetry is the same as the verb to breathe.

TOM ROBBINS

DEFINITION

- Acute respiratory failure (ARF) occurs when the body acutely fails to adequately eliminate carbon dioxide (CO_2) or to oxygenate the blood.
- As defined by arterial blood gas measurements, ARF is one or more of the following:
  1. An acute increase in the $PaCO_2$ to >50 mmHg
  2. An acute increase in $PaCO_2$ that produces a pH < 7.30
  3. An acute decrease in PaO_2 to <50 mmHg

EPIDEMIOLOGY AND PATHOPHYSIOLOGY

- The most common nonsurgical causes of ARF are drug overdoses, neuromuscular disease, adult respiratory distress syndrome (ARDS), chronic obstructive pulmonary disease (COPD), pneumonia, and cardiac failure.
- Pathophysiology. ARF results from the interrelated processes of hypercapnia and hypoxemia.
  1. Hypercapnia results from ventilation inadequate to eliminate the necessary amount of CO_2. Acutely, it is associated with a respiratory acidosis. The major physiologic causes include neuromuscular weakness, airflow obstruction, and increased pulmonary dead space.
  2. An increased production of CO_2 is frequently present in diseases leading to ARF.
  3. Hypoxemia has five possible physiologic causes:
     a. Decreased inspired oxygen tension
     b. Hypoventilation
     c. Ventilation-perfusion mismatch
     d. Shunt
     e. Diffusion limitation (rarely clinically significant)

DIFFERENTIAL DIAGNOSIS (Tables 18–1 and 18–2)

ARF can be separated into hypercapnic and hypoxemic ARF, but these conditions often occur together.

CLINICAL MANIFESTATIONS

- Symptoms
  1. Dyspnea is frequent but not universal.
  2. Hypercapnia may cause headache, mild sedation, and confusion, which may progress to coma.
  3. Symptoms associated with hypoxia include confusion, agitation, restlessness, and dizziness.
- Signs
  1. Signs associated with hypoxia include those of a sympathetic response such as tachycardia, hypertension, and peripheral vasoconstriction, as well as sympathetic decompensation such as bradycardia and hypotension.
  2. Signs of hypercapnia include vasodilation, diaphoresis, hypertension, and tachycardia.
  3. Additional physical findings depend on the etiology of the ARF.
     a. In COPD, ARF is associated with labored respirations and decreased breath sounds on auscultation. Wheezing may be minimal with severe airway obstruction.
     b. In neuromuscular disorders a decreased rate or depth of respirations may be apparent.

TABLE 18–1. Common Causes of Hypercapnia

1. Drug overdose
2. Myxedema
3. CNS dysfunction
   a. Stroke
   b. Brain tumor
   c. Head trauma
   d. Central hypoventilation
   e. Spinal cord disease: trauma, poliomyelitis, Guillain-Barré syndrome, and amyotrophic lateral sclerosis
4. Myasthenia gravis
5. Drug-induced neuromuscular disorders (e.g., due to aminoglycosides)
6. Muscular dystrophy
7. Chest wall abnormalities
   a. Flail chest
   b. Kyphoscoliosis
8. Airway obstruction
   a. Central (tracheal stenosis, vocal cord tumor)
   b. Peripheral (asthma, COPD)
9. Pulmonary edema

TABLE 18–2. Common Causes of Hypoxia

COPD/Asthma
Hypoventilation
ARDS
Pulmonary embolism
Pneumonia or atelectasis
Acute right-to-left shunt
Interstitial fibrosis

- Prognostic clinical indicators. Specific clinical signs that are predictive of eventual death or the need for mechanical ventilation are:
  1. Pulse >120 or <70 beats per minute
  2. Respiratory rate >30
  3. Palpable scalene muscle recruitment during inspiration
  4. Palpable abdominal muscle tensing during expiration
  5. Inability to perform vital capacity testing on command
  6. Irregularity of respiratory rhythm

RECOMMENDED DIAGNOSTIC APPROACH

- An arterial blood gas (ABG) sample in which PaO_2 and $PaCO_2$ approach 50 mmHg indicates possible ARF. If the abnormalities are acute and the pH is less than 7.30, the findings are consistent with ARF.
- Rule out life-threatening problems.
  1. Problems that produce an immediate threat to life through marked hypoxemia, hypercapnia, and acidosis must be ruled out.
  2. Patients should be evaluated for sufficient reserve to compensate for further deterioration in condition. Often ARF can be reversed with rapid therapy such as oxygen for hypoxemia or bronchodilators for airflow obstruction.
  3. If hypercapnia and hypoxia persist, intubation and mechanical ventilation are indicated.
- Evaluate other disease possibilities.
  1. The history and physical examination usually narrow etiologic possibilities to a few diseases or processes.
  2. Anemia must be ruled out. It can greatly increase the severity of ARF by producing tissue hypoxia and lactic acidosis.
  3. The chest X-ray helps to limit the differential diagnoses.
     a. Processes leading to ARF that are associated with "clear" chest X-rays include airflow obstruction, pulmonary embolism, and central or neuromuscular causes of hypoventilation.
     b. Infiltrates on the chest X-ray suggest pneumonia, atelectasis, pulmonary edema due to cardiac failure, ARDS, or pulmonary fibrosis.

4. An ECG helps to diagnose cardiac causes of respiratory failure such as acute myocardial infarction and severe arrhythmias.

Bibliography

Bartlett RH, et al. A prospective study of acute hypoxic respiratory failure. Chest 1986;89(5):684–689.

Moser KM. Acute respiratory failure with hypercapnia. In: Moser KM, ed. Respiratory Emergencies. St. Louis, C.V. Mosby, 1982, pp. 82–93.

Pontoppidan H, et al. Acute respiratory failure in the adult. N Engl J Med 1972;287:690–698.

Rosen RL. Acute respiratory failure and chronic obstructive lung disease. Med Clin N Amer 1986;70(4):895–907.

19

SOLITARY PULMONARY NODULE

JAMES TAYLOR

We should always presume the disease to be curable
until its own nature prove it otherwise.

PETER MERE LATHAM (1789–1875)

DEFINITION AND GENERAL COMMENTS

- A solitary pulmonary nodule (SPN) is a circumscribed
  round or oval intrapulmonary lesion up to 4 cm in diameter.
  The term circumscribed means the lesion is surrounded by
  air-filled lung. The margins may be smooth or irregular.
  Most patients are asymptomatic at the time their SPN is
  detected.
- Goals in the management of SPNs
  1. Resection of potentially curable primary lung cancers
     with minimal delay. Less than half of patients with
     bronchogenic carcinoma have resectable disease at the
     time of diagnosis.
  2. Resection of a solitary lung metastasis from an extra-
     thoracic site.
  3. Avoidance of lung resection for benign disease. For
     most benign processes, resection offers no therapeutic
     benefit to the patient.

DIFFERENTIAL DIAGNOSIS

- Although there are many causes of SPNs (Table 19–1), the
  central question in the evaluation of an SPN is whether or
  not the lesion is malignant. The frequency of malignancy
  varies from 5% in SPNs detected in radiologic surveys of
  the general population to 40 to 50% in patients referred for
  lung resection.
- The rate of malignancy varies with the definition of SPN; if
  lesions up to 6 cm are included, more lesions will be malignant.
- The standard has been to distinguish between small-cell
  and non–small-cell carcinoma prior to resection because it
  was not considered beneficial to resect small-cell tumors.
  Recent reports have shown improved survival with resection of isolated small-cell tumors combined with chemotherapy, making the distinction between small-cell and
  non–small-cell tumors prior to thoracotomy less important
  and perhaps immaterial.

TABLE 19–1. Causes of Solitary Pulmonary Nodules

I. Neoplastic
  A. Malignant
    1. Bronchogenic carcinoma (adeno carcinoma, squamous cell, small ("oat") cell, large cell)[a]
    2. Solitary metastasis (e.g., kidney, colon, breast, ovary, testis)[a]
    3. Bronchial adenoma (carcinoid, mucoepidermoid, cylindroma)
    4. Bronchoaveolar cell carcinoma
    5. Lymphoma
    6. Primary sarcoma of the lung
  B. Benign
    1. Hamartoma[a]
    2. Arteriovenous malformation[a]
    3. Chondroma
    4. Lipoma (usually pleural)
    5. Fibroma
    6. Leiomyoma
    7. Hemangioma
    8. Intrapulmonary lymph node
    9. Endometrioma
    10. Neural tumor
    11. Inflammatory pseudotumor (e.g., histiocytoma, plasma cell granuloma)
    12. Thymoma
II. Inflammatory
  A. Granuloma
    1. Tuberculosis[a]
    2. Histoplasmosis[a]
    3. Coccidioidomycosis[a]
    4. Cryptococcosis
    5. Nocardiosis
    6. Blastomycosis
    7. Gumma
    8. Sarcoidosis
    9. Q fever
    10. Atypical measles infection
  B. Abscess
  C. Hydatid cyst
  D. Bronchiectatic cyst (fluid-filled)
  E. Fungus ball
  F. Organizing pneumonia
  G. Inflammatory pseudotomor
  H. Mucoid impaction (asthma, allergic aspergillosis)
  I. Rheumatoid nodule
  J. *Dirofilaria immitis* (dog heartworm)
III. Vascular
  A. Infarct[a]
  B. Pulmonary vein varix or anomaly
  C. Wegener's granulomatosis
IV. Developmental
  A. Bronchogenic cyst (fluid-filled)
  B. Pulmonary sequestration
  C. Pericardial cyst

TABLE 19–1. Causes of Solitary Pulmonary Nodules *Continued*

V. Inhalation
    A. Silicosis (conglomerate mass)
    B. Lipoid granuloma
    C. Aspirated foreign body
VI. Other
    A. Hematoma
    B. Emphysematous bulla (fluid-filled)
    C. Extramedullary hematopoiesis
    D. Mimicking densities[a]
        1. Fluid in interlobar fissure (pseudotumor)
        2. Artifacts (buttons, snap, etc.)
        3. Nipple shadow
        4. Skin and subcutaneous lesions
        5. Pleural lesions

[a] More common causes of SPN.
Source: Modified by the author from Reed JC. Chest Radiology, Plain Film Patterns and Differential Diagnoses. Chicago, Year Book Medical Publishers, 1987.

EPIDEMIOLOGY

- Age. An SPN in a person under the age of 35 has a <1% probability of malignancy. After the age of 35 there is a steady increase in the percentage of nodules that are malignant (70 to 100% of all nodules appearing in the eighth decade of life are malignant).
- Exposures
  1. The use of cigarettes is the single most important exposure predisposing to malignancy.
  2. Exposure to asbestos raises the risk of bronchogenic carcinoma. The combination of cigarette and asbestos exposures has a multiplicative effect on cancer risk.
  3. Occupational exposure to uranium, plutonium, or nickel raises the likelihood of malignancy.
  4. Geographic exposures may suggest a fungal etiology for a nodule (coccidioidomycosis, histoplasmosis, and blastomycosis).
- Nonpulmonary malignancy. Even with a history of extrathoracic malignancy, a newly detected SPN is as likely to be a second primary as it is a single metastasis. Metastatic disease more commonly presents as multiple pulmonary nodules.

HISTORY AND PHYSICAL EXAMINATION

- Medical history. The history may be helpful but is rarely diagnostic.
  1. Bacterial pneumonia can resolve to leave a residual pulmonary pseudotumor.
  2. Trauma can leave pulmonary hematomas or scars that might appear as an SPN.

3. Rheumatoid lung disease can occasionally appear as a single nodule, as can mucoid impaction in a patient with asthma.
4. Use of oil-based nose drops or intranasal glycerine can lead to lipoid granulomatia.
5. Some patients may have been told years previously that they had an abnormality on their chest radiograph.

- Physical examination
  1. A careful breast, pelvic, genital, and rectal examination and a stool occult blood test help to exclude extrathoracic primaries.
  2. Lymphadenopathy and hepatosplenomegaly point to lymphoma or metastatic disease.
  3. Supraclavicular adenopathy or upper thoracic venous congestion (superior vena cava syndrome) suggests mediastinal involvement.
  4. Clubbing and weight loss suggest malignancy.

RADIOGRAPHIC FEATURES

- Size. The larger the lesion, the higher the likelihood of malignancy. Less than 10% of benign lesions are greater than 3 cm in size, while malignant nodules are evenly distributed in size from 1 to 6 cm.
- Calcification
  1. The most common patterns of calcification are strongly predictive of benignity; these include diffuse, laminated, "popcorn," and large central calcifications.
  2. Eccentric calcification can be seen with scar carcinomas. Rarely, malignant SPNs have small central calcifications. These patterns must be considered indeterminate.
- Nodule-lung interface. A lobulated or shaggy surface on the nodule suggests malignancy, while a smooth, sharp surface supports benignity.
- Doubling time
  1. The doubling time is the time it takes for a nodule to double in *volume*. When a nodule's diameter has increased by a factor of 1.26, the tumor has doubled in volume.
  2. The mean doubling times for primary lung carcinomas range from 1 to 15 months. Very rapid or very slow growth is more typical of benign processes.
  3. A lesion that doubles in less than a month is very likely infectious or related to lung infarction. Exceptions are metastatic lesions from rapidly growing extrapulmonary primaries such as testicular cancer, osteogenic sarcoma, chorionic carcinoma, or renal cell carcinoma.
  4. If a prior chest X-ray or CT scan is not available, the doubling time can only be determined by observing the lesion prospectively, and in many cases this is not appropriate.

RECOMMENDED DIAGNOSTIC APPROACH (Figure 19–1)

- All SPNs must be considered malignant unless benignity can be established with reasonable certainty.
- Step one
  1. Every effort should be made to obtain and review old chest films. A report of a negative chest radiograph is of little value since small pulmonary nodules are often missed.
  2. If the lesion has demonstrated no growth for at least 2 years, it is generally benign. Observation with serial chest X-rays annually for another 3 to 5 years is prudent.
  3. Other situations in which benignity can be reasonably assumed and observation recommended are:
     a. Age less than 35 years and no history of malignancy
     b. Nodule shows a benign pattern of calcification. Such patients should be reassessed with chest X-rays at 3-month intervals for the first year, at 6-month intervals for the second year, and annually for another 3 to 5 years.

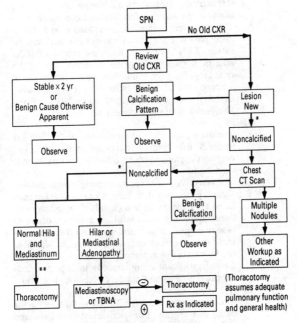

* Consider observation if patient less than 35 years old.
** Some would do TTNA or TBBX here.

Figure 19–1. Diagnostic approach to the patient with an SPN.

- Step two
  1. If benignity has not yet been established, a chest CT scan should be obtained. The CT scan is more sensitive than a chest radiograph in demonstrating calcifications, and a benign pattern will identify the lesion as nonmalignant. The CT scan may also demonstrate other pulmonary nodules not apparent on the chest radiograph.
  2. The CT scan identifies hilar or mediastinal adenopathy with a sensitivity of 80 to 90%. If adenopathy is not detected by CT, mediastinoscopy is generally not necessary at the time of surgery. If adenopathy is present, the patient very likely has unresectable carcinoma. Some patients with malignant pulmonary nodules will have nonmalignant adenopathy, thus the patient should not be denied a potentially curative resection until mediastinoscopy or transbronchial needle aspiration has confirmed malignant adenopathy. When evaluating possible lung malignancy, the chest CT should be extended to include the liver and adrenal glands to rule out metastatic disease at these sites.
- Step three
  1. Clinical practices diverge considerably at this point.
     a. If the CT scan shows normal hila and mediastinum, many would advise proceeding directly to thoracotomy for resection of the nodule, assuming adequate pulmonary function and general health.
     b. The reasoning behind this approach is as follows: if the patient undergoes transthoracic needle aspiration (TTNA) or bronchoscopic biopsy (TBBX) and the nodule is malignant, resection will be the next step. Surgery would only be averted if a convincing nonmalignant cause for the nodule were demonstrated by the biopsy procedure, and the likelihood of this is generally low.
  2. TBBX
     a. The diagnostic yield of bronchoscopy for SPNs is under 20% for lesions 2 cm or less in diameter. The diagnostic yield is 40 to 60% for lesions greater than 2 cm.
     b. The sensitivity of bronchoscopy is greater for malignant processes than benign ones. A lesion may be safely considered benign only if the biopsy was fluoroscopically successful, no evidence of tumor is seen pathologically, and material other than normal lung is seen to explain the lesion. Otherwise the biopsy is indeterminate.
     c. Complications of bronchoscopy include pneumothorax (3 to 5%) and massive bleeding (1 to 3%).
  3. TTNA
     a. The diagnostic yield for TTNA is 80 to 95% for malignant lesions, but such results are expected only with very experienced operators and pathologists.
     b. Benignity can be established in 50 to 85% of benign lesions if large enough specimens are obtained, but

an aspirate showing only normal cells generally must be interpreted as indeterminate.

c. Peripheral nodules have higher success rates than more central nodules.

d. Complications include pneumothorax (20 to 30%), one-third of which will require chest tubes and hemoptysis.

4. There are situations in which TTNA or TBBX is clearly advisable prior to or rather than thoracotomy:

    1. When there is strong evidence of nonresectability and a tissue diagnosis is needed to plan therapy.

    2. When the patient is not a candidate for surgery due to poor pulmonary function or other illness.

    3. When the patient is at high risk for surgery (e.g., advanced age or severe heart disease) and proof of malignancy is desired before recommending thoracotomy.

    4. When the patient has a peripheral nodule and a positive sputum cytology (uncommon with peripheral nodules) bronchoscopy is employed to rule out a coexisting central or upper airway lesion.

- Probability of malignancy

1. Bayes' theorem and decision analysis provide guidelines by which nodule size, patient age, and smoking history may be used to estimate the probability that a nodule is malignant (see Cummings et al., 1986a).

2. In using decision analysis to compare immediate thoracotomy to TTNA/TBBX to a period of observation, there was surprisingly little difference in the outcomes. There are several reasonable approaches to the diagnosis of SPNs, and patient preference should play a significant role in managing SPNs.

Bibliography

Baker RR, et al. The role of surgery in the management of selected patients with small cell carcinoma of the lung. J Clin Oncol 1987;5:697–702.

Cummings SR, et al. Estimating the probability of malignancy in solitary pulmonary nodules. Am Rev Resp Dis 1986a;134:449–452.

Cummings SR, et al. Managing solitary pulmonary nodules. Am Rev Resp Dis 1986b;134:453–460.

Inouye SK, Sox HC. Standard and computed tomography in the evaluation of neoplasms of the chest. Ann Int Med 1986;105:906–924.

Swensen SJ, et al. An integrated approach to evaluation of the solitary pulmonary nodule. Mayo Clin Proc 1990;65:173–186.

20

MEDIASTINAL MASSES

TERRY J. MENGERT

> Those diseases that medicine do not cure are cured by the knife. Those that the knife does not cure are cured by fire. Those that fire does not cure must be considered incurable.
>
> HIPPOCRATES

DEFINITION

- Anatomy. The mediastinum is the median region of the thorax separating the two pleural sacs. Its superior border is the thoracic outlet (the area defined by the first ribs and the first thoracic vertebra). Its inferior border is the diaphragm. Its lateral borders are the mediastinal parietal pleura. Anteriorly and posteriorly its borders are the sternum with its costal cartilages and the 12 thoracic vertebrae, respectively.
- Subdivisions (Table 20–1).
  1. Nearly 50% of mediastinal masses are not symptomatic and discovered fortuitously; of these, 10% are malignant.
  2. Of the 50% of mediastinal masses that are symptomatic, one-half are malignant.
  3. Because of the high risk of malignancy it is never appropriate to just "observe" a mass over time. A diagnosis must be sought.

DIFFERENTIAL DIAGNOSIS (Table 20–2)

Mediastinal masses may originate inside or outside of the mediastinum.

SIGNS AND SYMPTOMS (Table 20–3)

Nearly 50% of mediastinal masses are found incidentally on a chest radiograph and are without symptoms.

CLINICAL EVALUATION

- Chest X-ray. Evaluation of the mediastinum should begin with a posteroanterior and lateral X-ray.
- History. Direct questioning to elicit symptoms known to be associated with mediastinal masses (see Table 20–3) should be done.

TABLE 20–1. Subdivisions and Contents of the Mediastinum

Superior Mediastinum (area superior to the horizontal line that passes from the sternal angle to the lower border of the fourth thoracic vertebra)
  Thymus gland
  Transverse aorta and great vessels
  Part of the trachea and esophagus
  Nerves (vagi and phrenics most prominent)
  Lymph nodes
Anterior Mediastinum (area between the sternum and fibrous pericardium)
  Thymus gland
  Ascending aorta
  Vena cava and azygos vein
  Lymph nodes
  Fat and connective tissues
Middle Mediastinum (area between the anterior mediastinum and the anterior margin of the thoracic spine)
  Heart and pericardium
  Pulmonary vessels
  Trachea and major bronchi
  Vagus and phrenic nerves
  Lymph nodes
  Fat and connective tissues
Posterior Mediastinum (area posterior to the fibrous pericardium and anterior to the posterior rib cage and the spinal column)
  Descending aorta
  Posterior intercostal arteries
  Azygos and hemiazygos veins
  Esophagus
  Thoracic duct
  Sympathetic chain
  Lymph nodes

- Physical exam
  1. Head: look for Horner's syndrome, oral cancer, or infection (e.g., candidiasis).
  2. Neck: evaluate for nodes, venous distention, and palpable thyroid abnormalities.
  3. Chest: evaluate for supraclavicular nodes or masses, wheezing, rhonchi, and cardiac murmurs and rubs.
  4. Breasts: evaluate for gynecomastia, masses, tenderness, and discharge. Palpate both axilla for nodes or masses.
  5. Abdomen/Genital: palpate for masses and organomegaly. Check stool for occult blood.
  6. Neurologic: evaluate closely for evidence of myasthenia gravis (fatigability of muscle action and power on repeated testing, with ocular muscles frequently involved).

TABLE 20–2. Mediastinal Masses

Superior Mediastinum
    Thymic tumors or cysts
    Thyroid masses
    Parathyroid tumors
    Aneurysm or ectasia of aorta or other great vessels
    Lymphomas
    Lymphadenopathy (inflammatory or malignant)
    Lung cancer
    Tumors and other abnormalities of the trachea and
       esophagus
Anterior Mediastinum
    Thymic tumors or cysts
    Teratoma
    Thyroid masses
    Parathyroid tumors
    Lymphomas
    Lymphadenopathy
    Lung cancers
    Malignant germ cell neoplasms (e.g., seminoma)
    Mesenchymal neoplasms (e.g., lipoma)
Middle Mediastinum
    Lymphoma
    Lymphadenopathy (including that caused by sarcoidosis)
    Lung cancers
    Tumors and other abnormalities of the trachea
    Cysts (bronchogenic and pleuropericardial)
    Lipomas
    Vascular tumors
    Plasmacytoma
    Epicardial fat pads
    Hiatal hernia (through Morgagni's foramen)
    Granulomatous mediastinitis
Posterior Mediastinum
    Neurogenic tumors (e.g., neurofibroma, schwannoma,
       pheochromocytoma)
    Lymphoma
    Cysts (including thoracic duct, enteric, and bronchogenic)
    Esophageal tumors and other abnormalities
    Hiatal hernia (through foramen of Bochdalek)
    Aneurysm of descending thoracic aorta
    Lung cancer
    Thyroid masses
    Lymphadenopathy
    Diseases of the thoracic spine

- Blood tests
  1. A complete blood count and electrolyte panel are appropriate general studies.
  2. Additional studies should be obtained only as indicated by a patient's signs and symptoms, e.g., thyroid func-

TABLE 20–3. Signs and Symptoms of Mediastinal Masses

Chest: pain, fullness, tightness
Nonspecific: fevers, weight loss, malaise, anorexia
Compression/Displacement of Mediastinal Structures
    Tracheobronchial: cough, dyspnea, stridor, wheezing, recurrent respiratory infections
    Esophageal: odynophagia, dysphagia, reflux symptoms
    Vascular: superior vena cava syndrome
    Sympathetic ganglion: Horner's syndrome
    Recurrent laryngeal nerve: hoarseness, dysphonia
    Cardiac: tamponade, dysrhythmias
    Pulmonic stenosis: murmurs
Endocrine Abnormalities
    Cushing's disease
    Hypertension
    Hypoglycemia
    Gynecomastia
    Hypo- or hyperthyroidism
    Multiple endocrine abnormalities (Type I: includes parathyroid hyperplasia and adenoma, insulinoma, gastrinoma, and pituitary neoplasia)
Other Syndromes (not described above)
    Myasthenia gravis (thymoma)
    Red cell aplasia (thymoma)
    Autoimmune diseases (thymoma)
    Hypogammaglobulinemia (thymoma)
    Alcohol-induced lymph node pain (lymphoma)
    Neurofibroma-related osteoarthritis

Source: Adapted from Rosenberg JC. In: Devita VT, et al., eds. Cancer: Principles and Practices of Oncology, Vol. 1, 3rd ed. Philadelphia, J.B. Lippincott, 1989, p. 707.

tion; serum calcium, phosphorus, and magnesium in a patient with generalized weakness and suspicion of parathyroid dysfunction; serum alphafetoprotein and the beta subunit of human chorionic gonadotropin in the patient with suspected germ cell neoplasm.

FURTHER DIAGNOSTIC TESTS

- Thoracic computed tomography (CT)
    1. In most cases, the study to obtain after a chest X-ray will be a chest CT with contrast material (contrast is utilized to define vascular structures).
    2. The CT scan is able to accurately distinguish fatty, vascular, calcified, noncalcified, and cystic soft tissue masses. It cannot differentiate benign and malignant solid, nonfatty masses.
- Magnetic resonance imaging (MRI). MRI is an excellent technique for visualizing the mediastinum in detail. It is the modality of choice in the patient with a history of contrast

reactions. Its accuracy in visualizing mediastinal structures, however, is not better than CT.

- Angiography. In the setting of acute trauma, intraarterial digital or conventional angiography are the preferred techniques to assess mediastinal or pleural bleeding and the aorta and its branches.
- Percutaneous transthoracic needle biopsy
  1. Major indications include:
     a. Determine the etiology of a soft tissue mediastinal mass.
     b. Determine the diagnosis of a hilar mass in patients with negative bronchoscopy or no other evidence of an endobronchial lesion.
     c. Determine that a lung cancer is unresectable by demonstrating its spread to the mediastinum.
  2. Percutaneous transthoracic needle biopsy has a diagnostic accuracy of 80 to 95% for malignant lesions (but if a lymphoma is present, it will be adequately classified in only 50% of cases). The diagnostic accuracy for benign lesions is 70 to 80%.
- Mediastinoscopy. Utilizing a suprasternal notch incision and a tissue plane dissection, the mediastinoscope is passed anterior to the trachea and posterior to the aortic arch and great vessels down to the carina. Tissue from abnormal masses or nodes in the paratracheal, parabronchial (above the main stem), superior posterior mediastinum, and to a limited extent, the subcarinal and hilar regions may be obtained.
- Anterior mediastinotomy. Under general anesthesia, the aortopulmonary window area is accessed for tissue biopsy using an incision in the left second intercostal space just lateral to the sternum.
- Thoracotomy. In many circumstances a mediastinal mass will require surgery and a diagnostic thoracotomy.
- Other studies
  1. Iodine-131 thyroid scan may be indicated if clinical evidence indicates that the mediastinal mass may be a goiter (up to 10% of mediastinal masses).
  2. Esophagram is occasionally used to identify a hiatal hernia presenting as a mediastinal mass.
  3. Endoscopy
     a. Esophagoscopy may be utilized in the patient with esophageal symptoms.
     b. Bronchoscopy may be indicated in the setting of a mediastinal mass accompanied by atelectasis or when a bronchogenic carcinoma is likely (e.g., hemoptysis).

RECOMMENDED DIAGNOSTIC APPROACH

- Chest X-ray (posteroanterior and lateral views)
- History and physical examination. Specific tests will frequently be indicated by the clinical circumstances:
  1. Trauma patient with widened mediastinum—proceed with aortography.

2. Nontrauma patient with chest pain and widened mediastinum—proceed with chest CT and/or aortography.
3. Symptoms of hyper- or hypothyroidism and abnormally enlarged thyroid gland on physical examination—proceed with thyroid function tests and consider iodine-131 scan.
4. Middle mediastinal mass suspicious for a hiatal hernia on chest radiograph—proceed with esophagram.
5. Odynophagia and/or dysphagia—consider esophagram and esophagoscopy with biopsy as appropriate.
6. Hemoptysis—consider bronchoscopy and chest CT.
7. Myasthenia gravis, pure red cell aplasia, or hypogammaglobulinemia—proceed with chest CT in search of a thymoma.
8. Clinical presentation of sarcoidosis—proceed with biopsy of appropriate tissue (e.g., skin lesions, accessible abnormal lymph nodes, or transbronchial lung biopsy).

- Chest CT. In many cases the mediastinal mass is completely asymptomatic, or information from the history and physical exam does not give diagnostic guidance. In that setting, a contrast enhanced chest CT is the procedure of choice (consider MRI in the patient with a history of contrast reactions).

  1. If CT demonstrates mass is vascular or fatty tissue, biopsy is not indicated.
  2. If CT demonstrates mass is solid or cystic—tissue biopsy is required.

- Biopsy

  1. The choice of which procedure to use (e.g., percutaneous transthoracic needle biopsy, mediastinoscopy, anterior mediastinotomy, or thoracotomy) should be made in consultation with an interventional radiologist and surgeon.
  2. Thoroughly examine the patient in search of a readily accessible abnormal lymph node (e.g., supraclavicular node) or mass before a more invasive procedure is considered.

Bibliography

Casamassima F, et al. Magnetic resonance imaging and high-resolution computed tomography in tumors of the lung and mediastinum. Radiotherapy and Oncology 1988;11:21–29.

Mueller PR, vanSonnenberg E. Medical progress: Interventional radiology in the chest and abdomen. N Engl J Med 1990;322(19):1364–1374.

Nath PH, et al. Percutaneous fine needle aspiration in the diagnosis and management of mediastinal cysts in adults. S Med J 1988; 81(10):1225–1228.

Newell, JD. Evaluation of pulmonary and mediastinal masses. Med Clinics North Am 1984;68:1463–1480.

Platt JF, et al. Radiologic evaluation of the subcarinal lymph nodes: A comparative study. AJR 1988;151:279–282.

Thermann M, et al. Efficacy and benefit of mediastinal computed tomography as a selection method for mediastinoscopy. Ann Thorac Surg 1989;48:565–567.

21

ASTHMA

TIM OBERMILLER

Get your room full of good air, then shut up the windows and keep it. It will keep for years.

SIDNEY JOHNSON (1920–1987)

DEFINITION AND GENERAL COMMENTS

The American Thoracic Society defines asthma as a "disease characterized by an increased responsiveness of the trachea and bronchi to various stimuli, manifest by airway narrowing." Asthma is an episodic illness. Although airflow obstruction from asthma is usually reversible, occasionally in severe and prolonged asthma, airflow obstruction may become chronic. Asthma affects 4% of the U.S. population. Half of the cases occur in children; 75% occur before age 40. There is a group of late-onset asthmatics who have more severe disease.

PATHOPHYSIOLOGY

- All asthmatics have a nonspecific hyperresponsiveness of the tracheobronchial tree.
- Asthmatics develop reversible airflow obstruction in response to environmental stimuli, resulting in increased airway resistance, decreased expiratory flow rates, lung hyperinflation from air-trapping, increased work of breathing, and a ventilation-perfusion mismatch that causes hypoxia.
- Airflow obstruction has several different causes:
  1. Bronchospasm
     a. The key pathophysiologic finding in asthma is a reduction in airway caliber as the result of bronchial smooth muscle contraction.
     b. Respiratory smooth muscle tone is modulated by cholinergic fibers from the vagus nerve, which, when stimulated, cause cough and bronchoconstriction.
     c. Bronchospasm also results directly from chemical mediators such as histamine, arachidonic acid metabolites, and platelet activating factor (PAF).
  2. Mucus plugging. Mucus production is increased due to an increased number of goblet cells and hypertrophy of mucus glands.
  3. Inflammation
     a. Pulmonary mast cells are activated when specific antigens bind to IgE on their surface membranes.

b. The released chemical mediators cause bronchoconstriction and increased vascular permeability, which causes mucosal edema.

c. In many asthmatics, there is an influx of inflammatory cells responding to chemotactic factors. These cells release cytokines, which promote inflammation.

ASTHMA CLASSIFICATION

Although the traditional distinction between intrinsic and extrinsic asthma may not be valid (both groups can have elevated IgE and eosinophil levels), it remains clinically useful.

- Extrinsic (allergic) asthma. The majority of cases occur in the pediatric and young adult populations. Allergic asthma can be due to seasonal allergens or ubiquitous inhaled allergens such as dust, feathers, danders, and mold. It is associated with:
  1. A personal or family history of atopy with rhinitis, eczema, or urticaria.
  2. Positive immediate hypersensitivity reactions with a wheal and flare to intradermal injections of airborne antigens.
  3. Elevated serum IgE and eosinophil levels.
  4. A positive bronchial response to specific inhaled provocation tests.
- Intrinsic (idiopathic) asthma. These patients lack an allergic history and may develop asthma after an upper respiratory infection. Onset may be late in life, and management is often more difficult.

DIFFERENTIAL DIAGNOSIS

- Upper airway obstruction. Laryngeal edema may appear with stridor and harsh breath sounds.
- Localized wheezing suggests endobronchial pathology such as foreign body aspiration, neoplasm, or bronchial stenosis.
- Left ventricular failure ("cardiac asthma").
- Recurrent wheezing (episodic) can also be seen with carcinoid tumors, recurrent pulmonary embolism, and chronic bronchitis. Eosinophilic pneumonia and polyarteritis also occasionally involve asthmalike symptoms.

STIMULI THAT PRECIPITATE BRONCHOSPASM

- Airborne allergens. Airborne allergens are common culprits. The patient must be exposed to the allergens long enough to induce a state of sensitivity. Once that occurs, exposure to even very small amounts of allergens can cause bronchospasm.

- Medications
  1. Aspirin or nonsteroidal anti-inflammatory agents. This sensitivity often occurs in combination with nasal polyposis and sinusitis.
  2. Beta-blocking agents, including ophthalmic solutions, and food and drug additives (e.g., metabisulfites, tartrazine dyes).
- Environmental pollutants. Attacks may be related to inhalation of sulfur dioxide or other gases or particulate matter.
- Occupational asthma. Occupational asthma may be IgE mediated, related to direct release of bronchoconstrictors, or due to general airway irritation.
- Respiratory infections
  1. An upper respiratory infection is the most common event that exacerbates both intrinsic and extrinsic asthma.
  2. Sinusitis may initiate and perpetuate asthma.
  3. Allergic bronchopulmonary aspergillosis should be considered in patients with recurrent asthma, pulmonary infiltrates, and eosinophilia.
- Exercise. Activities in cold, dry air such as skiing are more provocative than swimming.
- Gastroesophageal reflux (GER). Bronchospasm may result from aspiration or through reflex mechanisms.
- Emotional stress. Psychologic factors may increase bronchospasm in certain individuals.

CLINICAL FEATURES

- History
  1. Patients classically complain of a triad of dyspnea, cough, and wheezing, which alternate with symptom-free periods. Cough or dyspnea may occur alone.
  2. At initial evaluation, the precipitating factors should be carefully elicited, with a particular search for an allergic component.
- Physical Examination
  1. During symptom-free periods, patients may be normal or have wheezing only during forced expiratory maneuvers.
  2. During acute attacks patients develop a sense of constriction in the chest and soon exhibit tachypnea and cough.
  3. Inspiratory and expiratory wheezing may be audible without a stethoscope.
  4. As obstruction worsens, patients use the accessory muscles of breathing and develop pulsus paradoxus from the large swings in pleural pressure.
  5. In critical situations, wheezing may lessen or disappear as a result of the marked decrease in airflow. These findings herald impending respiratory failure and the possible need for intubation and mechanical ventilation.

- Objective clinical measures of asthma severity
  1. Grading scale (Table 21–1). A score of 4 suggests severe asthma and may suggest the intensity of treatment required.
  2. Pulmonary function measures
     a. The forced expiratory volume in one second (FEV_1) or peak expiratory flow rate (PEFR) should be obtained in all patients with acute asthma to assess severity, guide therapy, and aid in disposition decisions.
     b. FEV_1 and PEFR correlate highly, and either is better than a combination of heart rate, respiratory, and pulsus paradoxus at predicting poor response to therapy.
     c. PEFR less than 16% of predicted (or less than 60 L/min) or FEV_1 less than 0.6 L should be considered severe asthma.

LABORATORY FINDINGS

- Blood studies. Blood and sputum eosinophilia occur often but are not universal or specific for asthma.
- Arterial blood gases (ABGs)
  1. During an acute exacerbation, the usual findings are hypoxia with a widened alveolar-arterial oxygen difference and a respiratory alkalosis.
  2. ABGs have little use in evaluating the severity of asthma. They provide little clinical information until the PEFR is less than 25% of predicted value. Oxygenation can be assessed inexpensively and noninvasively with pulse oximetry.
  3. In impending respiratory failure, ABGs must be ob-

TABLE 21–1. Asthma Severity Scoring System

FACTOR	VALUE FOR SCORE OF 0	VALUE FOR SCORE OF 1
Pulse rate (beats/min)	<120	>120
Respiratory rate (breaths/min)	<30	>30
Pulsus paradoxus (mmHg)	<18	>18
Peak expiratory flow rate (PEFR, L/min)	>120	<120
Dyspnea	Absent-mild	Moderate-severe
Accessory muscle use	Absent-mild	Moderate-severe
Wheezing	Absent-mild	Moderate-severe

Source: Adapted from Fischl MA, et al. An index predicting relapse and need for hospitalization in patients with acute bronchial asthma. N Eng J Med 1981; 305: 783–789.

tained to assess for respiratory acidosis and the need for mechanical ventilation. Since respiratory alkalosis is the usual derangement in asthma, a $PaCO_2$ that is increasing toward normal may indicate impending respiratory failure and the need for frequent monitoring of ABGs.

4. Metabolic acidosis is another ominous sign of impending respiratory failure resulting from lactic acidosis due to fatiguing respiratory muscles.

- Skin testing.   Patients with asthma may exhibit positive wheal and flare reactions to skin tests, but these results may not correlate with pulmonary symptoms.

- Chest X-ray

  1. X-rays are usually normal during symptom-free periods and show hyperinflation during an exacerbation.

  2. · They are not indicated unless asthma is severe and other diseases are suspected such as pneumothorax, cardiac asthma, or airway obstruction from a foreign body. Pneumonia is a rare finding in asthma.

- Pulmonary function tests. Bedside spirometry is the best method to evaluate the severity of an asthma attack and to monitor the patient's progress.

- Bronchial provocation tests

  1. These tests are useful to detect airway hyperresponsiveness. An aerosolized antigen or a bronchoconstricting agent is administered, followed by spirometry. A dose-response curve may be generated: patients with a greater response get bronchoconstriction with a lower dose.

  2. Inhalation of antigen extracts or industrial dusts may indicate specific reagin-mediated bronchospasm.

  3. A positive response to histamine or methacholine indicates nonspecific hyperresponsiveness. The histamine or methacholine tests are useful to evaluate patients with an equivocal history of asthma or those who have a chronic episodic cough but normal pulmonary function test results.

Bibliography

Boushey HA, et al. Bronchial hyperreactivity. Am Rev Resp Dis 1980;121:389.

Fischl MA, et al. An index predicting relapse and need for hospitalization in patients with acute bronchial asthma. N Engl J Med 1981;305:783–789.

Kelsen SG, et al. Emergency room assessment and treatment of patients with acute asthma. Am J Med 1978;64:622–628.

Nowak RM, et al. Arterial blood gases and pulmonary function testing in acute bronchial asthma: Predicting patient outcomes. JAMA 1983;249:2043–2046.

Shim CS, Williams MH, Jr. Evaluation of the severity of asthma: Patients versus physicians. Am J Med 1980;68:11–13.

22

CHRONIC OBSTRUCTIVE PULMONARY DISEASE

THOMAS R. MARTIN

When man grows old. . . . There is much gas within his thorax, resulting in panting and troubled breathing.

HUANG TI (The Yellow Emperor) (2697–2597 B.C.)

DEFINITION AND GENERAL COMMENTS

- The term "chronic obstructive pulmonary disease" (COPD) refers to a group of disorders characterized by chronic obstruction to expiratory airflow.
- Expiratory obstruction may occur because of intraluminal secretions, thickening of airway walls, or collapse of airway walls from loss of surrounding supporting structures.
- Most patients with COPD have some combination of chronic bronchitis and emphysema. Chronic asthma, cystic fibrosis, and chronic interstitial diseases can all be associated with chronic airflow obstruction.
- Chronic bronchitis
  1. Chronic bronchitis is defined clinically. The definition requires a productive cough that occurs on most days, for at least 3 months of the year, for 2 consecutive years.
  2. Chronic bronchitis is caused by chronic exposure to inhaled irritative agents, the most common of which is cigarette smoke. It is associated with mucus hypersecretion in the airways, but the gas exchange parenchyma of the lung is not disturbed.
  3. Most patients have subtle airflow obstruction, but a minority progress to disabling airflow obstruction.
- Emphysema. Emphysema is defined pathologically.
  1. Progressive destruction of terminal bronchioles and alveolar walls occurs, which destroys the gas exchange parenchyma. Airway obstruction occurs because of loss of the normal support structures that tether larger airways open during exhalation.
  2. Patients with pure emphysema complain of progressive dyspnea. In contrast to chronic bronchitis, cough is not a prominent symptom.
  3. Emphysema is thought to result from a disturbance in the balance between proteases and antiproteases in the

189

lung parenchyma. Patients with alpha$_1$-antitrypsin deficiency develop severe emphysema in the lung bases where blood flow is greatest.

- Epidemiology. COPD is common in smokers and rare in nonsmokers. Up to 27% of men and 13% of women in the general population have symptoms and/or spirometric abnormalities that suggest COPD.

PATHOPHYSIOLOGY

- Airflow obstruction
  1. Chronic airflow obstruction is caused by:
     a. Accumulation of excess secretions in the airway lumen.
     b. Thickening of the airway walls by glandular and muscular hyperplasia.
     c. Loss of the elastic recoil pressure of the lung parenchyma.
  2. Excess airway secretions and bronchial wall thickening are characteristic of chronic bronchitis. Loss of lung elastic recoil is the dominant feature of emphysema.
- Gas exchange
  1. Hypoxemia
     a. Hypoxemia in COPD occurs because airflow obstruction causes abnormalities in ventilation-perfusion (V_A/Q) relationships.
     b. In chronic bronchitis, airway obstruction causes maldistribution of inspired gas, but perfusion of the lung parenchyma is relatively unaffected.
     c. In emphysema, destruction of respiratory bronchioles and alveolar walls causes destruction of alveolar capillaries and enlargement of air spaces. Thus, V_A/Q mismatch may be relatively small until late in the course of the disease. Hypoxemia occurs late in emphysema and indicates severe loss of lung parenchyma.
  2. Hypercapnia
     a. Hypercapnia in COPD is caused by severe V_A/Q mismatch and/or abnormalities in ventilatory drive.
     b. COPD patients with acute respiratory failure and progressive hypercapnia usually have maximal neural output from their respiratory center. The hypercapnia is the result of dysfunction of the respiratory bellows. Fatigue of the ventilatory muscles is an important factor causing respiratory failure.
     c. Some patients with COPD have blunted ventilatory drives allowing hypercapnia.

CLINICAL FEATURES

- Chronic bronchitis
  1. Patients with chronic bronchitis complain of chronic

cough and phlegm production. Expiratory wheezing results from airway obstruction. Patients with significant chronic bronchitis become hypoxemic early in the course of the disease because of V_A/Q mismatching.

2. Chronic hypoxemia may cause erythrocytosis, pulmonary hypertension, and cor pulmonale.
   a. Clinical findings include plethora, cyanosis, dependent edema, elevation of venous pressure, right ventricular heave, accentuated pulmonic component of S_2, S_3 gallop, and hepatic congestion.
   b. Clubbing does not occur with chronic bronchitis. Its presence suggests an additional disorder.

- Emphysema
  1. Patients with pure emphysema complain of exertional dyspnea. Chronic cough and sputum production are rare if the patient does not smoke.
  2. The patients have signs of hyperinflation of the lungs, including flattened diaphragms, and increased resonance to thoracic percussion.
  3. The heart is usually small and in a midline position, with a subxiphoid point of maximal impulse. Clubbing does not occur in patients with pure emphysema.

LABORATORY FEATURES

- Chest X-ray
  1. The chest X-ray shows signs of hyperinflation of the lungs. These include flattened diaphragms and an increase in the retrosternal airspace.
  2. The cardiac silhouette may be small and midline in emphysema, but it is usually normal in patients with chronic bronchitis.
  3. When cor pulmonale occurs, the cardiac silhouette is enlarged and the pulmonary artery size increased.
- Pulmonary function tests (PFTs)
  1. PFTs show evidence of airflow obstruction and air trapping.
  2. The forced expiratory volume in one second (FEV_1) is less than 80% of predicted. The ratio of the FEV_1 to the forced vital capacity (FVC) is below 70%.
  3. Total lung capacity (TLC) and functional residual capacity (FRC) are increased because of gas trapped in the lungs.
  4. The vital capacity is usually reduced because of gas trapping.
  5. Patients in whom the FEV_1 increases more than 15% following an inhaled bronchodilator have partially reversible airflow obstruction.

CLINICAL COURSE

- Complications
  1. Respiratory failure. Respiratory failure in COPD oc-

curs when V_A/Q worsen in the lung (usually due to muscle fatigue from increased work of breathing), when the bellows function of the thorax fails, or when the central ventilatory drive is suppressed.

2. Cor pulmonale. In COPD patients, cor pulmonale occurs as a consequence of sustained pulmonary hypertension. The pulmonary hypertension is caused by the destruction of large portions of the pulmonary vascular bed, as in emphysema, or by pulmonary vasospasm caused by chronic hypoxemia.

3. Lung cancer. The incidence of lung cancer is high in patients with COPD because smoking is a common risk factor.

- Prognosis

1. The single best prognostic indicator is the postbronchodilator FEV_1. Patients whose FEV_1 improve significantly with bronchodilators have a better prognosis than patients who lack a bronchodilator response.

2. A single exacerbation of COPD does not have major effect on long-term survival. However, an episode of severe respiratory failure markedly worsens prognosis with an up to 50% 1-year mortality after an episode in which mechanical ventilation is required.

RECOMMENDED DIAGNOSTIC APPROACH

- Suspicion of the presence of COPD and the predominant type comes from the history and physical examination.
- Laboratory testing with PFTs makes the diagnosis by documenting the presence of airflow obstruction.
- Arterial PO_2 should be measured for therapeutic (rather than diagnostic) reasons.

Bibliography

Burrows B. Differential diagnosis of chronic obstructive pulmonary disease. Chest 1990;97(2 suppl):16S–18S.

Burrows B. Airways obstructive diseases: Pathogenetic mechanisms and natural history of the disorder. Med Clin North Am 1990;74: 547–559.

Flenley DC. Chronic obstructive pulmonary disease. Dis Mon 1988;34:537–599.

Martin TR, et al. The prognosis of patients with chronic obstructive pulmonary disease after hospitalization for acute respiratory failure. Chest 1982;82:310–314.

Nocturnal Oxygen Therapy Trial Group. Continuous or nocturnal oxygen therapy in hypoxemic chronic obstructive pulmonary disease. Ann Intern Med 1980;93:391–398.

23

PULMONARY EMBOLISM

JOSEPH J. CROWLEY

Definition of cough: A convulsion of the lungs velli-
cated by some sharp serosity.

SAMUEL JOHNSON (1755)

DEFINITION

1. Pulmonary embolism (PE) is the obstruction of a portion
   of the pulmonary arterial system, usually by a thrombus
   that has been dislodged from a site in the deep venous
   system.
2. Deep venous thrombosis (DVT) located in the popliteal,
   femoral, or iliac veins causes 90% of PE.

EPIDEMIOLOGY

1. The annual incidence of PE in the United States is 600,000
   cases, of which 10% are fatal.
2. Over 75% of PE fatalities occur within a few hours, and
   these deaths can only be prevented by avoiding DVT.

GENERAL COMMENTS

1. Three factors (Virchow's triad) contribute to thrombo-
   genesis: stasis, vessel intimal abnormalities, and alterations in coagulation. Certain conditions are associated
   with a higher risk of thromboembolism (Table 23–1). In
   the appropriate clinical setting, these conditions mandate
   measures to prevent DVT and raise the level of suspicion
   of PE.
2. Embolic obstruction produces an area of lung that is ven-
   tilated but not perfused. This "dead space" cannot partic-
   ipate in effective gas exchange.
3. The primary hemodynamic consequence of PE is a decrease in the cross-sectional area available for pulmonary
   arterial blood flow. Vascular obstruction must be greater
   than 50% to cause increased pulmonary arterial pressure
   and vascular resistance. Once this does occur, acute right
   heart failure or chronic pulmonary hypertension and right
   ventricular hypertrophy may develop.
4. The underlying cardiopulmonary status of the patient
   helps determine the clinical severity of an embolic event.

TABLE 23-1.   Risk Factors for Venous Thromboembolism

Stasis	Immobilization, obesity, chronic deep venous insufficiency, congestive heart failure, chronic pulmonary disease, occupation with prolonged venous stasis
Estrogens	Oral contraceptives
Malignancy	Adenocarcinoma of the lung and gastrointestinal tract
Trauma	Surgery (postoperative period), burns, pelvic or lower extremity fractures, postpartum period
Hypercoagulability	Deficiency of antithrombin III, protein S, and protein C, homocystinuria, lupus anticoagulant, plasminogen abnormalities, polycythemia
Other	Age >70 years, splenectomy

5. Pulmonary infarction rarely accompanies PE and usually occurs several hours after the event. In most cases of infarction, there is preexisting compromise of the bronchial arterial flow or airway flow to the area of embolism (e.g., left ventricular failure, mitral stenosis, and chronic obstructive pulmonary disease). Twenty percent of PE occurring in these individuals result in infarction.

HISTORY (Table 23-2)

1. The most common symptom of PE is sudden onset of dyspnea related to the increased alveolar dead space.
2. Pleuritic chest pain is less common than was once believed and is associated with atelectasis or infarction. The chest pain may be a dull, substernal discomfort related to increases in pulmonary arterial pressure or to right ventricular ischemia.

TABLE 23-2.   Symptoms in Patients with Pulmonary Emboli

COMMON (>50%)	OCCASIONAL (20–50%)	UNCOMMON (<20%)
Asymptomatic	Leg pain	Syncope
Dyspnea	Chest pain	Angina
Apprehension	Cough	Hemoptysis
	Palpitations	
	Sweats	

PHYSICAL EXAMINATION (Table 23–3)

1. Findings on physical examination are often minimal and nonspecific. A focal area of decreased breath sounds, rales, wheezing, or pleural friction rub may occur.
2. With extensive embolism, there may be cardiac findings of acute cor pulmonale.
3. DVT is an excellent indicator of concurrent PE, but objective evidence of DVT is present in only 70% of patients with PE.

LABORATORY STUDIES

1. Routine studies of blood chemistry and cell counts contribute little to the diagnosis of PE.
2. Arterial blood gases often indicate hypoxemia, hypocapnia, and respiratory alkalosis. Patients may hyperventilate to raise the arterial PO_2 (PaO_2), but there is a widening of the alveolar to arterial oxygen difference.
3. ECGs
   a. The usefulness of the ECG lies in ruling out myocardial infarction or pericarditis. More than half of the ECG changes disappear within 5 to 14 days.
   b. The majority of patients with PE simply have a sinus tachycardia. Few have atrial fibrillation or flutter.
   c. Classic, but less common, findings occur with right ventricular overload and may include S_1Q_3 pattern or right ventricular hypertrophy.
4. Chest X-ray
   a. The most common finding is a normal X-ray. Loss of surfactant or infarction may lead to:
      i. A pleural-based parenchymal infiltrate.
      ii. Evidence of pleural reaction or effusion.
      iii. Volume loss with elevation of the hemidiaphragm.
   b. Other findings include:
      i. Disparity in the size of comparable vessels.
      ii. Oligemia of a lung zone with hyperlucency

TABLE 23–3. Physical Signs in Patients with Pulmonary Emboli

COMMON (>50%)	OCCASIONAL (20–50%)	UNCOMMON (<20%)
No signs	Fever (<38°C)	Wheezing
Tachypnea (resp. rate >16/min)	Rales	Decreased breath sounds
Tachycardia (pulse >100/ min)	Phlebitis	Cyanosis
	Diaphoresis	Murmur
		S_3 gallop
		Loud P_2
		Jugular venous distention

(Westermark's sign) suggesting obstruction with increased flow to other areas.

c. Chest X-ray is helpful to exclude pneumothorax and congestive heart failure.

RECOMMENDED DIAGNOSTIC APPROACH

1. Although the clinical picture may be compelling for the diagnosis of PE, the history, physical examination, ECG, and chest X-ray are nonspecific. The diagnosis can only be made with a ventilation-perfusion (V_A/Q) scan and/or pulmonary angiography.

2. Since PE is usually a complication of DVT, demonstration of lower extremity thrombosis both corroborates the diagnosis and provides a clinical indication for anticoagulation.

3. The diagnostic approach is based on the clinical situation and the risks of the contemplated therapy. In a patient with a relative contraindication to anticoagulation, definitive diagnosis by pulmonary angiography may be needed.

4. Diagnosis of DVT (see Chapter 24)

   a. Contrast venography is the "gold standard" against which other techniques are measured.

   b. Radiofibrinogen leg scanning is very effective in demonstrating thrombi up to midthigh. It is ineffective if heparin therapy has been initiated. The combination of a normal radiofibrinogen and impedance plethysmography studies rules out a leg thrombus.

   c. Impedance plethysmography identifies most acute venous thrombi in the popliteal, femoral, or iliac (but not calf vein) systems. Normal impedance plethysmography examinations on days 1, 2, and 7 provide confidence that thigh thrombus is not present and that undetected calf thrombi are not progressing.

   d. Doppler/ultrasound (duplex) is increasingly utilized to detect above-knee thrombi. It has been well validated only in outpatient clinical settings.

5. The V_A/Q scan (Table 23–4)

   a. Some clinicians will not pursue the diagnosis of PE once a DVT has been demonstrated since the treatment of these conditions are similar.

TABLE 23–4. Interpretation of V_A/Q Scans

V_A/Q Scan Result	Chance of PE (%)
Normal perfusion scan	0
Segmental perfusion defect(s) with matched ventilation defects(s)	25
Subsegmental or smaller perfusion defect(s) with or without matched ventilation defect(s)	Indeterminate
Segmental or greater perfusion defect(s) with normal ventilation	90

b. Any parenchymal disease such as pneumonia, chronic obstructive pulmonary disease, or atelectasis with reduced ventilation may cause decreased blood flow. A ventilation scan assesses ventilation in the area of abnormal blood flow.

c. A normal 6-view perfusion scan excludes a PE.

6. Pulmonary angiography

a. This is the only means of obtaining anatomic information about the pulmonary vasculature.

b. It is usually well tolerated, particularly if selective injection of pulmonary arteries is done.

c. Artifacts may occur requiring repeated injections, and the ability to evaluate small vessels is limited. The examiner must also be familiar with the possible angiographic findings of abrupt cutoff of a vessel with or without complete obstruction and filling defects in which the clot creates a negative shadow as dye flows around it.

Bibliography

Hollerich VT, Wigton RS. Diagnosing pulmonary embolism using clinical findings. Arch Intern Med 1986;146:1699–1703.

Huisman MV, et al. Management of clinically suspected acute venous thrombosis in outpatients with serial impedance plethysmography in a community hospital setting. Arch Intern Med 1989;149:511–513.

Hull R, et al. Pulmonary angiography, ventilation lung scanning, and venography for clinically suspected pulmonary embolism with abnormal perfusion scans. Ann Intern Med 1983;98:891–899.

Lensing AWA, et al. Detection of deep vein thrombosis by real-time B-mode ultrasonography. N Engl J Med 1989;320:342–345.

Moser KN. Venous thromboembolism. Am Rev Respir Dis 1990; 141:235–249.

The PIOPED investigators. Value of the ventilation/perfusion scan in acute pulmonary embolism: Results of the prospective investigation of pulmonary embolism diagnosis (PIOPED). JAMA 1990;263:2753–2759.

24

ACUTE VENOUS THROMBOSIS

MILES CRAMER

Varicose veins are the result of improper selection of grandparents.

WILLIAM OSLER (1849–1919)

DEFINITION

Thrombosis (clot) of the venous system usually results from the interactive effects of blood flow stasis, hypercoagulability, and/or endothelial injury (Virchow's triad). Venous thrombosis can be superficial or deep, acute or chronic. In *deep venous thrombosis* (DVT), the inflammatory component is minimal. DVT most commonly involves the veins located from the knee to the abdomen (proximal veins) or to the veins of the calf (distal veins), or both.

EPIDEMIOLOGY

In the United States, of the 800,000 estimated patients with DVT each year:

1. 6% will have a fatal PE.
2. 20% will have a nonfatal PE.
3. 66% will experience chronic venous insufficiency leading to the postthrombotic syndrome (edema, hyperpigmentation, and ulceration; Table 24–1).

Approximately 60% of the female population who develop proximal DVT do so in connection with either hormone therapy or childbirth (23% with hormone therapy, 14% after cesarean section, and 23% after vaginal delivery).

PATHOLOGY

Acute DVT frequently begins in the venous sinuses of the calf and valve cusp pockets in the veins of the calf or thigh. Thrombi may also form in the iliofemoral segment. The incidence of left iliofemoral DVT is at least twice that for the right side. The thrombus may propagate proximally or distally, embolize, or, rarely, spontaneously lyse.

TABLE 24–1. Key Features of Natural History (Untreated)

A. 28% of general surgery patients develop calf vein thrombi.

B. 80% of calf vein thrombi spontaneously lyse, and up to 20% propagate into the popliteal vein.

C. 50% of popliteal thrombi cause clinically significant PE.

    1. 30% of patients with PE have *symptomatic* leg vein thrombi.

    2. Over 80% of patients with PE have *venographically documented* lower extremity thrombi.

D. Once the thrombus stabilizes, it is eventually covered by endothelium and becomes a permanent venous obstruction. Recanalization may occur in as many as 10% of patients, but there is usually damage to the venous wall and valves.

DIFFERENTIAL DIAGNOSIS

DVT is usually unilateral and rarely occurs spontaneously. It usually develops in the context of Virchow's triad (Table 24–2).

TABLE 24–2. Factors That Predispose to DVT

Alteration of Venous Flow (Stasis)
  Postoperative factors (general surgery): Age over 40 years, previous DVT, malignancy, obesity, severity of operation
  Congestive heart failure
  Prolonged bed rest
  Postpartum condition
  Prolonged travel in a sitting position
  Chronic debilitating conditions: e.g., after spinal cord injury
Hypercoagulability
  Malignancy
  Sepsis
  Oral contraceptives: risk of thromboembolism is 3.5 to 6 times greater for estrogen-therapy patients.
  Polycythemia
  Thrombocytosis
Injury to Vein Lining
  Trauma
  IV catheters or IV medications
  Previous DVT
  Systemic lupus erythematosus

CLINICAL FEATURES

Clinical assessment of venous thrombosis begins by excluding other causes of unilateral pain, tenderness, swelling, and erythema (Table 24–3).

- Superficial thrombophlebitis. Superficial thrombophlebitis is manifest by an area of localized tenderness, erythema, and induration, classically located over the greater saphenous vein and its tributaries. Superficial phlebitis is usually benign and is generally not thought to lead to pulmonary embolism.

- Deep Vein Thrombosis (Table 24–4)
    1. The symptoms of DVT are inaccurate for diagnostic purposes in 50% of the cases.
    2. The determination of proximal or distal DVT is critical to the type of diagnostic test ordered and to subsequent patient management.

DIAGNOSTIC STUDIES

Objective methods must be used to determine both the presence and extent of venous thrombi. Recent advances in noninvasive techniques, especially color-flow duplex ultrasound scanning, make them the method of screening patients for DVT.

- Noninvasive techniques
    1. Ultrasonic duplex scan
        a. This technique allows direct visualization of the calf, popliteal, femoral, iliac, and inferior vena

TABLE 24–3. Other Causes of Unilateral Leg Symptoms

CONDITION	RELATIVE INCIDENCE	CHARACTERISTICS
Cellulitis or lymphedema	Common	Edema usually extends onto dorsum of foot (rare in DVT)
		Edema responds poorly to leg elevation
		Cutaneous erythema and tenderness are usually more pronounced, as in a systemic response
		Lymphedema is often painless
Muscle cramps	Occasional	Localized muscular tightness
Arthritis	Rare	Joint pain; there may be joint effusion
Ruptured Baker's cyst	Rare	Rapid acute swelling of calf, ankle, and foot
		Initial location of pain in calf and/or popliteal fossa
Compression from pregnancy	Occasional	Partial compression of iliac veins may occur
		Edema is usually bilateral
Compression from renal transplant	Rare	Patient complains of groin pain
		Edema may be evident

TABLE 24–4. Signs and Symptoms of DVT

Unilateral lower extremity pain

Unilateral lower extremity edema (excluding dorsum of the foot); a difference between leg circumferences > 1 cm is significant.

Tenderness to palpation.

Low-grade fever.

Hemoptysis

Inability to fully extend the leg without pain in the calf or popliteal fossa region (Homans' sign)

Phlegmasia cerulea dolens (blue leg) due to extensive and diffuse involvement of both the deep and superficial veins and leading to massive swelling with impaired arterial inflow and cyanosis

Phlegmasia alba dolens (white leg) due to massive thrombosis that involves perivenous lymphatics. The leg turns white as result of extreme edema.

---

cava venous systems and is the noninvasive method of choice. Color-flow duplex is more accurate in determining calf vein patency than standard duplex ultrasound.

   b. Partial obstruction as well as total occlusion can be detected.

   c. It is highly accurate (sensitivity = 96%, specificity = 91%) and easily allows serial follow-up scans.

2. Doppler ultrasound

   a. This nonimaging modality is highly observer-dependent and assesses venous patency by listening to audible blood flow characteristics.

   b. In experienced hands, this test yields a sensitivity of 68% and specificity of 95% for DVT and fails to detect up to 50% of calf vein thrombi. It is insensitive to partial venous obstruction or duplicate venous systems.

3. Impedance plethysmography (IPG)/Strain gauge plethysmography (SPG)

   a. These commonly used indirect methods of assessing venous occlusion detect proximal venous occlusion by plotting the venous filling volume against the venous emptying rate.

   b. IPG and SPG have sensitivities of 97% and specificities of 87% but fail to detect up to 80% of calf vein thrombi and are insensitive to duplicate venous systems, partial venous obstruction, and extensive venous collateralization.

• Invasive techniques

1. Contrast venography

   a. This technique is the "gold standard" objective method of diagnosing both distal and proximal DVT.

   b. Up to 6% of patients develop a "chemical phlebitis" as a result of irritation of the vein endothelium by the contrast medium.

    c. Venographic criteria of thrombosis
      i. Termination of a column of contrast medium at a constant site with refilling at a site above termination
      ii. Nonfilling of a portion of the venous system
      iii. Diversion of flow into collaterals
      iv. Appearance of contrast medium on either side of a thrombus ("railroad tracking")

2. Radionuclide venography
    a. This technique detects only proximal venous occlusion. It usually cannot detect partial venous obstruction and is insensitive to calf vein thrombi.
    b. It has a lower risk and causes less pain to the patient than contrast venography.

3. Perfusion—ventilation lung scan
    a. This test is usually done in conjunction with a radionuclide venogram and is used to exclude PE.
    b. A negative perfusion scan is highly significant and accurate.
    c. A positive study has approximately 50% accuracy (see Chapter 22).

RECOMMENDED DIAGNOSTIC APPROACH (Figure 24–1)

If clinical suspicion is present, one or more of the following tests should be performed: duplex scan, Doppler studies, SPG, or IPG. Results may be negative (no further diagnostic tests are necessary), positive (proceed with treatment), or

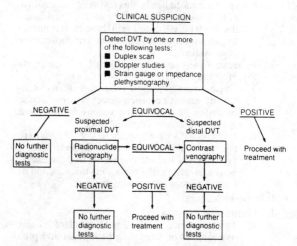

Figure 24–1. Approach to the patient with suspected deep vein thrombosis (DVT). (Modified from Cummins RO, Eisenberg MS. Blue Book of Medical Diagnosis. Philadelphia, W.B. Saunders Co, 1986, p. 30.)

equivocal (further studies are indicated as outlined in Figure 24-1). A positive duplex study is accurate enough to initiate treatment. However, Doppler should be combined with either of the plethysmographic techniques to ensure optimal diagnostic accuracy.

Bibliography

Cramer M, et al. The detection of proximal deep vein thrombosis by strain gauge plethysmography through the use of an outflow/capacitance discriminant line. Bruit 1983;VII:17–21.

Cronen JJ, et al. Deep venous thrombosis: US assessment using vein compression. Radiology 1987;162:191–194.

Dauzat MM, et al. Real-time b-mode ultrasonography for better specificity in the noninvasive diagnosis of deep vein thrombosis. J Ultrasound Med 1986;5:625–631.

Katz ML, et al. Technical aspects of venous duplex imaging. J Vasc Technol 1988;XII:100–102.

Nix ML, et al. Duplex venous scanning: image vs doppler accuracy. J Vasc Technol 1989;XIII:121–126.

Wright DJ, et al. Pitfalls in lower extremity venous scanning. J Vasc Surg 1990;11:675–679.

25

ADULT RESPIRATORY DISTRESS SYNDROME

RICHARD MAUNDER

Keep breathing.

SOPHIE TUCKER

DEFINITION AND GENERAL COMMENTS

- Definition. Adult respiratory distress syndrome (ARDS) is an acute respiratory failure that can occur following major trauma, aspiration of gastric contents, systemic infection, and a variety of other events.
- Pathophysiologic description. In patients with ARDS, inflammatory cells within the lung release mediators capable of tissue injury. Damage to the alveolar-capillary membrane alters lung vascular permeability, causing accumulation of protein-rich interstitial and alveolar edema fluid. Reduced lung compliance and impaired gas exchange are the physiologic hallmarks of ARDS. The initial injury in ARDS is often followed by impaired surfactant function, cellular proliferation, disruption of alveolar architecture, and eventual lung fibrosis.
- Criteria for diagnosis (Table 25–1). Generalized pulmonary infiltrates and hypoxemia are the key features of the syndrome. The onset is acute, usually related temporally to a catastrophic clinical event (Table 25–2). Alternative explanations for respiratory distress, such as cardiac failure, must be excluded.

DIFFERENTIAL DIAGNOSIS (Table 25–3)

- Misinterpretation of the chest X-ray. Chest X-rays of critically ill patients are difficult to interpret. Inadequate inflation or motion artifact may produce a picture resembling ARDS when no abnormality is present. Pleural fluid collections in a supine patient may confuse by producing diffuse haziness of the lung fields. Artifacts may appear due to subcutaneous emphysema or the presence of a body cast over the thorax.
- Chronic lung disease. Patients with interstitial fibrosis, lymphangitic carcinoma, chronic airflow obstruction, and other respiratory conditions may meet the criteria outlined in Table 25–1.
- Pulmonary infection. A variety of pathogens, most commonly viral, can produce diffuse pulmonary infiltrates and

TABLE 25–1. Diagnostic Criteria for ARDS

1. Respiratory distress
   Tachypnea > 25/min
   Labored respirations
2. Hypoxemia
   $PaO_2 < 75$ with $FiO_2 > 0.5$
   $PaO_2/F_1O_2 < 175$ or $PaO_2/P_AO_2 < 0.3$
3. Multilobar pulmonary infiltrates
4. Pulmonary artery wedge pressure < 18 mmHg
5. No alternative explanation for the above findings

PaO_2 = arterial oxygen tension in torr.
FiO_2 = inspired fraction of oxygen.
P_AO_2 = alveolar oxygen tension in torr.

hypoxemia, particularly in immunocompromised patients. In general, viral pneumonia is included as a cause of ARDS. Occasionally, however, a bacterial or fungal pneumonia may become generalized with endobronchial spread to produce a clinical picture resembling ARDS.

- Hydrostatic pulmonary edema (congestive heart failure). Pulmonary edema as a result of cardiac failure produces a clinical picture that often is indistinguishable from ARDS. The clinical setting, associated symptoms, and prior history may be helpful, but a firm diagnosis of ARDS requires documentation of a normal pulmonary artery wedge pressure. The cutoff in Table 25–1 (<18 mmHg) assures that lung edema is not entirely caused by elevated hydrostatic forces so that vascular permeability is definitely increased.

CLINICAL FEATURES OF ARDS

- History
  1. Clinical risk factors. Table 25–2 lists common causes of ARDS. Infrequent causes include drug overdose, pancreatitis, viral pneumonia, and inhaled toxins (including oxygen). In the absence of sepsis, shock is rarely if ever the only cause of ARDS.
  2. Symptoms. Alert patients complain of dyspnea, but there are no distinctive clinical features associated with ARDS. Mental status is often impaired.
  3. The earliest sign in virtually all cases is respiratory distress.

TABLE 25–2. Risk of ARDS After Predisposing Clinical Conditions

Sepsis syndrome	20–40%
Aspiration of gastric contents	30–35%
Multiple transfusions (>15 units/24 hr)	26%
Long bone fractures	5–8%
Pulmonary contusion	17%
Near-drowning	40%

TABLE 25-3. Differential Diagnosis in ARDS

1. Misinterpretation of chest X-ray
   Poor lung inflation
   Pleural effusions (in supine patient)
   Inadequate X-ray penetration
2. Chronic lung disease
   Scarring disorders (sarcoidosis, idiopathic pulmonary
      fibrosis, asbestosis)
   Allergic alveolitis
   Lymphangitic carcinomatosis
   Chronic obstructive pulmonary disease
3. Pulmonary infection
   Viral pneumonia
   Diffuse gram-negative pneumonia
   Tuberculosis
   Disseminated fungal infection
4. Hydrostatic pulmonary edema
   Cardiac failure
   Volume overload

4. Timing of ARDS
   a. Most patients who develop ARDS do so within 24
      hours after the inciting event.
   b. The natural history of ARDS is extremely
      variable.
      i. A third of patients respond to therapy and
         demonstrate steady improvement in pulmo-
         nary function and radiographic abnormalities
         in the first week.
      ii. One-third (usually those with ongoing illness
         such as systemic infection) show progression
         despite treatment and never recover
      iii. Another third show initial signs of stabili-
         zation and improvement but develop compli-
         cations, such as sepsis, which lead to clinical
         deterioration.
      iv. Mortality is approximately 60%.
5. Survivors of ARDS generally do well, but approximately 40% have residual abnormalities of pulmonary
   function, including airflow obstruction (25%), low diffusing capacity (23%), fall in PaO_2 with exercise (11%),
   and reduced lung volumes.

LABORATORY FEATURES OF ARDS

1. By definition, hypoxemia is present; hyperventilation is
   usually present in the early stages of ARDS. Since hypoxemia is predominantly caused by venoarterial shunting,
   PaO_2 improves minimally with increases in FIO_2. Long-
   term ARDS frequently leads to increased dead space,
   impairing CO_2 elimination and causing hypercarbia.
   Characteristically, there is dramatic improvement with
   the application of positive end-expiratory pressure
   (PEEP).

2. Most frequently, there is radiographic progression from a normal chest X-ray to a finely dispersed interstitial edema pattern, and eventually to generalized bilateral infiltrates. The process is "patchy" in 20 to 30% of cases. Large pleural effusions are unusual in ARDS and should raise the suspicion of pulmonary infection, traumatic hemothorax, or superimposed cardiac failure.
3. Reduced lung compliance occurs in most cases of established ARDS, but it may be normal in the early stages.
4. Pulmonary artery pressure is frequently elevated, particularly in ARDS caused by sepsis.

RECOMMENDED DIAGNOSTIC APPROACH

• Arterial blood gases. Measurement of arterial blood gases is required, since hypoxemia is one of the diagnostic criteria for ARDS (Table 25-1).
• Chest X-ray. Documentation of bilateral multilobar infiltrates is required for the diagnosis of ARDS.
• Edema fluid protein. If a sufficient volume of edema fluid can be obtained, the edema fluid : plasma protein ratio may help distinguish ARDS from cardiogenic edema. A ratio of greater than 0.7 indicates increased permeability, while one of less than 0.5 suggests edema caused by elevated hydrostatic pressures.

Bibliography

Hudson LD. Causes of the adult respiratory distress syndrome—clinical recognition. Clin Chest Med 1982;2:195–212.

Maunder RJ. Clinical prediction of the adult respiratory distress syndrome. Clin Chest Med 1985;6:413–426.

Montgomery AB, et al. Causes of mortality in patients with the adult respiratory distress syndrome. Am Rev Resp Dis 1985;132:485–489.

Rinaldo JE, Rogers RM: Adult respiratory distress syndrome—changing concepts of lung injury and repair. N Engl J Med 1982;306:900–909.

Wiedemann HP, et al., eds. Acute lung injury (symposium). Crit Care Clinics 1986;2:377–665.

26

CHRONIC INTERSTITIAL PNEUMONITIS

ROBERT DREISIN

Love, and a cough, cannot be hid.
GEORGE HERBERT (1593–1633)

DEFINITION AND GENERAL COMMENTS

Most patients with diffuse infiltrates on chest X-ray have acute illnesses (left ventricular failure, mitral valve disease, ARDS, and atypical pneumonias). Chronic interstitial pneumonitis refers to infiltration lasting more than 2 months without dramatic clinical and radiographic change (Table 26–1).

IMMUNOLOGIC AND HYPERSENSITIVITY REACTIONS

- Goodpasture's syndrome
  1. Definition. "Goodpasture's syndrome" is a distinct entity characterized by recurrent, acute pulmonary hemorrhage, rapidly progressive glomerulonephritis, and anemia.
  2. Etiology. Goodpasture's syndrome is defined by the presence of antibody directed at alveolar and glomerular basement membranes. In the absence of demonstrable circulating or tissue-bound antiglomerular basement membrane (anti-GBM) antibody, only a presumptive diagnosis of Goodpasture's syndrome can be made.
  3. Epidemiology. Goodpasture's syndrome is primarily a disease of young and middle-aged (median age 21) Caucasian men.
  4. Clinical presentation and course
     a. Recurrent hemoptysis is typical. It is accompanied by radiographic evidence of diffuse pulmonary infiltration, caused by intra-alveolar blood and mild alveolar septal thickening.
     b. Hematuria, proteinuria, and azotemia characteristic of a rapidly progressive glomerulonephritis become apparent in several weeks. The glomerulonephritis occasionally precedes the pulmonary hemorrhage.

TABLE 26–1. Immunologic and Idiopathic Causes of Chronic Pulmonary Infiltrates

Immunologic and hypersensitivity reactions
    Goodpasture's syndrome
    Hypersensitivity pneumonitis
    Connective tissue disease
        Rheumatoid arthritis
        Systemic lupus erythematosus
        Progressive systemic sclerosis
        Polymyositis-dermatomyositis
        Sjögren's syndrome
        Ankylosing spondylitis
Idiopathic
    Idiopathic pulmonary fibrosis
    Sarcoidosis
    Pulmonary alveolar proteinosis
    Wegener's granulomatosis

Source: Dreisin RB. Hypersensitivity pneumonitis (extrinsic allergic alveolitis). In: Mitchell RS, Petty TL, eds. Synopsis of Clinical Pulmonary Disease, 3rd ed. St. Louis, C.V. Mosby Company, 1982.

    c.   Course. The typical course of an untreated patient is inexorable progression. Usually, survival is less than 6 months, but prolonged, spontaneous remissions have been reported.

5.   Chest X-ray
    a.   There are diffuse alveolar infiltrates in a perihilar distribution. Initially, they may be localized, and fluctuate in severity.
    b.   The chest X-ray clears between episodes of bleeding, but the interstitium eventually becomes accentuated due to pulmonary hemosiderosis.

6.   Laboratory tests
    a.   Iron-deficiency anemia is almost always present at some point in the illness.
    b.   Elevated BUN and serum creatinine levels with proteinuria, hematuria, pyuria, and cylindruria characteristically develop after pulmonary symptoms start.
    c.   Hemosiderin-laden macrophages are seen by iron staining of sputum or bronchoalveolar lavage fluid.
    d.   The definitive diagnosis is established by demonstration of anti-GBM antibodies in renal or lung biopsies or serum. Negative tests should be repeated in more than one laboratory if clinical suspicion is high.

7.   Histopathology
    a.   Alveoli are filled with blood and hemosiderin-laden macrophages. The interstitium may be thickened by an infiltrate of mononuclear phagocytes, edema, and fibrosis.
    b.   Glomeruli show changes typical of rapidly progressive glomerulonephritis.
    c.   Immunofluorescent staining demonstrates immu-

noglobulin and complement deposition along the alveolo-capillary and glomerular basement membranes.

8. Recommended diagnostic approach
   a. Search for characteristic iron-deficiency anemia, azotemia, and microscopic hematuria.
   b. Anti-GBM antibody in tissue and serum is confirmatory.

- Hypersensitivity pneumonitis (extrinsic allergic alveolitis)
  1. Definition. Hypersensitivity pneumonitis is the lung's reaction to antigenic organic dusts, in most cases, a fungal spore (Table 26–2).
  2. Etiology. The condition is mediated by Types 3 (immune complex–mediated) and 4 (sensitized T-lymphocyte–mediated) hypersensitivity reactions.
  3. Epidemiology
     a. Patients are usually exposed to antigenic material in specific occupations or hobbies. Farmer's lung disease occurs in farmers exposed to fungally contaminated hay in silos. Pigeon fancier's disease may affect those exposed to droppings and dander.
     b. The source of exposure may be an otherwise innocuous environmental source, such as a contaminated air conditioner.
  4. Clinical presentation and course. The specific manifestations are more closely related to the intensity and duration of antigenic exposure than to the identity of the antigen.
     a. Acute form. The classic picture of acute hypersensitivity pneumonitis occurs when a sensitive farmer enters a silo with high concentrations of fungal spores. Within 4 to 6 hr, fever, chills, cough, dyspnea, and anorexia develop. Chest pain and hemoptysis are unusual. Generally, the symptoms last 24 to 48 hr. Rales are unusual, and wheezing is not heard unless the patient is atopic.
     b. Chronic form
        i. The patient may have experienced an acute reaction so mild that it was unrecognized. Cough and dyspnea develop insidiously.
        ii. The physical examination in these patients is similar to patients with COPD. Rales are less frequent.
        iii. The course may be progressive and irreversible unless antigen is avoided.
  5. Chest X-ray
     a. Acute form. Scattered soft alveolar infiltrates are seen. With massive antigenic exposure an ARDS-like pattern may occur.
     b. Chronic form. Hyperexpansion and increased interstitial markings are present.
  6. Laboratory data
     a. In the acute response, leukocytosis parallels the fever curve. In chronic disease there is no leukocytosis.

TABLE 26-2. Antigens, Their Sources, and Disease Entities That Can Produce Hypersensitivity Pneumonitis

DISEASE	SOURCE OF ANTIGEN	PRECIPITINS
Air conditioner and humidifier lung	Fungi in air conditioner and humidifiers	Thermophilic actinomycetes
Aspergillosis	Ubiquitous	*Aspergillus fumigatus, A. flavis, A. niger, A. nidulans*
Bagassosis (sugarcane workers)	Moldy bagasse	*Thermoactinomyces vulgaris*
Bird fancier's lung	Pigeon, parrot, or hen droppings	Serum proteins and droppings
Byssinosis	Cotton, flax, hemp	Unknown
Farmer's lung	Moldy hay	*Micropolyspora faeni, T. vulgaris*
Malt worker's lung	Moldy barley, malt dust	*A. clavatus, A. fumigatus*
Maple-bark pneumonitis	Moldy maple bark	*Cryptostroma corticale*
Mushroom worker's lung	Mushroom compost	*M. faeni, T. vulgaris*
"New Guinea" lung	Moldy thatch dust	Thatch of huts
Pituitary snufftaker's lung	Heterologous pituitary powder	Heterologous antigen of pituitary snuff
Sequoiosis	Moldy redwood sawdust	*Graphium aurea, basidium pullalans*
Sisal worker's lung	Unknown	Unknown
Smallpox handler's lung	Not yet demonstrated	Not yet demonstrated
Suberosis	Moldy oak bark, cork dust	Unknown
Wheat weevil disease	Infested wheat flour	*Sitophilus granarius*

    b. Precipitating antibodies to the offending antigen are demonstrable in 60 to 90% of affected patients but may be present in unaffected exposed workers as well.

    c. Bronchoalveolar lavage fluid contains disproportionate numbers of T-suppressor lymphocytes.

    d. Pulmonary function abnormalities are:

        i. In acute hypersensitivity pneumonitis a nonatopic person has a fall in FVC and FEV_1 (restrictive) peaking at 5 to 7 hr after exposure and resolving within 24 hr. An atopic individual has an immediate fall in FEV_1 (obstructive) lasting 30 to 60 min followed by a delayed response similar to that seen in a nonatopic person.

        ii. In chronic hypersensitivity pneumonitis, results are variable. Lung volumes are generally diminished. The diffusion capacity for carbon monoxide is impaired.

7. Histopathology

    a. In acute hypersensitivity pneumonitis, lung biopsy demonstrates interstitial infiltration by plasma cells, lymphocytes, and occasionally neutrophils. Foamy macrophages are seen within alveolar spaces and terminal airways, and an obliterative bronchiolitis may be present.

    b. In chronic hypersensitivity pneumonitis, bronchial fibrosis and centrilobular emphysema are found. Scattered but sparse granulomata are characteristic.

8. Recommended diagnostic approach

    a. A careful history in search of appropriate exposures is crucial.

    b. Circulating precipitating antibodies and T-suppressor cells in bronchoalveolar lavage fluid are suggestive but not diagnostic.

    c. In equivocal cases in which diagnostic certainty is necessary, open lung biopsy is the only path to a definitive diagnosis.

• Connective tissue disease

1. Rheumatoid arthritis. Radiographic evidence of interstitial pneumonitis is seen in 20% of patients, physiologic evidence in 40%, and pathologic evidence in 80%. Other intrathoracic diseases are:

    a. Pleural effusion or pleural thickening, seen in 20%, is not more prevalent in those with diffuse fibrotic disease.

    b. Rheumatoid pulmonary nodules occur in patients with high titers of rheumatoid factor who also have subcutaneous nodular disease. There is no significant association between rheumatoid nodules and interstitial pneumonitis.

2. Systemic lupus erythematosus. Pleural effusions are much more common than lupus pneumonitis. The interstitial pneumonitis is usually chronic and mild.

3. Progressive systemic sclerosis. Interstitial fibrosis is

present in 80% of lung specimens from autopsied patients with progressive systemic sclerosis. Pulmonary hypertension from intimal proliferation is seen in 20%.

4. Polymyositis-dermatomyositis. Interstitial pneumonitis with fibrosis occurs in fewer than 10% of patients. Concomitant bronchiolitis obliterans is seen in a higher percentage of patients than in the other connective tissue disorders.

5. Sjögren's syndrome may coexist with any of the other connective tissue diseases. When it occurs alone it is usually associated with a lymphocytic interstitial pneumonitis.

6. Ankylosing spondylitis. Patients with ankylosing spondylitis rarely develop fibrosis of one or both upper lung fields. The apical infiltration is usually out of proportion to the relatively mild disease in the lower lung fields. Infiltrates may cavitate in advanced cases. The apical infiltrates of ankylosing spondylitis only appear many years after the onset of the spondylitis.

7. Recommended diagnostic approach
   a. Diffuse interstitial pneumonitis/fibrosis in a patient with known connective tissue disease does not require further diagnostic work-up.
   b. Pleural effusions should be evaluated by thoracentesis, primarily to exclude coexistent infection or malignancy, all of which are seen more frequently in patients with interstitial disease of any etiology.
   c. Solitary (but not multiple) rheumatoid nodules may require resection to exclude malignancy.

IDIOPATHIC FORMS OF INTERSTITIAL LUNG DISEASE

• Idiopathic pulmonary fibrosis

1. Definition. Idiopathic pulmonary fibrosis refers to diffuse interstitial inflammatory conditions without a specific cause that develop into fibrosis. It is a diagnosis of exclusion.

2. Epidemiology. The mean age is 50 years, but all ages may be affected.

3. Clinical presentation and course
   a. Dyspnea with exertion is the most common initial symptom. Nonproductive cough occurs in 35% of patients.
   b. The mean survival from diagnosis until death in one series was 4.8 years. "Hamman-Rich syndrome" refers to the rare patient with a fulminant course leading to death within 6 months. More commonly, patients show some decrease in pulmonary function for a few months, then stabilize for many years, often in apparent response to corticosteroid and immunosuppressive therapy.

4. Chest X-ray
   a. The chest X-ray shows an increase in fine interstitial markings in a reticular pattern at the lung

bases. As the disease progresses, these irregularities increase in thickness and involve the rest of the lung, with eventual honeycombing.

    b. A pattern of bilateral triangular haziness extending from both hila to the costophrenic angles is seen in desquamative interstitial pneumonia (DIP), a variant of idiopathic pulmonary fibrosis.

5. Laboratory data

    a. Seventy percent of patients have polyclonal gammopathy, and 80% have an elevated erythrocyte sedimentation rate.

    b. There are positive antinuclear and rheumatoid factors in 10 to 40% of cases.

    c. Bronchoalveolar lavage shows an elevated percentage of neutrophils, lymphocytes, and/or eosinophils when compared with controls.

6. Histopathology

    a. Usual interstitial pneumonitis (UIP), the most common form, is characterized by a pleomorphic infiltrate of lymphocytes, plasma cells, eosinophils, and fibroblasts.

    b. DIP is characterized by engorgement of alveolar spaces by large alveolar macrophages with varying degrees of interstitial inflammation and fibrosis.

    c. Lymphocytic interstitial pneumonitis (LIP) is frequently associated with Sjögren's syndrome and macroglobulinemia. There is a monotonous interstitial infiltrate of normal-appearing lymphocytes.

7. Recommended diagnostic approach

    a. When characteristic clinical and radiographic alterations of an interstitial pneumonitis occur in a patient with restrictive lung disease of no obvious cause, a presumptive diagnosis is made. Rheumatoid factor and antinuclear antibodies must be absent or present in only low titer.

    b. Transbronchial biopsies help exclude sarcoidosis, lymphangitic carcinomatosis, and hypersensitivity pneumonitis.

    c. Open lung biopsy, if the patient can tolerate it, if the diagnosis is critical, or if the patient is being studied as part of a research protocol, is necessary for a definitive diagnosis.

• Sarcoidosis (see Chapter 27)

• Pulmonary alveolar proteinosis

1. Definition. Pulmonary alveolar proteinosis is a disease of unknown origin characterized by the diffuse filling of alveolar spaces by proteinaceous material.

2. Clinical presentation and course. Patients generally are seen with exertional dyspnea. Most patients have a spontaneous remission. Nocardial lung or brain abscess is an unusual complication.

3. Chest X-ray. Diffuse, bilaterally symmetric alveolar infiltrates are typical. Unilateral disease or an interstitial radiographic appearance are less frequent and hilar adenopathy is observed in a few cases.

4. Laboratory data. More than 80% of patients with pul-

monary alveolar proteinosis have an isolated elevation of lactate dehydrogenase (LDH).

5. Histopathology. There is deposition of a surfactantlike material that stains pink with eosin and is strongly positive in response to the periodic acid–Schiff (PAS) reaction. Mild interstitial inflammation and fibrosis may be seen but are less marked than the alveolar-filling process.

6. Recommended diagnostic approach
   a. Bronchoalveolar lavage yields characteristic surfactant "lamellar bodies."
   b. Transbronchial biopsy with PAS stain is usually diagnostic. Open lung biopsy is definitive in equivocal cases.

- Wegener's granulomatosis
  1. Definition. Wegener's granulomatosis is a necrotizing granulomatous vasculitis involving primarily the upper respiratory tract, lungs, and glomeruli. It is most common in the third to fifth decades, but may occur at any age.

  2. Clinical presentation and course
     a. Upper airway involvement includes ulcers, erosions, pseudotumors, saddle nose deformity, sinusitis, and bony erosion.
     b. Lung involvement consists of nodules and cavities, unilateral or bilateral.
     c. Renal involvement consists of focal glomerulitis, glomerulonephritis, and parenchymal masses.
     d. Less commonly involved sites include the joints (arthralgias), skin (palpable purpura, ulcerating infarct), eyes (granulomatous uveitis, orbital pseudotumor), ears (serous otitis media), heart (coronary vasculitis and pericarditis), and nervous system (mononeuritis multiplex, cranial neuritis).
     e. A limited form sparing the kidneys may occur.

  3. Chest X-ray. There are nodules or cavities, or both. True diffuse interstitial infiltration, except by multiple discrete nodules, is not seen.

  4. Laboratory data
     a. Anemia, leukocytosis, and hematuria are present.
     b. The antinuclear antibody or rheumatoid factor is positive in fewer than 10% of patients.
     c. Antineutrophil cytoplasmic antibodies (ANCA) are seen in 90% of cases.

  5. Histopathology. There is a diffuse granulomatous vasculitis involving the medium-sized vessels, with an associated disseminated small vessel leukocytoclastic vasculitis. The necrotizing granulomas in the lung are surrounded by a zone of what appears to be a usual interstitial pneumonitis.

  6. Recommended diagnostic approach
     a. The clinical presentation suggests the diagnosis.
     b. ANCA determination is sensitive and specific but is also new and subject to interlaboratory variation.
     c. Biopsy of nasal mucosa, lung, or kidney is usually necessary for definitive diagnosis.

Bibliography

Dreisin RB. Hypersensitivity pneumonitis. In: Mitchell RS, Petty TL, eds. Synopsis of Clinical Pulmonary Disease, 3rd ed. St. Louis, C.V. Mosby Company, 1982, pp. 126–135.

Noelle B, et al. Anticytoplasmic autoantibodies: Their immunodiagnostic value in Wegener granulomatosis. Ann Int Med 1989;111: 28–40.

27

SARCOIDOSIS

TIM OBERMILLER, *and*
GANESH RAGHU

It is not easy to show that any disease is absolutely local, on the one hand, or absolutely general, on the other.

ELISHA BARTLETT (1804–1855)

DEFINITION

Sarcoidosis is a multisystem granulomatous disorder of unknown etiology. The diagnosis is established when clinico-radiographic findings are supported by histologic evidence of at least noncaseating epithelioid cell granulomas in at least one organ or a positive Kveim-Siltzbach skin test.

EPIDEMIOLOGY

- Sarcoidosis occurs worldwide but with a variable geographical, sexual, and racial prevalence. In the United States, prevalence ranges from 11 to 71 per 100,000.
- It commonly affects those in their third or fourth decades, but has been reported in people as young as 3 months and as old as 80.
- It is 10 to 12 times more common in American blacks than whites. Black women are twice as prone as black men to develop sarcoidosis.

PATHOLOGY

- Histology
  1. The characteristic finding in sarcoidosis is the non-caseating granuloma, which can develop in nearly any organ and can be widespread despite a lack of signs or symptoms.
  2. In the lung, noncaseating granulomas are often present in the submucosa and peribronchial regions, and may be associated with interstitial pulmonary fibrosis.
  3. Noncaseating granulomas are not specific for sarcoidosis, and can be seen in other disorders including mycobacterial and fungal infections, lymphoma, foreign body reactions, berylliosis and in regional lymph nodes associated with neoplastic or inflammatory reactions.

- Immunologic features
  1. Abnormalities in the immune system include:
     a. Impaired cutaneous delayed hypersensitivity, though patients with active tuberculosis usually have a positive tuberculin skin test.
     b. Lymphopenia with decreased numbers of T lymphocytes that are not functionally normal.
     c. Humoral immunity is intact with normal to high numbers of circulating B lymphocytes and elevated IgG immunoglobulin levels, which are often elevated.
  2. Granulomas are the result of heightened cell-mediated immunologic events at the sites of disease activity. This is best characterized in the lung where an alveolitis/fibrosis is mediated by macrophage-lymphocyte activation (unknown antigen) and the effect of locally released cytokines.

DIFFERENTIAL DIAGNOSIS (Table 27–1)

Differential diagnosis varies with the affected sites and organs.

TABLE 27–1. Differential Diagnosis of Noncaseating Granulomas in the Lung

A. Infections
1. Bacterial
   Tuberculosis
   Tularemia
   Brucellosis
2. Fungi
   Blastomycosis
   Coccidioidomycosis
   Histoplasmosis
3. Other
   Toxoplasmosis
   Schistosomiasis
B. Hypersensitivity Pneumonitis
1. Inhaled antigens
   Farmer's lung
   Bird fancier's lung
   Maltworker's lung
2. Drugs, e.g.,
   methotrexate
C. Chemical Reactions
   Berylliosis
   Talc granulomatosis
D. Vasculitis
   Wegener's granulomatosis
   Churg-Strauss granulomatosis
   Lymphomatoid granulomatosis
   Bronchocentric granulomatosis
E. Miscellaneous
   Eosinophilic granuloma

CLINICAL FEATURES (Table 27–2)

- Since sarcoidosis may affect nearly any organ of the body, clinical features vary considerably depending upon the site(s) and extent of disease involvement.

TABLE 27–2. Frequency of Organ Involvement and Common Clinical Manifestations

ORGAN	FREQUENCY (%)	CLINICAL MANIFESTATIONS
Lung	95–100	Common: restrictive lung disease Uncommon: airflow obstruction from endobronchial disease, pleural effusions
Lymph nodes	73	Palpable adenopathy, usually nontender, movable, and symmetric
Liver	70	Asymptomatic infiltration, hepatomegaly, intrahepatic cholestasis, cirrhosis and portal hypertension
Skin	32	Erythema nodosum, lupus pernio (disfiguring bluish-purple plaques), nodules, papules, and plaques (may occur at scars)
Eye	21	Keratoconjunctivitis, uveitis, chorioretinitis, optic neuritis, lacrimal gland enlargement, conjunctival follicles
Spleen	18	Splenomegaly, rarely hypersplenism
Bone	14	Lytic or sclerotic lesions, usually of the small bones of hands and feet
Salivary glands	6	Parotid enlargement, sicca syndrome
Joints	6	Acute inflammatory arthritis, mono- or polyarthralgias
Heart	5	Cardiomyopathy, arrhythmias, cor pulmonale, conduction disturbances
Nervous system	5	Cranial nerve palsies, meningitis, space-occupying lesions, diabetes insipidus
Kidneys	4	Renal failure, calculi

- History
  1. Half of patients are asymptomatic when the disorder is first diagnosed.
     a. Patients may come to attention due to an abnormal chest X-ray or nonspecific constitutional symptoms such as fatigue, fever, malaise, anorexia, and weight loss, which occur in 20 to 30% of patients.
     b. Of patients with specific organ involvement, 90% present with lung disease manifest by cough, dyspnea, and wheezing.
     c. In fewer than 10% of patients, extrathoracic disease such as lymphadenopathy, skin lesions, ocular lesions, or splenomegaly is the stimulus for medical attention.
  2. Temporal patterns of presentation include:
     a. The acute sarcoid syndrome (Lofgren's syndrome): erythema nodosum, bilateral symmetrical hilar adenopathy, and arthralgias. It is rarely seen in the United States except in the Puerto Rican population of New York. Fever, uveitis, and arthritis are also manifestations of acute sarcoidosis.
     b. Patients that present with symptoms of a duration of less than 2 years are considered subacute, and those greater than 2 years chronic. Chronic disease is usually slowly progressive. In general the more chronic the disease, the worse the prognosis.
- Physical examination (Table 27–2)

LABORATORY STUDIES

- Serum calcium. 10% of patients with sarcoidosis develop hypercalcemia due to increased intestinal calcium absorption resulting from enhanced sensitivity to and increased levels of dihydroxyvitamin D_3.
- Twenty-four–hour urine calcium collection. Patients with a normal serum calcium should be screened for hypercalciuria, which is more frequent than hypercalcemia.
- Liver function tests. Serum alkaline phosphatase may be elevated with hepatic involvement; transaminases and bilirubin are increased less frequently.
- Serum angiotensin converting enzyme (ACE). Levels of this enzyme are elevated in 60% of patients with sarcoidosis, but can also be increased in diseases that mimic sarcoidosis.
- Kveim-Siltzbach test
  1. This diagnostic test may be helpful in selected patients in whom a tissue diagnosis is not possible. It is rarely used in the United States.
  2. A sample of tissue suspension from the spleens of patients with sarcoidosis is injected intradermally. A positive test means that a skin biopsy done 4 to 6 weeks later demonstrates a granulomatous reaction at the injection site.

3. Major disadvantages of this test are limited availability of the suspension, lack of purified antigen, lack of standardization, and the delay required for diagnosis.

- Pulmonary Function Tests (PFTs)
  1. Typically, pulmonary sarcoidosis causes a restrictive pattern with reduced lung volumes and a decrease in the diffusion capacity of carbon monoxide (DL_{co}).
  2. Occasionally airflow obstruction occurs from endobronchial or severe peribronchial disease and is manifest by a reduction in the FEV_1-to FVC ratio.
  3. Since PFTs measure physiologic derangement, they do not always correlate with clinical and radiographic findings.
  4. ABGs are useful when dyspnea is present and typically demonstrate a widened alveolar to arterial oxygen difference.

- Chest X-ray (Table 27–3)
  1. Bilateral symmetric hilar adenopathy, often associated with paratracheal and other mediastinal lymphadenopathy, is the most characteristic finding. When hilar adenopathy is bilateral and symmetric in a perfectly asymptomatic person, it is considered diagnostic.
  2. Although interstitial disease is more common, nodular and alveolar-filling patterns are also seen; an upper lobe reticulonodular pattern is a frequently seen parenchymal abnormality.
  3. The radiographic stages of sarcoidosis correlate with prognosis, but not with symptoms or functional impairment.

- Gallium scan. Gallium accumulates in areas of inflammatory foci including the lung parenchyma, lymph nodes, spleen, and other extrapulmonary sites in patients with sarcoidosis. In some cases it may help localize sites of extrapulmonary disease.

- Computed tomography (CT)
  1. CT is more sensitive than chest X-rays for detection of mediastinal lymphadenopathy and parenchymal abnormalities. Since most patients have abnormal chest X-rays, CT should be restricted to selected patients.
  2. High-resolution CT may identify characteristic peribronchial patterns of involvement in patients with sarcoidosis, but they are not yet specific enough to preclude biopsy.

- Bronchoalveolar lavage (BAL)
  1. Analysis of cells retrieved by BAL from the lower respiratory tract reveals an increase in alveolar T lymphocytes in typical patients with sarcoidosis. In those with active disease, the majority of lymphocytes are T-helper cells.
  2. Because the technique and cell analysis have not been standardized and the results of clinical studies have been controversial, it is not recommended for routine use.

- Transbronchial lung biopsy (TLB). Because of its safety, high yield (Table 27–4), and the high frequency of lung

TABLE 27–3. Radiographic Stages in Sarcoidosis

STAGE	RADIOGRAPHIC FINDINGS	FREQUENCY OF OCCURRENCE (%)	RESOLUTION RATE (%)	DIFFERENTIAL DIAGNOSIS
0	Normal	5–10		
1	Lymphadenopathy[a] alone	40	65	Lymphoma Fungal disease Bronchogenic cancer Metastatic cancer Primary tuberculosis Brucellosis
2A	Lymphadenopathy[a] with parenchymal infiltrates	25–30	45	Tuberculosis Lymphoma Lymphangitic carcinomatosis Fungal disease Silicosis Berylliosis
2B	Parenchymal infiltrates alone	10–20	20	Tuberculosis Fungal diseases All interstitial lung diseases Alveolar proteinosis
3	Pulmonary fibrosis (honeycombing, hilar retraction, bullous lesions)	15		All interstitial lung diseases Tuberculosis Fungal diseases Bronchiectasis

[a] Hilar, paratracheal, and/or mediastinal.

222

TABLE 27–4. Diagnostic Yield: Biopsy Site and Technique

Biopsy Site	Technique	Yield (%)
Lung	Open lung biopsy	100
	Mediastinoscopy	90–100
	Transbronchial biopsy	
	Stage I	60
	Stage II	80–95
Liver	Needle aspiration	70
Scalene node	Needle aspiration	50–80
Skin	Punch biopsy	35
Conjunctiva with follicles	Biopsy	25
Minor salivary glands	"Lip biopsy"	60

involvement, fiberoptic bronchoscopy with TLB is the most frequently used technique to obtain histologic evidence of sarcoidosis.

RECOMMENDED DIAGNOSTIC APPROACH

- Since the clinical manifestations of sarcoidosis are variable and can be mimicked by other disorders, it is a diagnosis of exclusion. The diagnosis requires compatible clinical and radiographic findings, exclusion of mycobacterial and fungal infection, and histologic evidence of noncaseating granulomas.
- Assessment should include:
  1. Physical examination (Table 27–2). Ophthalmology consultation is required.
  2. Pulmonary function tests. Obtain spirometry, lung volumes, DL_{co} and ABGs. Exercise testing may be useful to detect subtle disease when the diagnosis is in question.
  3. Serum calcium. Hypercalcemia can corroborate the diagnosis and may require therapy.
  4. Twenty-four–hour urine calcium. This should be checked if the serum calcium is normal.
  5. Liver function tests.
  6. ECG
  7. Skin tests. Tuberculin skin test with controls should be done.
- Biopsy. Noncaseating granulomas and the absence of infection are required for a confirmed diagnosis. In addition to special stains, all biopsied organs must be cultured to exclude fungal and mycobacterial infections.
  1. Biopsy sites (Figure 27–1)
     a. If any conjunctival, lymph node, or cutaneous lesions are present, biopsy may be diagnostic.
     b. The next procedure of choice is fiberoptic bron-

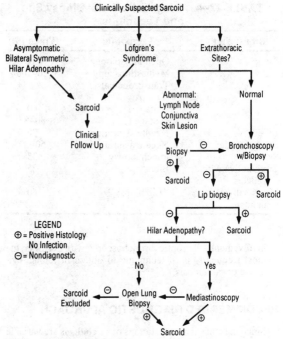

Figure 27–1. Algorithm to confirm diagnosis of sarcoidosis.

    choscopy with endobronchial and/or transbronchial lung biopsy.

  c. Random biopsy of minor salivary glands (lip biopsy) should be considered if the above procedures have not yielded a diagnosis.

  d. Mediastinoscopy is required to biopsy mediastinal or hilar adenopathy if the above procedures are nondiagnostic. Open lung biopsy is almost never needed to make a diagnosis, but its yield is nearly 100%, even in patients with stage I disease.

  e. Noncaseating granulomata in the liver and lymph nodes are less specific than in the lung, but may be diagnostic in the appropriate clinical setting (Table 27–4).

2. Biopsy is unnecessary. Certain clinical pictures are so distinctive that histologic confirmation is not essential.

Bibliography

DeRemee RA. The roentgenographic staging of sarcoidosis. Chest 1983;83:128.

Nosal A, et al. Angiotensin-1-converting enzyme and gallium scan in noninvasive evaluation of sarcoidosis. Ann Intern Med 1979;90:328.

Thomas PD, Hunninghake GW. State of art: Current concepts of the pathogenesis of sarcoidosis. Am Rev Respir Dis 1987;135:747.

Transactions of the New York Academy of Sciences. Seventh International Conference on Sarcoidosis and Other Granulomatous Disorders. Ann NY Acad Sci 1975;278:1.

Winterbauer RH, et al. A clinical interpretation of bilateral hilar adenopathy. Ann Intern Med 1973;78:65.

SECTION IV

RENAL

28

HEMATURIA

JANE LEMAIRE

The urine of man is one of the animal matters that have been the most examined by chemists. This liquid, which commonly inspires men only with contempt and disgust, which is generally ranked amongst vice and repulsive matters, has become, in the hands of the chemists, a source of important discoveries.

COUNT ANTOINE FRANCOIS DE FOURCROY
(1755–1809)

DEFINITION AND GENERAL COMMENTS

- Hematuria is divided into gross hematuria or microhematuria.
  1. Microhematuria is defined as 3 or more red blood cells (RBCs) per microscopic high-power field (HPF). When a patient has more than 100 RBCs/HPF, significant pathology is more likely.
  2. Many cases of hematuria are initially detected by a dipstick method.
     a. The peroxidase activity of hemoglobin or myoglobin react with the dipstick reagent to cause a color change.
     b. Ascorbic acid or a urine pH of less than 5.1 may cause a false-negative test (when compared to microscopic examination).
     c. Bacterial peroxidases, povidone-iodine, and hypochlorite bleaches may cause a false-positive test.
     d. The sensitivity of urine dipsticks is 91 to 100%. The specificity of a reaction that is "1+" or greater is 65 to 99%.
- Prior to diagnostic work-up, false hematuria should be excluded.
  1. Red urine that is negative for blood may be due to dietary factors (beets or berries), drugs (rifampin, phenytoin, phenazopyridine, methyldopa), or food dyes.
  2. Myoglobinuria from rhabdomyolysis and hemoglobinuria from intravascular hemolysis can cause a positive dipstick test for blood that is not associated with RBCs on microscopic exam.
  3. Vaginal bleeding may contaminate urine specimens and cause false hematuria.

DIFFERENTIAL DIAGNOSIS (Table 28–1)

The frequency of diseases found in patient series varies with the population.

CLINICAL FEATURES

- History. Characterization of the hematuria may provide diagnostic clues:
  1. Is it gross or microscopic hematuria (Table 28–2)?
     a. Initial hematuria suggests a urethral lesion.
     b. Terminal hematuria suggests a bladder neck or prostatic urethral source
     c. Total hematuria may result from a bladder, ureter, or kidney source.
  2. Infections
     a. Acute symptoms such as fever, dysuria, and urinary frequency suggest urinary tract infection as the source of hematuria. Prostatitis may additionally cause perineal, suprapubic, or low back pain.
     b. A history of a new sexual partner suggests STD.
     c. Schistosomiasis (*Schistosoma hematobium*) is the most common cause of hematuria worldwide.
     d. Patients with hematuria after an upper respiratory tract infection may have IgA nephropathy.
  3. Malignancy
     a. The most common urologic cancer is transitional cell carcinoma of the bladder, and 80% of patients have hematuria. Of patients with the second most common cancer, renal cell carcinoma, 60% have hematuria.
     b. Weight loss, anorexia, and flank pain are seen with malignancies of the genitourinary tract.
     c. Risk factors for urologic cancer include age greater than 60 years, tobacco or analgesic use, a history of pelvic irradiation or cyclophosphamide use, *Schistosoma hematobium* infection, and occupational exposure to certain dyes.
  4. Systemic illness
     a. Rash, fever, arthralgias or arthritis, and hemoptysis suggest connective tissue disease or vasculitis (Table 28–1).
     b. Bruising, petechiae, or other bleeding sources indicate a work-up for coagulopathy. Therapeutic anticoagulation does not usually cause hematuria.
  5. Medications. Prescription and nonprescription medications may be implicated (Table 28–1).
  6. Stone disease. A history of acute onset of flank and groin pain or a family history of stones suggest urolithiasis.
  7. Vascular disease. Damage to the kidney from renal vein thrombosis or renal infarction from emboli may cause hematuria.
  8. Both strenuous exercise and trauma can cause hematu-

TABLE 28-1. Differential Diagnosis of Hematuria

A. Infectious
   Urinary tract infection
      Urethritis
      Prostatitis
      Cystitis
      Pyelonephritis
      Perinephric abscess
   Tuberculosis
   Schistosomiasis
   Endocarditis
   Poststreptococcal glomerulonephritis (impetigo, pharyngitis)
B. Systemic
   Goodpasture's syndrome (anti-GBM syndrome)
   Systemic lupus erythematosus
   Polyarteritis nodosa
   Wegener's granulomatosis
   Coagulopathy
   Hypertension
   Diabetes
C. Malignancy
   Renal cell carcinoma
   Transitional cell carcinoma (ureter, bladder)
   Adenocarcinoma (prostate)
   Squamous cell carcinoma (urethra)
D. Toxins
   Papillary necrosis: analgesics, alcohol
   Hemorrhagic cystitis: cyclophosphamide, busulfan
   Interstitial nephritis: penicillins, rifampin, ibuprofen
      sulfonamides, phenytoin, lithium
   Glomerulonephritis: gold, penicillinamine, heroin,
      probenecid
   Loin pain—hematuria syndrome: oral contraceptives
E. Familial
   Hemoglobinopathy (e.g., sickle cell disease or trait)
   Polycystic kidney
   Medullary sponge kidney
   Alport's syndrome ("hereditary nephritis," associated
      with hearing loss)
   Vascular malformation
F. Urolithiasis
   Nephrolithiasis
   Bladder stone
   Prostate stone
G. Miscellaneous
   Exercise
   Trauma
H. Vascular
   Renal infarct
   Renal vein thrombosis
I. Primary renal disease
   Glomerulonephritis
   IgA nephropathy (Berger's disease)

TABLE 28–2. Frequency of Specific Causes of Hematuria

DIAGNOSIS	PERCENT OF PATIENTS WITH LISTED DIAGNOSIS	
	Microscopic hematuria	Gross hematuria
Urologic cancer	5	22
Bladder	4.0	15.0
Renal	0.5	3.6
Prostate	0.5	2.4
Ureteral	0.2	0.8
Other	0.2	0.6
Nephrolithiasis	5	11
Renal disease	2	0
Urinary tract infection	4	33
Prostatic hyperplasia	13	13
Other	28	13
No source found	43	8

Source: Adapted from Sutton JM. Evaluation of hematuria in adults. JAMA 1990; 263:2479.

ria. Exercise-induced hematuria may occur in up to 18% of people but resolves in 24 to 48 hours.
   9. Family history (Table 28–1) may identify inherited disorders associated with hematuria.
 • Physical examination. Although each patient should have a thorough examination, the clues provided in the history may direct the examination to specific areas.
   1. Blood pressure or funduscopic abnormalities may suggest hypertensive nephropathy.
   2. The cardiovascular exam may note an irregular rhythm or murmur that could indicate a source of emboli or vascular bruits to suggest vascular occlusive disease.
   3. Abdominal masses are seen with renal cell carcinoma or polycystic kidney disease. Costovertebral angle tenderness and fever suggest pyelonephritis.
   4. A prostatic nodule, bogginess, or enlargement suggests tumor, prostatitis, or benign prostatic hypertrophy, respectively.
   5. The urethral meatus should be examined for lesions. Pelvic examination may suggest that vaginal bleeding has caused false hematuria.

LABORATORY STUDIES

 • Urine studies
   1. The urinalysis may detect evidence of primary renal disease such as RBC casts or proteinuria. Some authors have found that dysmorphic RBCs (as examined by phase-contrast microscopy) suggest glomerular disease.

2. Infection is suggested by bacteriuria, pyuria, or white blood cell casts.
3. Urine eosinophils may be prominent in patients with interstitial nephritis.
4. Urine cytology has a sensitivity of 67% and a specificity of 96% in the diagnosis of malignancy. It is most effective in detecting poorly differentiated transitional cell carcinoma of the bladder, and may be more sensitive than cystoscopy in detecting in-situ lesions.

• Blood studies
1. BUN, serum creatinine, and electrolyte levels, and CBC should be determined. Patients with an abnormal serum creatinine level should have their creatinine clearance measured.
2. Clinical clues may suggest other studies (Table 28–3).

• Radiographic studies. These allow the urinary tract to be studied for tumors, stones, and cysts.
1. A "KUB" X-ray can identify radioopaque stones; 80% of stones contain calcium.
2. The intravenous pyelogram (IVP) evaluates the function and anatomy of the upper urinary tract and may detect masses, filling defects in the ureters or bladder (stones or tumors), papillary necrosis, hydronephrosis, or decreased renal function. Clinically apparent acute renal failure occurs in 0.15% of examinations, and death occurs in 1 to 7 per 100,000 contrast injections.
   a. If a patient is at risk for contrast nephropathy (multiple myeloma, diabetic with nephropathy, patients with depleted intravascular volume), a renal ultrasound can substitute for the IVP. It is also an excellent modality for visualizing renal cysts.
   b. A suspected renal mass can be further assessed by ultrasound or CT.
3. Retrograde pyelography may be done if contrast nephropathy is a significant risk or if abnormal function

TABLE 28–3. Blood Studies for Evaluation of Hematuria

Coagulation studies
Erythrocyte sedimentation rate
Antistreptolysin O titer
Antinuclear antibody
Serum protein electrophoresis
Hemoglobin electrophoresis
Serum acid phosphatase level
Tuberculin skin test
Chest X-ray
Blood cultures
Anti-GBM
Hepatitis B surface antigen
Serologic test for syphilis or the human immunodeficiency virus
Serum complement or cryoglobulin studies

limits the usefulness of an IVP. It requires cystoscopy and anesthesia.
4. Renal angiography or venography is usually reserved for preoperative evaluation of a known renal mass. They may be helpful if cystoscopy demonstrates active localized bleeding (i.e., from one ureter).
· Cystoscopy is used to evaluate pathology of the urethra, bladder, and lower ureters.

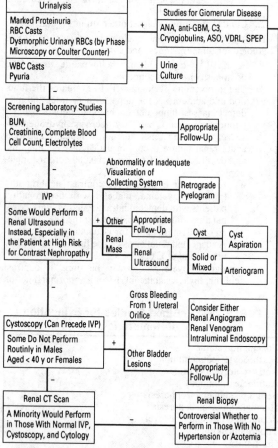

Figure 28–1. Evaluation of the patient with hematuria. RBC indicates red blood cell; WBC, white blood cell; ANA, antinuclear antibody; anti-GBM, antibody to glomerular basement membrane; C3, serum C3 complement; ASO, antistreptolysin O; SPEP, serum protein electrophoresis; BUN, serum urea nitrogen; IVP, intravenous pyelogram; and CT, computed tomography. (From Sutton JM. Evaluation of hematuria in adults. JAMA 1990;263:2477.)

1. Abnormalities may be safely biopsied through a cystoscope. The average sensitivity for bladder carcinoma is 87% but it is lower for in situ or flat lesions.
2. Urine cytology, when obtained via cystoscopic lavage, has a sensitivity of 80%.
3. Fiberoptic ureteroscopy may allow direct visualization of the ureters and renal pelvis.

- Indications for renal biopsy to evaluate a patient with hematuria remain controversial. Hypertension, proteinuria, or reduced creatinine clearance make a renal biopsy more likely to provide prognostic or therapeutic information.

RECOMMENDED DIAGNOSTIC APPROACH (Figure 28–1)

- The history, physical, and urinalysis direct further workup. False hematuria must be excluded. Use clinical information to classify a patient's risk for serious disease, especially urologic cancer.
- For low-risk patients, repeat the urinalysis. If asymptomatic microhematuria with 3 or more RBCs/HPF is present on 3 occasions, the patient should have IVP, cystoscopy, urine culture, and cytology. In this setting, cystoscopy has a low yield for patients less than 40 years old.
- All patients with gross hematuria or microhematuria greater than 100 RBCs/HPF should have IVP, cystoscopy, urine culture, and cytology performed regardless of risk.
- Patients with risk factors for urologic malignancy and any degree of microhematuria should have the same evaluation as above.
- If no diagnosis is made, repeat the urinalysis in 6 months. For persistent hematuria, repeat the urine cytology every 6 months, and the IVP and cystoscopy every year for 3 years.
- Routine screening for hematuria is not justified in healthy adults free of risk factors for urologic malignancy, with the possible exception of patients over 60 years of age.

Bibliography

Bartlow BG. Microhematuria: Picking the fewest tests to make an accurate diagnosis. Postgrad Med 1990;88(4):51–55.

Bauer DC. Evaluation of hematuria in adults. West J Med 1990;152:305–308.

Mohr DN, et al. Asymptomatic microhematuria and urologic disease. JAMA 1986;256:224–229.

Schoolwerth AC. Hematuria and proteinuria: Their causes and consequences. Hosp Pract 1987(Oct. 30):45–62.

Sutton JM. Evaluation of hematuria in adults. JAMA 1990;263:2475–2480.

Warshauer DM, et al. Detection of renal masses with sensitivities and specificities of excretory urography/linear tomography, US, and CT. Radiology 1988;169:363–365.

Woolhandler S, et al. Dipstick urinalysis screening of asymptomatic adults for urinary tract disorders. JAMA 1989;262:1214–1219.

29

ACUTE RENAL FAILURE

STUART L. BURSTEN

What is man, when you come to think upon him, but a minutely set, ingenious machine for turning, with infinite artfulness, the red wine of Shiraz into urine?

ISAK DINESEN

DEFINITION

- Acute renal failure (ARF) is a sudden fall in renal function characterized by azotemia. Urine output may be normal, increased, or decreased.
- Criteria for diagnosis. Initial criteria for ARF are rising blood urea nitrogen (BUN) and creatinine concentrations. There is extensive overlap among all forms of ARF. Transition between forms is common. For example, prerenal azotemia may progress to acute tubular necrosis (ATN). Late ATN may mimic chronic obstruction or chronic glomerulonephritis in that the patient is polyuric with salt-losing nephropathy.

DIFFERENTIAL DIAGNOSIS (Table 29–1)

- Prerenal ARF. This accounts for 40 to 60% of cases. It is caused by diminution in the renal blood flow. Major causes include:
  1. Cardiac. These include CHF, cardiogenic shock, and pericardial tamponade.
  2. Hepatic. Alcoholic hepatitis or cirrhosis produce a relative decrease in intravascular volume through accumulation of ascites or arteriovenous fistulae.
  3. Hemorrhage. Blood loss can produce acute hypovolemia that leads to ARF.
  4. GI losses. Diarrhea, vomiting, intraluminal fluid in bowel obstruction, and intraluminal gut fluid and bowel wall edema in inflammatory bowel disease may cause hypovolemia.
  5. Sequestration of intravascular volume. This may occur in patients with burns or pancreatitis.
  6. Medications
     a. Loop diuretics (furosemide, bumetanide) and thiazide diuretics may cause hypovolemia.
     b. Because of washout of the interstitial osmolar gradient, the prolonged use of diuretics results in loss of concentrating function. This is the setting in

TABLE 29–1. Diagnostic Features of the 4 Types of ARF

Prerenal
  Signs on physical examination of volume depletion or
    "third-spacing" of fluid
  Volume depletion by hemodynamic criteria such as
    pulmonary capillary wedge pressure
  Urinalysis and laboratory findings as in Tables 29–3 and
    29–4
  Response to volume repletion with reversal of azotemia
    plus, if oliguric, increase in urine output with
    normalization of urinary indices
  No evidence of obstruction on ultrasound if oliguria
    persists
Postrenal
  Laboratory indices similar to those in prerenal azotemia
    (see Table 29–4)
  Ultrasonographic evidence of bilateral hydronephrosis, or
    unilateral hydronephrosis if a single kidney is present,
    or evidence of intraabdominal, retroperitoneal, or
    pelvic obstructing masses
  Evidence of bilateral obstructed flow on radiohippurate
    scans
  Evidence of obstructed flow on retrograde pyelography
Intrarenal: primary parenchymal disease
  Urinalyses in accordance with Table 29–3
  Severe hypertension is common
  No evidence of obstruction on ultrasound if persistently
    oliguric
Intrarenal: acute tubular necrosis
  No signs, symptoms, or hemodynamic indications of
    ongoing hypovolemia or persistent ARF following
    correction of hypovolemia
  Urinalyses and laboratory findings in accordance with
    Tables 29–3 and 29–4
  No response to volume repletion or challenge with either
    resolution of azotemia or increased urine output
  No evidence of obstruction

which nonoliguric prerenal azotemia is most
common.

  c. Nonoliguric prerenal ARF may also be caused by
inhibition of the effect of antidiuretic hormone
(ADH, vasopressin) on the collecting duct by lithium or demeclocycline.

• Postrenal ARF. This category causes 2 to 15% of ARF
cases. Generally, the patient is oliguric or anuric. There
may be wide fluctuations in urine output due to changes in
the obstructing lesions with the patient's position.

  1. Intraureteric obstruction. Causes include (in order of
frequency) stones, clots, pus, or tissue (i.e., papillary
necrosis due to diabetes mellitus or analgesic drug
excess).

2. Extraureteric obstruction
   a. This is most commonly caused by tumors involving the retroperitoneal lymph nodes (e.g., lymphomas and testicular carcinomas). In women, 70% of cases of obstructive ARF are caused by pelvic tumors.
   b. In 5% of all patients with postrenal ARF, the cause is retroperitoneal fibrosis from ergot alkaloids or radiation therapy.
3. Lower urinary tract obstruction. Prostatic hypertrophy causes >80% of obstructive ARF cases in men.
- Intrarenal ARF (Table 29–2). Representing 30 to 50% of all ARF, this category may be further subdivided into primary renal parenchymal disorders and ATN.
   1. Primary renal parenchymal disease accounts for 10 to 20% of intrarenal ARF in adults.

TABLE 29–2. Causes of Intrarenal Acute Renal Failure

Primary renal disease
  Vascular
    Glomerulonephritis
    Vasculitis of polyarteritis nodosa
    Scleroderma
    Malignant hypertension
    Thrombotic thrombocytopenic purpura
    Hemolytic-uremic syndrome
    Renal embolization
  Tubulointerstitial diseases
    Medications (e.g., semisynthetic β-lactamase–resistant penicillins, nonsteroidal anti-inflammatory drugs)
    Hypercalcemia
    Hypokalemia (severe)
    Myeloma proteins
  Crystallization within the tubular lumen
    Oxalate crystals (ethylene glycol ingestion)
    Urate crystals (hyperuricemia greater than 18 to 20 mg/dl)
    Methotrexate derivatives
    Tumor lysis syndrome (urate and calcium phosphate deposition)
Acute tubular necrosis
  Ischemic ATN
    Hypotension
    Sepsis
    Aortic cross-clamping
    Prerenal azotemia (severe)
  Toxic ATN
    Heavy metals
    Halogenated alkanes
    Medications (e.g., aminoglycosides, radiographic contrast material)
    Myoglobin (rhabdomyolysis)
    Hemoglobin (extensive hemolysis)

2. Acute tubular necrosis (ATN). The term ATN is largely a misnomer, since tubular necrosis is almost never found. Vasomotor changes produce tubular ischemia, tubular dysfunction, and tubuloglomerular feedback, which in turn cause decreased glomerular filtration rates.

• Oliguric versus nonoliguric ARF
   1. ARF may initially be nonoliguric or oliguric. Oliguric ARF may become nonoliguric spontaneously or with volume or diuretic therapy.
   2. Nonoliguric renal failure accounts for 30 to 40% of intrarenal ARF and has a better prognosis. Nonoliguric ARF has a mortality of 30%, and oliguric ARF has a mortality of 60%.

CLINICAL FEATURES

• Prerenal ARF
   1. History. A history of dizziness, syncope, CHF, hepatic disease with ascites, chronic renal insufficiency, use of diuretics for any reason, or persistent vomiting or diarrhea suggests prerenal status.
   2. Physical examination
      a. Physical examination may reveal postural changes in pulse and blood pressure.
      b. A large weight loss may indicate volume depletion.
      c. Weight gain may accompany intravascular volume loss with total body volume overload. Signs include ascites, lower extremity or sacral edema, chronic stasis dermatitis, or ulcers in the lower extremities. Signs of congestive heart failure may be present.
   3. Hemodynamics. Trends must be followed to reach valid conclusions.
      a. A persistently low pulmonary capillary wedge pressure (PCWP) suggests hypovolemia, whereas a rising or high PCWP suggests cardiac failure and renal underperfusion.
      b. In patients with cardiac or pulmonary disease, physical signs may be confusing or absent and hemodynamic monitoring plays a larger role in diagnosis.

• Postrenal ARF
   1. History. Relevant historical features include:
      a. Nephrolithiasis
      b. Repeated pyelonephritis, or immune deficiency with fungal disease
      c. Hematuria, particularly gross hematuria
      d. Previous pelvic tumor or lymphoma
      e. Previous abdominal radiation treatment that may cause fibrosis
      f. Drug ingestion (e.g., treatment for migraine headaches with ergot alkaloids)

    g. Hesitancy, dribbling, incontinence, frequency, or dysuria suggesting prostatic disease

  2. Physical examination

    a. Bilateral flank pain and tenderness occurs in 70 to 80% of patients with obstruction. Costovertebral angle tenderness may suggest ascending infection.

    b. Signs of inferior vena cava or lymphatic obstruction (brawny edema or lymphedema in the lower extremities) or ascites may indicate tumor.

• Intrarenal ARF: primary parenchymal disease

  1. History

    a. A history of upper respiratory infection suggests postinfectious glomerulonephritis. Fever, rash, or pleuritic pain may point to vasculitis.

    b. Histories of drug use are important. Commonly implicated medications include NSAIDs, lithium, antibiotics, diuretics, chemotherapeutic agents (cyclophosphamide, methotrexate), anticoagulants, and cimetidine.

  2. Physical examination may find evidence of vasculitis. Hypertension is present in more than 85% of cases but is nonspecific. Rashes are often present. Sclerodactyly suggests scleroderma.

• Intrarenal ARF: acute tubular necrosis. Hypotension does not need to be documented in postsurgical patients, particularly those older than 60, in order for the physician to suspect ATN. A history of preexisting prerenal azotemia may point to progression to ATN. Other causes include:

  1. Sepsis. When ATN is present without a well-defined etiology, it is worthwhile to look for sepsis.

  2. Medications or toxins. Aminoglycosides and radiologic contrast material are common causes of ATN in hospitalized patients. Exposure to dry cleaning fluid or heavy metals is an often neglected historical item.

  3. Rhabdomyolysis. Persons found unconscious or with seizures may sustain rhabdomyolysis. Hypokalemia and hypophosphatemia may induce rhabdomyolysis.

  4. Hemolysis. Patients with hemolysis (transfusion reactions, microangiopathic hemolysis) may have ATN.

RECOMMENDED DIAGNOSTIC APPROACH (Tables 29–3 and 29–4)

• Urinalysis. If red blood cell casts are present, studies to evaluate autoimmune diseases may be indicated (Chapter 31).

• Urine osmolality. Urine osmolality (U_{osm}) should be measured. Specific gravity measurements are of limited utility in patients with ATN because it may be affected by dissolved substances such as glucose or protein.

  1. Prerenal azotemia. Ninety percent of patients have $U_{osm} \geq 500$ mOsm/L.

  2. Postrenal ARF. Initial U_{osm} resembles that of prerenal azotemia. Persistent obstruction leads to tubular damage and transition to a lower U_{osm}.

TABLE 29–3. Urinalysis in Diagnosis of Acute Renal Failure

	RBC	WBC (POLYS)	WBC	EPITHELIAL CELLS	PIGMENTED GRANULAR CASTS	RBC CASTS	WBC CASTS	CRYSTALS
Proliferative glomerulonephritis	++	+	0	0	0	++	+	0
Small vessel vasculitis	++	+	0	0	0	++	+	0
Obstructive uropathy	++	+ (esp. with infection)	0	+c	+	0	+	+ (urate crystals if stones)
Tubulointerstitial nephritis	+	+	++b	+	+	+	+	+
Acute tubular necrosis	++	+	0	++	++	0	+	+
Pyelonephritis	+	++	0	+	0	0	++	+
Preglomerular vasculitis	0	0	0	0	0	0	0	0
Scleroderma	0	0	0	0	0	0	0	0
Hemolytic-uremic syndrome	+	+	0	0	0	+	+	0
Tumor lysis syndrome	+	+	0	++	++	+	+	++

a All findings are transient; one must perform serial urinalyses.

b Eosinophiluria occurs in 65 to 85% of patients with tubulointerstitial nephritis but is easily missed, owing to transience.

c Inflammatory cells are common in obstruction; the physician should also look for tumor cells (i.e., lymphocytes in lymphoma or transitional cells in carcinoma).

Source: Bursten SL. Acute renal failure. In: Cummins RO, Eisenberg MS (eds.), Blue Book of Medical Diagnosis: W. B. Saunders, 1986. p. 202.

TABLE 29–4. Laboratory Findings in Acute Renal Failure

TEST	PRERENAL AZOTEMIA	ACUTE TUBULAR NECROSIS	POSTRENAL[a]
Osmolality	>500 mOsm/L	<350 mOsm/L	Initially >500 mOsm/L but decreases
U_{osm}/P_{osm}	>1.25	<1.07	Variable
BUN/CREAT (plasma)	>20/1	10/1	>20/1
U_{creat}/P_{creat}	≥20	≤10	Variable
U_{Na}	≤20	≥40	>100 in postobstructive diuretic phase
Fractional excretion of sodium FE_{Na}[b]	<1%	>2%	Variable

[a] Most laboratory test results are variable in postrenal acute renal failure depending on whether obstruction is complete, variable, or superimposed on an interstitial process.

[b] $FE_{Na} = (U_{Na}/P_{Na}) \times (P_{creat}/U_{creat})$.

3. ATN. Ninety percent of patients have $U_{osm} \leq 350$ mOsm/L (due to loss of concentrating ability with tubular dysfunction).

4. U_{osm}/P_{osm}
   a. The overlap range (U_{osm} 350 to 500 mOsm/L) is not diagnostically useful. The ratio of urine to plasma osmoles (U_{osm}/P_{osm}) is more useful and eliminates the error induced by azotemia.
   b. Ninety-five percent of patients with ATN have $U_{osm}/P_{osm} \leq 1.07$; 95% of patients with prerenal azotemia have $U_{osm}/P_{osm} \geq 1.25$.

- BUN and creatinine
  1. Creatinine. With complete cessation of glomerular filtration, serum creatinine increases by about 1 mg/dl/day. This daily increase is less in patients with decreased muscle mass (as in an older person) and more (up to 2.5 mg/dl/day) in young muscular males.
  2. Urea
     a. Urea is freely filtered and variably reabsorbed. Reabsorption is proportional to the flow of water in tubules, the presence of ADH, the local tubular pressure, and the peritubular blood flow.
     b. Production of urea is affected by hepatic disease and varies widely. Starvation, low-protein diet, and hepatic failure cause decreased production of BUN, whereas hypercatabolic states such as burns, sepsis, infection, glucocorticoid use, trauma, and postsurgical condition increase its production.
     c. The rate at which BUN rises with complete cessation of glomerular filtration ranges from 24 mg/dl/day to 60 mg/dl/day.

- Plasma BUN/creatinine ratio
  1. Reabsorption of urea is increased greatly in prerenal and postrenal azotemia.
  2. A BUN/creatinine ratio $\geq 20/1$ is present in more than 80% of cases of renal and postrenal azotemia.
  3. Intrarenal ARF and ATN are characterized by proportionate BUN/creatinine increments (10/1) because of a direct drop-off in filtration.

- Urine creatinine
  1. Urine creatinine (U_{creat}) is a marker of ability to concentrate urine, since creatinine is filtered without reabsorption and with only slight secretion.
  2. $U_{creat}/P_{creat} \leq 10$ is found in 85% of patients with ATN, whereas $U_{creat}/P_{creat} \geq 20$ is found in 85% of patients with prerenal ARF.

- Urine sodium (U_{Na})
  1. The ability to conserve sodium in proportion to the amount filtered is a marker of intact tubular function.
  2. $U_{Na} \leq 20$ mEq/L occurs in over 90% of prerenal azotemia cases, whereas a value ≥ 40 mEq/L is found in over 90% of patients with ATN.

- Fractional excretion of sodium (FE_{Na})
  1. A more sensitive test is the calculated FE_{Na}: $U_{Na}/P_{Na} \times P_{creat}/U_{creat}$.
  2. Over 90% of patients with prerenal azotemia have values < 1%, whereas over 90% of patients with ATN have values > 2%.
  3. A FE_{Na} of <1% is common in renal parenchymal disease, particularly glomerulonephritis, since the tubules retain function and attempt to compensate in response to diseased glomeruli and falling glomerular filtration rate.
- Other laboratory tests
  1. A clue to the presence of tubuloischemic necrosis may be hyperchloremic acidosis of rapid onset.
  2. Myoglobin levels in urine may confirm rhabdomyolysis.
  3. A severe anion gap metabolic acidosis with oxalate crystals in urine may indicate ethylene glycol toxicity.
  4. A hyperchloremic tubular acidosis with hyperkalemia occurs in 80% of patients with postobstructive diuresis.
- Ultrasound
  1. Ultrasonographic examination of the kidneys, ureters, and pelvis may reveal the presence and cause of obstruction in 85% of cases.
  2. If the index of suspicion of obstruction is high (as with preexisting tumor, abdominal mass, transplantation, or a single kidney), a retrograde pyelogram may be indicated.
- Nuclear studies
  1. Flow studies (pertechnetate, glucoheptonate) measure renal perfusion and may exclude vascular problems.
  2. Hippurate functional studies can measure continuing renal function, suggest or confirm the presence of acute tubular necrosis, diagnose obstruction, or suggest renal transplant rejection.
- IV urography is limited by the difficulty of giving dye to patients with marginal fluid status and by fear of exacerbating renal failure.
- Renal biopsy is rarely indicated in ARF. Biopsy is usually reserved for oligoanuria that persists for longer than 3 weeks or when a treatable disease (e.g., Goodpasture's syndrome, SLE) is strongly suspected.

Bibliography

Goldstein MB. Acute renal failure. Med Clin North Amer 1983; 67:1325–1341.

Levinsky NG, Alexander EA. Acute renal failure. In: Brenner BM, Rector FC Jr, eds., The Kidney. Philadelphia, W.B. Saunders, 1986.

Myers BD, Morna SM. Hemodynamically mediated acute renal failure. N Engl J Med 1986;314:97.

Spital A, et al. Acute idiopathic tubulointerstitial nephritis: Report of two cases and review of the literature. Am J Kid Dis 1987;9:71–78.

30

CHRONIC RENAL FAILURE

STUART L. BURSTEN

Superficially, it might be said that the function of the kidneys is to make urine; but in a more considered view one can say that the kidneys make the stuff of philosophy itself.

HOMER W. SMITH (1895–1962)

DEFINITIONS AND GENERAL COMMENTS

- Definition. Chronic renal failure (CRF) is defined as a long-term decline in kidney function.
- Criteria for diagnosis. The major criterion is a slow inexorable rise in the serum blood urea nitrogen (BUN) and creatinine levels.
  1. Most diseases that cause CRF usually appear as acute renal failure (ARF).
     a. A renal biopsy may be performed at the time that the patient is examined initially in ARF.
     b. When a chronic process is suspected, or the creatinine level is already greater than 5 mg/dl, a biopsy is seldom helpful and reveals nonspecific chronic GN or diffuse scarring.
  2. Ultrasound can examine renal size and estimate functional reserve: small, scarred, or contracted kidneys have little functional component remaining.
  3. Three phases of CRF may be identified:
     a. Renal insufficiency—malaise, nocturia, and mild anemia.
     b. Frank renal failure—progressive acidosis, hypocalcemia, hyperphosphatemia, and worsening anemia.
     c. Uremia or end-stage renal disease. The glomerular filtration rate is less than 5 cc/min, and severe symptoms and metabolic-endocrine disturbances require dialysis.

MAJOR CAUSES OF CRF

- Glomerular disease. Glomerular diseases cause 60% of CRF cases.
  1. Nephrotic causes: membranous glomerulonephritis (GN), focal glomerulosclerosis, membranoproliferative GN, and chronic nonspecific GN.

245

2. Nephritic causes: postinfectious GN, IgA nephropathy, Goodpasture's syndrome, idiopathic crescentic GN, and non-Goodpasture's anti-GBM disease.

- Vascular disease: diabetic nephropathy, malignant hypertension, bilateral renal artery stenosis, fibromuscular hyperplasia, polyarteritis nodosa, and Wegener's granulomatosis.

- Tubular disease: heavy metal poisoning from lead or cadmium, analgesic nephropathy, chronic hypercalcemia, chronic hypokalemia, Fanconi's syndrome, radiation nephritis, uric acid nephropathy, amyloidosis, and multiple myeloma.

- Intrinsic urinary tract disease: chronic pyelonephritis, chronic upper tract obstruction (stones, pus, clots, or tumors), and lower tract obstruction, most commonly prostatic.

- Collagen-vascular disease: SLE, scleroderma, and mixed cryoglobulinemia.

- Congenital processes: polycystic kidneys, medullary cystic disease, and hypoplastic kidneys.

- Causes of ARF. Any process that causes ARF may also advance to CRF if renal damage is sufficiently severe. (Although most ARF is reversible, an estimated 10 to 15% of cases advance to CRF and end-stage disease.)

FACTORS THAT ACCELERATE END-STAGE RENAL DISEASE

Patients with chronic renal insufficiency may have slow progression of their dysfunction. Any patient with a rapidly rising BUN and creatinine level, when previously the patient had a slow, defined rate of increase, should be evaluated for:

- Urinary tract obstruction. This is seen most often when obstruction was the original cause of the CRF. Uremic patients may also have bladder neck dysfunction and obstructive urethral edema after instrumentation. Signs and symptoms are frequently absent.

- Urinary tract infection. Virtually 100% of patients with CRF will be infected at some time and almost universally after instrumentation.

- Volume depletion. This is a relatively common problem in early renal insufficiency, when the ability to conserve sodium may be lost. Diuretic use and acute fluid loss from vomiting, diarrhea, fever, or exercise may contribute to sodium loss.

- Hypokalemia. This is also more common than is generally suspected in CRF. Potassium-excreting ability is preserved until quite late in the course of CRF, with hyperkalemia generally a sign of far-advanced uremia. Preservation of volume may dictate sacrifice of potassium homeostasis.

COMPLICATIONS OF CRF

- Anemia
  1. The anemia of CRF is usually normochromic and normocytic. It is primarily due to decreased erythropoietin production, but diminished maturation and faster turnover of RBC play a role.
  2. Anemia usually begins early in the course of renal insufficiency with hematocrits of 25 to 32%. With frank renal failure, the level drops to 19 to 25%.
  3. Occult bleeding may cause iron-deficiency anemia. Platelet and clotting disorders promote blood loss.
- Platelet and clotting disorders
  1. CRF is often accompanied by an acquired von Willebrand's disorder, with factor VIII and platelet dysfunction.
  2. These problems are generally observed in advanced uremia, in which the BUN is 100 to 150 mg/dl and creatinine is below 10 mg/dl. They are aggravated by aspirin and infection. Antibiotics that affect vitamin K–dependent factors (cefamandole, moxalactam, and cefoperazone) should not be administered.
- Peripheral neuropathy
  1. Peripheral neuropathy occurs in patients with advanced uremic renal failure. It is similar to the peripheral neuropathy of diabetes. It is probably toxin related and is partially reversible with dialysis.
  2. It may be diagnosed by careful evaluation of vibration sense, soft touch, and position sense. Nerve conduction studies are confirmatory.
- Aluminum toxicity dementia
  1. This degenerative disorder is due to deposition of aluminum in the CNS.
  2. Aluminum dementia may occur prior to dialysis in patients with advanced uremia if there have been months to years of consumption of aluminum-containing antacids for phosphate binding.
  3. Aluminum dementia is manifest by a stuttering dysphasia that progresses to aphasia, seizures, and disorientation. Hemodialysis may aggravate these findings.
  4. Serum aluminum levels are difficult to obtain, and their meaning is not fully understood.
- Renal osteodystrophy
  1. In young persons with uremia who have not yet had closure of the growth plates, the onset of osteodystrophy produces severe bone pain and growth retardation.
  2. In older patients, osteodystrophy is usually asymptomatic until it is far advanced and pathologic fractures develop.
  3. Uremic osteodystrophy varies widely from person to person, with respect to onset and patient response to vitamin D metabolites, calcium supplements, and aluminum.

- Metabolic complications
  1. Uremic patients develop a peripheral insensitivity to insulin causing glucose intolerance and hyperinsulinism.
  2. Inhibition of lipoprotein lipase by uremic toxins, plus hyperinsulinism, causes the hyperlipidemic state that is characteristic of uremia (increased VLDL).
  3. Diabetics whose condition progresses to CRF require less insulin because of reduced renal clearance.

- Vascular complications
  1. Hypertension. The hypertension in CRF is due to chronic volume overload and increased peripheral resistance from altered vascular tone. The blood pressure is often difficult to control until dialysis is initiated.
  2. Pericardial disease. Because of hemodialysis, with its intermittent anticoagulation and associated hemorrhage, pericardial disease has become common. Echocardiography may assist in the diagnosis of all pericardial conditions.
     a. Acute pericarditis. This common complication of uremia usually responds to dialysis. Symptoms include fever and pleuritic chest pain. A 2- or 3-component friction rub is present (even if intermittent) in all patients.
     b. Cardiac tamponade
        i. This may cause a significant fall in blood pressure during dialysis.
        ii. Neck veins are monophasically elevated, with distant heart sounds. A pulsus paradoxus (greater than 15 to 20 mmHg) is present in 75 to 80% of patients.
        iii. Right heart catheterization reveals equalization of diastolic pressures in all chambers.
     c. Chronic constrictive pericarditis
        i. In this condition, the neck veins are phasically elevated, demonstrating Kussmaul's elevation, a paradoxic rise during inspiration, which is not seen in pericardial tamponade.
        ii. There may be a pericardial knock caused by ventricular constriction at the end of diastole.
        iii. Pulsus paradoxus is rarely, if ever, present.
  3. Atherosclerosis. This results from a combination of factors found in end-stage disease: glucose intolerance, poorly controlled hypertension, hyperlipidemia, and the high prevalence of cigarette smoking (60 to 80% of cases) in patients with CRF.

- Infection
  1. Uremia predisposes to bacterial and viral infections through inhibition of phagocytic ability and T-cell deficiency.
  2. Fever is often suppressed in uremia. The most frequent

serious infections are staphylococcal septicemia, staphylococcal abscesses in the urinary tract (especially perinephric abscesses), osteomyelitis, infectious endocarditis, hepatitis B, and herpes zoster.

RECOMMENDED DIAGNOSTIC APPROACH

- Factors that accelerate CRF
  1. Urinary tract obstruction. Ultrasound examination of the kidneys, pelvis, and retroperitoneal area is indicated if the BUN or creatinine levels have suddenly increased.
  2. Urinary tract infection. Microscopic examination of clean-catch urine specimens for WBC, RBC, and bacteria is imperative. As renal failure progresses, urinalysis becomes less helpful.
  3. Volume depletion. Postural changes in blood pressure and pulse may suggest volume depletion. In patients with autonomic neuropathy (e.g., diabetics), this is a nonspecific finding.
- Complications of CRF
  1. Anemia
     a. The hematocrit should be followed closely for trends and changes. Microcytosis may reflect iron deficiency, but it may accompany normal iron status in the anemia of CRF.
     b. Serum iron and transferrin levels only reveal changes consistent with peripheral block to iron utilization. Ferritin usually accumulates in patients with CRF, but a low serum level (less than 20 to 30 ng/dl) suggests iron deficiency.
  2. Platelet and clotting disorders. These may be diagnosed by measuring the platelet count and the bleeding, prothrombin, and partial thromboplastin times.
  3. Peripheral neuropathy
     a. This may be suspected by clinical evaluation of vibration sense, soft touch, and position sense.
     b. Nerve conduction studies confirm the presence of a neuropathy.
  4. Aluminum toxicity dementia. This is a clinical diagnosis based on a compatible history and the findings of dysphasia or aphasia, seizures, and disorientation.
  5. Renal osteodystrophy
     a. In patients with persistent hypocalcemia and hyperphosphatemia, hand radiographs should be obtained to screen for the onset of osteodystrophy.
     b. Radioimmunoassay for *N-terminal* parathyroid hormone (PTH) may be obtained to demonstrate the secondary hyperparathyroidism.
     c. Definition of the degree and type of disease requires a bone biopsy with special stains for matrix and aluminum.

Bibliography

Brenner BM, Stein JH, eds. Chronic renal failure. In: The Contemporary Issues in Nephrology Series, No. 7. New York, Churchill-Livingstone, 1981.

Eknoyan G, ed. Chronic renal failure. In: Kurtzman NA, ed. Seminars in Nephrology, Vol. 1, No. 2. New York, Grune and Stratton, 1981.

Tzamaloukas AH. Diagnosis and management of bone disorders in chronic renal failure. Med Clin North Am 1990;74:961–974.

31

NEPHROTIC SYNDROME

ALAN WATSON

It is no exaggeration to say that the composition of the blood is determined not by what the mouth takes in but by what the kidneys keep.

HOMER W. SMITH (1895–1962)

DEFINITION

1. Nephrotic syndrome refers to a constellation of clinical and laboratory abnormalities that are the consequences of proteinuria in excess of 3.5 g/24 hr/1.73 m^2.*
2. The nephrotic syndrome is not an etiologic diagnosis but merely indicates abnormal glomerular permeability. This may be the consequence of a primary glomerular disease (primary or idiopathic nephrotic syndrome) or may represent a renal manifestation of a wide variety of disease processes (secondary nephrotic syndrome).
3. The four criteria generally regarded as necessary for the complete diagnosis of the nephrotic syndrome include:
   a. Proteinuria: >3.5 g/24 hr/1.73 m^2
   b. Hypoalbuminemia: <2.5 g/dl
   c. Edema
   d. Hyperlipidemia
4. Whether the latter 3 features actually develop in the setting of nephrotic-range proteinuria depends partly on factors such as the compensatory reserve of the liver to synthesize albumin (normal rate of synthesis is 12 to 14 g/day), the degree of increase in albumin catabolism by the kidney, and the avidity of salt retention.
5. From a practical point of view, a diagnosis of nephrotic syndrome is commonly made when proteinuria is greater than 3.5 g/24 hr/1.73 m^2 of body surface area and is, according to urine protein electrophoresis, composed predominantly of albumin. In some conditions (membranous nephropathy, diabetic nephropathy) the proteinuria may be nonselective, and a broad spectrum of serum proteins are filtered.

---

* A 70-kg, 175-cm (5′ 9″) person has a body surface area of 1.84 m^2, see Chapter 61 for nomogram).

EPIDEMIOLOGY

1. In the U.S. and European pediatric populations (under 16 years), the incidence of nephrotic syndrome is approximately 2 to 5 cases per 100,000 persons/yr, with a male-to-female predominance of 2 to 2.5 : 1. Minimal change disease accounts for over 60% of these cases and for over 90% of nephrotic syndrome as a result of primary glomerular disease in children between the ages of 2 and 6 years.
2. In adults, minimal-change disease is less common, the sex incidence is closer to unity, and secondary nephrotic syndrome is more frequently encountered. The increasing prevalence of diabetes mellitus in the adult population is largely responsible for the latter feature.

DIFFERENTIAL DIAGNOSIS

1. Renal biopsy makes it possible to classify idiopathic nephrotic syndrome into reasonably well-defined clinico-pathologic entities. The primary disorders and their relative frequencies in pediatric and adult populations are shown in Table 31–1.
2. The wide variety of disease states, chemical toxins, infections, and medications that can be associated clinically with the nephrotic syndrome are shown in Table 31–2.
3. The most frequent causes of secondary nephrotic syndrome are diabetes mellitus, multiple myeloma, neoplastic disease, and connective tissue diseases, particularly SLE. IV drug use (leading to heroin nephropathy) and associated infections, such as hepatitis B and HIV infection, are, in certain areas, commonly associated with the nephrotic syndrome.

TABLE 31–1. Prevalence of Primary Glomerular Disease in the Nephrotic Syndrome

Disease	Children (%)	Adults (%)
Minimal-change disease	60	20
Membranous glomerulonephritis	6	30
Proliferative glomerulonephritis	10	30
Focal glomerular sclerosis	8	8
Membranoproliferative glomerulonephritis	10	5
Mesangial proliferative glomerulonephritis	5	6
Miscellaneous	1	1

TABLE 31-2. Major Causes of Secondary Nephrotic Syndrome

Metabolic disease
  Diabetes mellitus
  Amyloidosis
Connective tissue disease
  SLE
  Polyarteritis
  Cryoglobulinemia
Infection
  Bacterial: subacute bacterial endocarditis, leprosy,
    syphilis
  Viral: hepatitis B, HIV, cytomegalovirus, Epstein-Barr
    virus
  Protozoal: malaria, toxoplasmosis
  Helminthic: filariasis, schistosomiasis
Neoplasia
  Lymphoma, leukemia, multiple myeloma
  Lung, colon, stomach, breast
Medication/Toxin
  Penicillamine, gold, captopril, heroin, NSAIDs
  Silver, bismuth, mercury
Heredofamilial
  Familial nephrotic syndrome
  Sickle cell disease
  α_1-Antitrypsin deficiency
  Fabry's disease
  Nail patella syndrome
Vascular
  Renal artery stenosis (rare)
  CHF
  Tricuspid incompetence
  Constrictive pericarditis
  Renal vein thrombosis
Miscellaneous
  Pregnancy
  Massive obesity
  Vesicoureteric reflux

CLINICAL FEATURES

Clinical features of the nephrotic syndrome arise as a direct result of abnormal glomerular permeability and the resultant massive proteinuria.

1. Edema: The hallmark sign of the nephrotic syndrome is edema, which reflects an increase in the interstitial component of the extracellular fluid compartment. Edema is usually localized to gravity-dependent areas, although in more severe instances it may become generalized (anasarca). Edema of internal organs may also give rise to symptoms such as anorexia, nausea, and vomiting that result from edema and dysfunction of the GI mucosa.

2. Malnutrition: Loss of lean body mass can result from a persistently negative nitrogen balance (decreased intake plus increased loss and increased catabolism of albumin), which in children may be great enough to induce marasmus. The concomitant presence of edema may mask weight loss resulting from malnutrition.

3. Susceptibility to infection: A diminution of humoral defense mechanisms (IgG, factor B, decreased opsonization) is regarded as responsible for the well-recognized susceptibility of patients with nephrotic syndrome to severe infections, notably caused by pneumococcus, *Klebsiella,* and coliform species.

4. Thromboembolic tendency
   a. Renal vein thrombosis occurs in 5 to 20% of cases. Patients are commonly asymptomatic, though flank pain, hematuria, loss of renal function, and pulmonary embolism may occur. Whereas in the past it was assumed that renal vein thrombosis was the causative factor in nephrotic syndrome, recent observations suggest that the syndrome precedes and predisposes to the development of renal vein thrombosis. Diagnosis is made noninvasively (ultrasound, CT) or by renal venography.
   b. Other complications occur in 20% of cases. Venous thrombotic complications affect the pulmonary veins and extremities. Arterial complications can affect the coronary, cerebral, and peripheral circulations.

5. Metabolic complications
   a. Accelerated atherosclerosis is related to lipid abnormalities.
   b. Osteomalacia is related to altered vitamin D metabolism.

6. Signs and symptoms of underlying disease. These include retinopathy and neuropathy in diabetes mellitus; bone pain and anemia in multiple myeloma; arthritis and rash in connective tissue disease; and periodic chills or fevers and a history of travel in malaria.

LABORATORY FEATURES

1. Proteinuria: The proteinuria is in excess of 3.5 g/24 hr/ 1.73 m^2 of body surface area and is predominantly albumin. The diagnosis of nephrotic syndrome relies heavily on the quantification of urinary protein in a 24-hr urine collection. It is well recognized that the amount of protein excreted can vary substantially from day to day and that errors in timing the 24-hr urine samples are common. Moreover, such collections are cumbersome and time-consuming.

   Several studies have demonstrated that a determination of the protein : creatinine ratio in single urine samples correlates well with the quantity of protein in timed urine collections and that a protein : creatinine ratio of greater than 3.5 represents nephrotic-range proteinuria. The protein:creatinine ratio of single urine samples may prove to be a satisfactory substitute for the determination of protein excretion in 24-hr urine collections.

2. Hypoalbuminemia. Serum albumin is usually less than 3.5 g/dl.

3. Hyperlipidemia. VLDL and LDL levels increase; HDL level decreases.

4. Hypocalcemia. The observed reduction in serum calcium is not solely a result of a decrease in the protein-bound fraction of calcium. Vitamin D–binding protein is lost in the urine causing a decrease in serum concentrations of $25(OH)D_3$ and $1,25(OH)_2D_3$ with a resultant decrease in calcium absorption and the ionized calcium fraction of the serum. For reasons that remain unclear, however, these changes are not observed in all patients with the nephrotic syndrome.

5. Thyroid function studies. Total thyroxine and thryoxine-binding globulin increase, but the level of free thyroxine is normal.

6. Coagulation factors. Factors V and VII and fibrinogen increase while antithrombin III decreases. The increase in fibrinogen is the most consistent and important abnormality.

7. Immunoglobulin. Low serum levels of immunoglobulin G may result from urinary losses and renal hypercatabolism.

8. Urinalysis. Proximal tubule dysfunction may cause glycosuria. Glycosuria alone does not necessarily indicate an impaired glucose tolerance in the setting of nephrotic syndrome. Oval fat bodies represent cholesterol esters, which appear as "Maltese crosses" on polarizing microscopy.

9. Miscellaneous findings. Hypokalemia, hypomagnesemia, and a proximal renal tubular acidosis may all occur.

RECOMMENDED DIAGNOSTIC APPROACH

The high incidence of minimal-change lesions as the cause of nephrotic syndrome in children allows presumptive diagnosis of this entity in the pediatric setting. A minimal-change lesion is even more likely if steroid therapy induces remission of proteinuria. In the occasional case in which steroid/cytotoxic drug therapy fails to improve the nephrotic syndrome, a renal biopsy is indicated.

In adults, a work-up of secondary causes of nephrotic syndrome includes a detailed clinical evaluation, serum and urine protein electrophoresis, a lupus screen, hepatitis B surface antigen and possibly HIV antibody status. Where a presumed cause such as diabetes or amyloidosis are detected, a renal biopsy is generally unnecessary unless the subsequent clinical course proves incompatible with the clinical diagnosis. In such circumstances, a renal biopsy should be performed. When no obvious cause is apparent, renal biopsy generally provides an accurate diagnosis and prognostic assessment and aids in the formulation of a rational therapeutic plan.

Bibliography

Cameron JS, Glassock RJ, eds. The Nephrotic Syndrome. New York, Marcel Dekker, Inc., 1988.

Carbone L, et al. Course and prognosis of human immunodeficiency virus-associated nephropathy. Am J Med 1989;87:389–395.

Dubrow A, et al. The changing spectrum of heroin-associated nephropathy. Am J Kid Dis 1985;5:36–41.

Glassock RJ, et al. Primary glomerular disease. In: Brenner B, Rector F, eds. The Kidney, 2nd ed. Philadelphia, W.B. Saunders, 1981.

Harrington JT, Kassirer JP. Renal vein thrombosis. Ann Rev Med 1982;33:255–262.

Keating MA, Althausen AF. The clinical spectrum of renal vein thrombosis. J Urol 1985;133:938–945.

ACUTE GLOMERULONEPHRITIS AND THE NEPHRITIC SYNDROME

JEFFREY B. KOPP

FALSTAFF: What says the doctor to my water?
PAGE: He said, sir, the water itself was a good healthy water; but, for the party that owed it, he might have more diseases than he knew for.

SHAKESPEARE (1564–1616)

INTRODUCTION TO GLOMERULOPATHY

- The term "glomerulopathy" refers to a group of disorders (with various causes and clinical manifestations) with a pathologically and functionally abnormal glomerulus.
- Damage to the glomerulus usually results in proteinuria, which is often the only marker of glomerular disease. With further damage, cells may appear in the urine: erythrocytes, leukocytes, tubular cells, and casts. Finally, diminished renal function occurs, manifest by azotemia and sodium retention.
- The clinical syndromes seen include:
  1. Nephritic syndrome
  2. Proteinuria and nephrotic syndrome (see Chapter 31)
  3. Hematuria
  4. Rapidly progressive nephritis with azotemia
  5. Chronic renal failure (see Chapter 30)
- The term glomerulonephritis (GN) is derived from pathology and refers to inflammatory cells within the glomerulus. Hence the diagnosis of GN in a strict sense can only be made from a renal biopsy. Patients with the histologic diagnosis of GN may have any of the syndromes of glomerular disease listed above.

THE NEPHRITIC SYNDROME

The nephritic syndrome consists of the following features:
- Hematuria
  1. Hematuria, defined as more than 2 RBC per high power field of spun sediment, is nearly always present in

patients with the nephritic syndrome. Gross hematuria occurs in about one-third of cases.

2. Hematuria usually results from nonglomerular pathology; the presence of RBC casts or proteinuria is the key evidence that implicates the glomerulus.

- RBC casts
    1. RBC casts are nearly pathognomonic for the nephritic syndrome.
    2. When red cells enter the tubular lumen proximal to the ascending limb of Henle's loop (the site of Tamm-Horsfall protein secretion), they may be incorporated into a protein matrix to form red cell casts.
    3. Because casts in urine may disintegrate if the specimen is agitated or allowed to sit for too long, clinicians must examine the urine themselves.
        a. First-void urine is the most productive, since it often has the highest osmolarity and the lowest pH, which are conditions that favor cast formation.
        b. The best place to look for casts is at the periphery of the coverslip, since casts are carried there by capillary action.

- Proteinuria
    1. Normal 24-hr protein excretion is less than 150 mg. Patients with the nephritic syndrome usually excrete 500 mg to 3.5 g daily, but some excrete less and others exhibit nephrotic-range proteinuria, defined as excretion of greater than 3.5 g/day.
    2. In the nephritic syndrome the serum albumin is rarely reduced to the low levels that are seen in the nephrotic syndrome.

- Renal insufficiency
    1. Half of patients have some elevation of the BUN or creatinine levels.
    2. One-quarter of patients are oliguric, producing less than 500 cc urine/day.

- Sodium retention
    1. A fall in glomerular filtration causes active tubular reabsorption of sodium.
    2. Edema is seen in 90% of patients. Facial edema is common, in contrast to the dependent edema that results from CHF.
    3. CHF is not seen in patients with the nephritic syndrome unless they have an underlying cardiomyopathy or severe oliguria.
    4. Mild hypertension is common, but moderate or severe hypertension occurs in only 10% of patients.

- Diagnostic criteria (Table 32–1)
    1. The diagnosis of acute nephritic syndrome can be made in patients with hematuria with either RBC casts or proteinuria in excess of 0.5 g/day.
    2. This identifies some but not all of the patients for whom the eventual histologic diagnosis is GN. The conditions of some patients fit both nephritic and nephrotic syndromes.

TABLE 32–1. Diagnostic Features of the Nephritic Syndrome

Hematuria
RBC casts in urine
Proteinuria (0.5 to 3.5 g/day)
Renal insufficiency
Sodium retention (edema, hypertension)

CLINICAL FEATURES

- History
  1. Patients with the nephritic syndrome may complain of dark urine (more often described as smoky or tea-colored than bloody), flank or loin pain, headaches, or edema. Many patients are asymptomatic.
  2. Patients with nephritis as a result of systemic illness may have nonrenal symptoms, including rash in SLE, abdominal pain in Henoch-Schoenlein purpura, or fever in subacute bacterial endocarditis.
- Physical examination. The most useful clinical signs result from extracellular volume excess: hypertension and edema.

LABORATORY FEATURES

- Initial laboratory evaluation
  1. Initial tests include measurement of BUN and creatinine, urinalysis, and a 24-hr urine collection for creatinine clearance and protein. The 24-hr urine creatinine excretion reflects the completeness of the collection: women should excrete 10 to 15 mg of creatinine/kg of body weight/day; men should excrete 15 to 20 mg of creatinine/kg of body weight/day.
  2. Complement levels help elucidate the cause of the nephritic syndrome. The initial screen should include at least serum complement (C3) and total serum hemolytic complement (CH_{50}). The fourth component of complement (C4) is useful in some cases (Table 32–2).
- Subsequent evaluation is guided by the results of complement testing.
  1. Low serum complement
     a. Systemic diseases. These disorders are usually apparent from the history and physical examination by the time the nephritic syndrome is manifest. Specific clues include SLE, subacute bacterial endocarditis, shunt nephritis, and cryoglobulinemia.
     b. Renal diseases. Clinical distinction between the diseases in this category may be difficult.
        i. Poststreptococcal GN
           (i) This occurs 1 to 4 weeks after pharyngitis or skin infection with group A beta-hemolytic streptococci. Nephritis usually lasts 3 to 8 weeks.

TABLE 32–2. Diseases Associated with the Nephritic Syndrome

Low Serum Complement
A. Systemic diseases
    1. SLE
        Focal proliferative GN (75%)
        Diffuse proliferative GN (90%)
    2. Subacute bacterial endocarditis (90%)
    3. Shunt nephritis (infected ventriculoatrial shunts) (90%)
    4. Cryoglobulinemia (85%)
B. Renal diseases
    1. Acute poststreptococcal GN (80 to 90%)
    2. Membranoproliferative GN (70%)
Normal Serum Complement
A. Systemic diseases
    1. Polyarteritis nodosa
    2. Allergic granulomatosis
    3. Hypersensitivity vasculitis
    4. Wegener's granulomatosis
    5. Henoch-Schoenlein purpura
    6. Goodpasture's syndrome
    7. Visceral abscess
B. Renal diseases
    1. IgG-IgA nephropathy
    2. Rapidly progressive GN (RPGN)
        RPGN associated with granular deposits
        Anti-GBM antibody-mediated RPGN
        RPGN without glomerular deposits

Percentages are the approximate frequencies of depressed complement in the given disease.

    (ii) Features may include oliguria, gross hematuria, edema, hypertension, and encephalopathy. Five percent of adult patients have intermittent or persistent abnormalities in urine samples or renal function. An even smaller number have rapidly progressive GN (see below).

    (iii) Throat or skin cultures frequently yield *Streptococcus*.

    (iv) The antistreptolysin O (ASO) titer rises above 200 units in most patients with pharyngeal infection but it takes 3 to 5 weeks, the rise may be blunted by prior antibiotic therapy, and titers change little with skin infection.

    (v) Complement activation in poststreptococcal GN occurs by the alternative pathway, resulting in a low C3 (generally less than 50% of normal values), a low CH_{50}, and a normal C4. The low complement levels almost always return to normal by 8 weeks, even when some urinary abnormalities remain.

(vi) Abnormal immunoproteins may occur including immune complexes, cryoglobulins, and C3 nephritic factor (a nephritic factor related to an autoantibody acting on the C3 convertase of the classic complement pathway).

ii. Membranoproliferative GN (mesangiocapillary GN)

(i) This is a heterogeneous group of disorders which typically affects individuals between 5 and 30 years of age.

(ii) At least 2 pathologic syndromes exist: type I (subendothelial deposit disease) and type II (dense deposit disease).

(iii) Half of the patients have the nephrotic syndrome, 30% have lesser degrees of proteinuria, and the remainder present with the nephritic syndrome. Hypertension is less common than in poststreptococcal GN. Azotemia is present in half of cases and indicates a worse prognosis.

(iv) In membranoproliferative GN, serum C3 and CH_{50} concentrations are consistently and chronically depressed. In type I, the serum C4 level may be normal or low (reflecting alternate or classical pathway activation respectively). In type II, the serum C4 level is normal. The alternate pathway may be activated by C3 nephritic factor.

(v) Only 20% of patients have an elevated ASO titer (unlike poststreptococcal GN).

(vi) The distinction between the types of membranoproliferative GN is only possible by examination of a renal biopsy.

(vii) The clinical course is often progressive but the rate of progression is variable. After 10 years half of patients have end-stage renal disease.

2. Normal serum complement

a. Systemic diseases. Involvement of other organ systems helps guide the clinician in evaluating this group of patients. Associated systemic diseases and their signs and symptoms include:

i. Polyarteritis nodosa. Hypertension, arthralgias, eosinophilia, and gastrointestinal and neurologic symptoms.

ii. Allergic granulomatosis. Asthma and pulmonary infiltrates.

iii. Wegener's granulomatosis. Sinusitis and pulmonary infiltrates.

iv. Henoch-Schoenlein purpura. Arthritis, purpura, abdominal pain, and gastrointestinal bleeding.

    v. Goodpasture's syndrome. Pulmonary hemorrhage.

  b. Renal diseases. In renal diseases the time course of the illness is a useful discriminant.

    i. Idiopathic IgG-IgA nephropathy (Berger's disease, benign recurrent hematuria)

      (i) These patients have hematuria that is frequently gross, follows minor viral infection, either respiratory or gastrointestinal, and resolves in 2 to 6 days. Malaise, low-grade fever, and flank pain may occur.

      (ii) Blood pressure is usually normal and edema is absent.

      (iii) Twenty percent of patients have a slow progression to renal failure.

    ii. Rapidly progressive glomerulonephritis (RPGN)

      (i) This is a heterogeneous group of disorders which cause the nephritic syndrome with rapid loss of renal function. Typically the serum creatinine doubles in a 3-month period, and some patients (untreated) develop renal failure within weeks to months. Oliguria and azotemia are common at presentation.

      (ii) Since renal biopsy commonly demonstrates cellular crescents within Bowman's space, the pathologic term "crescentic GN" is sometimes used as a synonym for the clinical term RPGN.

      (iii) The diagnostic approach to the patient with this syndrome must include prompt renal biopsy, since therapy that is initiated early is more effective.

· Final evaluation: renal biopsy (see below).

RECOMMENDED DIAGNOSTIC APPROACH

· The clinical history, physical examination, and complement level measurements often indicate the diagnosis. A renal biopsy may only be needed if several diagnostic possibilities remain that involve different therapies or prognoses.

· In some cases, the rapid tempo of the disease makes such a delay for complement values unacceptable. Indications for hospitalization include oliguria, elevated creatinine level, malignant hypertension, or symptomatic fluid overload.

· Patients with the nephritic syndrome in whom renal function is deteriorating rapidly should be evaluated for other causes of renal dysfunction such as hypovolemia, nephrotoxins, and urinary obstruction. If these causes have been ruled out, such patients generally require a renal biopsy to identify RPGN.

Bibliography

Cohen AH, et al. Clinical utility of kidney biopsies in the diagnosis and management of renal disease. Am J Nephr 1989;9:309–315.

Glassock RJ, et al. Primary and secondary glomerular diseases. In: Brenner BM, Rector FC, eds. The Kidney. Philadelphia, W.B. Saunders, 1986, pp. 929–1084.

Madaio MP, Harrington JT. The diagnosis of acute glomerulonephritis. N Engl J Med 1983;309:1299–1302.

West CD. The complement profile in clinical medicine. Complement Inflamm 1989;6:49–64.

33

UROLITHIASIS

RAYMOND G. RAMUSACK

Never accept a drink from a urologist.

ERMA BOMBECK'S FATHER

DEFINITIONS AND GENERAL COMMENTS

- Urolithiasis (nephrolithiasis, renal calculi, kidney stones) denotes a condition characterized by the presence of concretions (calculi, stones) within the urinary tract.
- Stones are typically located within the renal calicies or pelvis. They may become lodged in the ureter or bladder, causing excruciating pain, obstruction, hematuria, or infection.
- Urolithiasis should be distinguished from nephrocalcinosis, which is a generalized calcification of the renal parenchyma.
- Patients may be categorized by their stone disease activity and composition (Table 33–1):
    1. First-time stone former. The first episode of symptomatic stone disease or an asymptomatic, incidentally discovered stone.
    2. Surgically active stone disease. Stone-related pain, obstruction, or infection is present. The stone causing symptoms may have been generated years before and remained stable over time until the onset of symptoms. Therapeutic intervention (medical or surgical) may be necessary.
    3. Metabolically active stone disease. There is evidence of new stone-forming activity, stone growth, or the passage of documented gravel within the past year. This designation requires adequate imaging studies within the prior year.
    4. Metabolically indeterminate stone disease. Insufficient imaging or clinical information is available to determine stone disease activity.
    5. Recurrent stone former. More than one episode of surgically active stone disease or evidence of metabolically active stone disease.
    6. Active stone disease. New stones are forming or preformed stones are growing, as confirmed by radiographic studies.
    7. Inactive urolithiasis. No change in stone-forming activity over the prior year by imaging and clinical criteria.
    8. Latent stone formers. This designates the 15 to 20% of

TABLE 33–1. Composition and Frequency of Renal Stones

COMPOSITION	FREQUENCY (%)
Calcium oxalate	30–35
Calcium oxalate/phosphate mixture	30–35
Calcium phosphate	10
Magnesium ammonium phosphate (also called struvite)	5–10
Uric acid	<5
Cystine	1
Xanthine	<1

normal subjects who are at risk to generate stones under situations of metabolic stress such as dehydration, immobilization, or malabsorption.

- Epidemiology
    1. Urolithiasis is the third most common disorder of the urinary system after urinary tract infections and benign prostatic hypertrophy.
    2. Stone disease has an annual estimated incidence of 7 to 21 cases per 10,000. Its estimated lifetime prevalence is 5% for women and 12% for men by age 75 years. Eighty percent of patients are men with a peak onset at age 20 to 30 years.
    3. The incidence of urolithiasis is greatest in the summer months and in the southeastern United States.

DIFFERENTIAL DIAGNOSIS

Many conditions may cause flank or lower abdominal pain. The differential diagnosis includes:

- Gastrointestinal diseases
    1. Appendicitis
    2. Peptic ulcer
    3. Intestinal obstruction
    4. Mesenteric adenitis
    5. Irritable bowel syndrome
    6. Inflammatory bowel disease
    7. Acute diverticulitis
    8. Gastroenteritis
- Gynecologic diseases
    1. Salpingitis
    2. Ectopic pregnancy
- Hepatobiliary diseases
    1. Cholecystitis
    2. Pancreatitis
- Vascular diseases
    1. Mesenteric infarction
    2. Aortic dissection

CLINICAL FEATURES

- Natural history
  1. Urolithiasis is a chronic disease marked by frequent recurrences. Most of the conditions associated with urolithiasis are lifelong.
  2. Urolithiasis has a 70 to 80% recurrence rate, with an average interval to recurrence of 7 years for women and 9 years for men. Fifteen to twenty percent of stone recurrences occur in the first 2 years. Sixty percent of first-time stone formers will be stone-free for 10 years.
  3. In patients with recurrent stones, the interval between successive episodes tends to remain constant or decrease.
  4. Urolithiasis is a common cause of morbidity but is a rare cause of chronic renal failure or death.
- Clinical classification of urolithiasis is based on knowledge of the crystal composition of the stone (and other laboratory parameters) and known associated metabolic, anatomic, and infectious diseases (Table 33–2).
- Acute stone passage
  1. Symptoms. The most common presentation of urolithiasis is pain of abrupt or rapid onset due to ureteral obstruction.
     a. Stone pain is severe and may persist for hours to days, and may not be colicky in nature.
     b. The classic pain distribution is from the flank or costovertebral angle (CVA) to the groin or genitals.
     c. Pain and other symptoms may vary according to the anatomic location of the stone as it traverses the urinary tract (Table 33–3).
     d. Anterior abdominal pain is an extremely unusual presenting sign, and other causes should be considered (Table 33–4).
     e. Atypical patients (often with staghorn calculi) have chronic flank or back discomfort, suggesting other visceral or musculoskeletal disorders.
     f. Pain is more severe than accompanying symptoms such as nausea.
     g. Occasional patients only pass small, sandlike concretions with relatively little pain.
     h. Other symptoms of urolithiasis include acute, persistent, or recurrent urinary tract infection (UTI) or hematuria.
  2. Historical data
     a. Sickle cell disease, analgesic abuse, recurrent UTIs with papillary necrosis, or clot formation in the urinary tract can cause symptoms similar to acute stone passage.
     b. A history of hypercalcemia, medication use (vitamins, antacids, acetazolamide, calcium supplements, high-dose vitamin C, thiazides, or allopurinol), UTI, or knowledge of a personal or family history of one of the diseases known to be associated with urolithiasis may aid evaluation.

Text continued on page 272

TABLE 33–2. Stone Type and Metabolic Abnormalities

STONE TYPE	PERCENT OF ALL STONES	DIAGNOSTIC CRITERIA	CLINICAL FEATURES
Calcium stones	70–80		Age at peak incidence: men 20–40, women 40–60
A. Hypercalciuric states	45–90	Urine Ca (24 hr): >300 mg for men, >250 mg for women, >4 mg/kg for either gender	
1. Idiopathic hypercalciuria (absorptive or resorptive)		Normal serum calcium; diagnosis of exclusion; separation of absorptive vs. resorptive requires fasting and calcium loading test and is usually not clinically helpful; more useful approach: measure and identify risk factors promoting stone formation (hyperoxaluria, hyperuricosuria, hypocitraturia, low urine pH, low urine volume)	Autosomal dominant heredity; peak age 30–50, female and male; no bone disease or distinguishing clinical features
2. Primary hyperparathyroidism	5–10	Unexplained increased serum Ca; inappropriately high immunoreactive parathormone level	Most common hypercalcemic cause of stones; 15% have stones, often Ca phosphate; two-thirds have bone disease; hyperuricemia or hyperuricosuria may coexist

(Table continued on following page)

267

TABLE 33–2. Stone Type and Metabolic Abnormalities Continued

	STONE TYPE	PERCENT OF ALL STONES	DIAGNOSTIC CRITERIA	CLINICAL FEATURES
3.	Hypercalcemic or normocalcemic causes: hypo/hyperthyroidism, malignancy, sarcoidosis, hypervitaminosis D, Cushing's syndrome, Paget's disease, immobilization, milk-alkali syndrome, acromegaly	5–10	Increased serum Ca; diagnosis made by specific lab tests or clinical setting	Clinical features suggest underlying disorder; malignancy is common cause of hypercalcemia but rare cause of stones
4.	Antacid-induced hypophosphatemia	small	Chronic, excessive ingestion of phosphate binding antacids; low serum phosphate	Osteomalacia may be present
5.	Distal renal tubular acidosis (RTA)	rare	Hyperchloremic acidosis; hypokalemia; minimum urine pH >5.5 and serum bicarbonate level <19 mEq/L after ammonium chloride (100 mg/kg) oral challenge test in absence of bacteriuria (which may change pH)	70% of patients with distal RTA get stones; stones not caused by proximal and type IV RTA; associated diseases: dysproteinemia, Sjögren's syndrome, jejunoileal bypass surgery, amphotericin B, lithium, acetazolamide, medullary sponge kidney; clues: nephrocalcinosis,
6.	Incomplete distal RTA		Systemic acidosis absent but minimal	

		urine pH >5.5 after ammonium chloride challenge test	recurrent Ca phosphate stones, papillary tip calcification, fasting urine pH >6.0 in absence of infection, hypocitraturia (<150 mg/24 hr), osteomalacia
B. Hyperuricosuric calcium oxalate urolithiasis	10–20	Urine uric acid >750 mg/24 hr for women, >800 mg/24 hr for men; 30–50% have hypercalciuria	This class has 20% of calcium oxalate stone formers; most do not have gout; uric acid crystals form nidus for Ca oxalate precipitate; usually due to excess dietary purine intake; risk of both uric acid and Ca oxalate stones is increased in patients with gout
C. Hyperoxaluric states	2	Urine oxalate >60 mg/1.73 m²/24 hr; majority of patients with Ca oxalate stones have normal urine oxalate	
1. Enteric hyperoxaluria	2	History of fat malabsorption or ileal disease: resection, jejunoileal bypass, small bowel Crohn's disease, bacterial overgrowth, chronic biliary or pancreatic disease	Does not occur with ileostomies
2. Primary hyperoxaluria	rare	Increased urinary oxalic and glycolic acids (type I) or increased urinary oxalic and L-glyceric acids (type II)	Fulminant stone disease and nephrocalcinosis, renal insufficiency, and generalized oxalosis may occur at an early age

(Table continued on following page)

TABLE 33–2. Stone Type and Metabolic Abnormalities Continued

STONE TYPE	PERCENT OF ALL STONES	DIAGNOSTIC CRITERIA	CLINICAL FEATURES
3. Miscellaneous		History of dietary excess, high-dose vitamin C (several g/day), drugs (see above), pyridoxine deficiency	Drug causes: ethylene glycol, methoxyflurane, vitamin C
D. Idiopathic calcium lithiasis	15–20	All serum and urine concentrations normal	Tendency toward recurrent stones
Uric acid lithiasis	<10		
A. Hyperuricemia		Hyperuricemia and increased urine uric acid: >800 mg/24 hr (men); >750 mg/24 hr (women)	25% with gout form uric acid stones, higher risk while taking uricosuric agents; 25% with uric acid stones have gout; low urine output is a risk factor for urolithiasis; dietary protein excess is frequent
B. Idiopathic		Persistent acidic urine; serum and urine uric acid levels are normal	Recurrent stones; tends to occur with gout; associated with chronic dehydration (hot climates)
Infection stones (struvite lithiasis)	10–15	Stones made of magnesium ammonium	Requires UTI with urea-splitting

		phosphate; urine pH is persistently alkaline; culture stone material (for fastidious organisms: *Ureaplasma urealyticum, Corynebacterium* sp.) if conventional culture negative	bacterium (*Proteus, Pseudomonas, Klebsiella, Staphylococcus aureus*, anaerobes); culture-negative cases may be due to fastidious organism; *E. coli* does not produce urease; often form staghorn calculi; half of patients have underlying metabolic or anatomic abnormality
Cystine lithiasis	1–3	Occurs only in cystinuria; homozygotes excrete >250 mg cystine/24 hr; screen urine with sodium nitroprusside test	Pathophysiology is renal tubular defect in cystine resorption; 10% of stones formed by cystinuric patients do not have cystine
Renal structural abnormalities	?	Usually struvite or Ca phosphate stones; probably infection associated	Associated with medullary sponge kidney, ectopic kidney, horseshoe kidney, polycystic kidney
Foreign body stones	<1	Drug components or metabolites	History of triamterene or other drug use

TABLE 33–3. Symptoms of Renal Stone by Location in Urinary Tract

LOCATION OF STONE	TYPICAL SYMPTOMS
Small caliceal stone	Asymptomatic
Obstructing caliceal stone	Flank pain, recurrent UTI, hematuria
Renal pelvis	Asymptomatic
Ureteropelvic junction	Flank or CVA pain, severe pyelonephritis
Proximal ureter	Acute, severe flank pain, hematuria
Ureter at pelvic brim	Pain migrates to lateral flank and abdomen; nausea and emesis
Ureterovesical junction	Irritative urinary symptoms (dysuria, urgency, frequency)

3. Physical examination
   a. Tachycardia, mild hypertension, diaphoresis, and tachypnea may accompany the severe pain of stone passage. Fever is not present in uncomplicated urolithiasis and suggests coexistent pyelonephritis or another diagnosis.
   b. Abdominal examination is remarkable for the absence of peritoneal findings. Bowel sounds are hypoactive, and distention may be present from re-

TABLE 33–4. Differentiation Between Urolithiasis and Peritoneal Pain

FINDING	UROLITHIASIS	PERITONITIS
Patient appearance	Tossing about	Avoids movement
Onset	Sudden	Gradual
Location of pain	CVA, flank	Anterior
Radiation of pain	To groin or genitals	Not usual
Fever	Only if infected	Usual
Associated symptoms	Nausea, vomiting, abdominal distention	Vomiting, constipation
Physical signs	Flank or CVA tenderness	Abdominal rigidity, guarding, rebound
Blood leukocyte count	Normal unless infected	Usually elevated
Urinalysis	Usually hematuria	Usually normal

flex gastric ileus due to acute renal pelvis dilatation.

LABORATORY FEATURES

- Urinalysis is the most important initial study.
  1. Gross or microscopic hematuria is usually present, but its absence does not exclude urolithiasis.
  2. Mild degrees of glycosuria and proteinuria may reflect tubular dysfunction from obstruction.
  3. An acid pH essentially excludes renal tubular acidosis. An alkaline pH suggests the possibility of a urea-splitting bacterial infection.
  4. Crystalluria may be helpful in predicting stone composition and the risk of recurrence.
     a. Cystine crystals are diagnostic of cystinuria but occur in a minority of patients. Their absence does not exclude the diagnosis.
     b. Struvite crystals are highly predictive of stone formation due to infection.
     c. Other common types of crystals (Ca oxalate, Ca phosphate, uric acid) are often found in both stone formers and non–stone formers.
- Blood studies
  1. The evaluation of all first stone episodes and most recurrent episodes should include a complete blood count (CBC) and serum calcium, sodium, chloride, potassium, bicarbonate, and creatinine level determinations.
  2. Conclusions about underlying causes should be made cautiously, as acute obstruction may result in transient abnormalities unrelated to stone formation. Further metabolic evaluation should be delayed for 6 to 8 weeks after an acute episode to allow return of baseline renal metabolic function.
- Radiographic evaluation allows definitive diagnosis of urolithiasis.
  1. "Flat plate" of the abdomen (KUB), as an isolated study, has low sensitivity and specificity for urolithiasis.
  2. The radiographic study of choice is the intravenous pyelogram (IVP).
     a. A dense nephrogram on the affected side is most common, and a dye column may be cut off or display a stone shadow.
     b. A marked delay in visualization indicates a complete or nearly complete ureteral obstruction.
     c. False-negative IVPs may result from passage of the stone due to increased luminal pressure generated by the study.
  3. For patients with contraindications to IVP dye, renal ultrasound, unenhanced renal CT, or radionuclide renal scanning may aid diagnosis.
     a. False-negative results with ultrasound are not

common but tend to occur with lower ureteral stones. High false-positive rates have been noted.

   b. All types of calculi, including uric acid stones, are easily visible on CT scanning. CT has the advantage of excellent overall visualization of the kidney and other retroperitoneal structures.

- Composition of renal stones. Calcium-containing stones account for 70 to 80% of stones and are principally composed of calcium oxalate and calcium phosphate, usually occurring as mixtures (see Table 33–1).

RECOMMENDED DIAGNOSTIC APPROACH

- Diagnosis of urolithiasis
   1. The definitive diagnosis of urolithiasis requires stone passage itself or radiographic evidence of the stone and its attendant urinary obstruction.
   2. Most stones that are less than 5 mm in diameter will pass spontaneously, usually within 48 to 72 hr. Stones larger than 5 mm have a much smaller chance of spontaneous passage.
   3. Analysis of the stone provides the crystal composition and is the most important clue to underlying disorders and appropriate therapy.
- Metabolic evaluation of patients with urolithiasis. The yield and appropriateness of an extensive metabolic evaluation of patients with stone disease is controversial:
   1. Only a basic evaluation is recommended for the patient with a first stone. Multiple stones or recurrent disease (i.e., surgically or metabolically active) require more complex evaluation.
   2. Basic (limited) evaluation
      a. Medical history. Identify possible medical or environmental risk factors: family history of stone disease, estimation of frequency of previous stones, fluid intake or restriction, urine volume, climatic and geographic variables, occupation, immobilization, diet, and medications.
      b. Examination. Evidence of malignant neoplasm, skeletal disease, inflammatory bowel disease, intestinal bypass, or UTI should be sought.
      c. Laboratory studies
         i. Urinalysis and urine culture
         ii. Determinations of serum electrolyte, calcium, phosphate, creatinine, and uric acid concentrations
         iii. Qualitative urine screening for cystinuria when the composition of the stone is unknown
         iv. Hypercalcemia warrants a serum parathyroid hormone assay.
      d. Imaging studies
         i. KUB and IVP should be performed (unless contraindicated) to identify obstruction and

allow definition of existing stones and the anatomy of the collecting system.

    ii. Renal tomograms are very sensitive for visualizing stones.

    iii. IVPs done during an acute stone episode are often of poor quality, and some clinics may repeat a high-resolution IVP with or without tomograms to adequately exclude medullary sponge kidney in patients with apparent idiopathic hypercalciuria.

  e. Confirmatory laboratory studies ideally should not be done during illness or recent recovery from a stone episode or surgery (6 to 8 weeks). Rather, follow-up studies should be on outpatients in their basal state of health and on their usual diet.

3. Complex (extensive) evaluation

  a. All patients should have a 24-hr urine collection for analysis of volume, pH, and calcium, phosphate, sodium, uric acid, oxalate, citrate, and creatinine contents.

  b. Specialized testing is reserved for patients with recalcitrant disease.

    i. Provocative acid-loading tests, oral calcium deprivation and loading studies, determination of urinary inhibitor concentration, or calculation of urinary saturation indices may be indicated.

    ii. Serum parathyroid hormone levels may be indicated in patients with high-normal or marginally elevated ionized calcium levels.

Bibliography

Coe FL, Parks JH. Nephrolithiasis: Pathogenesis and Treatment, 2nd ed. Chicago, Year Book Medical Publishers, 1988.

Maxwell MH, Kleeman CR, Narins RG, eds. Clinical disorders of fluid and electrolyte metabolism, 4th ed. McGraw-Hill, 1987.

National Institutes of Health Consensus Conference. Prevention and treatment of kidney stones. Jour Am Med Assoc 1988;260:978–981.

Preminger GM. The metabolic evaluation of patients with recurrent nephrolithiasis: A review of comprehensive and simplified approaches. J Urol, part 2 1989;141:760–763.

Stewart C. Nephrolithiasis. Emerg Med Clin North Amer 1988;6:617–630.

Wilson DM. Clinical and laboratory approaches for evaluation of nephrolithiasis. J Urol, part 2, 1989;141:770–774.

Yendt ER, Cohanim M. Clinical and laboratory approaches for evaluation of nephrolithiasis. J Urol, part 2 1989;141:764–769.

SECTION V

GASTROINTESTINAL

34

ABDOMINAL PAIN

JOHN HALSEY *and* MICHAEL KIMMEY

Dyspepsy and cheerfulness do not go together.

JAMES JACKSON (1777–1867)

GENERAL COMMENTS

- Abdominal pain accounts for 5% of emergency room visits.
- Diagnostic principles
  1. Abdominal pain may be well localized if somatic afferent nerves (abdominal skin, wall musculature, or parietal peritoneum) are stimulated. It may be less well localized and referred to uninvolved parts of the body if visceral afferent nerves (abdominal organs) are stimulated.
  2. Repeated patient examinations over time are diagnostically valuable.
  3. Definitive diagnosis may not be reached in up to 40% of cases of acute abdominal pain.
  4. The incidence of various causes of abdominal pain varies with the population studied.

DIFFERENTIAL DIAGNOSES (Table 34–1)

- Multiple classifications. Classification schemes of abdominal pain may be based on pain duration (acute versus chronic), location, abruptness of onset, and pathogenesis (inflammatory, obstructive, or ischemic).
- Diagnostic clues in selected causes of abdominal pain
  1. The clinical features of gastroenteritis, cholecystitis, pancreatitis, inflammatory bowel disease, nephrolithiasis, and pyelonephritis are covered elsewhere.
  2. Appendicitis
     a. Patients with acute appendicitis have moderate to severe (95%) steady (60%) pain that begins in the periumbilical region and then localizes to the right lower quadrant (RLQ) (75%). Pain precedes other symptoms in over 90% of patients.
     b. Other symptoms include nausea (75%), vomiting (60%), anorexia (75%), and diarrhea (20%).
     c. Physical examination shows temperature greater than 38° C (45%), rebound tenderness and guarding (70 to 80%) usually in the RLQ (65%), and right lateral rectal wall tenderness (30 to 40%).
     d. The WBC count is greater than 10,000 in 90% of

TABLE 34–1. Causes of Abdominal Pain Grouped by Location and Rate of Onset

	Onset		
Location and Disorder	**Sudden**	**Rapid (min)**	**Gradual (hr)**
Right upper quadrant (RUQ)			
Cholecystitis and biliary colic	*	**	*
Perforated duodenal ulcer			
Hepatitis			*
Hepatic congestion (vascular)			*
Perihepatitis (Fitz-Hugh-Curtis syndrome)			*
Retrocecal appendicitis		*	
Pyelonephritis			*
Pneumonia			*
Epigastric (may also be RUQ or LUQ)			
Pancreatitis		*	*
Peptic ulcer		*	*
Gastritis			*
Myocardial infarction	**	*	
Left upper quadrant (LUQ)			

Splenic rupture or infarction	*		*
Splenic enlargement	*		
Colonic perforation (tumor, foreign body)			**
Pyelonephritis			*
Pneumonia			
Right lower quadrant (RLQ)			
Appendicitis		**	***
Mesenteric adenitis		**	*
Regional enteritis			***
Diverticulitis (cecal, Meckel's)		*	
Left lower quadrant (LLQ)			
Diverticulitis (sigmoid)		*	**
Irritable bowel syndrome			*
RLQ or LLQ (depending on side involved)			
Ruptured ectopic pregnancy	**	*	* (before rupture)
Ruptured ovarian cyst	*		
Ovarian torsion		**	*
Salpingitis		**	*
Mittelschmerz	*	**	*
Ureteral calculi			*

Table continued on following page

TABLE 34–1. Causes of Abdominal Pain Grouped by Location and Rate of Onset Continued

LOCATION AND DISORDER	ONSET		
	Sudden	Rapid (min)	Gradual (hr)
Incarcerated inguinal hernia	**	**	*
Ruptured aortic aneurysm		*	* (before rupture)
Diffuse pain			
Gastroenteritis			**
Peritonitis		(see underlying cause)	
Early appendicitis	*		*
Intestinal obstruction		*	*
Intestinal infarction			*
Diabetic ketoacidosis		**	*
Sickle cell crisis		*	**
Acute intermittent porphyria			*
Lead intoxication			*
Narcotic withdrawal			*

** Signifies a more common type of onset if mode of onset is variable.

patients. In 80% of patients, the WBCs include more than 75% neutrophils.

   e. Abnormal abdominal X-rays (appendicolith, localized ileus, increased RLQ soft tissue density) occur in half of patients but are not specific for appendicitis.

   f. Compression ultrasonography may confirm the clinical impression by showing a thickened appendiceal wall or yield an alternative diagnosis in ambiguous cases.

3. Peptic ulcer disease

   a. Compared with patients with duodenal ulcer (DU) and those with dyspepsia and no ulcer, patients with gastric ulcer (GU) tend to be older and to have more pain that occurs sooner after meals and is less likely to be relieved by antacids.

   b. Epigastric pain (60 to 80% of cases) that is relieved by antacids (40 to 80%) and radiates to the back (20 to 30%) is characteristic of ulcer patients. Anorexia (30 to 60%), nausea (50 to 70%), and vomiting (30 to 70%) are common.

   c. Epigastric tenderness is present in 50% of cases.

   d. Contrast radiography or endoscopy is needed to distinguish between GU, DU, and nonulcer dyspepsia.

   e. Patients with *perforated ulcers* have sudden onset of severe (95%) steady (95%) pain that often has a generalized distribution (50%). Diminished bowel sounds (50 to 90%), abdominal rigidity (80%), and free subdiaphragmatic air on upright abdominal X-ray are characteristic of perforation.

4. Bowel obstruction

   a. Patients with small bowel obstructions have periumbilical (40%), crampy (90%), severe (60%) abdominal pain that precedes vomiting (90%). Eighty percent of patients have a history of prior abdominal surgery.

   b. Physical examination reveals hyperperistaltic bowel sounds in 50% of cases but diminished or absent sounds in 25%. Abdominal distention is common but may be absent early in the illness.

   c. WBC counts greater than 10,000 (60%) and dilated bowel loops with air-fluid levels on abdominal X-rays are useful findings but are not necessary to make the diagnosis.

5. Diverticulitis

   a. Ten percent of people in the United States have diverticula, and 10 to 20% of these develop diverticulitis at some time in their lives. Patients are generally elderly (70% are over age 60).

   b. Patients with diverticulitis have pain that is steady (40%) or cramping (30%), of moderate severity (60%), and located in the left lower quadrant (LLQ) (25%) or generally in the lower half of the abdomen (35%).

   c. Patients with diverticulitis may have nausea

(50%), vomiting (30%), diarrhea (30%), constipation (40%), and rectal bleeding (25%).

d. Abdominal rebound, rigidity, and guarding are infrequent (30%), and tenderness (20%) or a mass (10%) may be found on rectal examination.

e. Leukocytosis is seen in over 90% of cases.

6. Vascular diseases

   a. Abdominal aortic aneurysm (AAA)

      i. Most patients with an AAA are asymptomatic, and 85% are unaware of the presence of an aneurysm at the time of rupture.

      ii. All patients with a ruptured or leaking aneurysm have pain that is felt in either the back (35%), abdomen (30%), or both the abdomen and back (35%). The pain has been present over 24 hr in 50%.

      iii. A pulsatile abdominal mass is palpable in 90%, and abdominal X-rays show an aneurysm in 75% of cases. Early diagnosis is crucial to a successful surgical outcome.

   b. Intestinal angina

      i. Intermittent dull or cramping midabdominal pain beginning 30 min after a meal and lasting for 1 to 2 hr is characteristic. Steatorrhea may be present.

      ii. Physical examination often reveals an abdominal bruit, but this is not diagnostically useful. Definitive diagnosis requires angiography.

   c. Mesenteric arterial occlusion

      i. Severe midabdominal pain that is initially colicky, periumbilical, and with severity out of proportion to physical findings is seen in intestinal infarction. Over several hours the pain becomes generalized.

      ii. With progression, systemic signs including fever and hypotension develop.

      iii. Laboratory findings include metabolic acidosis, leukocytosis (often with WBC count greater than 30,000), and, occasionally, elevated amylase.

      iv. The same clinical findings in a patient with valvular heart disease or atrial fibrillation should suggest the presence of a superior mesenteric artery embolus, which may be amenable to surgical removal.

7. Irritable bowel syndrome

   a. This syndrome is a benign intestinal motor disturbance that affects 15 to 20% of the general population and is the most frequent cause for gastroenterologic consultation.

   b. The abdominal pain has a variable quality. It is usually lower abdominal, relieved by defecation in 50% of patients, and rarely awakens the patient at night.

   c. A history of both diarrhea and constipation, excessive flatulence, and mucus in stools is frequent.

     d.   Laboratory and radiographic studies are normal.

- Lower abdominal pain in women. In addition to the usual causes of abdominal pain, special consideration must be given to disorders of the female reproductive system.

  1. Ectopic pregnancy

     a. One-fourth of patients with an ectopic pregnancy have a history of pelvic inflammatory disease (PID). Other risk factors include prior ectopic pregnancy, IUD use, and prior tubal sterilization surgery (7% of all ectopic pregnancies).

     b. Over 90% of patients with an ectopic pregnancy have abdominal pain that initially is mild, crampy, and unilateral (75% of cases). Pain may generalize and produce shoulder pain and orthostatic dizziness when the fallopian tube ruptures.

     c. Eighty-five percent of patients have a history of a recently missed menstrual period, and 80% have irregular, usually mild, vaginal bleeding.

     d. Pelvic examination may reveal cervical motion or adnexal tenderness, but a mass is often not found.

     e. A serum pregnancy test is positive in >95% of cases and is preferred to urine pregnancy tests, which may be negative especially during early pregnancy.

     f. Graded compression ultrasonography and endovaginal sonography are helpful in visualizing early ectopic pregnancies.

     g. Culdocentesis and laparoscopy may be useful if the clinical diagnosis of ectopic pregnancy is not confirmed by ultrasound.

  2. Ovarian cysts

     a. Cysts commonly occur in mid to late cycle (follicular cysts) and in early pregnancy (corpus luteum cyst).

     b. The cysts may rupture, causing acute severe lower abdominal pain, often with peritoneal signs. The pain resolves spontaneously over 6 to 24 hr.

     c. Cysts greater than 6 cm in size may undergo torsion. In this case pain does not resolve, and 80% of patients have a palpable adnexal mass.

     d. WBC are usually not seen on Gram's stain of cervical mucus. Diagnostic laparoscopy should be used early if torsion is suspected.

  3. PID

     a. Lower abdominal pain (94% of cases), increased vaginal discharge (55%), and irregular vaginal bleeding (36%) are seen in women with pelvic inflammatory disease.

     b. Signs include a temperature above 38° C (41%), and right upper quadrant (RUQ) tenderness (30%).

     c. Leukocytosis (50%) and WBCs on a Gram's stain of cervical mucus are often seen.

     d. Since the clinical diagnosis of PID may be wrong in 35% of cases, liberal use of diagnostic laparoscopy is recommended.

CLINICAL MANIFESTATIONS

- History
  1. Character of pain. Severity, rate of onset, location, duration, frequency, radiation, and aggravating and alleviating factors should be sought.
     a. Sudden onset of pain. Sudden onset of pain that does not diminish suggests perforated viscus, embolism, torsion, or hemorrhage.
     b. Crampy pain. This suggests biliary colic, renal colic, intestinal obstruction, gastroenteritis, or ectopic pregnancy.
     c. Severe pain. The most severe pains are seen with renal colic, intestinal infarction, dissecting aortic aneurysm, and perforated ulcer.
  2. General review of systems. This should cover potential sources of referred pain (myocardial or pulmonary) and metabolic causes (ketoacidosis or hyperlipidemia).
  3. Medical history. A history of drug and alcohol use, prior abdominal surgery, concurrent medical problems including atherosclerotic disease, and family history of similar problems (may suggest porphyria, familial Mediterranean fever, or sickle cell anemia) should be sought.
- Physical examination
  1. General examination. Look for signs of increased autonomic activity (flushing, diaphoresis, tachycardia, or mydriasis), fever, postural hypotension, heart failure, and pneumonia.
  2. Body posture
     a. Patients with renal, biliary, or intestinal colic move frequently, often in a writhing motion.
     b. Those with peritonitis lie quietly on their backs, often with hips and knees flexed.
     c. Patients with pancreatitis prefer a sitting posture, usually leaning forward.
  3. Abdominal examination
     a. Inspection. Distention, dilated veins, an enlarged organ or mass, and visible peristalsis may be present.
     b. Auscultation. Bowel sounds (useful if absent or if high-pitched rushes are heard), bruits (present in the epigastric area of 20% of normals), friction rubs, venous hums, and presence of a succussion splash should be evaluated.
     c. Palpation
        i. The examination should begin with light touch with one finger before examining for deep tenderness, masses, and organomegaly.
        ii. Local and remote rebound tenderness, involuntary guarding, and tenderness to light percussion signify underlying inflammation or peritonitis.
        iii. Femoral and inguinal canals should be examined for hernias.
     d. Percussion. Liver and spleen sizes should be esti-

mated. Costovertebral angle tenderness should be noted.

e. Rectal examination. Rectal examination for a mass or tenderness is mandatory in all patients, as are pelvic examination in women and testicular examination in men.

LABORATORY EVALUATION

Essential Screening Tests

- Hematology
  1. The hematocrit is a useful index of bleeding. The patient's state of hydration is important in the interpretation of results.
  2. An elevated WBC count suggests an inflammatory disease; however, a normal count does not eliminate any diagnostic possibility. In general, the WBC differential is useful only when a low or elevated total count is found.
  3. Screening coagulation tests (prothrombin time and platelet count) are important if bleeding or liver disease is suspected.
- Urinalysis
  1. This is a useful screening test for urinary tract pathology and diabetic ketoacidosis.
  2. Urine specific gravity is an indicator of intravascular volume.
  3. Inflammatory processes in the urinary system or near the ureter (e.g., appendicitis or acute diverticulitis) may produce pyuria.
- Serum electrolytes and creatine and BUN. These tests are widely ordered and useful if renal disease or significant vomiting or diarrhea are present. They usually do not make the diagnosis.
- Serum amylase
  1. This test remains the most common screening test for pancreatitis. Elevations may be caused by nonpancreatic disease, usually from an elevated salivary isoenzyme.
  2. Half of patients with acute alcohol intoxication have an elevated total serum amylase level, but only one-fourth of these have an elevated pancreatic isoenzyme level.
- Serum bilirubin
  1. Jaundice is detectable at serum bilirubin levels above 3 to 4 mg/dl.
  2. Seven percent of the normal population have Gilbert syndrome and may have a serum bilirubin level up to 5 mg/dl. The bilirubin is primarily unconjugated, and this finding is not related to abdominal pain.
- Serum pregnancy test. Women of reproductive age with lower abdominal pain should have an ectopic pregnancy excluded.

- Abdominal X-rays. Significant abnormalities are not missed if this examination is limited to patients with moderate or severe abdominal pain and those with high clinical suspicion of renal or biliary calculi, bowel obstruction, ischemia, or trauma.
- Additional tests
  1. Chest X-ray, EKG, and measurement of liver enzymes may be useful in certain cases.
  2. GI endoscopy, radiographic contrast examination, ultrasound, CT, biliary scintigraphy, and abdominal angiography are useful adjunctive measures in selected clinical settings.

RECOMMENDED DIAGNOSTIC APPROACH

A single diagnostic approach cannot be recommended in the evaluation of a patient with abdominal pain. Laboratory and procedural investigation is different in each case and should be directed by the physician's diagnostic impressions after a complete and careful history and physical examination have been performed.

Bibliography

Brewer RJ, et al. Abdominal pain: An analysis of 1000 consecutive cases in a university hospital emergency room. Am J Surg 1976;131:219–223.

Eisenberg RL, et al. Evaluation of plain abdominal radiographs in the diagnosis of abdominal pain. Ann Intern Med 1982;97:257–261.

Hickey MS, et al. Evaluation of abdominal pain. Emerg Clin North Am 1989;7(3):437–452.

Silen W. Cope's Early Diagnosis of the Acute Abdomen, 17th ed. New York, Oxford University Press, 1987.

Staniland R, et al. Clinical presentation of acute abdomen: Study of 600 patients. Br Med J 1972;3:393–398.

Way LW. Abdominal pain. In: Sleisinger MH, Fordtran JS, eds. Gastrointestinal Disease, 4th ed. Philadelphia, W.B. Saunders, 1989, pp. 238–250.

35

GASTROINTESTINAL BLEEDING

GEOFFREY JIRANEK

We all need someone we can bleed on.

MICK JAGGER

GENERAL COMMENTS AND EPIDEMIOLOGY

- Bleeding is a cardinal manifestation of pathology in the GI tract. Occult bleeding may be the only clue to the presence of GI cancer.
- There are approximately 350,000 hospital admissions yearly in the United States for upper GI bleeding with an associated mortality of 10%.

DIFFERENTIAL DIAGNOSIS

- Bleeding can be categorized by location (Table 35–1).
- Most bleeding significant enough to cause hospitalization originates in the esophagus, stomach, or duodenum.
  1. Peptic ulcers are a common cause of acute and chronic bleeding. Ulcers from caustic substances and infections, such as cytomegalovirus, are rare.
  2. Severe stress such as sepsis, shock, and burns can cause a diffuse hemorrhagic gastritis, but significant bleeding is usually due to areas where submucosal vessels have been exposed by ulceration. Ethanol can cause a hemorrhagic gastritis, but the blood loss is seldom severe.
  3. Portal hypertension
     a. Varices may bleed acutely but do not generally cause chronic occult bleeding. The most frequent location is the esophagus.
     b. Portal hypertensive gastropathy may also occur causing hemorrhage.
  4. Mallory-Weiss tears usually bleed acutely and often stop bleeding spontaneously unless there is portal hypertension.
  5. Vascular malformations (vascular ectasia, telangiectasia, angiodysplasia, angioma) can cause acute large-volume bleeding and chronic occult bleeding.
     a. The stomach and duodenum are affected much more often than the esophagus.

TABLE 35–1. Differential Diagnosis of GI Bleeding

Esophagus, stomach, and duodenum
  Ulcer
  Hemorrhagic gastritis
  Varices
  Mallory-Weiss tear
  Vascular malformation
  Neoplasm
  Ischemia
  Linear erosion in a hiatal hernia
  Arterial-enteric fistula
  Foreign body trauma
  Hemobilia
Jejunum and ileum
  Neoplasm
  Vascular malformation
  Diverticula (including Meckel's)
  Crohn's disease
  Intussusception
  Radiation enteritis
  Ischemia
  Vasculitis
  Infection
  Varices
  Foreign body trauma
Colon
  Vascular anomaly
  Diverticula
  Inflammatory bowel disease
  Infectious colitis
  Ischemia
  Vasculitis
  Neoplasm
  Solitary rectal ulcer
  Varices
Anus
  Hemorrhoid
  Fissure
  Neoplasm

    b. Gastric antral vascular ectasia, also known as "watermelon stomach," can cause chronic bleeding.
    c. A Dielafoy's lesion is an aberrant submucosal ectatic artery that can suddenly and massively bleed.
  6. Neoplasms (e.g., adenocarcinoma of the esophagus or stomach) occasionally cause acute or chronic bleeding.
  7. Ischemia is rare in the esophagus, stomach, and duodenum.
  8. Large hiatal hernias have been associated with intermittent linear erosions, which can cause chronic occult blood loss.

9. The distal duodenum is the most frequent site for an aorto-enteric fistula from a graft used to repair an abdominal aortic aneurysm.
   a. Bleeding can range from small amounts (herald bleeds) to massive bleeding.
   b. Arterial-enteric fistulae can very rarely develop from native aneurysms and communicate with adjacent gut structures anywhere from the esophagus to the rectum.
10. Bleeding can result from ingested sharp foreign bodies such as toothpicks and chicken bones.

- Jejunal and ileal causes of acute and chronic bleeding are much less common than upper GI tract and colonic causes.
  1. In adults the 3 most common lesions are neoplasm (such as leiomyoma, lymphoma, carcinoma, hemangioma, metastasis, and sarcoma), vascular malformation, and Crohn's disease.
  2. In children, intussusception, Meckel's diverticulum, and Crohn's disease are the more common causes of acute bleeding.

- Colon
  1. Neoplasms such as larger adenomas and adenocarcinomas are important causes of chronic occult bleeding.
     a. Thirty to fifty percent of the population develop adenomas, and 6% develop adenocarcinomas.
     b. Acute small-quantity bleeding and chronic occult bleeding are frequent presentations. Massive bleeding is much less common.
  2. Angiodysplasia is the most common vascular malformation occurring in the colon. It is typically located in the right side of the colon.
  3. Although diverticula are more common in the left colon, diverticula in the right colon are more likely to bleed. Bleeding is generally acute and not chronic or occult.

- Hemorrhoids and fissures are common causes of bleeding when the quantity is very small.

CLINICAL FEATURES

- History
  1. Character of bleeding
     a. Hematemesis implies that the bleeding site is proximal to the ligament of Treitz (duodenojejunal junction). Red blood indicates more active bleeding than "coffee ground emesis."
     b. Bleeding from the upper GI tract typically produces black stool (melena), while lower-tract bleeding produces red to maroon stool. Red to maroon-colored stool may occur with large volume upper GI bleeding.
     c. Bleeding of long duration is less likely to stop spontaneously. Melena that lasts for several days does not necessarily imply ongoing bleeding.

      d. Apparent GI bleeding may instead result from oronasopharyngeal, pulmonary, and, in women, vaginal and urinary bleeding.

2. Past history of GI bleeding. Many lesions that bled previously are apt to bleed again.

3. Abdominal pain
   a. Crampy discomfort is typical during transit of larger amounts of blood through the intestines.
   b. Dyspeptic symptoms suggest peptic ulcer disease, but many ulcers bleed without preceding dyspepsia.
   c. Significant abdominal discomfort with bleeding is unusual and suggests neoplasm, inflammatory bowel disease, or ischemia.

4. Diarrhea may occur with infections, ischemia, inflammatory bowel disease, and radiation enteritis.

5. History of nausea, retching, or vomiting is a clue to a possible Mallory-Weiss tear, but tears may occur without such history.

6. Risk factors for human immunodeficiency virus (HIV). These raise the possibility of Kaposi's sarcoma, lymphoma, or cytomegalovirus-related ulceration.

7. History of liver disease suggests the possibility of varices.

8. Prior surgical history. An aortic vascular graft in the abdomen or chest may erode into the GI tract (aorto-enteric fistula).

9. Medications
   a. Aspirin and nonsteroidal anti-inflammatory agents can cause gastric ulcers and are associated with an increased risk of bleeding from peptic ulcers.
   b. Prednisone and other catabolic steroids may increase the risk of peptic ulcers.
   c. Coumadin and heparin increase the risk of GI bleeding.
   d. Bismuth subsalicylate and iron can cause black stools that test negative for occult blood. Beets can cause red stool that does not contain blood.

10. Family history. Many lesions have some inherited component including peptic ulcers, inflammatory bowel disease, colon cancer, and rare vascular disorders such as hereditary hemorrhagic telangiectasia.

- Physical examination
  1. Vital signs provide a guide to the amount of volume loss and the cardiovascular response. Postural vital signs should be checked if the patient is not clearly intravascularly depleted.
  2. Skin
     a. Pallor and perfusion provide guides to anemia and circulatory response.
     b. Jaundice, spider angiomata, and palmar erythema may indicate liver disease.
     c. Mucocutaneous telangiectasias are associated with similar lesions which bleed in the GI tract (e.g., hereditary hemorrhagic telangiectasia).

d. Characteristic lesions of the very rare inherited syndromes such as blue rubber-bleb nevus syndrome, pseudoxanthoma elasticum, and Ehlers-Danlos syndrome may be found.

e. Erythema nodosum, erythema multiforme, and pyoderma gangrenosum may be associated with inflammatory bowel disease.

f. Acanthosis nigricans is a rare skin lesion found in the axilla, which is associated with internal malignancies including GI adenocarcinoma.

3. Nose and throat. Epistaxis can be confused with upper-tract bleeding in patients who swallow blood. Mucosal hyperpigmented spots may indicate Peutz-Jeghers syndrome associated with hamartomas which can bleed in the GI tract.

4. Abdomen

a. Hepatomegaly, a hard small liver, splenomegaly, ascites, and a caput medusa may all indicate liver disease.

b. Abdominal masses may indicate a neoplasm.

c. An aortic aneurysm raises the possibility of an aorto-enteric fistula.

5. Rectal. The color and occult blood test of stool should be determined. Digital exam may reveal a neoplastic mass.

LABORATORY FEATURES

- Blood studies

1. Recent bleeding requires 12 to 36 hr before intravascular volume equilibration allows the hematocrit to accurately reflect the amount of bleeding.

2. Coagulation parameters should be checked.

3. A ratio of BUN to serum creatinine greater than 50 favors an upper GI tract source.

4. Elevations of serum bilirubin, alkaline phosphatase, and transaminases or a decreased albumin suggest liver disease.

- Diagnostic imaging

1. Plain chest and abdominal X-rays are seldom useful.

2. Barium contrast studies of the upper or lower GI tract have no role in the diagnosis of acute bleeding. They can be useful with chronic bleeding or in evaluating the small bowel where endoscopy is cumbersome.

3. Nuclear medicine studies

a. Scans that use radionuclide-labeled RBC ("tagged red blood cell scan") can be used to localize bleeding. They can detect bleeding rates as low as 0.1 cc/min.

b. Meckel's scan. Most Meckel's diverticula that bleed contain ectopic parietal cells. Localization of Tc-99m pertechnetate in the RLQ constitutes a positive scan.

4. Angiograms can be performed to localize the bleeding and identify the lesion. Bleeding rates as low as

1 cc/min can be detected, and therapy with vasoactive medications and embolization is possible.

- Procedures
  1. A gastric lavage tube can be passed through the mouth or nose to aspirate for blood. This can be very helpful in:
     a. Defining the location (proximal to the ligament of Treitz)
     b. Assessing activity (occasionally misses active duodenal bleeding)
     c. This procedure should be performed on almost every patient when the location or activity of bleeding is uncertain.
  2. Esophagogastroduodenoscopy
     a. This is a relatively accurate procedure which can determine the activity and type of bleeding lesions.
     b. Certain findings predict the risk of further bleeding from peptic ulcers (Table 35–2).
  3. Lower GI endoscopy
     a. Sigmoidoscopy allows examination for anal lesions, rectosigmoid neoplasms, and colitis (infectious, idiopathic, and ischemic). Rigid sigmoidoscopy can usually be performed rapidly at the bedside with inexpensive disposable equipment.
     b. Anoscopy can be done if the anus was not well examined sigmoidoscopically or if sigmoidoscopy is not immediately available.
     c. Colonoscopy requires preparation with cathartics in order to investigate bleeding.
        i. For chronic or occult bleeding it accurately examines for neoplasms, colitis, and vascular malformations.
        ii. For recent active bleeding that has stopped, colonoscopy can also be useful.

RECOMMENDED DIAGNOSTIC APPROACH

- A clinical assessment of the volume, activity, and level of bleeding should be made by a thorough history, examination, and gastric lavage.
  1. Suspected upper GI bleeding—hospitalized patients

TABLE 35–2. Endoscopic Predictors of Further Bleeding from Peptic Ulcers

LESION AT ULCER BASE	RISK OF FURTHER BLEEDING (%)
Visible vessel—spurting	85
Visible vessel—not bleeding	50
Adherent clot	25
No vessel	<5

a. A hospitalized patient with suspected upper GI bleeding should have gastric lavage performed.

    i. If blood is found, then the site of bleeding is proximal to the duodenal-jejunal junction.

    ii. If fresh red bleeding does not clear with lavage, then urgent endoscopy is required to guide specific hemostatic therapy.

    iii. If the blood clears with lavage, then upper endoscopy can be performed electively during hospitalization.

b. If varices are a strong possibility, then urgent endoscopy is indicated even if the blood clears during gastric lavage because 50 to 70% of patients with bleeding varices rebleed from them with a mortality rate of 30% during the hospitalization. Endoscopic therapy reduces the rate of rebleeding from varices.

c. If bleeding was abrupt and massive (>4 units), and blood clears during gastric lavage, urgent endoscopy should be considered.

d. If the patient has an aortic vascular graft, emergent evaluation is necessary.

    i. A patient with an abdominal aortic graft who does not stabilize because of continuing massive blood loss may need emergent laparotomy.

    ii. If the patient stabilizes, upper GI endoscopy should be done to exclude an alternative bleeding source. If none is found, the graft should be searched for in the distal duodenum, but endoscopy often misses an aorto-enteric fistula. If the graft is seen in the distal duodenum, immediate surgery is indicated.

    iii. If endoscopy is negative, a CT scan should be performed. Since a CT scan can also miss an aorto-enteric fistula, an exploratory laparotomy should be considered in some situations.

2. Suspected lower GI bleeding—hospitalized patients

a. Lower GI bleeding is suspected when there is hematochezia.

b. Anoscopy should be performed to exclude an anal source of active bleeding.

c. Sigmoidoscopy is sometimes useful at this point (especially if there is some diarrhea) by diagnosing colitis and neoplasms.

d. Unless the bleeding quantity is small, gastric lavage and possibly upper GI endoscopy should be performed.

e. If these tests do not reveal a bleeding lesion and the patient appears to be bleeding, a tagged RBC scan should be performed.

    i. If the scan is positive, angiographic or surgical therapy can be planned.

    ii. Colonoscopy can be done after preparing the colon with cathartics if the patient is not actively bleeding.

- Chronic or occult GI bleeding
  1. When stool positive for occult blood is detected in a patient who is at risk for colon neoplasia, colonoscopy (or flexible sigmoidoscopy and barium enema) is recommended.
  2. In the absence of symptoms or risk factors for pathology in the upper GI tract, no further work-up is generally necessary. Otherwise, upper endoscopy is advised.
  3. If there are persistent unexplained abdominal symptoms or if anemia is present from GI blood loss then additional tests may include:
     a. Barium upper GI with small bowel series
     b. Enteroclysis (barium through a small bowel feeding tube with cellulose as a contrast agent)
     c. Angiography
     d. Small bowel endoscopy with a prototype instrument or long endoscope during an open laparotomy
     e. Meckel's scan
     f. Tagged RBC scan during suspected active bleeding episodes
     g. Laparotomy

Bibliography

Aldridge MC, Sim AJW. Colonoscopic findings in symptomatic patients without x-ray evidence of colonic neoplasms. Lancet 1986;2:833–835.

Cameron AJ, Higgens JA. Linear gastric erosion. A lesion associated with large diaphragmatic hernia and chronic blood loss anemia. Gastroenterology 1986;91:338–341.

Forde KA. Colonoscopy in acute rectal bleeding. Gastroint Endo 1981;27:219–220.

Gilliam JH, et al. The "watermelon" stomach. Gastroenterology 1985;88:1394–1398.

Kierman PD, et al. Aortic-enteric fistula. Mayo Clin Proc 1980;55:731–738.

Markisz JA, et al. An evaluation of 99m-Tc-labeled red blood cell scintigraphy for the detection and localization of GI bleeding. Gastroenterology 1982;83:394–398.

Quintero E, et al. Upper GI bleeding caused by gastroduodenal malformations. Dig Dis Sci 1986;31:897–901.

Snook JA, et al. Value of a simple biochemical ratio in distinguishing upper and lower GI hemorrhage. Lancet 1986;2:1064–1066.

Storey DW, et al. Endoscopic prediction of recurrent bleeding in peptic ulcers. N Engl J Med 1986;305:915–919.

Veldhuyzen van Zanten SJO, et al. Recurrent massive hematemesis from Dielafoy vascular malformation—a review of 101 cases. Gut 1986;27:213–218.

36

UPPER GASTROINTESTINAL DISORDERS

GEORGE J. COX, JR.

Anyone who believes that the way to a man's heart is through his stomach flunked geography.

ROBERT BYRNE

ESOPHAGEAL DISEASES

Clinical Features

- Pyrosis (heartburn), odynophagia (pain on swallowing), or true dysphagia suggest esophageal inflammation, spasm, or obstruction. Heartburn, most often described as a "hot" or "burning" sensation, is the most common symptom.
- Some esophageal diseases can produce chest pain that is similar to ischemic cardiac pain.
- Gastroesophageal reflux disease may cause hoarseness, nocturnal wheezing, or repetitive throat clearing.
- The history is of great importance. For example, further evaluation is not necessary when classical symptoms of reflux disease are present, dysphagia is not present, and symptoms resolve with antireflux maneuvers (head-of-bed elevation; avoiding alcohol, cigarettes, and nonsteroidal anti-inflammatory agents; and stopping oral intake several hours before lying down), and possibly short-term therapy to suppress gastric acid production.
- The evaluation depends on the acuteness of onset, duration of symptoms, and the ability to handle oral intake. The presence of risk factors for development of UGI malignancy, a history of exposure to a caustic agent (bleach, lye, or ammonia), or the presence of immunodeficiency may accelerate the work-up.

Differential Diagnosis (Table 36–1)

Major categories include esophagitis, esophageal obstruction, and motor disorders.

Laboratory Evaluation

- UGI barium examination and provocation testing
  1. Barium esophagraphic examination and provocation

TABLE 36–1. Differential Diagnosis of Esophageal Diseases

Esophagitis
  Acid reflux disease
  Infectious (viral or fungal)
  Caustic injury (including pills such as tetracycline, potassium chloride, ferrous sulfate, acetylsalicylic acid, or quinidine)
Obstructing lesions
  Rings (Schatzki's) and webs
  Diverticula (Zenker's, traction, and epiphrenic types)
  Benign tumors (leiomyoma, lipoma, papilloma, granular cell tumor)
  Malignant tumors
  Foreign body
Esophageal motor disorders
  Achalasia
  Diffuse spasm
  "Nutcracker" esophagus
  Nonspecific esophageal motility dysfunction
Chest pain of nonesophageal origin
  Coronary ischemia
  Musculoskeletal

---

    testing with esophageal acid perfusion (Bernstein test) have good sensitivities in the diagnosis of esophagitis.

2. The Bernstein test, the poorer of these methods, has a sensitivity of 59% and a positive predictive value of 57%.

3. These diagnostic methods are often used rather than esophagogastroduodenoscopy (EGD) when evaluating for probable mild reflux disease.

- Endoscopy

1. When symptoms suggest moderate to severe reflux disease, symptoms have been present for an extended period of time, odynophagia or dysphagia are present, or when symptoms develop in an immunocompromised host, a definitive diagnosis should be sought with endoscopy and biopsy.

2. Friability and ulceration are the most sensitive endoscopic findings to suggest reflux disease.

3. In Barrett's disease, where esophageal squamous epithelium is replaced by columnar-type epithelium, there is an increased risk of esophageal adenocarcinoma (40- to 60-fold).

    a. Malignancy is already present at the time of diagnosis in 9 to 26% of Barrett's patients.

    b. Current recommendations are for annual EGD with biopsy every 2 to 3 cm throughout the Barrett's segment.

4. Using small-caliber endoscopes, EGD is the most direct approach to assess injury from bleach, ammonia, or other caustic agents.

- pH monitoring
  1. The sensitivity of extended intraesophageal pH monitoring (with correlation to symptoms) is 79 to 95% with a specificity of 87 to 100%.
  2. The Tuttle test (short-term pH monitoring) has a false-positive rate of 31% and false-negative rate of 8%.
  3. In interpreting intraesophageal pH testing, the criteria for separation of normal from abnormal studies are not universally accepted. Furthermore, the presence of esophagitis is not always dependent on acid (as demonstrated in the achlorhydric patient with esophagitis due to bile acids, pepsin, or pancreatic secretions).
  4. The specificity of extended pH monitoring is comparable to that of EGD and manometry. Extended pH monitoring is less costly than EGD in screening for reflux disease.
  5. Patients should be tested in both upright and recumbent positions, in an ambulatory state, and without change in their usual dietary habits, including cigarette smoking. The percentage of time the pH is less than 4 is the most important variable in the diagnosis of reflux disease.
  6. When possible, simultaneous Holter monitoring should be considered to help identify individuals with cardiac or coexisting cardiac origin of their pain.
- Manometry
  1. Motor disorders of the esophageal body and lower sphincter are best defined with intraluminal pressure recordings. Disorders of the upper sphincter are diagnosed more satisfactorily with cinefluoroscopy.
  2. Radiographic examination is most often used for screening purposes since both motor dysfunction and mucosal diseases can be assessed. Inflammatory diseases are often not detected on X-ray examination since mucosal lesions smaller than 0.5 cm are often missed.
- Other tests. The Tensilon test (edrophonium IV injection) and provocation testing with intraluminal balloon dilatation are useful adjuncts in assessing patients with suspected esophageal origin of their chest pain. They are poor in discriminating motor dysfunction from esophagitis.

Recommended Diagnostic Approach

In approaching possible esophageal pain, the following sequence should be used:

- Exclude cardiac disease by ECG and/or treadmill testing.
- Identify structural GI disease by UGI series, EGD, and, possibly, abdominal ultrasound.
- Identify gastroesophageal reflux by pH monitoring. Consider an empiric trial of histamine₂ receptor antagonists.
- Identify esophageal motility disorders and irritable esophagus by manometry or provocative testing.

GASTRIC AND DUODENAL DISEASE

Clinical Features

- Dyspepsia is upper abdominal discomfort with or after eating, often associated with bloating or nausea.
    1. Dyspepsia is the most common symptom leading to diagnostic evaluation of the gastroduodenal region.
    2. Seventy percent of patients respond to empiric therapy within 2 weeks, and further diagnostic evaluation is not needed.
- The pain of peptic ulcer disease is classically epigastric and relieved by food, but this is inconsistent. The pain is often episodic, with individual episodes lasting several minutes.
- The Zollinger-Ellison (ZE) syndrome is present in 0.1 to 1.0% of patients with peptic ulcer disease. It should be considered when duodenal ulcer disease is recurrent, multiple, or in unusual locations, or in patients with multiple endocrine neoplasia type I (parathyroid, pituitary, and pancreatic islet cell neoplasia).

Differential Diagnosis (Table 36–2)

Laboratory Evaluation

- Radiographic imaging
    1. When compared with EGD, a barium UGI series requires less time, is less expensive, and does not require premedication. It is still considered the initial examination in patients with suspected ulcer disease. Double contrast X-rays can miss lesions smaller than 0.5 cm.
    2. Gastric ulcer
        a. Folds radiating to the edge of an ulcer crater, presence of Hampton's sign (a radiolucent line that traverses the orifice of the ulcer), and penetration of an ulcer beyond the gastric lumen on X-ray all suggest a benign ulcer.
        b. Three to seven percent of benign-appearing ulcers are malignant.
        c. Radiographic features that suggest malignant disease include:
            i. Ulcer located completely within the gastric wall or intraluminal mass
            ii. Nodularity of ulcer base or adjacent mucosa
            iii. Large ulcer
        d. Ulcers with malignant characteristics on UGI series should undergo EGD exam at the time of diagnosis.
        e. It is accepted practice for a radiographically benign-appearing ulcer to be examined by EGD after 8 weeks of treatment when healing would be expected, though some recommend universal EGD.
        f. Healing should be documented regardless of findings on initial radiographic or endoscopic evaluation.
    3. Gastritis may be suspected on double contrast UGI

TABLE 36–2. Differential Diagnosis of Gastric and Duodenal Disease

Gastritis
  Nonerosive (peptic disease, postgastrectomy, infection, malignancy, pernicious anemia)
  Erosive/hemorrhagic (drugs, ischemia, idiopathic)
Ulcer disease
  Peptic ulcer disease
  Caustic injury
  Malignancy
  Infection
Zollinger-Ellison (ZE) syndrome
Gastric outlet obstruction
  Recurrent ulcer disease
  Postoperative scarring
  Bezoar
  Foreign body
  Malignancy
Gastric or duodenal perforation
  Ulcer disease
  Ischemia
  Perioperative event
  Intestinal obstruction
  Diverticular disease
  Volvulus
Gastric-emptying disorders
  Gastroparesis
  Dumping syndromes

___

study, but many cases can only be diagnosed endoscopically.
4. The rarity of malignant duodenal ulcers makes biopsy after demonstration by UGI series only rarely needed.
5. ZE syndrome classically shows (on UGI series) prominent gastric folds or small bowel folds that are thickened or widened.
6. Gastroparesis, often seen in patients with diabetes, uremia, scleroderma, polymyositis, and narcotic use may be disclosed by UGI barium study. It may show retained or residual food and gastric secretions (despite prolonged fasting), poor peristalsis, gastric distention, or prolonged retention of barium.
7. Gastric outlet obstruction and gastroenterocolic fistulas, as well as penetration of ulcers into the pancreas, biliary tree, pericardium, and pleural space are not uncommon complications of ulcer disease. These are best approached with radiographic UGI examination with a water-soluble agent, such as Gastrografin. Nasogastric decompression may be required after examination.

- EGD
  1. Use of small-caliber flexible instruments has made this an extremely safe (mortality is 0.0004%) and well-

tolerated procedure. It requires air insufflation and is contraindicated if perforation is suspected.

2. EGD is generally considered the gold standard of anatomic UGI diagnosis, but precise guidelines for its indications are controversial and in a state of flux due to expanding therapeutic techniques.

3. The ability to obtain tissue for diagnosis is often critical. Examples include biopsies to exclude malignancy or dysplasia and analysis for infectious agents (e.g., *Helicobacter pylori,* the suspected causative agent of chronic type B gastritis).

- Radionuclide imaging

  1. This is the method of choice in assessing symptoms due to delayed or rapid emptying of gastric contents.

  2. Technetium-99m is bound to sulfur colloid and used to label chicken liver. The liver is ingested and scanning is performed to calculate the percentage of gastric emptying with time.

  3. Medications such as narcotics, cigarette smoking, body position, duodenal reflux disease, the size, consistency, and caloric content of the radiolabeled meal, and metabolic imbalance (e.g, sepsis, parenteral nutrition) can affect gastric emptying.

  4. Typically, test results are reproducible within 10 to 15% on a day-to-day basis, and radionuclide imaging can be used to assess response to therapy.

- Serum gastrin (Table 36–3)

  1. Radioimmunoassay of serum gastrin level is useful for screening for ZE syndrome.

     a. The normal level is <100 pg/ml, and patients with ZE syndrome usually have levels >200 pg/ml, and often much higher.

     b. After feeding, gastrin levels are unchanged in patients with ZE syndrome.

  2. Greatest success with the lowest rate of false positives for identifying patients is with the intravenous secretin test. The normal response is no rise of gastrin level, while patients with ZE syndrome show a rise within 2 to 10 min.

Recommended Diagnostic Approach

- The preferred initial diagnostic test for imaging the UGI tract depends on the likely diagnosis, availability and expertise, and relative cost.

- A double contrast UGI series is often the first test of choice. EGD is preferred if nonulcer mucosal lesions are likely or biopsy/therapeutic capability is desired.

- The indications for EGD developed by the American Society for Gastrointestinal Endoscopy are listed in Table 36–4. Recommendations for screening for GI malignancy are contained in Table 36–5.

TABLE 36–3.   Indications for Measuring Serum Gastrin

Family history of peptic ulcer
Ulcer associated with hypercalcemia or other
  manifestations of multiple endocrine neoplasia type I
Multifocal peptic ulcer
Peptic ulceration of postbulbar duodenum or jejunum
Peptic ulceration associated with diarrhea
Chronic unexplained diarrhea
Enlarged gastric folds on UGI X-ray
Before surgery for "intractable" ulcer
Recurrent ulcer after ulcer surgery

Source: Reprinted with permission from Wyngaarden JB, Smith LH, eds. Cecil Textbook of Medicine, 18th ed. Philadelphia, W.B. Saunders, 1988, p. 698.

TABLE 36–4.   Indications for EGD in Evaluation of UGI Disorders

Upper abdominal distress that persists despite an
  appropriate trial of therapy.
Upper abdominal distress associated with signs suggesting
  serious organic disease (e.g., anorexia and weight loss)
Dysphagia or odynophagia
Esophageal reflux symptoms that are persistent or
  progressive despite appropriate therapy
Persistent vomiting of unknown cause
Radiographic findings of:
   A neoplastic lesion, for confirmation and specific
      histologic diagnosis
   Gastric or esophageal ulcer
   Evidence of upper tract stricture or obstruction
   Mass
GI bleeding
   As the first procedure in most actively bleeding patients
   When surgical therapy is contemplated
   When rebleeding occurs after acute, self-limited blood
      loss
   When portal hypertension or aortoenteric fistula is
      suspected
   For endoscopic therapy of UGI bleeding
   For presumed chronic blood loss and iron-deficiency
      anemia when colonoscopy findings are negative

Source: Adapted with permission from Wyngaarden JB. Smith LH. eds. Cecil Textbook of Medicine, 18th ed. Philadelphia, W.B. Saunders, 1988, p. 669. American Society for Gastrointestinal Endoscopy, 1986.

TABLE 36–5. Screening for GI Malignancy

PRIMARY DISEASE	RISK	SCREENING RECOMMENDATIONS
Achalasia	Increased risk of esophageal cancer after 15 years of disease	Yearly endoscopy starting 15 yr after onset
Barrett's esophagus	8.6% incidence of adenocarcinoma	Yearly EGD with biopsy
Chronic atrophic gastritis, type B	10% risk of developing gastric cancer	EGD with biopsies every 6 to 12 months
Celiac disease	Increased risk of GI lymphoma and carcinoma	No surveillance in asymptomatic patient
Familial polyposis	High rate of gastric, periampullary, and duodenal carcinoma arising from adenomas	Annual endoscopy with polypectomy
Gastric polyps	Gastric carcinoma associated with adenomatous and hyperplastic types	Endoscopic surveillance every 1 to 2 yr after discovery of adenomatous polyp, no surveillance recommendations for hyperplastic polyps
Pernicious anemia (chronic type A atrophic gastritis)	10% incidence of gastric cancer	Annual endoscopy for patients with dysplasia
Plummer-Vinson syndrome	Associated with cancer of cervical esophagus	Yearly EGD
Scleroderma	Associated with esophageal dysplasia and cancer	Yearly EGD for the symptomatic patient
Tylosis	Up to 95% risk of developing esophageal cancer	Yearly EGD
Esophageal lye stricture	A 0.8 to 4.0% risk of developing cancer at stricture site	Yearly EGD starting 10 yr after injury
Head and neck cancer	A 1.0% incidence of synchronous or metachronous lesions of the esophagus	Esophagoscopy at time of presentation
Gastric resection	A 2 to 5% risk of stump carcinoma after 15 to 25 yr	EGD to screen symptomatic patients

Bibliography

Habr-Gama A, Waye JD. Complications and hazards of gastrointestinal endoscopy. World J Surg 1989;13:193–201.

Kahn KL, et al. The use and misuse of upper gastrointestinal endoscopy. Ann Intern Med 1988;109:664–670.

Rosen SN, Pope CE. Extended esophageal pH monitoring: An analysis of the literature and assessment of its role in the diagnosis and management of gastroesophageal reflux. J Clin Gastro 1989;11:260–270.

Schrock TR, ed. Surgical endoscopy. Surg Clin North Am 1989;69(6):1123–1357.

Sleisinger MH, Fordtran JS, eds. The esophagus: Anatomy, physiology, and disease. In: Gastrointestinal Disease: Pathophysiology, Diagnosis, and Management, 4th ed. Philadelphia, W.B. Saunders, 1989.

Sleisinger MH, Fordtran JS, eds. The stomach and duodenum: Anatomy, physiology, and disease. In: Gastrointestinal Disease: Pathophysiology, Diagnosis, and Management, 4th ed. Philadelphia, W.B. Saunders, 1989.

37

MALABSORPTION

JOHN HALSEY, *and* MICHAEL KIMMEY

I have finally kum to the konklusion that a good reliable sett ov bowels iz worth more tu a man than any quantity ov brains.

HENRY WHEELER SHAW ("Josh Billings") (1818-1885)

GENERAL COMMENTS

The prevalence of malabsorption syndrome in the general population is unknown.

DIFFERENTIAL DIAGNOSIS

- Irritable bowel syndrome
  1. Patients with vague abdominal pain, fatigue, and alteration in bowel habits are frequently thought to have the irritable bowel syndrome. The physician must be alert to clues that suggest malabsorption in these patients.
  2. Weight loss, muscle wasting, and edema are symptoms of advanced malabsorption but may also be caused by poor nutrition, severe depression, and occult malignancy, which should be excluded.
- Various causes of maldigestion and malabsorption (Table 37–1)

CLINICAL MANIFESTATIONS

- History
  1. Weight loss. This may be absent in early malabsorption; however, with time, weight loss usually becomes evident. Muscle wasting resulting from impaired protein metabolism may also be prominent.
  2. Appetite
     a. Most patients with small intestinal disease have poor appetite and decreased food intake, often because food exacerbates abdominal pain and diarrhea.
     b. Patients with pancreatic insufficiency may have hyperphagia and eat large quantities of food.
     c. Patients with iron deficiency may have a peculiar craving, or pica, for clay or ice.
     d. Patients with lactase deficiency often deduce that dairy products exacerbate their symptoms.

Text continued on page 315

TABLE 37–1. Classification and Clinical Findings in the Malabsorption Syndrome

| | | | | | LABORATORY TESTS | |
CAUSE	HISTORY	PHYSICAL EXAM	Fecal Fat Normal <6 g/day	D-Xylose	Jejunal Biopsy	Other
I. Intraluminal pancreatic enzyme deficiency						
A. Chronic pancreatitis	Recurrent episodes of acute pancreatitis, weight loss (95%), abdominal pain	Signs of weight loss, abdominal tenderness, edema/ ascites (10%)	Abnormal (30–40 g/ day)	Normal	Normal	Abnormal Schilling (40%), abnormal triolein breath test (95%), abnormal secretin stimulation test
B. Pancreatic resection	History of surgery	See above	See above	Normal	Normal	See above
C. Pancreatic carcinoma	Abdominal pain, weight loss	Abdominal mass, jaundice	See above	Normal	Normal	See above
D. Cystic fibrosis (CF) (Accounts for 95% of cases of pancreatic insuff. in children; 80% of children with CF have pancreatic insufficiency.)	Recurrent respiratory tract symptoms (90%), oily stools, failure to thrive	Smaller than expected for age (wt & ht), pulmonary findings	Abnormal (20–30 g/ day)	Normal	Normal	Elevated sweat chloride (98%)

Table continued on following page

307

TABLE 37–1. Classification and Clinical Findings in the Malabsorption Syndrome *Continued*

CAUSE	HISTORY	PHYSICAL EXAM	Fecal Fat Normal <6 g/day	D-Xylose	Jejunal Biopsy	Other
			LABORATORY TESTS			
II. Intraluminal bile salt deficiency						
A. Bile duct obstruction	Jaundice	Hepatomegaly	Abnormal (40 g/day with complete obstruction, 15–20 g/day with partial obstruction)	Normal	Normal	Elevated bilirubin, alkaline phosphatase
B. Hepatic insufficiency (generally chronic diseases, esp. cirrhosis)	Weakness (40%), Encephalopathy (40%), Anorexia (40%), Abdominal pain (30%)	Hepatomegaly (70%), ascites (60%), jaundice	Abnormal (10–20 g/day)	Normal	Normal	Prolonged prothrombin time, low albumin
C. Small intestinal bacterial overgrowth (blind loops, diverticula, motor abnormalities, scleroderma, diabetes, pseudo-obstruction)	Prior surgery, abdominal pain and distention in pseudo-obstruction, arthritis/skin changes in scleroderma	Surgical scars, findings of scleroderma or diabetes	Abnormal (15–20 g/day)	May be abnormal due to bacterial xylose metabolism	Normal	Abnormal Schilling, small bowel X-ray to R/O anatomic defects, abnormal bile acid breath test

			Fecal fat		Biopsy	Other tests
D. Defective ileal bile salt absorption						
1. Ileal resection (generally greater than 100 cm to give symptoms)	Prior surgery	Surgical scar	Abnormal (20–25 g/day)	Normal	Normal	Abnormal Schilling, abnormal bile acid breath test, gallstones (30%)
2. Ileitis	Diarrhea (90%), abdominal pain (80%)	Perianal disease (20%), arthritis (20%)	Abnormal (15–20 g/day)	Normal	May be abnormal (granulomas)	Abnormal Schilling, abnormal bile acid breath test, gallstones (30%)
III. Small intestinal disease						
A. Mucosal cellular defects						
1. Disaccharidase deficiency Lactase—common Maltase—uncommon Sucrose—rare	Diarrhea, flatulence, pain after ingestion of involved sugar (usually milk)	Usually normal	Normal		Normal histology	Abnormal sugar tolerance tests, assay enzymes in jejunal biopsy
2. Abetalipoproteinemia (rare childhood disease)	Failure to thrive, family history (autosomal recessive), cardiac arrhythmias	Ataxia, nystagmus retinitis pigmentosa, congestive heart failure	Abnormal (10–15 g/day)	Normal	Characteristic lipid vacuoles; normal villi	Low cholesterol and triglyceride levels

TABLE 37-1. Classification and Clinical Findings in the Malabsorption Syndrome Continued

			LABORATORY TESTS			
CAUSE	HISTORY	PHYSICAL EXAM	Fecal Fat Normal <6 g/day	D-Xylose	Jejunal Biopsy	Other
B. Lymphatic obstruction 1. Intestinal lymphangiectasia (Unusual)	Progressive edema and anasarca beginning in first two decades of life	Edema, ascites	Abnormal (15–20 g/ day)	Normal	Characteristic dilated lacteals; may be patchy	Hypoproteinemia, Intestinal protein loss
2. Lymphoma—malabsorption unusual with localized or secondary lymphoma; common with primary diffuse lymphoma	Abdominal pain, weight loss, ethnic history (Sephardic Jews, Arabs)	Clubbing, peripheral edema, abdominal mass (10–20%)	Abnormal (30–40 g/ day)	Abnormal	Characteristic but patchy lesions seen in 50–70% of diffuse cases	Hypoproteinemia, IgA heavy chains in serum (uncommon)
C. Other small intestinal defects 1. Celiac sprue (gluten-sensitive enteropathy)	Typical malabsorption symptoms, extra-intestinal symptoms may be prominent, childhood or adult onset	Clubbing, edema, dermatitis herpetiformis in a minority	Abnormal (25–30 g/ day)	Abnormal	Diffuse villous flattening with lymphocyte infiltration	Reversion to normal of jejunal biopsy after dietary gluten elimination

Disease	Clinical symptoms	Systemic/associated features	Fecal fat	D-xylose	Biopsy	Diagnosis
2. Tropical sprue	Prolonged (>1 yr) residence in tropical countries, malabsorptive symptoms with prominent anorexia	Weight loss, glossitis (25%)	Abnormal (15–20 g/day)	Abnormal	Abnormal; similar to celiac sprue	Clinical and biopsy, response to folate and tetracycline therapy, megaloblastic anemia (95%), rule out parasites
3. Whipple's disease	Arthritis (75%), fever (50%), CNS abnormalities (uncommon), recurrent pleuritis	Arthritis, lymphadenopathy, dementia, cranial nerve abnormalities (uncommon)	Abnormal (30–40 g/day)	Abnormal	Characteristic PAS positive macrophages in lamina propria	Iron deficiency anemia, clinical and usually biopsy, response to antibiotics
4. Eosinophilic gastroenteritis	Food allergies, abdominal pain, intermittent nausea and vomiting, asthma, allergic rhinitis (50%)	Eczema, urticaria	Abnormal (10–15 g/day)	Usually abnormal with mucosal disease	Patchy infiltration with eosinophils	Eosinophilia hypoalbuminemia, negative intestinal parasites
5. Amyloidosis (intestinal involvement in 70% systemic cases; malabsorption in 5%)	Abdominal pain, abdominal distention, vomiting	Macroglossia (20%), hepatosplenomegaly, peripheral neuropathy, arthritis	Abnormal (10–15 g/day)	Abnormal	Patchy amyloid deposition, especially in blood vessels	Abnormal rectal or subcutaneous fat biopsy (80%); thickened folds on X-rays

TABLE 37-1. Classification and Clinical Findings in the Malabsorption Syndrome Continued

| | | | | LABORATORY TESTS | | |
CAUSE	HISTORY	PHYSICAL EXAM	Fecal Fat Normal <6 g/day	D-Xylose	Jejunal Biopsy	Other
IV. Multiple defects						
1. Zollinger-Ellison syndrome	Peptic ulcer disease, diarrhea (30%)	Usually normal	Abnormal in 25% (15–20 g/day)	Normal	Usually normal; patchy microulcers may be present	High serum gastrin
2. Postgastrectomy	Prior gastric surgery (esp. Billroth II anastomosis)	Abdominal surgical scar	Abnormal (10–15 g/day)	Normal	Normal	Iron deficiency anemia (50%), osteomalacia (30%)
3. Radiation enteritis	Prior abdominal radiation (>4000 rads), watery diarrhea, tenesmus	Usually normal	Abnormal (10–15 g/day)	May be abnormal with small bowel involvement	Abnormal, although nonspecific changes	Sigmoidoscopy may show proctitis, small intestinal X-ray: fistulas, ulcers, strictures; bile acid breath test to R/O bacterial overgrowth

V. Uncertain etiology					
1. Immunodeficiency	Recurrent intestinal infections	Usually normal	Abnormal (10–20 g/day)	May be abnormal	Abnormal: May show absence of plasma cells of nodular lymphoid hyperplasia	Hypogammaglobulinemia or isolated immunoglobulin deficiency; *Giardia* cysts in stool
2. Carcinoid syndrome	Cutaneous flushes (head and neck), episodic abdominal cramps and diarrhea, wheezing	Hepatomegaly, tricuspid murmurs	May be abnormal (10–15 g/day)	Usually normal	Usually normal	Increased urinary 5-hydroxyindoleacetic acid
3. Parasitoses (*Giardia lamblia*, Coccidia, *Strongyloides, Capillaria, mycobacterium avium–intracellulare* (MAI), and ancylostomiasis may produce malabsorption)	Loose, mucusy stools. Fever and headache with coccidiosis; borborygmi and abdominal distention with capillariasis	Usually normal	May be abnormal (10–15 g/day)	Usually	Nonspecific changes or may see *Giardia* oocysts or MAI on acid-fast stains.	Stool for ova and parasites, eosinophilia with strongyloides

TABLE 37-1. Classification and Clinical Findings in the Malabsorption Syndrome Continued

| | | | | LABORATORY TESTS | | |
| | | | Fecal Fat Normal <6 g/day | D-Xylose | Jejunal Biopsy | Other |
CAUSE	HISTORY	PHYSICAL EXAM				
4. Diabetes mellitus (approx. 10% with diarrhea and 5% with steatorrhea)	Diarrhea often nocturnal. Renal, ocular, vascular disease often present	Peripheral neuropathy; retinopathy; often signs of weight loss	Abnormal (20–25 g/day)	May be normal or abnormal	Normal	Hyperglycemia, abnormal bile acid breath test due to bacterial overgrowth in minority
5. Other endocrinopathies (hyperthyroidism, hypothyroidism, hypoadrenocorticism)	Findings of specific endocrinologic disorder		Abnormal (15–20 g/day)	May be normal or abnormal	Normal	Check specific hormone levels

R/O = rule out

Source: Adapted from Kimmey, MB. Malabsorption. In: Cummins RO, Eisenberg MS. Blue Book of Medical Diagnosis. Philadelphia, W.B. Saunders, 1986, pp. 472–475.

3. Stool character and frequency
   a. Bowel movements may be normal or increased in frequency. The earliest change is often a marked increase in the bulk of stools. Oily, rancid stools are found in advanced cases.
   b. Floating stools correlate with gas, not fat, content. Excessive flatulence may indicate carbohydrate malabsorption.
   c. Bloody stools are seen predominantly with inflammatory bowel disease, infection, and ischemia.
4. Pain
   a. Most malabsorptive states are not accompanied by abdominal pain.
   b. Patients with Crohn's disease or radiation enteritis may have aching or cramping periumbilical or RLQ pain.
   c. Back pain may be seen with chronic pancreatitis.
   d. Patients with vascular insufficiency of the intestine often have severe, poorly localized pain that typically occurs 30 to 60 min after eating.
5. Other symptoms potentially caused by malabsorption
   a. Bruising and easy bleeding may be signs of vitamin K malabsorption.
   b. Night blindness and dry eyes may signify vitamin A insufficiency.
   c. Bone pain, tetany, and paresthesias may be caused by abnormal calcium metabolism from vitamin D and calcium malabsorption.
   d. Malnutrition and weight loss may also lead to pituitary dysfunction, loss of libido, or amenorrhea.
6. Prior medical history and other factors. Medical history (prior surgery, medications, alcohol use, ulcer disease, other medical problems such as arthritis and skin problems, and prior radiation), family history (cystic fibrosis, inflammatory bowel disease, and sprue), and ethnic background are all relevant and may provide etiologic clues.

• Physical examination
1. Vital signs. Hypotension and tachycardia may be caused by volume depletion or simply by severe malnutrition. Fever usually indicates the presence of infection or tumor.
2. Abdominal examination
   a. Abdominal distention may be caused by ascites or excessive intestinal gas. Bowel sounds are not diagnostically helpful.
   b. Hepatosplenomegaly may be seen with amyloidosis and occasionally with lymphoma.
   c. Abdominal masses may be felt in Crohn's disease, carcinoma, diverticulitis, and lymphoma.
   d. Significant abdominal tenderness is unusual in most diseases that cause malabsorption.
3. General physical examination
   a. Signs of malabsorption. These may include muscle wasting, edema, Trousseau's and Chvostek's

signs, skeletal deformities, bruises and purpura, glossitis, peripheral neuropathy, and clubbing.

b. Signs suggestive of underlying cause include:

    i. Thickened skin, especially over the fingers (scleroderma)

    ii. Grouped vesicles, especially on extensor skin surfaces (gluten sensitive enteropathy with dermatitis herpetiformis)

    iii. Wheezing (eosinophilic gastroenteritis or carcinoid syndrome)

    iv. Urticaria and flushing (systemic mastocytosis)

    v. Retinopathy and neuropathy (diabetes mellitus)

    vi. Arthritis (inflammatory bowel disease, Whipple's disease, amyloidosis, and hypogammaglobulinemia)

    vii. Signs of hypo- and hyperthyroidism

LABORATORY EVALUATION

- Routine tests. Screening tests include:

  1. Hematocrit with RBC indices (macrocytosis due to folate or vitamin B_{12} deficiency; microcytosis from iron deficiency)

  2. Serum carotene (fat malabsorption or dietary deficiency)

  3. Prothrombin time (vitamin K malabsorption or liver disease)

  4. Serum calcium (vitamin D or calcium malabsorption; hypoparathyroidism)

  5. Serum albumin (protein malabsorption, protein loss, or liver disease)

  6. Erythrocyte sedimentation rate (inflammatory bowel disease, lymphoma)

  7. Serum vitamin B_{12} and folate levels (useful to determine the cause of macrocytic anemia)

  8. Serum cholesterol (low in fat malabsorption)

- Fecal fat determination

  1. Qualitative

     a. Staining of a smear made from a routine stool specimen with Sudan stain and acetic acid provides a qualitative estimate of steatorrhea.

     b. The number and size of fat droplets correlate with the quantitative fat determination in adults who excrete greater than 12 to 15 g of fat/day.

     c. False-negative results are seen with low-fat diets, in children, and in mild degrees of steatorrhea (6 to 12 g of fecal fat/day).

  2. Quantitative

     a. Since normal fat digestion and absorption involves all phases of the digestive process, this test provides the most sensitive evaluation of the overall process.

   b. The patient is placed on a standard diet containing 80 to 100 g of fat/day. After 2 days, stool collection is begun and continued for 72 hr. Collection can be facilitated by using a paint can that is kept sealed between uses.
   c. Excretion of greater than 6 g of fat/24 hr is abnormal (2 standard deviations above the mean).
   d. Fecal fat quantitation does not distinguish the causes of malabsorption. If results are abnormal, further testing should be done to define the specific defect present.
   e. Potential errors and disadvantages of the test include:
      i. Inadequate stool collection
      ii. The necessity of patient cooperation
      iii. A defined, usually unsupervised diet over a 5-day period
      iv. Stool collection and analysis are unpleasant
      v. Laxatives such as mineral oil and castor oil cause falsely elevated values
      vi. A normal test result does not exclude malabsorption of substances other than fat (such as carbohydrates and vitamins).
   3. Simplified (24-hr) fat determination. The collection of stool for 24 hr, while the patient is on his or her regular diet, is often sufficient to diagnose steatorrhea and is much easier to perform than the standardized 72-hr stool collection.
- D-xylose test
   1. D-xylose is a 5-carbon sugar that is absorbed in the duodenum and proximal jejunum, is not metabolized by man, and is excreted unchanged in the urine.
   2. The test is performed by having the patient drink a solution of 25 g of the sugar in 500 ml of water.
   3. A plasma specimen 1 hr after ingestion should have greater than 20 mg/dl of xylose. Urine collected for 5 hr should contain over 4 g of xylose.
   4. Low xylose concentrations are seen with:
      a. Inadequate intestinal absorption caused by a decreased absorptive surface (in celiac sprue or intestinal resection)
      b. Infiltrative intestinal diseases if these are extensive (regional enteritis, lymphoma, or amyloid)
      c. Bacterial overgrowth states (due to bacterial metabolism of the xylose)
   5. Falsely low urine, but not serum, values are seen with massive ascites and decreased renal function.
- Breath tests
   1. Triolein breath test
      a. The triolein breath test screens for fat malabsorption by measuring $^{14}CO_2$ exhaled after ingestion of the carbon-14–labeled triglyceride triolein. If normal digestion and absorption are present, the triolein is metabolized with subsequent circulation and exhalation of $^{14}CO_2$.

b. Nonobese patients with steatorrhea exhale less $^{14}CO_2$ than nonobese patients without steatorrhea.

c. Results correlate well with quantitative fecal fat determination (100% sensitivity, 96% specificity). False-positive results are seen in 25% of obese patients and potentially in situations of delayed gastric emptying and obstructive pulmonary disease.

d. Although currently not widely available, this test may eventually become a more usable test for fat malabsorption than quantitative fecal fat determination. The specific defect causing fat malabsorption is not defined by this test.

2. Bile acid breath test

a. Orally ingested conjugated bile acids labeled with ^{14}C-glycine normally undergo enterohepatic circulation with minimal deconjugation.

b. In the presence of small intestinal bacterial overgrowth or ileal dysfunction or resection, bile acids are deconjugated, and when the glycine is metabolized, $^{14}CO_2$ is released and measured in the exhaled breath.

c. The bile acid breath test detects bacterial overgrowth with a sensitivity of 70% and a specificity of 90%. It is most useful when the pretest probability of bacterial overgrowth is intermediate, such as in diarrhea or steatorrhea of unknown cause, diabetes with diarrhea, and scleroderma.

- Schilling test (Table 37–2)

1. The Schilling test is used to determine the etiology of vitamin B_{12} (cobalamin) malabsorption. The standard (stage 1) Schilling test measures vitamin B_{12} absorption and is used to detect intrinsic factor deficiency in patients with pernicious anemia.

2. In stage 1, 100 μg of nonlabeled cobalamin is given IM to saturate the B_{12}-binding sites.

a. One μg of ^{57}Co-cyanocobalamin is administered orally and the subsequent 24-hr urinary excretion of radioactive cobalamin measured.

b. If less than 8% of the total radioactivity administered is excreted, then B_{12} malabsorption is established.

3. In stage 2, stage 1 is repeated with the addition of intrinsic factor.

a. If malabsorption is corrected, then pernicious anemia is established as the diagnosis.

b. If malabsorption of B_{12} persists after the addition of intrinsic factor, then stage 3 is accomplished by administering ^{57}Co-cyanocobalamin with pancreatic enzymes. Correction of malabsorption establishes pancreatic insufficiency as the diagnosis.

4. If malabsorption of B_{12} persists after stage 3, a trial of antibiotics should be administered on the presumption that bacterial overgrowth is present.

a. Tetracycline 500 mg 4 times daily or metronidazole 250 mg 3 times daily for a week is usually adequate.

TABLE 37–2. The 4-Stage Schilling Test

CONDITION	STAGE 1 (B₁₂ ONLY)	STAGE 2 (IF)	STAGE 3 (PANCREATIC ENZYMES)	STAGE 4 (AFTER ANTIBIOTICS)
B_{12} malabsorption	Decreased			
Deficient intrinsic factor a. Pernicious anemia b. Gastrectomy	Decreased	Normal		
Pancreatic insufficiency Chronic pancreatitis	Decreased	Decreased	Normal	
Bacterial overgrowth Intestinal stasis	Decreased	Decreased	Decreased	Normal
Terminal ileal disorders a. Resection b. Nontropical sprue c. Regional enteritis	Decreased	Decreased	Decreased	Decreased

Source: Modified from Ramano TJ, Dobbins JW. Evaluation of the patient with suspected malabsorption. In: Fisher RL, ed. Malabsorption and Nutritional Status and Support. Gastroenterology Clinics of North America, Philadelphia, W.B. Saunders, 1989. Copyright © W.B. Saunders.

319

    b. Stage 1 is then repeated, and if B_{12} malabsorption persists, ileal resection or disease is present.

  5. False-positive Schilling tests may occur with renal dysfunction, H_2-receptor blocker therapy, or inactive intrinsic factor. False-negatives may occur with achlorhydria or in concurrent B_{12} and folate deficiency.

- Small intestinal biopsy
  1. Peroral suction biopsy of the small intestinal mucosa is a safe procedure that provides useful diagnostic information in patients with evidence of intestinal malabsorption.
  2. Biopsy findings are usually diagnostic in celiac sprue, immunodeficiency, Whipple's disease, and abetalipoproteinemia. The biopsy is abnormal in celiac sprue, but is often not diagnostic.
  3. Small intestinal biopsy may be diagnostic in other diseases with a patchy distribution, including amyloidosis, systemic mastocytosis, eosinophilic enteritis, lymphoma, parasitic infestation, intestinal lymphangiectasia, and radiation enteritis.
  4. Nonspecific or normal findings are usually found in regional enteritis, tropical sprue, and conditions of bacterial overgrowth.
- Small intestinal X-rays
  1. This noninvasive test is most useful in defining abnormal anatomic details, including diverticula, congenital anomalies, enteroenteric fistulas, and postsurgical changes.
  2. Nonspecific abnormalities such as delayed transit time, thickened mucosa, increased intestinal fluid, and small bowel dilatation may be seen in other diseases with malabsorption.
  3. This test is frequently done early in the diagnostic evaluation because it is easy and noninvasive; however, it is rarely, by itself, sufficient to yield the underlying diagnosis.
- Secretin test
  1. The secretin test is a reliable quantitative pancreatic stimulation test that assesses pancreatic exocrine function. The test is cumbersome and, because of the large pancreatic reserve, requires greater than 75% of pancreatic function to be lost before results are abnormal.
  2. A tube is placed fluoroscopically in the second part of the duodenum and the collected aspirates analyzed for volume, bicarbonate, and pancreatic enzymes after intravenous administration of secretin and cholecystokinin.
- Other. Imaging procedures such as ultrasound, computed tomography, and endoscopic retrograde cholangiopancreatography, and the clinical response to oral pancreatic enzyme supplementation are also used in the evaluation of pancreatic insufficiency.

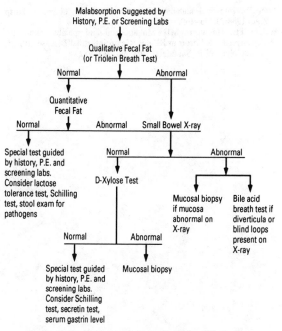

Figure 37–1. Diagnostic evaluation of malabsorption.

RECOMMENDED DIAGNOSTIC APPROACH
(Figure 37–1)

- The history, physical examination, and screening laboratory tests (hematocrit, prothrombin time, calcium, and albumin) suggest which patients should undergo specific laboratory testing.

- A diagnostic principle is to first define specific nutrient malabsorption (fecal fat, D-xylose, Schilling, and carbohydrate tolerance tests) and then to proceed to evaluation of the specific cause of the malabsorption (jejunal biopsy, pancreatic function tests, bile acid breath test, and small intestinal X-ray).

Bibliography

Greenberger NG, Isselbacher KJ. Disorders of absorption. In: Wilson JD, et al., eds. Harrison's Principles of Internal Medicine, 12th ed. New York, McGraw-Hill, 1990, pp. 1252–1268.

Ramano TJ, Dobbins JW. Evaluation of the patient with suspected malabsorption. In: Fisher RL, ed. Gastroenterology Clinics of North America: Malabsorption and Nutritional Status and Support. Philadelphia, W.B. Saunders, 1989, vol. 18, pp. 467–484.

Trier JS. Intestinal malabsorption: Differentiation of cause. Hosp Pract 1988;23:153–169.

Wright TL, Heyworth MF. Maldigestion and malabsorption. In: Sleisenger MH, Fordtran JS, eds. Gastrointestinal Disease, 4th ed. Philadelphia, W.B. Saunders, 1989, pp. 263–282.

38

IDIOPATHIC INFLAMMATORY BOWEL DISEASE

CHRISTINA M. SURAWICZ

Man should always strive to have his intestines relaxed
all the days [of his life] and that [bowel function] should
approximate diarrhea. This is a fundamental principle
in medicine, [namely] whenever the stool is withheld or
is extruded with difficulty, grave illnesses result.

MOSES BEN MAIMON (MAIMONIDES) (1135–1204)

DEFINITION AND GENERAL COMMENTS

There are two types of idiopathic inflammatory bowel disease
(IIBD): ulcerative colitis and Crohn's disease. These two diseases of unknown origin are distinct from inflammatory bowel
disease due to specific causes, such as infection, ischemia, or
antibiotics.

- Ulcerative colitis
  1. Ulcerative colitis is a diffuse mucosal inflammation
     that can involve the entire length of the colon, includ-
     ing the rectum, or any part of the colon.
  2. The term ''ulcerative proctitis'' refers to ulcerative
     colitis that is limited to the distal 10 cm of rectum, with
     no progression to the rest of the colon over a 1-year
     period.
- Crohn's disease
  1. Also called granulomatous ileocolitis, regional enteri-
     tis, and segmental colitis, Crohn's disease causes seg-
     mental and transmural inflammation that can involve
     any part of the GI tract from the mouth to the anus.
  2. Fistulae frequently form between the bowel and adja-
     cent organs or between segments of bowel.
     a. Crohn's colitis (27% of cases; solely colonic in-
        volvement).
     b. Isolated Crohn's disease of the small intestine
        (28%; also called regional enteritis).
     c. Crohn's ileocolitis (41%; the colon and ileum—
        usually the terminal ileum—are both involved).
     d. Isolated anorectal Crohn's disease occurs in 4% of
        patients.
- Epidemiology. Both ulcerative colitis and Crohn's disease
  appear most often in young adulthood. There is a smaller

second peak time of incidence in the 55- to 65-year age group. Jews have a higher prevalence of IIBD than the general population.

- Etiology
  1. No known cause exists for IIBD, but most investigators consider it an immunologically mediated disease.
  2. The high concordance rate in monozygotic twins and an increased incidence in families suggest that genetic factors play a role.
  3. The rising incidence of IIBD in industrialized nations points to environmental factors. Strains of mycobacteria, including *M. paratuberculosis*, have been isolated from diseased tissues of some patients with Crohn's disease, but definitive evidence of an infectious cause is lacking.

DIFFERENTIAL DIAGNOSIS (Table 38–1)

- Infectious colitis (Table 38–2). This usually has a self-limited course of less than 4 weeks.
  1. Bacterial. Forty to sixty percent of patients with an acute colitis syndrome have stool cultures that are positive for *Campylobacter, Salmonella,* or *Shigella.* Less common pathogens include *Escherichia coli,* including *E. coli* 0157 : H7 and *Yersinia.*
  2. Parasitic. Infection with amebae or schistosomiasis (from endemic areas) is possible.
  3. Homosexual men may have other pathogens such as *Neisseria gonorrhoeae, Chlamydia trachomatis,* syphilis, or herpes simplex virus type 2.
- Ischemic colitis usually occurs in older patients. Splenic flexure involvement is common (watershed area). No good diagnostic methods exist.
- Pseudomembranous colitis is usually associated with recent use of antibiotics. *Clostridium difficile* and its toxin are detected in the stool. Diagnostic pseudomembranes are observed at sigmoidoscopy.
- Cancer. A mass lesion can be detected by sigmoidoscopy, barium enema, or colonoscopy.

TABLE 38–1. Differential Diagnosis of IIBD

Infections (see Table 38–4)
Ischemia
Radiation enteritis
Collagenous colitis
Pseudomembranous colitis (*C. difficile*)
Solitary rectal ulcer syndrome
Drug-induced, i.e., gold, ampicillin (non–*C. difficile*)
Diversion colitis
Diverticulitis
Eosinophilic colitis
Graft-versus-host disease (GVHD)

TABLE 38–2. Infectious Diarrhea

BACTERIA	VIRUSES	PARASITES
Campylobacter spp.	Rotavirus	*Giardia lamblia*
Salmonella spp.	Norwalk virus	*Cryptosporidium*
Shigella spp.	Enteric adenoviruses	*Entamoeba histolytica*
Invasive *E. coli*	Cytomegalovirus	
Toxigenic *E. coli*	Herpes simplex virus (type 2)	
Noncholera *Vibrio*		
Aeromonas		
Vibrio cholera		
Clostridium difficile		
Yersinia enterocolitica		

- Radiation colitis. This condition occurs after radiation therapy, usually in women treated for gynecologic malignancies.
- Collagenous colitis causes watery diarrhea, usually in middle-aged women. The diagnosis is made by colorectal biopsy.

CLINICAL FEATURES (Table 38–3)

- Ulcerative colitis. The most common symptoms are bloody diarrhea, tenesmus, and crampy abdominal pain. Weight loss, anorexia, fever, nausea, and vomiting may also be present.
- Crohn's disease. The symptoms are often the same as in ulcerative colitis. Diarrhea is frequent. Abdominal pain

TABLE 38–3. Comparison of Ulcerative Colitis and Crohn's Disease

FEATURES	ULCERATIVE COLITIS	CROHN'S DISEASE
Distribution	Colon, diffuse	Entire GI tract, segmental
Inflammation	Superficial	Transmural
Ulcers	Microscopic	Macroscopic
Strictures	Rare	Common
Rectal sparing	Almost never	Common
Fistulae	Never	Can occur
Histology		
Granulomas	Never	Common
Focal disease	Rare	Common

occurs in 55 to 65% of patients and malnutrition in 12 to 22%. Fever, nausea and vomiting, and anorexia may also be prominent symptoms.

- Complications (Table 38–4). Many extraintestinal manifestations occur in both ulcerative colitis and Crohn's disease.
  1. Arthritis associated with IIBD. Two types of arthritis can occur in association with IIBD in up to 25% of patients.
     a. Axial arthritis, also known as the ankylosing spondylitis type, is associated with HLA-B27. The arthritic flares are unrelated to exacerbations of bowel disease.
     b. Peripheral "colitic" arthritis is monoarticular, usually affecting knees, ankles, wrists, and fingers. Arthritic flares are associated with exacerbation of bowel disease.
  2. Skin. Complications include oral aphthous ulcers (5 to 10%), erythema nodosum (3%, especially in Crohn's disease), and pyoderma gangrenosum (1 to 4%, especially in ulcerative colitis).
  3. Eye. Iritis occurs in 5 to 10% of cases. Episcleritis and uveitis can also occur.
  4. Hepatic lesions. Manifestations include pericholangitis, fatty liver, chronic active hepatitis, and cirrhosis. Sclerosing cholangitis is a complication of ulcerative colitis.
  5. Cancer. The incidence of colon cancer is increased significantly in patients with ulcerative colitis, usually after more than 7 years of disease. It may be multifocal. Dysplasia evident on colonic biopsy is a precursor of cancer. There is also an increase in intestinal cancer in Crohn's disease, but not as high as in ulcerative colitis.
  6. Complications in Crohn's disease. Some complications occur only with Crohn's disease. Cholesterol gallstones (from bile salt malabsorption) occur in 30% of cases. Oxalate renal stones (from fat malabsorption), amyloidosis, and right hydronephrosis (due to an obstruction by a RLQ mass) also occur.

TABLE 38–4. Complications of Crohn's Disease by Site of Involvement

	SMALL INTESTINAL DISEASE	ILEOCOLITIS	COLITIS
Rectal bleeding	10	22	46
Rectal fistula	5	21	19
Intestinal obstruction	35	44	17
Internal and cutaneous fistulae	17	34	16
Perianal fistula	14	38	36

- General physical examination
  1. Abdominal tenderness, especially in the LLQ or RLQ (with ileocecal involvement in Crohn's disease), is particularly common.
  2. Some findings strongly suggest Crohn's disease, including RLQ mass (ileocecal involvement) and perianal fistulae (however, fissures or abscesses can occur in ulcerative colitis or without IIBD).
  3. Aphthous mouth ulcers are frequent but nonspecific. Splenomegaly and clubbing of the nails each occur in 10% of patients.
- Rectal examination. A nodular rectal mucosa suggests Crohn's disease. Occult blood is often present in the stool.
- Sigmoidoscopy. Laxatives in suppository form or enemas should be avoided prior to sigmoidoscopy because they damage the mucosa and cause confusing artifacts. If needed, a tap water enema can be used to cleanse the mucosa.
  1. Ulcerative colitis
     a. The rectum is almost always diffusely involved.
     b. Mucosal edema obscures the normal vascular pattern. When the mucosa is friable, it bleeds spontaneously or when wiped. In more severe cases, there is loss of normal mucosa.
     c. Pseudopolyps are islands of normal mucosa surrounded by ulceration; they look like polyps but are only inflamed colonic mucosa.
  2. Crohn's disease. Often the rectum is normal. Aphthous ulcers or discrete linear ulcers with normal surrounding mucosa may occur. Mucosal involvement is usually not diffuse.

DIAGNOSTIC TESTING IN INFLAMMATORY BOWEL DISEASE

- Laboratory studies
  1. Anemia. Anemia is common. It is often microcytic as a result of iron deficiency or chronic disease. In Crohn's disease, B_{12} deficiency may cause macrocytic anemia.
  2. Hypokalemia may occur secondary to severe diarrhea.
  3. Hypoalbuminemia can result from intestinal albumin loss.
  4. Erythrocyte sedimentation rate (ESR) may be increased, although this is nonspecific.
  5. Superinfection. Superinfection can occur, usually with *Salmonella* or *Campylobacter*.
  6. Stool occult blood. Stool occult blood tests are often positive. Stool fat is increased in Crohn's disease only if malabsorption from small intestinal disease is present.
- Barium enema (BE) is indicated if sigmoidoscopy is equivocal or to document the extent of disease.
  1. Ulcerative Colitis. The BE can be normal in mild disease, but diffuse colonic involvement with shallow ul-

ceration is common. In chronic disease the haustral pattern of the transverse colon is lost. The colon may appear shortened and smooth.

2. Crohn's disease. The BE may show nondiffuse involvement ("skip areas") with discrete ulcers or fistulae. The terminal ileum may be contracted or stenosed ("string sign"). In isolated small intestinal disease, the BE is normal.

- Small bowel X-ray is useful in Crohn's disease to assess involvement of the ileum, or less commonly, jejunum or duodenum (3% of patients). The "string sign" of Crohn's disease (15% of patients) in the terminal ileum is due to transmural thickening and spasm.

- Colonoscopy is useful to diagnose the presence of disease, to differentiate ulcerative colitis from Crohn's disease, to assess severity, and to take biopsies for screening ulcerative colitis patients for precancerous dysplasia.

- Colorectal biopsy is indicated in most cases and can often distinguish between ulcerative colitis and Crohn's disease. Rectal biopsy can detect dysplasia, which may indicate development of colon cancer in either type of IIBD.

- Abdominal CT scan is useful to evaluate suspected complications such as abscess and fistula formation. In general, contrast radiography is superior to abdominal CT in evaluation of IIBD.

- Radionuclide scans are an adjunct to X-ray and colonoscopy in the evaluation of IIBD. Indium-111–labeled leukocyte scans are helpful in evaluating the terminal ileum.

RECOMMENDED DIAGNOSTIC APPROACH

1. A thorough history and physical exam including a stool test for occult blood is important. CBC, serum electrolytes, and ESR should be obtained.

2. If the stool has blood in it, the following tests are necessary:
   a. Stool culture (*Campylobacter, Salmonella, Shigella, Yersinia*) and examination for ova and parasites (especially amebae).
   b. Amebic serologies should be done for patients with chronic diarrhea.
   c. A stool sample should be cultured for *C. difficile* and assayed for *C. difficile* toxin.
   d. Male homosexuals should have tests done for gonorrhea, *Chlamydia,* syphilis, and herpes virus infection.

3. If cultures are negative, sigmoidoscopy (rigid or flexible) should be performed without a bowel preparation. A rectal biopsy should be considered, even if the mucosa is normal, to look for evidence of Crohn's disease or collagenous colitis.

4. If results of sigmoidoscopy are normal or equivocal, BE or colonoscopy should be considered. If these are not diagnostic, an UGI series with small bowel follow-through should be done to evaluate the ileum.

Bibliography

Farmer RG, et al. Clinical patterns in Crohn's disease: A statistical study of 615 cases. Gastroenterology 1975;68:627–635.

Greenstein AJ, et al. Extraintestinal complications of Crohn's disease and ulcerative colitis: Study of 700 patients. Medicine 1976;55:401–412.

Hampson SJ, et al. Mycobacteria and Crohn's disease. Gut 1988;29:1017–1019.

Kirsner JB, Shorter RG. Recent developments in "nonspecific" inflammatory bowel disease. N Engl J Med 1982;306:775–785, 837–848.

Lubat E, Balthazar EJ. The current role of computerized tomography in inflammatory disease of the bowel. Am J Gastroenterol 1988;83:107–113.

Navab F, et al. Early and delayed indium 111 leukocyte imaging in Crohn's disease. Gastroenterology 1987;93:829–834.

Prior A, et al. Is biopsy necessary if colonoscopy is normal? Dig Dis Sci 1987;32:673–676.

Rickert R. The important "imposters" in the differential diagnosis of inflammatory bowel disease. J Clin Gastroenterol 1984;6:153–163.

Surawicz CM, Belic L. Rectal biopsy helps to distinguish acute self-limited colitis from idiopathic inflammatory bowel disease. Gastroenterology 1984;86:104–113.

39

COLORECTAL CANCER

GEOFFREY JIRANEK

He sows hurry and reaps indigestion.

ROBERT LOUIS STEVENSON (1850–1894)

INTRODUCTION AND EPIDEMIOLOGY

- Colorectal cancer is the second leading cause of cancer death in the United States. In 1987, there were 145,000 new cases and 61,000 deaths from colorectal cancer. The lifetime risk that an individual will develop colorectal cancer is about 5 to 6%.
- There is indirect evidence that colorectal adenocarcinomas arise from adenomas. The chance that a 1-cm adenoma will evolve into a carcinoma has been estimated as 5 to 10%. Screening strategies that identify and remove adenomas should help reduce the number of colorectal cancer cases.
- The prognosis of colorectal cancer depends on its stage (Table 39–1).

RISK FACTORS FOR DEVELOPMENT OF COLORECTAL CANCER

- Age. Colon cancer is uncommon before the age of 40 unless there is a positive family history of colon cancer. Ninety percent of colorectal cancer occurs after the age of 50, and two-thirds of cases occur in patients aged 60 and older.
- Family history. Persons with a first-degree relative with colon cancer have a lifetime risk of colon cancer of 10 to 15% (increased 2- to 3-fold). Specific hereditary syndromes are associated with a much higher risk of colon cancer (Table 39–2).
- History of inflammatory bowel disease
  1. If ulcerative colitis affects the entire colon, there is an increased risk of colon cancer after an interval of 8 or more years after the onset of the colitis. The risk of colon cancer, after 40 years, is approximately 10 to 40%.
  2. If ulcerative colitis affects only the left side of the colon, the risk of colon cancer is less and increases after an interval of 15 or more years.
  3. Crohn's disease of the colon increases the risk of colon cancer, but the added risk is less well documented than with ulcerative colitis.

TABLE 39–1. Prognosis of Colorectal Cancer

STAGE	5-YEAR SURVIVAL (%)
Local invasion into bowel wall only (Dukes A and B)	80
Spread to regional lymph nodes (Dukes C)	45
Spread to distant sites (Dukes D)	5

TABLE 39–2. Hereditary Colon Cancer Syndromes

Familial adenomatous polyposis: Subtypes are known as familial adenomatous coli and Gardner's syndrome (adds other features such as osteomas, soft tissue tumors, dermoid tumors, and small bowel neoplasia)
1. Autosomal dominant, 90 to 100% penetrance
2. Many polyps throughout the colon, average number 1000
3. Typically a 10- to 15-year lag between onset of polyps and cancer
4. Cancer onset usually 20 to 40 years of age, average 30
5. One-third of cases are new mutations
6. Greater than 90% have hypertrophic pigmented retinal spots
7. Gene is on the long arm of chromosome 5
8. Accounts for 0.5% of total colorectal cancer cases

Hereditary nonpolyposis colorectal cancer: Also known as hereditary site specific colon cancer (Lynch I) and cancer family syndrome (Lynch II)
1. Autosomal dominant, penetrance 90%
2. Cancer arises with no or few other colorectal polyps
3. Diagnosis of syndrome sometimes unclear, depends on evaluation of an extended pedigree
4. Average age of cancer detection 44 years old
5. Synchronous cancer rate 15% (vs. 2% for noninherited colon cancer)
   Metachronous cancer rate 40% by 10 years (vs. 4% for noninherited colon cancer)
6. Location of cancer is often more proximal than typical cases: 60% proximal to hepatic flexure (vs. 25%), 20% in rectosigmoid (vs. 55%)
7. Lynch II includes endometrial, ovarian cancer, and probably breast, pancreatic, brain, bile duct, duodenal cancer
8. Accounts for up to 5% of total colorectal cancer cases

- Prior history of colorectal adenoma or adenocarcinoma increases the risk of recurrent adenomas and adenocarcinomas.
- Prior history of breast, uterine, or ovarian cancer may double the risk of colon cancer.

CLINICAL FEATURES

- Symptoms
  1. Blood in the stool
     a. Although nonspecific, this is often the presenting symptom of colon cancer.
     b. Hemorrhoids and anal fissures often cause fresh red blood in the stool but should not be presumed to be diagnostic in a patient at risk for colon cancer.
     c. Maroon and melenic stools can occasionally result from bleeding from proximal colon cancers.
  2. Anemia symptoms. The symptoms referable to anemia are diverse and include fatigue, dyspnea, angina, and peripheral edema.
  3. Abdominal pain and alteration of bowel habits
     a. Colon cancers can obstruct or perforate. Obstruction can occur acutely, causing significant abdominal pain with abdominal distension. Gradual obstruction may cause variable abdominal pain and either constipation, diarrhea, or both.
     b. Acute perforation with peritoneal signs is uncommon. Chronic perforation is more common and can result in variable abdominal pain, sometimes with an appreciable mass.
     c. Fistula formation may cause pneumaturia, dysuria, urinary frequency, fecal vaginal discharge, or fecal cutaneous drainage.
- Physical examination
  1. Skin. Pallor may indicate anemia resulting from bleeding from colon cancer. Acanthosis nigricans is a rare lesion in the axilla which can be associated with an internal malignancy.
  2. Lymph nodes. Infiltration of supraclavicular and inguinal lymph nodes with adenocarcinoma is a late sign of colon cancer.
  3. Abdomen. Masses and liver nodules from colorectal metastasis can occasionally be palpated.
  4. Rectal. Polyps and masses are occasionally palpable. The stool may contain gross or occult blood.

LABORATORY FEATURES

- Complete blood count. Anemia may be an important clue to a bleeding colon cancer.
- Serum iron, total iron-binding capacity, and ferritin. In patients over 40 with an unexplained iron deficiency, colon cancer is an important consideration.

- Serum bilirubin and liver enzyme (transaminase, alkaline phosphatase) levels. These tests can be elevated in patients with liver metastasis but are neither very sensitive nor specific.
- Serum carcinoembryonic antigen (CEA) level is elevated in many patients with colorectal cancer, but is too nonspecific to be used as a screening test. Its sensitivity is 36% in Dukes stage A and B lesions versus 74% in Dukes C and 83% in Dukes D lesions.
- Blood cultures positive for *Streptococcus bovis* or *Clostridium septicum* suggest the presence of concurrent colorectal cancer.
- Fecal occult blood test (FOBT)
    1. The guaiac-based Hemoccult II® is widely used as it is easy to perform and inexpensive. The sensitivity of Hemoccult II® for the detection of colorectal cancer is about 50%.
        a. In order to optimize sensitivity and specificity, the subject must avoid red meat, horseradish, radishes, melons, and vitamin C for 3 days before and during the stool testing. The cards should not be rehydrated and should be processed within a few days of collection.
        b. Newer methods such as HemoQuant® (measures hematoderived porphyrins) and HemeSelect® (measures hemoglobin with a specific antibody) are more cumbersome to perform but may have improved sensitivity and specificity. These have not been thoroughly tested in clinical trials.
    2. Trials of Hemoccult II® screening found a 2% rate of positivity in patients over 45 years old.
        a. The patients with positive tests had a 10% rate of colorectal cancer and a 30 to 40% rate of adenomas.
        b. When colorectal cancers were discovered as part of initial Hemoccult II® screening, the prognosis was often quite favorable because the stage was early.
        c. So far, no trial has shown a significant reduction in colorectal cancer death rate from screening with FOBTs, but the final results of these trials are still several years away.
- Radiographic studies
    1. Barium enema
        a. Double contrast barium enemas (with air) are superior to single contrast studies in detecting colorectal neoplasms.
        b. The sensitivity of double contrast barium enemas for colorectal cancers varies with the skill of the radiologist but is 85 to 95% with a specificity of 90 to 95%. For adenomas, the sensitivity is 70 to 80%.
        c. The bowel perforation rate is about 1 in 10,000.
    2. Abdominal ultrasound and CT scans are insensitive in detecting primary colorectal cancers but are useful to detect liver metastasis.

- Endoscopic studies
    1. Sigmoidoscopy
        a. After preparation with an enema, sigmoidoscopy can be performed with either rigid or flexible instruments. The latter is preferred owing to greater insertion distance and less patient discomfort.
        b. Approximately 30% of colorectal neoplasms develop within the reach of a 25-cm rigid sigmoidoscope; 55% can be reached with a 60-cm flexible sigmoidoscope.
        c. The sensitivity of biopsies for cancers and adenomas within these ranges is 85 to 95% for both techniques with no false-positives.
        d. In asymptomatic individuals over the age of 50 with average risk, flexible sigmoidoscopy yields approximately 0.2 to 0.4% colorectal cancers and 5 to 15% colorectal adenomas. When adenomas are found on flexible sigmoidoscopy screening, the usual recommendation is to perform complete colonoscopy with removal of all adenomatous polyps.
    2. Total colonoscopy
        a. Colonoscopy can be performed to the cecum in 95% of patients. Discomfort is typically moderate and can be lessened by routine IV sedation and analgesia.
        b. The sensitivity of colonoscopic biopsies for colorectal neoplasia is 90 to 95% with no false-positives.
        c. The perforation rate of diagnostic colonoscopy is about 1 in 1000.
        d. A key advantage to the use of colonoscopy for diagnosis of colorectal neoplasms is that therapeutic polypectomy and accurate histology can be performed.

RECOMMENDED DIAGNOSTIC APPROACH

- Colon cancer screening in asymptomatic patients
    1. Very high risk groups
        a. Familial adenomatous polyposis: flexible sigmoidoscopy yearly, start age 15 and continue to age 40 (colectomy is recommended if multiple adenomas are found).
        b. Familial nonpolyposis colorectal cancer syndrome: colonoscopy every 2 years, start at age 30 or 10 years younger than the index case in the family (subtotal colectomy is recommended if cancer is found).
        c. Universal ulcerative colitis for >8 years: colonoscopy with multiple biopsies every 1 to 2 years (colectomy is recommended if high grade dysplasia is found).

2. Increased risk groups
   a. Previous history of colon cancer removal: colono-scopy 1 year after resection; every 3 years thereafter.
   b. Previous history of colon adenoma removal: colonoscopy 1 to 3 years after resection; every 3 to 5 years thereafter.
   c. Left-sided ulcerative colitis for >15 years: colonoscopy with multiple biopsies every 1 to 2 years (colectomy is recommended if high-grade dysplasia is found).
   d. Previous history of breast, ovarian, or uterine cancer: starting at age 50, FOBT every year and flexible sigmoidoscopy every 3 to 5 years.
   e. First-degree relative with colorectal cancer: starting at age 40, FOBT every year and flexible sigmoidoscopy every 3 to 5 years.
3. Average risk individuals: starting at age 50, FOBT every 1 to 2 years and flexible sigmoidoscopy every 5 years.

- When the FOBT is positive, a full colon investigation is needed.
  1. Colonoscopy is generally preferred over barium enema because there is often a need for biopsy and/or polypectomy.
  2. When flexible sigmoidoscopy reveals an adenomatous polyp, then complete colonoscopy with polypectomy is generally indicated.
  3. If the sigmoidoscopy reveals a hyperplastic polyp, many authorities believe that colonoscopy is not needed, but this is controversial.

- When signs and symptoms suggest the possibility of colorectal cancer, the work-up should be individualized.
  1. If the suspicion of colorectal neoplasia is low (e.g., vague abdominal pain or a change in bowel habits), then a flexible sigmoidoscopy and a barium enema are good choices.
  2. If the suspicion is higher, expectation of finding colorectal neoplasia (e.g., intermittent gross blood in the stool with newly diagnosed iron-deficient anemia), then colonoscopy is preferred.
  3. Local expertise and patient preference are also factors to consider in the selection between barium enema and colonoscopy.

Bibliography

Aldridge MC, Sim AJ. Colonoscopy findings in symptomatic patients without X-ray evidence of colonic neoplasms. Lancet 1986;ii:833–834.

Allison JE, et al. Hemoccult® screening in detecting colorectal neoplasm: Sensitivity, specificity and predictive value. Ann Intern Med 1990;112:328–333.

American Cancer Society. Guidelines for detection of colorectal cancer. Cancer 1989;39:317.

Durdey P, et al. Colonoscopy or barium enema as initial investigation of colonic disease. Lancet 1987;ii:549–551.

Eddy DM. Screening for colorectal cancer. Ann Intern Med 1990;113:373–384.

Eddy DM, et al. Screening for colorectal cancer in a high-risk population. Gastroenterology 1987;92:682–692.

Fleischer DE, et al. Detection and surveillance of colorectal cancer. JAMA 1989;261:580–585.

Goulston KJ, et al. How important is rectal bleeding in the diagnosis of bowel cancer and polyps? Lancet 1986;ii:261–264.

Knight KK, et al. Occult blood screening for colorectal cancer. JAMA 1989;261:587–593.

Kronborg O, et al. Repeated screening for colorectal cancer with fecal occult blood test. Scand J Gastroenterol 1989;24:599–606.

Lynch HT, et al. Hereditary nonpolyposis colorectal cancer: Lynch syndromes I and II. Gastro Clin North Am 1988;17:679–712.

Selby JV, Friedman GD. Sigmoidoscopy in the periodic health examination of asymptomatic adults. JAMA 1989;261:595–601.

40

PANCREATITIS

JOHN HALSEY *and* MICHAEL KIMMEY

Remember that exploratory incisions should not be made a cloak for diagnostic incompetence.

RUTHERFORD MARISON (1853–1939)

DEFINITION

- Acute pancreatitis
  1. Acute pancreatitis is a process of pancreatic auto-digestion.
  2. The clinical diagnosis is based on a combination of physical, laboratory, and radiologic findings.
- Chronic pancreatitis
  1. Chronic pancreatitis is a continuing inflammatory process of the pancreas characterized clinically by recurrent or persisting episodes of abdominal pain and evidence of functional insufficiency such as steatorrhea or diabetes.
  2. Morphologically, chronic pancreatitis is characterized by irregular sclerosis of the gland with inflammation and destruction of exocrine tissue.

EPIDEMIOLOGY

- Acute pancreatitis. The annual incidence is 10 to 30 per 100,000 people. Countries with a higher alcohol consumption have a higher incidence of acute pancreatitis.
- Chronic pancreatitis. The incidence of chronic pancreatitis in the general population is unknown. Estimates vary from 3.5 to 27 per 100,000 population per year.

DIFFERENTIAL DIAGNOSIS

- Other causes of acute abdominal pain: peptic ulcer disease, nonulcer dyspepsia, acute cholecystitis, reflux esophagitis, bowel infarction, dissecting aortic aneurysm, acute pyelonephritis, pneumonia, and myocardial infarction.
- Other causes of chronic abdominal pain: pancreatic pseudocyst, abscess, or carcinoma, recurrent biliary colic, and irritable bowel syndrome.
- Other causes of hyperamylasemia (Table 40–1)

TABLE 40–1. Causes of Hyperamylasemia

Pancreatic disease
  Acute pancreatitis (65 to 75%)
  Chronic pancreatitis
  Pseudocyst
  Carcinoma
Disorders of nonpancreatic origin (mechanism known)
  Renal insufficiency (uncommon; rarely over twice
    normal)
  Malignant tumor (lung, ovary, thymoma, prostate)
  Salivary gland lesions
    Mumps (80%)
    Calculus
    Drugs (phenylbutazone)
  Macroamylasemia
Diseases of complex origin (mechanism uncertain)
  Intraabdominal diseases other than pancreatitis
    Perforated peptic ulcer (0 to 6%)
    Intestinal obstruction (20%)
    Ruptured ectopic pregnancy
    Mesenteric infarction (30%)
    Peritonitis (70%)
    Acute appendicitis
  Cerebral trauma
  Burns and traumatic shock
  Diabetic ketoacidosis
  Pneumonia
  Total parenteral nutrition

Percentages refer to the frequency of hyperamylasemia in the specific condition.

- Conditions associated with acute pancreatitis (Table 40–2)
  1. Alcohol. A history of prolonged excessive alcohol consumption is present in 50 to 60% of cases of acute pancreatitis in the United States, especially in urban populations.
  2. Gallstones
     a. This is the most common cause of acute pancreatitis in populations with low alcohol consumption. Chronic pancreatitis rarely develops.
     b. Recurrence occurs in half of patients if the stones are not surgically removed.
     c. Some patients have very high amylase levels that are out of proportion to the degree of pain or illness.
     d. Common duct stones are found in only one-third of cases, but ultrasound detects coexistent gallbladder stones in approximately 90% of these patients.
  3. Idiopathic. No cause is found in 10 to 20% of cases. Recurrence is seen in about one-quarter of these patients.
  4. Abdominal trauma
     a. Direct or penetrating blows to the epigastrium, (e.g., hitting automobile steering wheel) causes 3

TABLE 40–2. Conditions Associated with Pancreatitis

Acute Pancreatitis
  Alcohol
  Gallstones
  Idiopathic
  Trauma
  Postsurgical
  Drugs
  Metabolic
    Hypertriglyceridemia
    Hypercalcemia
  Hereditary
  Ductal manipulation
  Ductal obstruction
    Crohn's disease
    Duodenal diverticulum
    Pancreatic divisum
    Annular pancreas
    Afferent loop obstruction (postgastrojejunostomy)
  Infection
    Mumps
    Coxsackievirus B
    Mycoplasma pneumonia
    Hepatitis A
    Ascaris lumbricoides
    Clonorchis sinensis
  Miscellaneous
    Pregnancy (90% from gallstones)
    Penetrating duodenal ulcer
    Vasculitis
      Systemic lupus erythematosus
      Thrombotic thrombocytopenic purpura
      Henoch-Schoenlein purpura
Chronic Pancreatitis
  Alcohol (75% of cases)
  Tropical diseases
  Metabolic
    Hypertriglyceridemia
    Hypercalcemia
  Hereditary
  Traumatic
  Pancreatic divisum
  Idiopathic

to 5% of cases of acute pancreatitis. Trauma is the most common cause of acute pancreatitis in children.

  b. Pseudocysts (2 to 10%) and chronic pancreatitis (3%) may develop. Hyperamylasemia is seen acutely in only 25% of cases of blunt trauma–induced pancreatitis.

  5. Postsurgical

    a. Postsurgical pancreatitis is seen after surgery near the pancreas (0.8% after gastrectomy, 0.2 to 0.4%

after biliary tract surgery). Because hyperamylasemia is nonspecific postoperatively, this condition is difficult to diagnose and has a high mortality (25 to 40%).

   b. It also may be seen after cardiopulmonary bypass, perhaps due to prolonged ischemia.

   c. Pancreatitis after renal transplantation (2 to 7%) is often late (50% after 6 months) and has a multifactorial origin (drugs, infection, and metabolic conditions).

6. Drug-related pancreatitis. Medications associated with pancreatitis include: azathioprine, estrogens (including oral contraceptives), furosemide, sulfonamides, tetracycline, thiazides, and valproic acid.

7. Metabolic disorders

   a. Hypertriglyceridemia. Patients with familial hypertriglyceridemia who develop triglyceride levels greater than 2000 mg/dl (often associated with alcohol ingestion, untreated diabetes mellitus, estrogen therapy, or hypothyroidism) may develop pancreatitis. The serum is grossly lipemic with these levels of triglycerides.

   b. Hypercalcemia. Isolated cases of pancreatitis have been reported with hyperparathyroidism and with other causes of hypercalcemia.

8. Pancreatic duct manipulation. Hyperamylasemia is seen in up to 50% of patients after endoscopic retrograde cholangiopancreatography (ERCP). However, only 3% develop clinical pancreatitis.

• Conditions associated with chronic pancreatitis (see Table 40–2). Three-fourths of cases of chronic pancreatitis occur in heavy drinkers and alcoholics.

CLINICAL MANIFESTATIONS

• History (Table 40–3). The presence of risk factors that suggest the cause should be ascertained (see Table 40–2).

1. Patients with acute pancreatitis usually have a gradual onset of epigastric (70%) continuous (85%) pain that may radiate to the back (30%). Food may exacerbate symptoms, but patients are generally anorectic or vomiting.

2. Over 90% of patients with chronic pancreatitis have abdominal pain.

   a. The pain varies from mild continuous epigastric pain that is exacerbated by eating to an intermittent, excruciating, deep, boring type of pain that may radiate to the back. Patients often assume a sitting posture with forward flexion at the waist to reduce pain.

   b. Approximately one-third of patients are narcotic addicts.

   c. Steatorrhea and symptoms of glucose intolerance are common.

TABLE 40–3. Clinical Findings in Pancreatitis

Acute Pancreatitis
  Symptoms
    Abdominal pain (98%)
    Vomiting (50%)
    Hematemesis (2%)
    Mental confusion (25%)
  Signs
    Fever (80%)
    Hypertension (40%)
    Hypotension (25%)
    Abdominal distention (60%)
    Pleural effusion (15%)
    Ascites (2%)
    Grey Turner's sign (1%)
    Cullen's sign (1%)
    Necrotic skin nodules (1%)
Chronic Pancreatitis
  Symptoms
    Abdominal pain (90%)
    Weight loss (95%)
    Gastrointestinal bleeding (10%)
  Signs
    Jaundice (25%)
    Ascites (2%)
    Palpable abdominal mass (5%)
Pseudocyst
  Symptoms
    Abdominal pain (95%)
    Nausea or vomiting (60%)
    Weight loss greater than 10 pounds (50%)
  Signs
    Fever (20%)
    Abdominal mass (50%)
    Abdominal tenderness (70%)
    Ascites (20%)
    Jaundice (10%)

Percentages refer to the frequency of the specific finding in patients with definite pancreatitis.

- Complications of pancreatitis
  1. Pancreatic pseudocysts (see Table 40–3)
     a. These collections of fluid and necrotic debris develop 1 to 4 weeks after an episode of acute pancreatitis in about 5% of cases.
     b. A pseudocyst should be suspected if a palpable mass is found on abdominal examination and if clinical pancreatitis or hyperamylasemia do not resolve within 1 week.
  2. Pancreatic abscess
     a. Abscesses occur in 3 to 10% of cases of acute pancreatitis.

b. An abscess should be suspected in patients with persistent fever, tachycardia, leukocytosis, and signs of toxicity, especially if deterioration occurs after a period of initial improvement.

LABORATORY EVALUATION

- Amylase (see Table 40–1)
    1. Three-fourths of patients with acute pancreatitis have an elevated total serum amylase level that occurs within 24 hr of onset and returns to normal within 3 to 5 days. Severe pancreatitis may be present with a normal serum amylase level.
    2. The utility of total serum amylase activity in the diagnosis of pancreatitis has been overrated.
        a. Since 60% of the normal total serum amylase has a salivary gland origin, many cases of hyperamylasemia are caused by nonpancreatic disorders.
        b. Up to 50% of unselected acutely alcohol-intoxicated patients have an elevated total serum amylase level, but fewer than 20% of these have elevated pancreatic isoamylase levels.
        c. Numerous diagnostic errors occur in this setting because of too much reliance on total amylase level. Fractionation of the total amylase into pancreatic and salivary components greatly improves the specificity of this test.
    3. Urinary amylase and ratios of amylase to creatinine clearance are nonspecific and add little to the diagnosis.
- Lipase
    1. Serum lipase determination exhibits good sensitivity (70 to 85%) and excellent specificity (99%) for acute pancreatitis.
    2. It is normal in several disorders associated with hyperamylasemia.
    3. It remains elevated after the total serum amylase has returned to normal in acute pancreatitis. It is an excellent test, especially in confusing or delayed situations.
- Miscellaneous
    1. The hematocrit may be elevated as a result of hemoconcentration or decreased due to blood loss.
    2. A leukocytosis (15,000 to 24,000/mm^3) is frequent.
    3. Hyperglycemia (25%), hypocalcemia (25%), hypertriglyceridemia (10 to 20%), and hypoxemia (25% with partial pressure of oxygen < 60 mmHg) may be seen in acute pancreatitis.
    4. Ten percent of patients have serum bilirubin > 4 mg/dl. Liver enzymes are elevated in 60% of gallstone-associated cases, but only in 10% of alcohol-associated cases.
- Pancreatic function tests
    1. Serum amylase and lipase activities are usually normal in chronic pancreatitis.

2. Diagnosis often depends on the demonstration of loss of exocrine function.
   a. Increased stool fat is seen after 90% of pancreatic function has been lost.
   b. The secretin-stimulation test is the most sensitive test and may give the only abnormal finding in patients with abdominal pain caused by chronic pancreatitis. Approximately 75% of pancreatic function must be lost before the secretin test result is abnormal.
   c. An abnormal Schilling test result that is corrected by oral administration of pancreatic enzymes is found in 40% of patients with chronic pancreatitis.

- Imaging studies
  1. X-rays
     a. Plain abdominal X-rays show abnormal findings (colonic dilatation, obscured psoas margins, small intestinal effusion, or pancreatic calcification) in 40 to 50% of patients with acute pancreatitis.
     b. Radiographs are often helpful in excluding ruptured hollow viscus or other intraabdominal catastrophes in possible cases of acute pancreatitis.
     c. Pancreatic calcification is present in about 30% of people with chronic pancreatitis and generally signifies advanced disease.
  2. Ultrasound has a 90% accuracy in detecting pseudocysts. Abscesses, gallstones, and pancreatic calcification may also be seen. Follow-up of pancreatic fluid collections and guided needle aspiration of those fluid collections can be accomplished in persistent cases.
  3. CT scan is the imaging modality of choice for patients with clinically severe pancreatitis who fail to respond to conservative therapy or remain diagnostic dilemmas.
  4. ERCP is the only method for directly outlining the pancreatic duct system and can thus aid in the differential diagnosis of pancreatic disease. It is helpful in planning surgical procedures and may be useful for diagnosis and treatment in patients with severe gallstone pancreatitis.

RECOMMENDED DIAGNOSTIC APPROACH

- Acute pancreatitis
  1. Patients whose history and physical examination are compatible with acute pancreatitis should have laboratory tests, including CBC, serum glucose, electrolytes, calcium, and amylase.
  2. Serum pancreatic isoamylase or lipase should be used to confirm the diagnosis.
  3. Abdominal X-rays should be done if pain is severe, primarily to rule out other pathology.
  4. Patients without a history of alcohol ingestion should undergo abdominal ultrasonography for the detection of gallstones.

5. Ultrasound examination is also useful later in the course of illness if a pseudocyst or abscess is suspected.

- Chronic pancreatitis
  1. Patients with a history and physical examination compatible with chronic pancreatitis should be tested for hyperglycemia, fat malabsorption (qualitative or quantitative stool fat), and pancreatic calcification on abdominal X-ray.
  2. If the diagnosis is still in question, a secretin test should be performed.
  3. ERCP is useful in patients for whom surgery is contemplated or if the diagnosis is unclear and the presence of pancreatic structural anomalies (annular pancreas, pancreatic divisum) is suspected.

Bibliography

Freeny PC, ed. Radiology of the Pancreas. The Radiologic Clinics of North America. Philadelphia, W.B. Saunders Company, 1989, Vol. 27, pp. 1–193.

Greenberger NJ, Toskes PP. Approach to the patient with pancreatic disease. In: Wilson JD, et al., eds. Harrison's Principles of Internal Medicine, 12th ed. New York, McGraw-Hill, 1990, pp. 1369–1372.

Greenberger NJ, et al. Diseases of the pancreas. In: Wilson JD, et al., eds. Harrison's Principles of Internal Medicine, 12th ed. New York, McGraw-Hill, 1990, pp. 1372–1383.

Reber HA, ed. The Pancreas. Surgical Clinics of North America. Philadelphia, W.B. Saunders Company, 1989, Vol. 69, pp. 447–686.

Soergel KH: Acute pancreatitis. In: Sleisenger MH, Fordtran JS, eds. Gastrointestinal Disease, 4th ed. Philadelphia, W.B. Saunders Company, 1989, pp. 1814–1842.

SECTION VI

HEMATOLOGY

41

ANEMIA

THOMAS R. KLUMPP

She was very anaemic. Her thin lips were pale, and her skin was delicate, of a faint green colour, without a touch of red even in the cheeks.

W. SOMERSET MAUGHAM (1874–1965)

DEFINITION

Anemia is a decrease in the red cell mass leading to a loss of oxygen-carrying capacity in the blood. Anemia in males is defined as a hematocrit less than 40% or a hemoglobin less than 14 g/dl; in females, the respective values are 37% and 12 g/dl.

DIFFERENTIAL DIAGNOSIS (see Table 41–1)

HISTORY

- Symptoms
  1. Orthostatic dizziness, dyspnea, chest pain, or poor urine output suggest the need for urgent treatment (i.e., transfusion). Interpretation of serum iron, iron-binding capacity, ferritin, B_{12}, and folate may be impossible after a transfusion; blood for these tests should be obtained prior to transfusion.
  2. Weakness, fatigue, headache, and insomnia are common, but less ominous, symptoms of anemia. A history of fever, night sweats, or weight loss suggest an underlying disease causing anemia of chronic disease.
  3. A change in skin color may not be obvious in a dark-skinned patient. Direct questioning may yield a history of subtle yellowing from jaundice caused by hemolysis.
- History
  1. A history of preexisting infectious, inflammatory, or neoplastic disease may suggest anemia of chronic disease. A history of peptic ulcer disease, colonic polyps, or prosthetic heart valves may direct the work-up.
  2. A history of significant cardiac, pulmonary, or cerebrovascular disease may suggest a more urgent workup and/or the need for a lower threshold for transfusion.

TABLE 41–1. Causes of Anemia

Decreased production
  Anemia of chronic disease
    Chronic inflammatory disease
    Infection
    Cancer
    Renal failure
    Hypothyroidism
  Nutritional deficiency states
    Vitamin B_{12} deficiency
    Folate deficiency
    Iron deficiency
  Bone marrow suppression
    Toxins, e.g., ethanol, lead
    Drugs, e.g., anti-cancer drugs, chloramphenicol
    Bone marrow infection, e.g., parvovirus, tuberculosis
    Marrow infiltration by tumor, e.g., breast, prostate
  Primary bone marrow disorders
    Leukemia
    Myelodysplastic syndromes
    Myeloproliferative syndromes
Increased destruction or loss
  Hemolytic anemia—destruction of red cells within the
    bloodstream, spleen, or bone marrow
    Idiopathic autoimmune hemolytic anemia
    Disseminated intravascular coagulation
    Inherited hemolytic anemia, e.g., sickle cell anemia,
      thalassemia, spherocytosis
    Hypersplenism, e.g., due to congestive heart failure,
      lymphoma
    Prosthetic heart valves
    Thrombotic thrombocytopenic purpura
  Blood loss anemia—if chronic, often accompanied by
    iron-deficiency anemia
    GI—e.g., colonic neoplasms, duodenal ulcers
    GU—e.g., glomerulonephritis, GU tumor
    Pulmonary—e.g., Goodpasture's syndrome, tumors
    Trauma

- Drug history
  1. Intensive exposure to antineoplastic drugs can cause a permanent underproduction anemia due to destruction of erythroid progenitors.
  2. Many other drugs can cause marrow suppression. Chloramphenicol causes a dose-dependent reversible suppression and, more rarely, an idiosyncratic, often irreversible, aplastic anemia. Antithyroid drugs commonly cause marrow suppression.
  3. Several drugs cause peripheral immune hemolysis. Alpha-methyl dopa, penicillin, sulfa-containing drugs, and quinidine are common offenders.
- Social history. A history of ethanol abuse is associated with GI blood loss, nutritional deficiency, and direct bone mar-

row toxicity. Hypersplenism due to liver disease can contribute to anemia.

* Family history. A number of specific causes of anemia carry a genetic predisposition, including sickle cell anemia, glucose-6-phosphate dehydrogenase deficiency, thalassemia, and acute leukemia.

PHYSICAL EXAMINATION

* Vital signs
  1. The only anemia which commonly causes hypotension is acute blood loss. In the first few hours following whole blood loss, the degree of anemia noted may significantly underestimate the actual volume loss.
  2. Fever can be a clue to the underlying cause of the anemia, often anemia of chronic disease.
* Head and neck
  1. Lymphadenopathy has a wide differential diagnosis; most are associated with anemia of chronic disease.
  2. Scleral icterus is a clue to possible hemolysis.
* Chest. A hyperdynamic precordium and a benign systolic flow murmur are often appreciated.
* Abdomen
  1. Hepatomegaly may suggest infectious, inflammatory, or neoplastic causes for anemia of chronic disease.
  2. Splenomegaly can result from significant hemolysis; a spleen enlarged by other causes can decrease red cell survival.
  3. Contraindications to rectal examination are severe neutropenia or thrombocytopenia, due to the risk of causing bacteremia or serious bleeding, respectively. In these cases stool should be obtained for occult blood testing, but the rectal examination itself can be deferred.
* Neurologic. Severe anemia can cause lethargy or confusion or may aggravate underlying neurologic problems such as focal atherosclerotic vascular insufficiency or seizure disorders.

LABORATORY EVALUATION

* Red cell indices. The mean corpuscular volume (MCV) is the most useful.
  1. Low MCV. An important clue to the presence of iron deficiency or thalassemia, but also consistent with anemia of chronic disease, sideroblastic anemia, and lead poisoning.
  2. Normal MCV. This finding is of little diagnostic help, since most anemias, including iron deficiency, B_{12} deficiency, and folate deficiency, can present with a normal MCV.
  3. High MCV. Most suggestive of B_{12} or folate deficiency, but another important cause is hemolysis, due

to the presence of increased numbers of reticulocytes, which are larger than normal red cells. A high MCV in the absence of actual anemia can be a clue to vitamin B_{12} deficiency.

- Reticulocyte count
    1. The reticulocyte count distinguishes the "decreased-production" anemias from the "increased-destruction-or-loss" anemias. It is most useful when it is significantly elevated, i.e., greater than 5% of red cells. In this situation it is a reliable indicator of bone marrow response to blood loss or destruction.
    2. When mildly to moderately elevated (2 to 5%), the reticulocyte count is less useful and often indicates a suboptimal bone marrow response to red cell loss or destruction, i.e., a multifactorial anemia.

- Peripheral blood smear
    1. Schistocytes, or "bite cells," are red cells which appear to have a bite taken out of the cytoplasm. Even a small number (2 to 3 per high-power field) suggests mechanical hemolysis such as caused by disseminated intravascular coagulation, prosthetic heart valves, or thrombotic thrombocytopenic purpura.
    2. Hypochromia is an increase in the area of central pallor in the red cells. This finding suggests iron deficiency, particularly in the presence of significant anisocytosis (variation in red-cell size) and poikilocytosis (variation in red-cell shape).
    3. Spherocytes appear uniformly red because they have lost their area of central pallor. Two common causes are autoimmune hemolytic anemia and congenital spherocytosis. An elevated mean cell hemoglobin concentration (MCHC) may be seen.
    4. Nucleated red blood cells. The finding of even one nucleated red blood cell on a smear is highly suggestive of a serious marrow disorder such as a myeloproliferative syndrome or infiltration of the bone marrow by cancer.
    5. Basophilic stippling refers to the presence of multiple small black or purple inclusions within the red cells. It is a nonspecific finding in most cases. Coarse stippling suggests lead poisoning, which can be confirmed by an elevated plasma lead level and an elevated free erythrocyte protoporphyrin.
    6. Target cells have a central "target" of hemoglobin within the area of central pallor. They are seen in liver disease or thalassemia, but a number of other anemias can be associated with target cells as well.
    7. The appearance of the leukocytes should always be noted. A preponderance of virtually any type of WBC other than normal neutrophils can be a sign of possible leukemia.

- Vitamin B_{12} and folate. It is reasonable to obtain B_{12} and folate levels in cases of macrocytic anemia or in cases of otherwise unexplained normocytic anemia. Serum folate may be falsely normalized by short-term improvements in nutrition. The red-cell folate can be more sensitive in recently hospitalized homeless or alcoholic patients, whose nutritional status sometimes improves quickly after admission.

SPECIFIC DIAGNOSES

- Anemia of chronic disease
  1. Anemia of chronic disease is extremely common. It can be associated with virtually any inflammatory, infectious, or neoplastic condition, as well as with renal failure, liver disease, and hypothyroidism. The diagnosis is one of exclusion, since there is no specific laboratory test. Anemia of chronic disease is often a complicating factor in other anemias of specific cause, such as iron deficiency or B_{12} deficiency.
  2. In order to exclude other common problems, the reticulocyte count, iron, iron-binding capacity, B_{12}, folate, and stool occult blood determinations should be obtained. An elevated erythrocyte sedimentation rate is suggestive of this diagnosis, but is not sensitive or specific.
  3. In a patient with a hematocrit less than 30%, the diagnosis of anemia of chronic disease should usually not be made without a bone marrow examination.
- Iron deficiency
  1. This diagnosis is suggested by a low MCV, a low reticulocyte count, hypochromia on the blood smear, or a high platelet count.
  2. The optimal set of confirmatory tests in the setting of suspected iron deficiency is controversial.
     a. A low ferritin level is highly suggestive of iron deficiency. However, the ferritin level may be falsely normal as a result of the presence of inflammatory processes, hepatic or renal disease, or neoplasms. Iron deficiency is very unlikely in the face of a normal ferritin *if* the ESR is normal.
     b. A markedly decreased serum iron (Fe) in the face of an increased total iron-binding capacity (TIBC) is quite suggestive of iron deficiency, but other combinations of Fe and TIBC do not rule out iron deficiency.
     c. A bone marrow examination for stainable iron is considered to be the "gold standard" for iron deficiency. However, a therapeutic trial of iron of *defined duration*, e.g., 4 weeks, is reasonable prior to resorting to a bone marrow biopsy.
  3. Gastrointestinal malignancy *must* be actively searched for in the patient with unexplained iron deficiency.
- Folate deficiency
  1. Folate deficiency is seen most commonly in malnourished patients, e.g., alcoholics, the homeless, and illicit drug users.
  2. An elevated MCV is often but not always present.

3. Low serum folate or RBC folate is often found.
4. A therapeutic trial of folate is safe and inexpensive in an otherwise compatible setting.

- Vitamin B_{12} deficiency
  1. A normal MCV does not rule out this diagnosis. Thus it is reasonable to order a B_{12} level in a patient with otherwise unexplained normocytic anemia, or in a patient with compatible neurologic findings, such as unexplained ataxia or distal neuropathy. The diagnosis can usually be confirmed with a low serum vitamin B_{12} level.
  2. The Schilling test should be obtained in patients who have a low serum vitamin B_{12} level. The basic test involves the administration of radioactive vitamin B_{12} and the subsequent measurement of radioactivity excretion in the urine.
  3. In pernicious anemia, the most common form of vitamin B_{12} deficiency in the United States, the stomach does not excrete intrinsic factor, which is required for vitamin B_{12} absorption in the ileum. In this situation, the Schilling test shows a decrease in radioactivity excretion, which can be corrected by the addition of intrinsic factor.

- Hemolytic anemia
  1. A brief laboratory screen for hemolytic anemia is reasonable in most patients with anemia that remains unexplained after the initial history, physical, and laboratory screen discussed above. It should include a reticulocyte count, lactate dehydrogenase (LDH) level, a bilirubin, and a haptoglobin.
  2. Assuming that blood loss has been ruled out, a high reticulocyte count in combination with significant elevations in the LDH or bilirubin, or a decreased haptoglobin, suggests hemolysis. A high percentage of indirect-reacting bilirubin is suggestive of hemolysis, but a low fraction does not exclude it.
  3. The appropriate confirmatory test depends on the type of hemolysis suspected.
     a. For example, in a young black patient with a family history of sickle cell anemia, a hemoglobin electrophoresis or a "sickle screen" is a reasonable next step.
     b. In an otherwise healthy adult with a new onset of unexplained hemolysis, a positive Coombs' test can suggest the diagnosis of autoimmune hemolytic anemia. The peripheral smear should always be examined in cases of suspected hemolysis.
     c. Spherocytes suggest immune hemolytic anemia or congenital spherocytosis, while schistocytes suggest the possibility of disseminated intravascular coagulation (DIC), thrombotic thrombocytopenic purpura (TTP), or prosthetic heart valve hemolysis.

- Disseminated intravascular coagulation (DIC)
  1. DIC presents as a combination of hemolytic anemia,

thrombocytopenia, and an elevated prothrombin time or partial thromboplastin time.

2. Confirmatory tests include the fibrinogen and fibrin-split products.

- Thalassemia

1. The thalassemias, a group of disorders characterized by an imbalance in the synthesis of the α and β chains of hemoglobin, are the only common cause of microcytic anemia other than iron deficiency itself.

2. The diagnosis should be considered in cases of microcytic anemia when iron indices are normal. A markedly depressed MCV, out of proportion to the degree of anemia, is often seen.

3. The confirmatory test is the hemoglobin electropheresis. An elevated hemoglobin A_2, to 5% or more, is sufficient for a presumptive diagnosis of β-thalassemia minor, the most common type.

- Myelophthisic anemia

1. Myelophthisic anemia results from a "crowding out" of the normal bone marrow progenitors by other cells, most commonly metastatic cancer. Among the most common offenders are breast, lung, and prostate cancer.

2. An important early clue is the finding of nucleated RBCs or early leukocyte forms (a "leukoerythroblastic" picture) on the peripheral smear, but the only diagnostic test is examination of the bone marrow itself.

- Primary bone marrow disorders

1. Primary disorders of the bone marrow include the leukemias, the myeloproliferative syndromes, and the myelodysplastic syndromes.

2. In most cases the diagnosis is made by examination of the bone marrow in a patient whose anemia remains undiagnosed after the usual screening tests covered above. In some cases a first clue will be the appearance in the peripheral blood of immature or abnormal cells from any of the three major cell lines, including myeloblasts, pro- or meta-myelocytes, nucleated RBCs, or giant platelets.

RECOMMENDED DIAGNOSTIC APPROACH

- The initial work-up consists of a history and physical examination, including a stool test for occult blood, and a review of the MCV and the peripheral blood smear. An abnormally low MCV suggests iron deficiency or thalassemia as the two most likely possibilities. An abnormally high MCV suggests vitamin B_{12} or folate deficiency.

- If the possibilities cannot be narrowed after the above steps, the stool occult blood examination should be repeated and the reticulocyte count determined. A marrow that is not responding appropriately will continue to generate only the "normal" percentage of reticulocytes.

- A "normal" reticulocyte count with significant anemia suggests that the anemia is due to decreased production. A cost-effective initial screen in this situation includes an ESR (usually elevated in anemia of chronic disease), and serum ferritin, B_{12}, and folate levels.

- A reticulocyte count greater than 5% suggests blood loss or destruction. An initial screen in this situation includes serial stool examinations for occult blood, a urinalysis, and a serum bilirubin, LDH, and haptoglobin. Negative stool occult blood examinations and urinalysis essentially rule out unrecognized blood loss. An elevated bilirubin and LDH and/or a decreased haptoglobin are nearly always present in significant hemolysis.

- A reticulocyte count in the intermediate range, i.e., 1 to 5%, is compatible with decreased production, increased destruction or loss, or a combination of the two. In this situation a combination of the above screens is suggested.

- Patients with a hematocrit less than 30% require a bone marrow examination unless the anemia has an obvious cause and responds promptly to appropriate treatment.

- Many anemias are multifactorial. For example, slow GI blood loss from an early colonic neoplasm may be compensated by increased production by the bone marrow, going unrecognized until iron deficiency supervenes. Similarly, a well-compensated hemolytic anemia may not become evident until the bone marrow is suppressed by drugs or infection.

Bibliography

Beissner RS, Trowbridge AA. Clinical assesment of anemia. Postgrad Med 1986;80(6):83–95.

Beutler E. The common anemias. JAMA 1988;259:2433–2437.

Bunn HF. Pathophysiology of the anemias. In: Wilson J et al., eds. Principles of Internal Medicine. New York, McGraw-Hill, 1991, pp. 1514–1518.

Erslev AJ. Erythrocyte disorders: Classification and manifestations. In: Williams WJ, et al., eds. Hematology. New York, McGraw-Hill, 1990, pp. 423–429.

Guyatt GH, et al. Diagnosis of iron-deficiency anemia in the elderly. Am J Med 1990;88:205–209.

Nardone DA, et al. Usefulness of physical examination in detecting the presence or absence of anemia. Arch Intern Med 1990;150:201–204.

Simmons JO, et al. Does review of peripheral blood smears help in the initial workup of common anemias? J Gen Intern Med 1989;4:473–481.

42

ERYTHROCYTOSIS

RICHARD C. CHERNY

Yet who would have thought the old man to have had
so much blood in him?

SHAKESPEARE (1564–1616), Macbeth V,i

DEFINITION

Erythrocytosis (polycythemia) is an increase in the total RBC
mass. The condition is often first discovered on routine laboratory screening. In men, a hemoglobin concentration greater
than 17.5 g/dl [hematocrit (Hct) > 52%] and in women, a
hemoglobin concentration greater than 16.0 g/dl (Hct > 47%)
is elevated and necessitates further investigation.

CLASSIFICATION (Table 42–1)

1. Relative (apparent) erythrocytosis refers to a "relative"
   hematocrit elevation due to decreased plasma volume.
   Within this category are a group of patients that fall under
   the heading of spurious polycythemia, precise cause is
   unknown.
2. True erythrocytosis is unequivocally determined by an
   elevated total RBC mass, measured by chromium-51 labeling of red blood cells.
   a. Primary erythrocytosis, including polycythemia
      vera, is due to unchecked clonal pleuripotential stem
      cell proliferations.
   b. Secondary polycythemias are states of erythrocy-
      tosis due to elevated EPO levels.
      i. "Appropriate" polycythemias result from a high
         erythropoietin (EPO) level produced by a normal
         physiological response (see Table 42–1).
      ii. States of excessive endogenous EPO are "inap-
          propriate" or noncompensatory polycythemias.

CLINICAL FEATURES

Relative Polycythemia
(Spurious Polycythemia)

These patients are usually asymptomatic. Many are middle-
aged, overweight male smokers in stress-filled environments
or with chronic anxiety disorders.

TABLE 42–1. Classification of Erythrocytosis

A. Relative (apparent erythrocytosis)
   1. Dehydration, diuretics, extensive burns
   2. Spurious (stress, smokers, Gaisböck's)
B. Absolute (true erythrocytosis)
   1. Primary
      a. Polycythemia vera
      b. Erythremia
   2. Secondary
      a. Appropriate (compensatory)
         (1) Hypoxemia
            a. High altitude exposure
            b. Pickwickian syndrome
            c. Cardiopulmonary disorders
         (2) Abnormal hemoglobin function
            a. High-affinity hemoglobinopathies
            b. Carboxyhemoglobinemia
            c. Methemoglobinemia
            d. Sulfhemoglobinemia
      b. Inappropriate (noncompensatory)
         (1) Renal tumors and cysts, renal artery stenosis
         (2) Hepatomas
         (3) Cerebellar hemangioblastomas
         (4) Uterine myomas
         (5) Endocrine disorders
            a. Pheochromocytomas
            b. Aldosterone-producing adenomas
            c. Bartter's syndrome
            d. Cushing's disease
            e. High dose-adrenocortical steroids
            f. Androgen therapy

Polycythemia Vera

1. The signs and symptoms of polycythemia vera (Table 42–2) result from impaired blood flow and decreased tissue oxygenation of all organ systems. Pruritus, often problematic after a hot shower or bath, is also common.
2. Peptic ulcer disease occurs with 4 or 5 times the usual incidence.
3. One-third of patients suffer thrombosis or hemorrhage.
   a. Peripheral venous thrombosis, cerebral vascular accidents, and ischemic coronary artery disease are most frequent.
   b. Epistaxis, gingival bleeding, and upper GI bleeding are frequently encountered hemorrhagic complications.
   c. More than 75% of patients with uncontrolled polycythemia vera undergoing surgery develop hemorrhagic or thrombotic complications and about one-third of these patients die as a result.
4. Plethora, arterial hypertension, and splenomegaly are the common physical findings.

TABLE 42–2. Symptoms of Polycythemia Vera

SYMPTOM	PERCENT OF PATIENTS
Headache	48
Weakness	47
Pruritus	43
Dizziness	43
Sweating	33
Visual changes	31
Weight loss	29
Paresthesias	29
Dyspnea	26
Joint symptoms	26
Epigastric distress	24

Secondary Polycythemia

The signs and symptoms of secondary polycythemia reflect the consequences of hypervolemia and hyperviscosity, as in primary polycythemia. Other clinical features are due to the underlying disease, such as cyanotic congenital heart disease or chronic obstructive lung disease.

LABORATORY FEATURES (Table 42–3)

Relative Polycythemia

With the exception of an elevated hematocrit, most hematologic parameters are normal. In heavy smokers, carboxyhemoglobin levels are increased (>4%), which may explain the erythrocytosis. Measured plasma volume is usually decreased. EPO levels are normal.

TABLE 42–3. Laboratory Findings in Patients with Increased Hematocrit

FINDING	POLYCYTHEMIA VERA	SECONDARY POLYCYTHEMIA	RELATIVE POLYCYTHEMIA
RBC volume	Increased	Increased	Normal
Arterial oxygen saturation	Normal	Decreased or normal	Normal
Serum vitamin B_{12}	Increased	Normal	Normal
Serum vitamin B_{12} binding capacity	Increased	Normal	Normal
Leukocyte alkaline phosphatase	Increased	Normal	Normal
EPO level	Decreased	Increased	Normal

Source: Murphy S. Polycythemia vera. In: Williams WJ, et al., eds. Hematology, 4th ed., New York, McGraw-Hill, 1990, p 198.

Polycythemia Vera

1. Total red cell mass (measured by chromium-51 labeling) is elevated in patients with polycythemia vera. Plasma volume is usually normal or slightly increased. Erythrocytes are morphologically normal unless iron deficiency occurs.

2. As polycythemia vera progresses to the "spent" phase, ineffective intramedullary and extramedullary hematopoiesis leads to morphologic changes with marked anisocytosis and poikilocytosis (ovalocytes, elliptocytes, tear drops), and an increased number of nucleated red cells.

3. Moderate leukocytosis (12 to 25 × 10^9/L) occurs in two-thirds of patients, but neutrophil function is normal.

4. Thrombocytosis (450 to 800 × 10^9/L) occurs in half of patients. Initially, the bleeding time is normal but may become prolonged during the spent phase when ineffective platelet production is combined with platelet dysfunction.

5. Bone marrow examination reveals hyperplasia of all cellular elements with pronounced erythroid hyperplasia. Megakaryocytes are increased in size and number with increased ploidy. Iron staining demonstrates reduced or absent iron stores. Fibrosis often accompanies the spent phase of the disease.

6. Other lab features include:
   a. A serum B_{12} level above 900 pg/ml in one-third of patients.
   b. Hyperuricemia and hyperuricosuria, a result of rapid cellular proliferation, is present in 40% of patients, but gout is uncommon.
   c. Serum iron and ferritin levels are often decreased due to increased utilization or concurrent blood loss (e.g., phlebotomy).

TABLE 42–4. Criteria for Diagnosis of Polycythemia Vera

Eligibility: 1. No previous treatment except phlebotomy
2. Disease disgnosed no longer than 4 yr ago
3. Fulfillment of the following criteria:

Category A[a]	Category B[a]
1. Total red cell mass: male >36 ml/kg female >32 ml/kg	1. Thrombocytosis: platelet count >400 × 10^9/L
2. Arterial oxygen saturation >92%	2. Leukocytosis (no fever or infection): >12 × 10^9/L
3. Splenomegaly	3. Leukocyte alkaline phosphatase score >100
	4. Serum B_{12} >900 pg/ml or unbound serum B_{12} binding capacity (>2200 pg/ml)

[a] Polycythemia vera is present if the following combinations exist: A1 + A2 + A3 or A1 + A2 + any two from category B.

7. Arterial oxygen saturation is >92% and serves as a distinguishing feature from other forms of polycythemia.

8. The normal range for EPO is 10 to 30 mU/ml with the lower limit of sensitivity being 2 to 3 mU/ml. Very low (<3 mU/ml) EPO levels are a hallmark of polycythemia vera.

9. In patients with polycythemia vera, erythroid precursors grow spontaneously in vitro on semisolid tissue culture media. These erythroid colony-forming units (CFU-E) grow without exogenous EPO. This characteristic, unique to polycythemia vera, aids in definitive diagnosis in otherwise ambiguous cases.

10. In 1968, the National Polycythemia Vera Study Group adopted criteria for diagnosis (Table 42–4.)

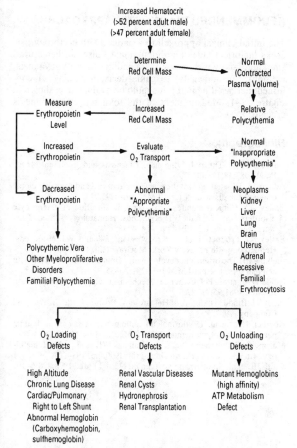

Figure 42–1. Evaluation of increased hematocrit. (Adapted from Adamson JW. The polycythemias: Diagnosis and treatment. Hosp Pract 1983;18:49.)

Secondary Polycythemia

1. Once an elevated erythrocyte volume is determined, measurement of arterial oxygen saturation separates primary ($>92\%$) from secondary polycythemia ($<92\%$).
2. Arterial oxygen (O_2) saturation is normal in carboxyhemoglobinemia, and measurement of the carboxyhemoglobin level ($>4\%$ is abnormal) is necessary.
3. Determining the P_{50} (partial pressure of oxygen at which the hemoglobin is 50% saturated) is useful in identifying patients with high-affinity hemoglobinopathies.
4. EPO levels are high in most types of secondary polycythemias. The frequency of paraneoplastic erythrocytosis varies with the type of tumor: 1 to 5% with renal cell carcinoma, 5 to 10% with hepatomas, and 15 to 20% with cerebellar hemangioblastomas.

RECOMMENDED DIAGNOSTIC APPROACH

The initial clinical approach to a patient with erythrocytosis seeks historical clues (cardiopulmonary disease, hematuria, smoking, family history) or exam findings (obesity, cyanosis, plethora, splenomegaly) to guide decision making. A confirmed increased hematocrit should be evaluated as shown in Figure 42-1. Measurement of the total red cell volume is crucial.

Bibliography

Adamson JW. The polycythemias: Diagnosis and treatment. Hosp Pract 1983;18(12):49–57.

Adamson JW, et al. Polycythemia vera: Stem-cell and probable clonal origin of the disease. N Engl J Med 1976;295:913.

Erslev AJ. Clinical manifestations and classification of erythrocyte disorders. In: Williams WJ, et al., eds. Hematology, 4th ed. New York, McGraw-Hill, 1990, pp. 414–429.

Erslev AJ. Production of erythrocytes. In: Williams WJ, et al., eds. Hematology, 4th ed. New York, McGraw-Hill, 1990, pp. 389–397.

Fialkow PJ. The origin and development of human tumors studied with cell markers. N Engl J Med 1974;291:26–35.

Golde DW, et al. Polycythemia: Mechanisms and management. Ann Int Med 1981;95:71–87.

Jandl JH. Blood: Textbook of Hematology. Boston, Little, Brown, and Company, 1987.

Koeffler HP, et al. Erythropoietin radioimmunoassay in evaluating patients with polycythemia. Ann Int Med 1981;94:44–47.

Murphy S. Polycythemia vera. In: Williams WJ, et al., eds. Hematology, 4th ed. New York, McGraw-Hill, 1990, pp. 193–202.

Smith JR, et al. Smokers' polycythemia. N Engl J Med 1978;298:6–10.

43

HEMOSTATIC DISORDERS

STEPHEN PETERSDORF

If you prick us, do we not bleed?

SHAKESPEARE (1564–1616)
The Merchant of Venice III, i, 65

BLEEDING DISORDERS

General Comments

- Disorders of primary hemostasis involve increased fragility of small blood vessels, decreased platelet count, or platelet function abnormalities. Bleeding from mucous membranes, petechiae, or superficial purpura result from abnormal primary hemostasis.
- Coagulation disorders (secondary hemostasis) are characterized by delayed, recurrent oozing from wounds as well as hematoma formation and are usually due to decreased clotting factors.
- Hemostatic defects can be congenital or acquired. Most patients with inherited defects start bleeding in childhood and have a family history of bleeding while acquired defects are usually noted when the patient is an adult and are often associated with an underlying disorder.

History

The following specific details should be determined:

1. Type of bleeding (e.g., epistaxis, petechiae, bleeding during menses, bleeding after dental extraction, generalized oozing, or bleeding into joints).
2. Onset of bleeding problem (lifelong history versus recent onset).
3. Nature of the inciting event, i.e., bleeding caused by trauma versus spontaneous bleeding.
4. Family history of bleeding.
5. Underlying systemic illnesses, particularly liver disease.
6. Medications, including nonprescription aspirin-containing compounds.

Physical Examination

Useful clinical abnormalities include the presence of petechiae, ecchymosis, or hemarthroses.

- Petechiae are dot hemorrhages that do not blanch with pressure. Their presence is characteristic of thrombocytopenia, dysfunctional platelets, or vasculitis. If petechiae are present primarily in the lower extremities or mucous membranes, thrombocytopenia is usually the cause of the bleeding. The presence of petechiae along with abnormalities in other organ systems suggests vasculitis as a cause of the bleeding.

- Disorders of secondary hemostasis are often manifest by ecchymoses, hemarthroses, or continued bleeding after trauma.

- Examination often reveals abnormalities characteristic of defects in both primary and secondary hemostasis such as the patient who has both petechiae and bruising.

Laboratory Evaluation

Laboratory evaluation is essential to define the etiology of the bleeding diathesis.

LABORATORY EVALUATION OF PRIMARY HEMOSTASIS

- Platelet count. A normal platelet count is $250,000/mm^3$ with a range of $150,000/mm^3$ to $350,000/mm^3$. Clinical bleeding rarely develops until the platelet count is less than $50,000/mm^3$.

- Bone marrow aspiration and biopsy. Thrombocytopenia is caused by decreased bone marrow production of platelets or increased peripheral destruction. If megakaryocytes are rarely seen in the bone marrow aspirate, then decreased production is the most likely cause of thrombocytopenia. If megakaryocytes are present in normal or increased numbers, the thrombocytopenia is due to increased peripheral destruction.

- Bleeding time
  1. The bleeding time (BT) is the best screening test of platelet function. The test is performed by making a reproducible skin incision 1 mm deep and several millimeters long on the forearm below a blood pressure cuff inflated to greater than 40 mmHg pressure.
  2. A platelet count of $75,000/mm^3$ is required to ensure a normal BT. A BT greater than 20 min or bleeding that needs to be stopped by local pressure is indicative of a clinically significant abnormality in platelet function. A moderately prolonged bleeding time may be difficult to interpret as the prolonged BT may result from operator error rather than a clinically significant problem.

- Platelet aggregation studies. When there is evidence of platelet dysfunction, platelet aggregation studies help determine whether the platelet dysfunction is due to abnormal adhesion, aggregation, or release. These tests are useful to diagnose aspirin exposure and rare defects such as Bernard-Soulier syndrome, Glanzmann's thrombasthenia, and storage pool deficiency.

- Von Willebrand's disease studies. Von Willebrand's disease (vWD) is the most common inherited defect of platelet function. Two of the most common tests of von Willebrand's factor are von Willebrand factor antigen (vWF Ag) and von Willebrand factor activity.

LABORATORY EVALUATION OF SECONDARY HEMOSTASIS

- Common screening tests for coagulation disorders typically include the prothrombin time (PT), thrombin time (TT), partial thromboplastin time (PTT), and fibrinogen level. A prolonged PT or PTT may be due to a decreased concentration of a clotting factor or a circulating factor inhibitor.
  1. The PT, TT, and PTT are prolonged only if an individual factor level is less than 20% of normal.
  2. If the prolonged test is corrected by incubating the patient's plasma with an equal volume of normal plasma, then the abnormality is due to a factor deficiency. If the addition of normal plasma fails to correct the abnormality, then a factor inhibitor is present. This test is often referred to as a 1 : 1 mix.
  3. Most patients with clinical bleeding have at least one abnormal screening test. Disorders that might lead to excessive bleeding with normal screening tests include Factor XIII deficiency, mild hemophilias (Factor VIII or IX deficiency), mild von Willebrand's disease, α_2-antiplasmin deficiency, platelet factor 3 deficiency, and scurvy.
- Prothrombin time (PT)
  1. The PT measures the clotting initiated by the extrinsic and common pathways and is thus dependent on Factor VII as well as Factors X, V, II, and fibrinogen.
  2. An abnormal PT is determined by comparing the value to that of a control plasma. In most laboratories, a clinically important factor deficiency prolongs the PT by more than 3 sec.
  3. An isolated prolongation of the PT may be caused by early liver disease, early warfarin effect, fat malabsorption with vitamin K deficiency, and factor VII deficiency.
- Partial thromboplastin time (PTT)
  1. The PTT measures clotting initiated by the intrinsic pathway (kallikrein, kininogen factors, XII, XI, VIII, IX) and common pathway (X, II, thrombin, and fibrinogen).
  2. The normal values for the PTT vary with each laboratory depending on the reagent used but are generally about 25 to 40 sec. The PTT is an effective screening test for all clotting factors except Factors VII and XIII, and will generally be prolonged if the factor levels are less than 20% of normal.
  3. A clinically important factor deficiency usually prolongs the PTT by 8 to 12 sec.

- Thrombin Time (TT)
  1. The TT measures the clotting time of plasma after the addition of thrombin. The TT is a more sensitive measurement of fibrin formation than the PT and PTT.
  2. The TT is useful to screen for abnormalities of fibrin formation caused by fibrin degradation products, myeloma paraproteins, congenital dysfibrinogenemias, or heparin contamination.
- Fibrinogen
  1. The fibrinogen concentration is determined by comparing the clotting time of plasma after thrombin is added to the clotting time of samples with known fibrinogen levels.
  2. Clinically significant bleeding occurs if the level is below 50 to 80 mg/dl. The fibrinogen level is decreased in patients with disseminated intravascular coagulation (DIC), afibrinogenemia, or patients receiving thrombolytic therapy.
- Second-level tests of hemostasis
  1. Coagulation factor assays. If an isolated factor deficiency is suspected after an abnormal screening test is detected, specific factor levels can be assayed. They are usually reported as a percent of the normal factor present in the plasma.
  2. Clot stability test
     a. The clot stability test evaluates the function of factor XIII.
     b. Factor XIII deficiency is not detected by the PT or PTT. The clot stability test is useful to evaluate bleeding in those patients with a bleeding diathesis who have normal screening tests.
  3. Fibrin degradation products. Measuring the fibrin degradation products (FDPs) is the screening test of fibrinolysis. FDPs are elevated in states such as disseminated intravascular coagulation where there is ongoing plasmin digestion of fibrin.

DIFFERENTIAL DIAGNOSIS

Primary Hemostasis

Disorders of primary hemostasis usually present with bleeding from the skin and mucous membranes. They are due to thrombocytopenia or decreased platelet function.

- Thrombocytopenia (Table 43–1)
  Clinical bleeding from thrombocytopenia is usually manifest as petechiae, epistaxis, bleeding from mucous membranes, and menorrhagia. It may develop when the platelet count is less than $50,000/mm^3$ and is common when the platelet count is less than $20,000/mm^3$. The severity of the bleeding is also affected by associated platelet dysfunction or coagulation disorders.

TABLE 43-1. Thrombocytopenia

A. Thrombocytopenia due to decreased marrow production (decreased bone marrow megakaryocytes)
   1. Viral infection
   2. Alcohol
   3. Drugs (e.g., thiazide diuretics)
   4. Disorders associated with marrow invasion (e.g., leukemia, metastatic carcinoma, infection)
   5. Disorders associated with defective myelopoiesis (e.g., aplastic anemia, myelodysplasia, Fanconi's syndrome, paroxysmal nocturnal hemoglobinuria)
B. Thrombocytopenia due to increased peripheral platelet destruction (normal to increased number of megakaryocytes)
   1. Immune-mediated destruction
      a. Immune thrombocytopenic purpura (ITP)
      b. Neonatal alloimmune purpura
      c. Posttransfusion purpura
      d. Drug-induced thrombocytopenic purpura (commonly implicated drugs include quinine, quinidine, gold, and heparin)
   2. Nonimmunologic destruction
      a. Hypersplenism
      b. Disseminated intravascular coagulation
      c. Thrombotic thrombocytopenic purpura (TTP)
      d. Hemolytic-uremic syndrome (HUS)
      e. Giant cavernous hemangioma (Kasabach-Merritt syndrome)
C. Congenital thrombocytopenia
   1. May-Hegglin anomaly
   2. Wiskott-Aldrich syndrome
   3. Fanconi's anemia

PLATELET DYSFUNCTION

- Patients who have a normal platelet count and yet have evidence of impaired primary hemostasis usually have a disorder of platelet function, which is detected by a prolonged bleeding time. Defects in platelet function may be due to impaired platelet adhesion to the subendothelium, aggregation with adjacent platelets or impaired secretion of platelet products. The most common cause of platelet dysfunction is aspirin ingestion (Table 43-2).

Secondary Hemostasis

Congenital defects typically involve only one coagulation factor. Acquired disorders usually involve a decrease in several coagulation factors.

- Congenital disorders. Factor VIII deficiency (hemophilia A), Factor IX deficiency (hemophilia B), and von Willebrand's disease account for greater than 95% of inher-

TABLE 43–2. Disorders Associated with Platelet Dysfunction

A. Congenital disorders of platelet function
 1. Defective adhesion to subendothelium: Von Willebrand's disease, Bernard-Soulier syndrome
 2. Defective platelet aggregation: Glanzmann's thrombasthenia, afibrinogenemia
 3. Defective platelet secretion: gray platelet syndrome
B. Acquired disorders of platelet function
 1. Uremia
 2. Multiple myeloma with paraproteinemia (may also have prolonged TT)
 3. Myeloproliferative diseases
 4. Drug-induced (e.g., aspirin, penicillin, thiazide diuretics)

---

ited deficiencies of coagulation. Hemophilia A and B have sex-linked inheritance. Von Willebrand's disease may have dominant or recessive inheritances. All of the other inherited factor deficiencies are rare and inherited in an autosomal recessive manner.

1. Factor VIII deficiency (hemophilia A)
 a. This is the most common deficiency (prevalence 100/million). It presents with hemarthroses, hematomas, and prolonged postoperative bleeding.
 b. Severe hemophiliacs have less than 1% of normal Factor VIII levels. Moderate hemophiliacs have 1 to 5% Factor VIII levels and have fewer spontaneous bleeding episodes, and mild hemophiliacs (5 to 20% Factor VIII) usually bleed only after surgery. Laboratory abnormalities: prolonged PTT, decreased Factor VIII levels.
2. Von Willebrand's disease
 a. Prevalence is 100/million.
 b. Presents with epistaxis, gingival bleeding, easy bruising, postoperative bleeding, and menorrhagia. Patients have platelet dysfunction and a Factor VIII abnormality. Laboratory abnormalities: prolonged bleeding time, prolonged PTT, decreased vWF antigen and activity.
3. Factor IX deficiency (hemophilia B or Christmas disease)
 a. Prevalence is 20/million.
 b. Clinical presentation is similar to Factor VIII deficiency.
 c. Laboratory abnormalities: prolonged PT and PTT, decreased Factor IX level.
4. Factor I (fibrinogen) deficiency
 a. Prevalence is 1/million.
 b. Clinical presentation is notable for prolonged bleeding at the umbilical stump at birth.
 c. Laboratory abnormalities: prolonged PT, PTT, and TT, and decreased fibrinogen level.

5. Factor II, V, and X deficiency
   a. Prevalence 1/million.
   b. Clinical presentation is similar to Factor VIII deficiency.
   c. Laboratory abnormalities: prolonged PT and PTT, decreased factor levels.
6. Factor XI deficiency
   a. Prevalence is 1/million.
   b. Presents as a mild bleeding diathesis.
   c. Laboratory abnormalities: prolonged PTT, decreased Factor XI level.
7. Factor XII deficiency
   a. Prevalence is 1/million.
   b. No clinical bleeding occurs.
   c. Laboratory abnormalities: prolonged PTT, decreased Factor XII level.

- Acquired disorders of coagulation (Table 43–3). Like the congenital deficiencies, patients may present with ecchymoses, hemarthroses, prolonged bleeding from wounds, and genitourinary and gastrointestinal tract bleeding. Acquired bleeding disorders are usually due to vitamin K deficiency, an acquired coagulation factor inhibitor, or a consumptive coagulopathy.
  1. Vitamin K deficiency
     a. Vitamin K is required for carboxylation of Factors II, VII, IX, and X. This process is critical for the clotting function of these factors.
     b. Warfarin anticoagulants act by interfering with the vitamin K–dependent synthesis of these factors. Vitamin K deficiency can also be caused by a dietary deficiency of vitamin K, intestinal malabsorption, biliary tract obstruction, low body stores of vitamin K at birth (in the neonate), and broad-spectrum antibiotics.
     c. Laboratory evidence of vitamin K deficiency includes a markedly prolonged PT (decreased Factors II, VII, and X) and a prolonged PTT from Factor IX deficiency.
  2. Acquired inhibitors of clotting factors
     a. Inhibitors or circulating anticoagulants directly inhibit coagulation factors. Inhibitors are usually antibodies to coagulation factors and often develop after patients receive replacement factors. They may develop spontaneously in patients who do not have an underlying factor deficiency.
     b. Factor VIII inhibitors are the most common inhibitors and are associated with hemophilia A, the postpartum state, and immunologic disorders such as rheumatoid arthritis.
     c. The lupus anticoagulant inhibits the phospholipid-dependent coagulation steps and is characterized by an isolated prolongation of the PTT that does not correct with a 1:1 mix. It occurs in 10% of patients with systemic lupus erythematosus (SLE) and in patients with other syndromes such as drug-induced SLE, rheumatoid arthritis, and AIDS.

TABLE 43–3. Common Hemostatic Disorders and Laboratory Abnormalities

Condition	Abnormal Tests	Normal Tests	Confirmatory Tests
Vitamin K deficiency	PT (PTT if IX is low)	PTT, TT, Plt	II, VII, IX, and X
Liver disease			
early	PT, PTT	TT, fibrinogen Plt	II, VII, IX, and X
chronic	PT, PTT, TT, fibrinogen, Plt		II, VII, IX, and X (decreased) FDP (increased)
DIC	PT, TT, PTT, fibrinogen, Plt		FDP
Heparin contamination	PTT, TT	PT	Protamine will correct
Lupus anticoagulant	PTT	PT, TT, Plt	PTT will not correct

Plt = Platelet count.

368

The lupus anticoagulant is not associated with abnormal bleeding but may be associated with arterial and venous thrombosis.
3. Consumptive coagulopathy
   a. Consumptive coagulopathy or DIC is a process that may result from diseases such as infection or malignancy.
   b. The common event is the pathologic generation of thrombin which leads to the activation of platelets. Fibrinogen is converted to fibrin thrombi, and Factors V and VIII are consumed. Activation of the fibrinolytic system leads to thrombocytopenia, decreased clotting factor levels, and increased FDPs.
   c. Because the platelet count is decreased and the clotting times are prolonged, symptoms include bleeding from wounds, epistaxis, gingival bleeding, and petechiae.

RECOMMENDED DIAGNOSTIC APPROACH

The history and physical examination provide clues to the type of bleeding. Appropriate laboratory evaluation is shown in Figures 43–1 and 43–2.

THROMBOSIS

General Comments

The development and propagation of thrombi is usually moderated by the balance between procoagulant factors in the blood and the fibrinolytic system that breaks down clots. There are a variety of mechanisms and diseases associated with excessive thrombosis (Table 43–4). Normal antithrombotic mechanisms include:

1. Clearance of activated coagulation factors by the liver and dispersal in the blood.
2. Inactivation of activated Factors XIa, IXa, Xa, and thrombin by antithrombin III.
3. Inactivation of Factors VIIIa and Va by activated protein C which also requires protein S as a cofactor.

Clinical Features

- History
  1. Arterial thrombosis can only occur at sites of underlying vessel wall disease such as at atherosclerotic plaques or prosthetic valves. The clinical manifestations are specific to the organ involved.
  2. Venous thrombosis does not require underlying vessel wall damage as stasis and increased viscosity increase the risk of thrombosis.
     a. Venous thrombosis typically occurs in the lower extremities or pelvic veins but may occur in the upper extremities, particularly in patients with a central venous catheter.

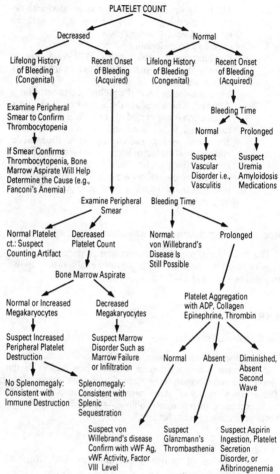

Figure 43–1. Evaluation of the patient with a clinically suspected disorder of primary hemostasis.

b. Symptoms frequently associated with venous thrombosis include pain, erythema, warmth, and swelling in the area of the clot.

c. If the clot is dislodged, a pulmonary embolism may result causing symptoms including chest pain, shortness of breath, cough, hemoptysis, and cardiac symptoms such as palpitations.

3. Acquired conditions that predispose to thrombosis may change the local venous environment or produce the tendency towards coagulation systemically.

a. A patient with recurrent episodes of venous thrombosis or a thrombotic disorder at a young age

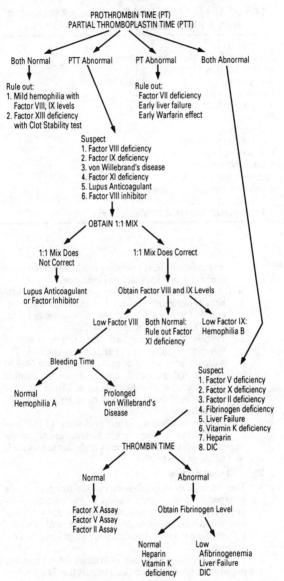

Figure 43–2. Evaluation of the patient with a clinically suspected abnormality in secondary hemostasis.

who has no predisposing conditions should be evaluated for a congenital thrombogenic condition, antithrombin III deficiency, protein C deficiency, protein S deficiency, and dysfibri-

**TABLE 43–4. Acquired Conditions Associated
with an Increased Risk of Thrombosis**

Trauma
Previous venous thromboembolism
Immobilization
Malignancy
Obesity
Varicose veins
Pregnancy
Estrogens
Nephrotic syndrome
Congestive heart failure
Lupus anticoagulant
Hematologic disorders
   Acute promyelocytic leukemia
   Myeloproliferative disorders
   Paroxysmal nocturnal hemoglobinuria

     nogenemia. These disorders can be inherited or be
     the result of a spontaneous mutation.

  b. Antithrombin III deficiency is inherited in an auto-
     somal dominant manner. The inherited defect ac-
     counts for 2 to 4% of venous thrombotic episodes
     in patients less than 45 years old.

  c. Protein C deficiency accounts for 5 to 8% of
     thrombotic episodes in patients less than 45. The
     patients have levels of protein C that are 50% of
     normal and the defect appears to be transmitted
     via heterozygous autosomal gene. The prevalence
     of protein C deficiency may be as high as 1 in 300
     individuals.

  d. Protein S deficiency is less prevalent (1 : 15,000—
     20,000) but its frequency in patients under the age
     of 45 with thrombotic events is similar to protein C
     deficiency (5 to 8%).

- Physical examination

  1. The findings associated with venous thrombosis are
     nonspecific and include edema of the extremity in-
     volved, tenderness to palpation, discoloration, venous
     distension, and occasionally a palpable cord. The de-
     finitive diagnosis of thrombosis requires imaging pro-
     cedures.

  2. The clinical manifestations of arterial thrombosis are
     organ specific and depend on the part that is affected.

Laboratory Evaluation

- Blood tests. There are no blood tests that can diagnose a
  blood clot in the circulation. Some tests may indicate patients who are predisposed to thrombosis.

  1. CBC (including review of the smear) may suggest
     chronic myelogenous leukemia, polycythemia vera, or
     essential thrombocytosis.

2. A PTT that is prolonged and does not correct with a
   1 : 1 mix suggests the lupus anticoagulant.
3. A prolonged TT suggests a dysfibrinogenemia.

- If there is a family history of thrombosis or the patient has
  recurrent thrombotic episodes, especially at a young age,
  more specific tests may be indicated.

   1. Antithrombin III level. A functional assay should be
      performed. Symptomatic patients have antithrombin
      III levels that are 40 to 60% of normal.
   2. Protein C and protein S activity. Functional and immu-
      nologic assays should be obtained. Often, these pa-
      tients will be taking warfarin, which also depresses
      protein C and S levels. In these cases, the finding of
      lowered ratios of protein C or S to Factor II or X is
      considered diagnostic for protein C or protein S defi-
      ciency.

- Imaging evaluation (see Chapter 24)

Bibliography

Bachmann F. Diagnostic approach to mild bleeding disorders. Semin
   Hematol 1980;17:292–305.
Colman RW, et al. Hemostasis and Thrombosis. Philadelphia, J.B.
   Lippincott, 1987.
Comp PC. Hereditary disorders predisposing to thrombosis. Prog He-
   mostasis Thrombosis 1986;8:71–102.
Comp PC. Overview of the hypercoagulable states. Semin Thrombosis
   Hemostasis 1990;16:158–161.
Gastineau DA, et al. Lupus anticoagulant: An analysis of the clinical
   and laboratory features of 219 cases. Am J Hematol 1985;19:
   265–275.
Hirsh J., ed. Venous thromboembolism: Prevention, diagnosis and
   treatment. Chest 1986;89(Suppl. 5):369–437.
Karpatkin S. Autoimmune thrombocytopenic purpura. Semin Hema-
   tol 1985;22:260–288.
Malpass TW, Harker LA. Acquired disorders of platelet function.
   Semin Hematol 1980;17:242–258.
Mammen EF. Congenital coagulation disorders. Semin Thrombosis
   Hemostasis 1983;9:1–22.
Rao AK, Holmsen H. Congenital disorders of platelet function. Semin
   Hematol 1986;23:102–118.

44

LYMPHADENOPATHY

OLIVER W. PRESS

> With the help of a surgeon, he might yet recover.
>
> SHAKESPEARE (1564–1616)
> A Midsummer Nights Dream, V, 1

DEFINITION

Lymphadenopathy is a pathologic enlargement of lymph nodes (generally >1 cm) or hard fixed nodes of any size.

DIFFERENTIAL DIAGNOSIS

- Infections are responsible for 65 to 70% of lymphadenopathy cases in a primary-care setting. In an additional 25 to 30% of cases, no specific cause is found. The relative frequencies of various infections in cases of cervical adenitis are shown in Table 44–1.
- Neoplasms cause approximately 1% of all cases of lymphadenopathy, but are found in 30 to 40% of nodes excised. The types of malignancies are shown in Table 44–2.
- Other causes of lymphadenopathy include: angioimmunoblastic lymphadenopathy, acquired immunodeficiency syndrome (AIDS) or other conditions related to HIV, storage diseases (Gaucher's disease, Niemann-Pick disease), drug reactions (phenytoin, hydralazine), serum sickness, collagen vascular diseases (e.g., SLE), skin diseases (eczema) with dermatopathic nodes, sarcoidosis (3.1% of biopsies), masses confused with lymphadenopathy (thyroglossal duct cysts, branchial pouch cysts, dermoid cysts, lipomas, submaxillary salivary gland enlargement).

CLINICAL FEATURES

History

- Inflammatory nodes are usually tender, mobile, arise acutely, and resolve rapidly (in less than 2 weeks)
- Lymph nodes that contain malignancy usually are nontender, may become fixed or matted, and arise insidiously with progressive enlargement.
- Inquiry should be made with regard to associated fever, chills, sweats, pruritus, weight loss, rashes, arthralgias,

TABLE 44–1. Relative Frequency of Infections in Cervical Adenitis

INFECTIONS	PERCENT OF CERVICAL ADENITIS
Bacterial	
Streptococci	40
Staphylococci	10–15
Mycobacteria (scrofula)	0–6
Brucellosis	<1
Viral	
Infectious mononucleosis	0–20
Cytomegalovirus	?
Rubella	?
Varicella	?
Measles	?
Cat scratch fever	3
Herpes simplex (1 and 2)	?
Protozoal infections	
Toxoplasmosis	<1
Fungal infections	
Histoplasmosis	<1
Coccidioidomycosis	<1
Sporotrichosis	<1

jaundice, purulent node drainage, pharyngitis, cough, hemoptysis, and stool changes.
- Medical history may divulge a history of tuberculosis, venereal disease, SLE, dental caries, scalp wounds, breast cancer, or alcohol and cigarette use (associated with head and neck, esophageal, and lung carcinomas).
- Environmental exposures to measles, mumps, rubella, chickenpox, mononucleosis, cats (toxoplasmosis or cat scratch fever), or ingestion of unpasteurized milk (brucellosis or mycobacterial disease) or anticonvulsants should be considered.
- Geographic considerations are important in assessing the likelihood of histoplasmosis (occurring in the Midwest) or coccidioidomycosis (occurring in the Southwest).
- A history of homosexual behavior, IV drug use, or hemophilia should arouse suspicion of AIDS or AIDS-related complex (ARC) commonly associated with persistent generalized lymphadenopathy (PGL).
- The risk of neoplastic lymphadenopathy is highly dependent on the age of the patient and the site of lymphadenopathy, as shown in Table 44–3.

Physical Examination

- The size, consistency, tenderness, warmth, fixation, fluctuance, and distribution of nodes should be noted.

TABLE 44–2. Types of Malignancies Found in Biopsies

Site	Number of Specimens	Benign (%)	Squamous Cell Carcinoma (%)	Adenocarcinoma (%)	Anaplastic Carcinoma (%)	Lymphoma (%)
Neck	234	63	6	8	6	18
Supraclavicular	187	37	13	18	23	9
Axillary	141	60	1	11	5	23
Groin	84	71	8	8	5	8

**TABLE 44–3. Risk of
Neoplastic Lymphadenopathy**

Characteristic	Risk of Malignancy (%)
All patients with adenopathy	1.1
Patients >40 yr old with adenopathy	4.0
Patients <40 yr old with adenopathy	0.4
Supraclavicular adenopathy	50
Age >40 and supraclavicular adenopathy	90

- Extensive otolaryngologic evaluation of the upper aerodigestive tract is mandatory in evaluating cervical nodes suspected of harboring malignancy.
- Detection of hepatosplenomegaly, abdominal masses, jaundice, tonsillitis, pharyngitis, and rashes is important.
- A careful search for malignancy is essential. This includes detection of breast masses, oral lesions, and stool with occult blood.

Laboratory Studies

Laboratory studies are unnecessary in the majority of cases of lymphadenopathy, since an inflammatory origin is usually obvious. However, in instances in which the etiology of lymph node enlargement remains obscure after careful history and physical examination, the following laboratory tests may be illuminating.

- CBC may reveal circulating malignant cells (in leukemia or lymphoma) or atypical lymphocytes indicative of mononucleosis.
- A chest X-ray may reveal mediastinal adenopathy (e.g., lymphoma or sarcoidosis) or pulmonary infiltrates (sarcoidosis, tuberculosis, AIDS-related *Pneumocystis* infection).
- Serologic testing may reveal evidence for infectious mononucleosis (the ''heterophile'' antibody), toxoplasmosis, AIDS (antibodies to the HIV virus), syphilis (VDRL), SLE (antinuclear antibodies), or hepatitis B (hepatitis B surface antigen).
- Cultures of symptomatic sites may document underlying infections such as pharyngeal streptococcal infection, lymphogranuloma venereum (*Chlamydia*), or tuberculosis.
- Fine needle aspiration of lymph nodes has gained popularity in the past decade because it affords a rapid, inexpensive, nonoperative means of providing a pathologic diagnosis of adenopathy.
  1. The sensitivity and specificity of this technique are alleged to be 93% and 95%, respectively, in the hands of an experienced cytopathologist. Nevertheless, this

approach remains controversial because of difficulties in diagnosing some entities (e.g., Hodgkin's disease) with this technique.

2. This approach is probably most useful in confirming metastatic disease to lymph nodes in patients with previously diagnosed carcinomas. It also is useful in patients with intraabdominal adenopathy who may be spared laparotomy if a percutaneous lymph node aspiration is diagnostic.

- Lymph node biopsy is the definitive diagnostic procedure for evaluating lymphadenopathy.

1. The excised node should be examined by frozen section, routine histology, and special stains (Gram's, fungal, and Ziehl-Neelsen) and should be cultured for aerobic, anaerobic, fungal, and mycobacterial organisms. In special cases, surface marker studies should be performed by immunofluorescence or immunoperoxidase methods (e.g., lymphomas), and electron microscopy should be considered (e.g., to detect characteristic granules in small-cell carcinoma of the lung).

2. Excisional biopsy of an entire node is far superior to needle biopsy in assessing lymphomas, since node architecture is essential for subclassification of lymphoid neoplasms.

3. It cannot be overemphasized that cervical lymph node biopsy should never be undertaken in an adult unless a detailed otolaryngologic evaluation has been performed previously to exclude intraoral, laryngeal, and nasopharyngeal lesions.

RECOMMENDED DIAGNOSTIC APPROACH

Following is a suggested approach to the evaluation of patients with lymphadenopathy according to the site of nodal involvement.

- Anterior and posterior neck nodes. Enlarged cervical nodes are found in 56% of patients with lymphadenopathy and are usually due to minor local infections.

1. Consider facial, dental, pharyngeal, and ear infections. Throat cultures, CBC, and serologic tests for mononucleosis may be indicated.

2. If the above tests are unproductive and the patient is nontoxic, further evaluation should be deferred for 1 to 2 weeks to permit benign inflammatory lymphadenopathy to recede before extensive testing is done.

3. If the lymph nodes remain enlarged after 1 to 2 weeks, the tests for mononucleosis should be repeated, and serologic studies for cytomegalovirus and toxoplasmosis, tuberculin skin test, and a chest X-ray should be performed.

4. If a diagnosis still has not been reached, a thorough otolaryngologic evaluation should be done to rule out a head and neck tumor, and then an excisional biopsy should be performed.

- Supraclavicular lymphadenopathy. Isolated supraclavicular adenopathy occurs in <1% of cases and usually is caused by metastatic malignancy from the thorax (breast or lung) or abdomen (stomach or colon). Chest X-ray should be done followed by early node biopsy.

- Axillary lymphadenopathy. This condition occurs in 4% of cases and should prompt a careful search for scratches, bites, infections, or lymphadenitis of the hands and arms as well as careful breast examination.

  1. If none of these examinations show an abnormality, and the patient is nontoxic, further evaluation should be deferred, and the patient should be reexamined in 1 to 2 weeks. Isolated axillary node enlargement is unusual for mononucleosis.

  2. If the mass persists longer than 1 to 2 weeks, serologic tests for mononucleosis, cytomegalovirus, and toxoplasmosis, a tuberculin skin test, and a chest X-ray should be done. A node biopsy should be scheduled.

- Inguinal lymphadenopathy occurs in 16% of cases. In the absence of obvious infection or tumor of the lower extremities or genitals, serologic studies for syphilis and lymphogranuloma venereum should be performed, followed by the tests described for axillary lymphadenopathy after a 1- to 2-week waiting period. Inguinal nodes are often difficult to assess because of the frequency with which they are enlarged in normal individuals ("dermatopathic nodes").

- Generalized lymphadenopathy occurs in 24% of cases. It is commonly caused by viral diseases, systemic illnesses, ARC, or drug reactions. If an acute viral illness is known to be present, no work-up is indicated. Otherwise, testing should follow the sequence outlined here:

  1. Cessation of drugs capable of causing lymphadenopathy (e.g., phenytoin, allopurinol, hydralazine)

  2. Serology for HIV, mononucleosis, cytomegalovirus, and toxoplasmosis.

  3. Other tests include blood cultures (for endocarditis), tuberculin skin testing, antinuclear antibodies (for SLE), chest X-ray (for sarcoidosis, tuberculosis, Hodgkin's disease), CBC blood and smear, liver function tests.

  4. Node biopsy. The advisability of node biopsy in patients with ARC and PGL is controversial. Biopsies in most of these patients reveal follicular hyperplasia and do not affect patient management. However, in a minority of patients, neoplasms (lymphomas, Kaposi's sarcoma) or opportunistic infections will be detected (e.g., tuberculosis, atypical mycobacteria, histoplasmosis). Indications for biopsy of lymph nodes related to PGL include:

     a. Marked constitutional symptoms
     b. Localized adenopathy
     c. A disproportionately enlarging node
     d. Bulky mediastinal or abdominal adenopathy
     e. Cytopenias with an elevated sedimentation rate and otherwise negative evaluation
     f. Patient reassurance

Bibliography

Abrahms DI. AIDS-related lymphadenopathy: The role of biopsy. J Clin Oncol 1986;4:126–127.

Allhiser JN, et al. Lymphadenopathy in a family practice. J Fam Pract 1981;12:27–32.

Berkheiser SW. A survey of cervical lymph node biopsies. Penn Med 1988;91:64–66.

Bottles K, et al. Fine-needle aspiration biopsy of patients with the acquired immunodeficiency syndrome (AIDS): Experience in an outpatient clinic. Ann Int Med 1988;108:42–45.

Fijten GH, Blijham GH. Unexplained lymphadenopathy in family practice. J Fam Pract 1988;27:373–376.

Greenfield S, Jordan MC. The clinical investigation of lymphadenopathy in primary care practice. JAMA 1978;240:1388–1393.

Kardos TF, et al. Fine needle aspiration biopsy in the management of children and young adults with peripheral lymphadenopathy. Cancer 1989;63:703–707.

Lee Y-T, et al. Lymph node biopsy for diagnosis: A statistical study. J Surg Oncol 1980;14:53–60.

Linet OI, Metzler C. Incidence of palpable cervical nodes in adults. Postgrad Med 1977;62:210–213.

Saltzstein SL. The fate of patients with nondiagnostic lymph node biopsies. Surgery 1965;58:659–662.

Slap GB, et al. When to perform biopsies of enlarged peripheral lymph nodes in young patients. JAMA 1984;252:1321–1326.

Sundaresh HP, et al. Etiology of cervical lymphadenitis in children. Am Fam Phys 1981;24:147–151.

45

LEUKEMIA

DAVID BOLDT

Of direst cruelty; make thick my blood.
SHAKESPEARE (1564–1616)
Macbeth I,V, 38

DEFINITION

- General

Leukemias are characterized by uncontrolled proliferation of bone marrow cells. In this chapter, 4 types are considered: acute myeloid leukemia (AML); acute lymphocytic leukemia (ALL); chronic myelocytic leukemia (CML); and chronic lymphocytic leukemia (CLL).

The prompt and precise diagnosis of leukemia, especially acute leukemia, is essential. More than half of children with ALL can be long-term survivors (probably cured). Seventy-five percent of patients with AML achieve temporary remissions of the disease, and 15 to 20% may be long-term (5-year) survivors with standard therapy. Intensive-dose chemotherapy or high-dose chemo/radiotherapy followed by bone marrow transplantation may yield disease-free survival rates of 40 to 50% at 2 years.

- Criteria for diagnosis. Diagnosis of leukemia, although frequently inferred from clinical and peripheral blood findings, requires bone marrow examination. Cytochemical, cytogenetic, and cell surface marker analyses may also be required for precise diagnosis and classification.

  1. AML
     a. AML is diagnosed when bone marrow is infiltrated by >30% myeloblasts. The presence of Auer rods in blast cells, seen in 50% of cases, is pathognomonic for AML.
     b. There are 7 subtypes of AML (designated M1 to M7) determined by morphologic and cytochemical features of the blast cells according to the French-American-British (FAB) classification. To date, the FAB classification has not been useful in assessment of prognosis or choice of therapy.
     c. Most cases of AML display abnormal cytogenetic features. Application of cytogenetic analysis has permitted recognition of several distinct AML syndromes with unique clinical behaviors.
  2. ALL is diagnosed when the bone marrow has >30% lymphoblasts. Over 90% are positive for the enzyme terminal deoxynucleotidyl transferase (TDT) and may

express lymphocyte differentiation markers. Most notable is the presence of the common ALL antigen (CALLA) on surfaces of lymphoblasts in 50 to 75% of all patients. FAB classification of ALL denotes three subtypes (termed L1 to L3) and does have prognostic utility.

3. CML

   a. The diagnosis of CML is not based on identification of a predominance of one specific cell type in bone marrow or blood. It is manifest by excessive granulocyte production in the peripheral blood and bone marrow. Leukocytosis is profound (average WBC is 75,000/mm³). All stages of granulocyte development from blast to mature polymorphonuclear leukocyte are expanded in bone marrow, and all are present in peripheral blood. Confirmatory findings include splenomegaly, a decreased leukocyte alkaline phosphatase (LAP) score in peripheral cells, and basophilia.

   b. The diagnosis of CML is established conclusively by demonstrating the Philadelphia chromosome in bone marrow cells. The Philadelphia chromosome is a reciprocal translocation between the long arms of chromosomes 9 and 22 resulting in the formation of a new fusion gene, termed *bcr-abl,* on chromosome 22. Ten to fifteen percent of patients with CML lack the Philadelphia chromosome. In many of these cases, sensitive molecular techniques can be used to demonstrate presence of the *bcr-abl* fusion gene or its protein product.

4. CLL is diagnosed when a peripheral blood lymphocytosis >15,000/mm³ and lymphocytic marrow infiltration of >40% are present. CLL cells have morphologic characteristics of mature small lymphocytes. In 95% of cases the lymphocytes have monoclonal immunoglobulin markers. In 5% of cases T-cell surface markers can be found.

EPIDEMIOLOGY

• Demographic features

1. AML represents 40% of all leukemias. It is predominantly a disease of adults. Whereas 85% of acute leukemias in individuals over age 25 are AML, only 18% in younger individuals are AML.

2. ALL makes up 20% of all leukemias and is the predominant leukemia of children. Its incidence peaks between ages 2 and 6.

3. CML makes up 15% of all leukemias. The median age of onset is the fourth decade.

4. CLL represents 25% of all leukemias in the Western Hemisphere. It is uncommon in Asian populations. The median age of onset is the sixth and seventh decades, and CLL does not occur in children and adolescents. There is a 2:1 male-to-female predominance.

- Etiologic considerations
  1. Associated factors. Recent evidence strongly links an RNA retrovirus, human T-cell leukemia virus (HTLV), to the development of one uncommon type of leukemia, adult T-cell leukemia. In general, however, the cause of leukemia is unknown.
  2. Siblings of patients with leukemia have a 4-fold increased risk of developing the disease. In patients with ALL under age 10, there is a 20% concordance among identical twins. Hereditary diseases such as trisomy 21, Bloom syndrome, Fanconi's anemia, and ataxia-telangiectasia are associated with an increased risk of leukemia.
  3. Ionizing radiation is a leukemogenic agent in man. Japanese survivors of atomic bombings have dose-related increased incidences of AML, ALL, and CML but not of CLL. Exposure to therapeutic X-rays also carries a markedly increased risk of leukemia for radiologists working in the era before adequate shielding, patients with ankylosing spondylitis treated with spinal radiation, and individuals who received thymic irradiation during infancy.
  4. Drugs and chemicals. Benzene, toluene, cancer chemotherapeutic agents, chloramphenicol, and phenylbutazone are all associated with increased incidences of leukemia, usually AML. The increased incidence of AML now recognized in patients treated for Hodgkin's disease (as high as 5 to 10% of patients surviving after combination chemotherapy), multiple myeloma (risk as high as 20% 5 years after diagnosis), and polycythemia vera (15%) may represent therapy-associated leukemia.
  5. Association with certain hematologic diseases. Other hematologic diseases have a high risk for subsequent development of leukemia. These include refractory anemia with excess blast cells (30%), myeloproliferative syndromes (15%), acquired sideroblastic anemia (5 to 10%), and aplastic anemia (5%).

DIFFERENTIAL DIAGNOSIS

- Leukemia vs. leukemoid reactions. The myeloid leukemias (AML and CML) must be distinguished from exuberant reactive leukocytoses termed leukemoid reactions. Leukemoid reactions are caused most commonly by infections or malignancies and less commonly by immunologic diseases. Total leukocyte counts $>50,000/mm^3$ or blasts in the peripheral blood, or both, strongly suggest leukemia. Features that favor a diagnosis of CML include low LAP score, basophilia, and elevated serum vitamin B_{12} levels. Bone marrow morphology and cytogenetics are diagnostic.
- Leukemia vs. other malignancies. Metastatic carcinoma or myelofibrosis or, rarely, infections invading the bone marrow may provoke a leukoerythroblastic peripheral blood picture with anemia, luekocytosis, immature leukocytes,

and nucleated erythrocytes. Clinically affected patients may experience weight loss and fatigue similar to those of leukemia patients. Definitive diagnosis is established by bone marrow biopsy.

- ALL vs. benign lymphocytosis and lymphadenopathy. Careful examination of peripheral smears usually distinguishes atypical lymphocytes from the lymphoblasts of ALL. In other cases the occurrence of characteristic serologic findings is diagnostic. Differential diagnosis includes infectious mononucleosis, cytomegalovirus infection, toxoplasmosis, acute infectious lymphocytosis, other viral infections, immunologic disorders such as SLE, and juvenile rheumatoid arthritis.

- CLL vs. other lymphoid malignancies. In middle-aged to elderly adults a peripheral blood lymphocytosis in which the cells resemble normal mature lymphocytes is CLL until proved otherwise. The chief consideration of differential diagnosis is to distinguish CLL from other lymphoid malignancies such as hairy cell leukemia, lymphosarcoma cell leukemia, Waldenström's macroglobulinemia, and the Sézary syndrome.

- Leukemia vs. other hematologic disorders. In as many as 50% of patients with ALL, leukemia may present as pancytopenia with few or no peripheral blasts. Other hematologic causes of pancytopenia, such as aplastic anemia, myelofibrosis, refractory anemia with excess blasts, sideroblastic anemia, and deficiencies of vitamin B_{12} or folic acid, may be distinguished by bone marrow examination.

CLINICAL MANIFESTATIONS

- Acute leukemias
  1. Bone marrow failure. Patients with acute leukemias most commonly have signs and symptoms of bone marrow failure.
     a. Anemia occurs in 98% of cases, producing easy fatigability, weakness, orthostasis, and pallor.
     b. Granulocytopenia occurs in 75% of cases and may be present even with a high WBC count. Patients with granulocytopenia, especially with absolute granulocyte counts $<500/mm^3$, are susceptible to infection and may have fever and signs referable to local or systemic infection.
     c. Thrombocytopenia occurs in 80 to 90% of cases. Characteristic clinical findings include petechiae, purpura, and mucous membrane bleeding. Individuals with platelet counts $<20,000/mm^3$ are at risk for developing spontaneous intracranial hemorrhage.
  2. Organ infiltration. Leukemic cells can infiltrate virtually any tissue. Clinical findings seen commonly in acute leukemias because of organ infiltration include hepatosplenomegaly and lymphadenopathy (70% of ALL patients; 30 to 40% of AML); nodular skin lesions (5% of ALL; 10% of AML); bone pain and arthralgias

(50% of ALL); gingival hypertrophy (characteristic of monocytic AML variants); and headaches, blurred vision, papilledema, seizures, or cranial nerve dysfunction caused by meningeal leukemia (5 to 10% of ALL; 1% of AML).

3. Disseminated intravascular coagulation (DIC) is seen frequently in association with the acute promyelocytic variant of AML.

4. Time course. In most patients with acute leukemia, the time course of illness is short, progressing rapidly over days to weeks. By contrast, in elderly patients disease onset may be more insidious, occurring over many months, with the so-called "smoldering" acute leukemia.

- Chronic leukemias

  1. Insidious onset. Chronic leukemias are most likely to develop insidiously. Thirty percent of cases of CLL and 10% of CML cases are diagnosed incidentally during evaluation of unrelated complaints or during routine medical examinations.

  2. Nonspecific symptoms. Patients with CML frequently have easy fatigability, fever, and weight loss. Splenomegaly is found in 90% of patients and may produce symptoms such as LUQ pain or early satiety. Bone pain is seen in 30 to 40% of cases, and sternal tenderness can often be elicited. Infection is not a problem because mature granulocytes are present in markedly increased numbers. Platelets are usually normal or increased in numbers, and bleeding is uncommon despite platelet dysfunction in most patients.

  3. The clinical course of CML is unique among all the leukemias. Following a median 3 to 4 years of stable disease, virtually all patients enter a phase of accelerated leukemia activity. This phase has been termed blast crisis, metamorphosis, or transformation. The clinical picture may resemble acute leukemia, or, alternatively, progressive bone marrow failure may ensue. Bone marrow transplantation for appropriately selected patients during the chronic stable phase of CML produces long-term disease-free survival in 50 to 65% of patients and may be curative. However, therapy for CML in the accelerated phase is ineffective, and median survival from onset of this stage is 6 to 8 months.

  4. Clinical features of CLL most commonly reflect organ involvement by leukemia cells. The Rai staging system (Table 45–1) is useful for assessing prognosis.

  5. Immunologic phenomena. CLL is unique in its association with a variety of immunologic phenomena. These include hypogammaglobulinemia (50% of cases), autoimmune hemolytic anemia (10 to 25%), and immune thrombocytopenia.

LABORATORY TESTS

- CBC, platelet count, and examination of peripheral blood smear

TABLE 45-1. Rai Staging System

Stage 0: Peripheral blood (>15,000/mm³) and bone marrow
lymphocytosis (>40%)
Median survival 12.5 yr
20% of patients

Stage I: Lymphocytosis plus lymphadenopathy
Median survival 6 to 8 yr
25% of patients

Stage II: Lymphocytosis plus lymphadenopathy plus
splenomegaly or hepatomegaly
Median survival 4 to 5 yr
25% of patients

Stages III and IV: Lymphocytosis plus lymphadenopathy
plus splenomegaly but with (stage III) anemia
(hemoglobin <12 g%) or (stage IV) thrombocytopenia
(platelets <100,000/m³)
Median survival 1.5 yr
30% of patients

- Bone marrow aspiration and biopsy. Cytogenetic analysis should be included. Cultures should be performed when infection is considered possible.
- Cytochemical tests on blood or bone marrow smears. These include:
  1. Peroxidase: AML
  2. Sudan black B: AML
  3. Specific and nonspecific esterases: AML
  4. Periodic acid—Schiff: ALL
  5. TDT: ALL
  6. Leukocyte alkaline phosphatase: CML
- Surface markers and other specialized tests
  1. Lymphocyte markers: CALLA and T- and B-cell markers
  2. Myeloid differentiation antigens
  3. Lysozyme is positive in monocytic types of AML
  4. DNA restriction enzyme analyses to detect immunoglobulin or T-cell receptor gene rearrangements. These rearrangements can be indicative of B- or T-lymphocyte lineage.
- Blood chemistry and miscellaneous laboratory tests
  1. Metabolic derangements. Possible associations with leukemia include hyperuricemia, hyper- and hypokalemia, hyper- and hypocalcemia, and hypophosphatemia.
  2. Coagulation screen for DIC. PT, PTT, TT, fibrinogen, and fibrinogen-fibrin degradation products should be measured.
  3. CLL
     a. Serum protein electrophoresis may find hypogammaglobulinemia. There is a monoclonal spike in 15% of cases.

b. Coombs' test and reticulocyte count are used to evaluate autoimmune hemolytic anemia.
4. Lumbar puncture in ALL. This is used to evaluate meningeal leukemia.

RECOMMENDED DIAGNOSTIC APPROACH

As a general rule, the critical diagnostic decisions are first to diagnose acute leukemia and second to differentiate ALL from AML. Therapy must be instituted promptly.

* Morphology. Careful morphologic assessment of peripheral blood smears and bone marrow preparations establishes a diagnosis of acute leukemia in virtually all cases, but the differentiation between ALL and AML may be more difficult.
* Morphologically undifferentiated acute leukemia. Twenty-five percent of acute leukemia cases are morphologically undifferentiated. Tests to distinguish between ALL and AML include:
  1. Cytochemistry including TDT determination. Ninety percent of ALL but only 10% of AML are positive for TDT. Most undifferentiated acute leukemias are resolved by cytochemical tests.
  2. Serum or urine lysozyme. This is positive in monocytic variants of AML.
  3. Analyses for expression of lymphoid or myeloid differentiation antigens
  4. DNA restriction endonuclease analyses
* Diagnosis of chronic leukemias should be made promptly but does not have the same urgency as diagnosis of acute leukemias. The differentiation of CLL from other lymphoid leukemias is beyond the scope of this manual. CML is differentiated from leukemoid reactions as discussed earlier. The presence of the Philadelphia chromosome or the *bcr-abl* fusion gene is diagnostic of CML.

Bibliography

Bennett JM, et al. Criteria for the diagnosis of acute leukemia of megakaryocyte lineage (M7): A report of the French-American-British Cooperative Group. Ann Intern Med 1985;103:460–462.

Champlin R, Gale RP. Acute lymphoblastic leukemia: recent advances in biology and therapy. Blood 1989;73:2051–2066.

Cheson BD, et al. Guidelines for clinical protocols for CLL: Recommendations of the NCI-sponsored working group. Am J Hematol 1988;29:152–163.

Clift RA, et al. The treatment of acute nonlymphoblastic leukemia by allogeneic marrow transplantation. Bone Marrow Transplant 1987;2:243–258.

Freeman AS, Nadler LM. Cell surface markers in hematologic malignancies. Semin Oncol 1987;14:193–212.

Gale RP, Foon KA. Acute myeloid leukemia: Recent advances in therapy. Clinics Haematol 1986;15:781–810.

Gehan EA, et al. Prognostic factors in acute leukemia. Sem Oncol 1976;3:271–282.

Koeffler HP. Syndromes of acute nonlymphocytic leukemia. Ann Intern Med 1987;107:748–758.

Korsmeyer SJ. Antigen receptor genes as molecular markers of lymphoid neoplasms. J Clin Invest 1987;79:1291–1295.

Kurzrock R, et al. The molecular genetics of Philadelphia chromosome-positive leukemias. N Engl J Med 1988;319:990–998.

Rai KR, et al. Clinical staging of chronic lymphocytic leukemia. Blood 1975;46:219–234.

Shaw MT. The cytochemistry of acute leukemia: A diagnostic and prognostic evaluation. Sem Oncol 1976;3:219–228.

Sweet DL Jr., et al. The clinical features of chronic lymphocytic leukemia. Clin Haematol 1977;6:185–202.

46

LYMPHOMAS

DAVID BOLDT

Diagnosis precedes treatment.

RUSSELL JOHN HOWARD (1875–1942)

DEFINITION

- General. Lymphomas are malignant disorders characterized by uncontrolled proliferation of lymphocytes, lymphocyte precursors, or certain other cell types normally
  involved in immune reactions. There are two large groups
  of lymphomas: Hodgkin's disease (HD) and non-
  Hodgkin's lymphoma (NHL).

- Diagnostic Criteria. Precise classification of lymphomas
  requires microscopic examination of an intact lymph node.
  Thus, excisional biopsy is generally the best approach.
  Because reactive hyperplasia is often present in inguinal
  and femoral lymph nodes, biopsy of these nodes should be
  avoided.

  1. Diagnosis of HD requires demonstration of Reed-
     Sternberg cells in the appropriate cellular milieu.
  2. Diagnosis of NHL is made when lymph nodes show
     replacement of normal architecture by relatively uni-
     form populations of lymphoid cells. Reed-Sternberg
     cells are not present.

- Classification. Both HD and NHL are divided into subtypes based on histopathologic features. These subtypes
  have both prognostic and therapeutic implications.

  1. Four subclasses of HD are recognized. They are:
     a. Lymphocyte predominance (10 to 15% of cases),
        with the most favorable prognosis
     b. Nodular sclerosis (30 to 40%), with an interme-
        diate prognosis
     c. Mixed cellularity (30%), with an intermediate
        prognosis
     d. Lymphocyte depletion (5 to 15%), with the least
        favorable prognosis
  2. Classification of NHL is in a state of flux. Two classi-
     fications that are widely used are the Rappaport Classi-
     fication and the NCI Working Group Classification
     (Table 46–1). Both classifications facilitate identifica-
     tion of favorable and unfavorable histologic subtypes.
     a. Favorable histologic NHL subtypes (low grade)
        are characterized by indolent disease courses (me-
        dian survival 7 to 8 years) and high rates of respon-

TABLE 46–1. Classification of the Non-Hodgkin's Lymphomas

NCI WORKING FORMULATION	RAPPAPORT CLASSIFICATION
Low grade	
Small lymphocytic	Diffuse lymphocytic, well differentiated
Follicular, small cleaved cell	Nodular lymphocytic, poorly differentiated
Follicular, mixed small cleaved and large cell	Nodular, mixed lymphocytic-histiocytic
Intermediate grade	
Follicular, large cell	Nodular histiocytic
Diffuse, small cleaved cell	Diffuse lymphocytic, poorly differentiated
Diffuse, mixed small cleaved and large cell	Diffuse mixed lymphocytic-histiocytic
Diffuse, large cell (cleaved and noncleaved)	Diffuse histiocytic
High grade	
Large cell immunoblastic	Diffuse histiocytic
Lymphoblastic (convoluted and nonconvoluted)	
Small noncleaved cell (Burkitt and non-Burkitt)	Diffuse undifferentiated

Source: Portlock CS. Introduction to neoplasms of the immune system. In: Wyngaarden JB and Smith LH, eds. Cecil Textbook of Medicine, 18th ed. Philadelphia, W.B. Saunders, 1988, pp. 1007–1009.

siveness to therapy (80 to 85%). Paradoxically, although a favorable subtype NHL may be controlled by therapy for prolonged periods of time, it is seldom, if ever, cured.

b. Unfavorable histologic NHL subtypes (intermediate and high grades) pursue aggressive disease courses (median survival of untreated patients less than 1 year), but approximately 50% of cases may be curable if they are treated vigorously with appropriate chemotherapy.

3. Seventy-five percent of NHLs are of B-lymphocyte origin. The cutaneous lymphoma mycosis fungoides and Sézary syndrome usually originate from T-lymphocytes. Fewer than 1% of all lymphomas are derived from macrophages. The term "histiocytic lymphoma" is a misnomer, since the malignant cells in this disorder are activated lymphocytes or immunoblasts.

EPIDEMIOLOGY

- Demographic features
  1. HD accounts for 1% of human malignancies. It displays a unique biomodal age-specific incidence curve. One peak occurs between ages 15 and 35 years and a second after age 50. Overall, the incidence is higher in males, but in the 15- to 35-year age range it is identical in both sexes. Favorable histologic subtypes are more prevalent in young patients.
  2. NHL makes up 2 to 3% of human malignancies. It may occur at any age, but incidence peaks between ages 40 and 60. There is no sex predilection.

- Etiologic considerations
  1. Viruses. Viruses are strongly implicated as causes of at least two human lymphomas: Epstein-Barr (EB) virus in Burkitt's lymphoma and human T-cell leukemia virus (HTLV) in adult T-cell leukemia-lymphoma.
  2. Disorders of immunoregulation. Both inherited (severe combined immunodeficiency disease, Wiskott-Aldrich syndrome, ataxia-telangiectasia, and others) and acquired (drug-induced immunosuppression as in renal transplant recipients; AIDS) immunodeficiency syndromes are associated with increased incidences of malignant lymphomas. Risks range from 40 to 100 times those expected in renal transplant recipients to 10,000 times those expected in some patients with hereditary immunodeficiency. Five percent of AIDS patients develop lymphomas. Certain autoimmune diseases are associated with increased incidences of lymphomas.
  3. Hereditary factors. A 3- to 7-fold increase of HD has been noted in siblings and close relatives of affected patients. An association exists between HD and human leukocyte antigen (HLA) types A1, B1, B6, and B15.

CLINICAL MANIFESTATIONS

- Lymphadenopathy. The majority of patients with lymphomas first seek medical attention because of lymphadenopathy (90% of HD, 67% of NHL). In HD, adenopathy is most likely to be localized and central in location (mediastinal adenopathy in up to 60%). In NHL, it is most likely to occur at multiple sites and to be peripheral in location (epitrochlear, popliteal, or mesenteric nodes; Peyer's patches; and Waldeyer's ring). In both HD and NHL, cervical adenopathy is the most common site of nodal involvement (60 to 70%)

- Constitutional symptoms. These are prominent features of both HD and NHL. Fever, sweats, and weight loss are present in 20 to 25% of patients at diagnosis. In a minority of this group constitutional symptoms may occur in the absence of detectable lymphadenopathy. HD may also occur with pruritus (10 to 15% of cases) or with a peculiar alcohol pain syndrome in which pain occurs in involved lymph nodes shortly after alcohol ingestion.

- Extranodal disease. Less than 1% of HD patients have extranodal primary sites, and only 10% have disease widely disseminated to visceral sites (most commonly liver, bone marrow, lung, and pleura). By contrast, 25% of NHL occurs with extranodal primary sites and 50 to 60% of patients have disease disseminated to viscera. The liver (20 to 50% of patients) and bone marrow (30 to 50%) are the most common sites of involvement and are involved most frequently in favorable histologic subtypes. GI involvement is present initially in 15% of NHL and is important to document because of its association with GI bleeding and perforation. CNS involvement is uncommon at examination but should be carefully excluded in patients with unfavorable subtypes of NHL as it ultimately develops in 15–20% of these individuals.

DIFFERENTIAL DIAGNOSIS (see also Chapter 44)

- Differential diagnosis of lymphadenopathy
  1. Infections can be bacterial, mycobacterial, fungal, viral, or parasitic.
  2. Immunologic diseases include collagen vascular diseases, sarcoidosis, serum sickness, and drug reactions.
  3. Malignancies include lymphomas and metastatic cancer.
  4. Miscellaneous or of unknown cause. Angioimmunoblastic lymphadenopathy, dermatopathic lymphadenopathy, and persistent generalized lymphadenopathy associated with HIV infection should be considered in the differential diagnosis.
- Diagnostic considerations
  1. The likelihood of a malignant cause of lymphadenopathy increases with age. Diagnostic lymph node biopsy specimens are malignant in 20% of patients younger than 30 years and in 60% of those older than 50. Among young patients, malignant nodes are 2 to 3 times more likely to be lymphoma than carcinoma. In older patients the statistics are exactly reversed.
  2. The likelihood that biopsy will reveal a malignancy is two-thirds for supraclavicular nodes and one-third for cervical, axillary, or inguinal nodes.
  3. The consistency of lymph nodes on palpation may be helpful in differential diagnosis. Nodes containing lymphoma are "rubbery," whereas those involved by carcinoma are rock-hard. Tender warm erythematous nodes associated with fluctuance or lymphangitic streaking are characteristic of regional infections.
  4. The presence of nodal tenderness alone or fluctuation in size of lymph nodes over weeks to months is not a reliable sign by which to assess whether lymphadenopathy is benign or malignant.

RECOMMENDED DIAGNOSTIC APPROACH

- Regional lymphadenopathy
  1. Chest X-ray. If hilar or mediastinal adenopathy is present, lymph node biopsy is indicated.
  2. Supraclavicular area. Biopsy should be done.
  3. Cervical area
     a. Evaluation and treatment should be done for local infections of the oropharynx, ear, and face. Evaluation for infectious mononucleosis syndromes (EB virus, toxoplasmosis, or cytomegalovirus) should be performed as discussed in Chapter 77.
     b. If results of these are negative and nodes persist for 2 weeks, or if the patient's condition is deteriorating, lymph node biopsy is indicated. A careful otolaryngologic examination should precede the biopsy.
  4. Axillary area
     a. Evaluation should be done for local trauma or infections of hands and arms.
     b. Breast examination is performed in women.
     c. If the above measures are negative and nodes persist for 2 weeks, or if the patient's condition is deteriorating, proceed to lymph node biopsy.
  5. Inguinal area
     a. Evaluation is done for local trauma or infections of feet and legs. The perineal area is examined for lesions of herpes simplex type 2, lymphogranuloma venereum, syphilis, and other infections (see Chapter 69).
     b. If these measures are negative and nodes persist for 2 weeks, of if the patient's condition is deteriorating, proceed to lymph node biopsy.
- Generalized lymphadenopathy (see Chapter 44)
- Principles of lymph node biopsy. Careful planning of lymph node biopsy, including the advice of the pathologist, is critical. Considerations for optimal processing of node biopsies are as follows:
  1. Excisional biopsy of an intact lymph node including the capsule is optimal.
  2. The node is bisected and smears and cultures for bacteria, mycobacteria, and fungi are obtained.
  3. Lymph node imprints are prepared.
  4. Frozen section determines the need for further specimens or special studies.
     a. If frozen section shows carcinoma in a male, the specimen is placed in formalin for routine permanent sections. In a female, part of the fresh node should be processed for steroid receptor studies if breast carcinoma is a possibility.
     b. If undifferentiated malignancy is evident on frozen section, part of the specimen should be placed in glutaraldehyde for electron microscopy, and part should be processed for lymphocyte marker studies.

    c. If frozen section shows reactive hyperplasia or is nondiagnostic but malignancy is strongly suspected, a second node biopsy should be done. Up to 25% of patients with lymphoma require multiple biopsies to establish a diagnosis.

5. The remaining specimen is placed in fixative for routine permanent sections.

6. The average yield for lymph node biopsies in establishing diagnosis is 60%. Follow-up studies of patients with nondiagnostic lymph node biopsies reveal that half will develop either a malignancy or a collagen vascular disease within the ensuing decade.

- Staging evaluation in lymphomas. Staging evaluation should be undertaken to determine the extent of disease involvement. Stage of disease for either HD or NHL may be assessed by means of the Ann Arbor staging classification (Table 46–2).

1. In HD, prognosis relates directly to Ann Arbor stage, and precise staging is critical for designing optimal therapy. Staging evaluation may require a variety of clinical, laboratory, X-ray, and surgical procedures designed to provide maximal information about disease extent. Decisions about staging procedures are individualized and are based on the extent to which results will influence management of each patient.

2. In NHL prognosis does not relate so clearly to Ann Arbor stage, and treatment options are usually based on histologic subtype (favorable vs. unfavorable) rather than anatomic extent of disease. Therefore, in NHL staging evaluation is less aggressive than in HD and is used primarily to document response to therapy or disease progression.

TABLE 46–2. Ann Arbor Staging Classification

STAGE	EXTENT OF DISEASE
I	Single lymph node region or single extralymphatic site (IE)
II	Two or more lymph node regions on same side of diaphragm (II) or single extralymphatic site plus one or more lymph node regions on same side of diaphragm (IIE)
III	Lymph node regions on both sides of diaphragm alone (III) or plus single extralymphatic site (IIIE), the spleen (IIIS), or both (IIISE)
IV	Diffuse or disseminated involvement of extralymphatic organs
A category	No symptoms; denotes favorable prognosis
B category	Unexplained weight loss > 10% of body weight; unexplained fever > 38°C; night sweats; denotes unfavorable prognosis

Bibliography

Boldt DH. Lymphadenopathy and splenomegaly. In: Stein JH, ed. Internal Medicine, 3rd ed. Boston, Little, Brown & Company, 1990, pp. 1023–1030.

Fauci AS, et al. Acquired immunodeficiency syndrome: Epidemiologic, clinical, immunologic, and therapeutic considerations. Ann Int Med 1984;100:92–106.

Greenfield S, Jordan MC. The clinical investigation of lymphadenopathy in primary care practice. JAMA 1978;240:1388–1393.

Kaplan HS. Hodgkin's Disease, 2nd ed. Cambridge, MA, Harvard University Press, 1980.

Lee YT, et al. Biopsy of peripheral lymph nodes. Am J Surg 1982;48:536–539.

Lester EP, Ultmann JE. Non-Hodgkin's lymphoma. In: Williams WJ, et al., eds. Hematology, 3rd ed. New York, McGraw-Hill, 1983, pp. 1035–1056.

Non-Hodgkin's lymphoma pathologic classification project. National Cancer Institute–sponsored study of classifications of non-Hodgkin's lymphomas: Summary and description of a working formulation for clinical usage. Cancer 1982;49:2112.

47

MULTIPLE MYELOMA

JULIA PHISTER

Thy bones are marrowless.

SHAKESPEARE (1564–1616) Macbeth III, iv, 94

DEFINITIONS

- Multiple myeloma (MM) is a malignancy of plasma cells. Most patients are older than 40 years, and 99% secrete electrophoretically detectable amounts of a single immunoglobulin or light chain (M-spike) into the serum or urine. Myeloma's manifestations are caused by plasma cell infiltrates in the bone or bone marrow, or other organs.
- Waldenström's macroglobulinemia (WM) is a malignancy of IgM-producing lymphocytes with plasmacytoid features that behaves more like a lymphoma than myeloma. It presents with nonspecific weakness and symptoms attributable to hyperviscosity (headaches, visual or auditory symptoms, congestive heart failure, or a bleeding diathesis) rather than bony pain.
- Monoclonal gammopathy of unknown significance (MGUS), formerly called benign monoclonal gammopathy, is a fortuitously detected M-spike that is not associated with symptoms or signs or other laboratory or X-ray manifestations. It is frequently found in the elderly (2% of 50- to 79-year-olds, 16% of 80- to 90-year-olds). Over 10 years, only 20% progress to a more malignant disease (80% MM, 10% WM, and 10% amyloidosis).

DIFFERENTIAL DIAGNOSIS

- The symptomatic presentations of MM are protean, but it must be considered in an elderly patient with new back or axial skeletal pain, lytic bone lesions, anemia, unexplained renal insufficiency, or frequent infections.
- Lytic bone lesions in the elderly most often result from metastatic carcinoma. Such lesions are rarely purely lytic and are uniformly associated with a positive bone scan and usually an elevated alkaline phosphatase.
- Solitary plasmacytoma may cause a lytic bone lesion with normal urine and serum electrophoreses.
- The differential diagnosis of a monoclonal gammopathy includes
  1. Chronic inflammatory processes

2. Non–B-cell malignancies
3. Autoimmune diseases such as cold agglutinin disease and Sjögren's syndrome
4. Lymphoproliferative diseases such as WM, chronic lymphocytic leukemia, and non-Hodgkin's lymphoma. These secondary gammopathies are usually due to IgM.
5. MGUS, which is a diagnosis of exclusion based on clinical, laboratory, and radiographic criteria

CLINICAL FEATURES (Table 47–1)

- Symptoms
  1. Weakness and fatigue occurs in most patients and may be associated with anemia, renal failure, hypercalcemia, hyperviscosity, or renal failure.
  2. Bone pain (especially back and rib) occurs in 70%.
  3. Infections are present in 25% of patients at diagnosis and are the leading cause of death. Herpes zoster, pneumococcus, and Hemophilus are common early pathogens.
  4. Neurologic symptoms at disgnosis include:
     a. Obtundation due to hypercalcemia
     b. Myelopathy or cranial neuropathy due to plasmacytoma
     c. Carpal tunnel syndrome due to amyloidosis
     d. Sensorimotor neuropathy due to light chain deposition
  5. Bleeding can be due to quantitative or qualitative platelet defects, specific anticoagulants, or vascular purpura from amyloidosis or cryoglobulins.
  6. Congestive heart failure can result from severe anemia, an elevated plasma volume from the paraproteinemia, and occasionally from hyperviscosity or an amyloid-associated restrictive cardiomyopathy.
  7. GI manifestations include oral symptoms from bony involvement of the jaw and maxilla, nausea or constipation with hypercalcemia, or malabsorption because of amyloidosis.
- Signs
  1. Fever is almost always associated with infection.
  2. Orthostasis may be due to hypercalcemia-related dehydration, sepsis, or amyloid-related neuropathy.
  3. Ocular findings may include hemorrhages and exudates from severe anemia or hyperviscous sludging in the retinal vessels.
  4. Oral findings include macroglossia associated with amyloidosis. Local plasmacytoma may cause bony masses or loose teeth.
  5. Hepatosplenomegaly and lymphadenopathy can be seen in patients with IgD MM, WM, and amyloidosis.
  6. Palpable plasmacytomas or areas of focal tenderness are common over the vertebrae, rib cage, and proximal long bones.

TABLE 47–1. Clinical Features of Selected Monoclonal Gammopathies

CLINICAL FEATURE	MGUS	MM	WM
Prevalence	1% at age 60 3% at age 75	3–4 per 100,000	0.5 per 100,000
Mean age at diagnosis		60–65	60–65
Symptoms at diagnosis	—	+	+
Symptoms progress with time	—	+	+
Lymphadenopathy	—	rare	40%
Hepatosplenomegaly	—	rare	25%
Hyperviscosity	—	2–5%	40%
Anemia	variable	60%	70–90%
Neutropenia or thrombocytopenia	—	15%	10%
Lytic lesions	—	60%	very rare

	5–10% plasma cells (normal)	>15% plasma cells (often abnormal)	20–30% have abnormal infiltrates of plasmacytoid cells
Bone marrow			
M-spike (prevalence/usual amount at diagnosis)			
IgG	65%/<2–3 g	52%/>2–3 g	—
IgA	25%/<1g	22%/>1 g	—
IgM	10%/<1–2 g	very rare	100%/>1–2 g
Prevalence of Bence-Jones proteinuria	Rare	50–70%	10%
Bence-Jones proteinuria only	Very rare	25%	—
Natural history	20% develop malignant lymphoproliferative disorder at 10 years	30-month mean survival	50-month mean survival

7. Dermatologic changes include amyloid papules and purpura. The purpura is nonpalpable when associated with thrombocytopenia, hyperviscosity, or amyloidosis, and palpable when associated with cryoglobulinemia.
8. Neurologic signs include metabolic encephalopathy, peripheral neuropathy, radiculopathy, and spinal cord compression.

LABORATORY STUDIES

- Common laboratory tests
    1. Hyponatremia with normal osmolarity may result from high serum protein concentrations.
    2. A low anion gap (<7) is common because the M-spike is negatively charged.
    3. Renal dysfunction occurs in 15 to 50% at diagnosis.
        a. Renal failure is the second leading cause of death but is often treatable.
        b. Most frequently, it is due to light chain deposition and cast formation with tubular damage. This damage is potentiated by hypercalcemia, dehydration, and nephrotoxins, especially radiographic contrast dye.
        c. Rarely, patients present with nephrotic syndrome, which almost always represents secondary amyloidosis causing glomerular rather than tubular disease.
    4. Hypercalcemia (above 11 mg/dl) is present in 30% of patients at diagnosis.
    5. The total serum protein is elevated in 75% of patients with MM when compared with previous levels. The rest are nonsecretors or secrete only light chains, which do not elevate the serum protein significantly.
    6. Anemia is present in 60% at diagnosis, and results from decreased production and crowd-out. It is frequently less severe than it appears because of paraprotein-associated hypervolemia and hemodilution.
    7. Mild neutropenia and thrombocytopenia are found in 15% of patients at diagnosis.
    8. Occasional plasma cells are found peripherally in 15% of patients. Plasma cell leukemia, with more than 1000 plasma cells/mm^3, is unusual and carries a dismal prognosis.
    9. The erythrocyte sedimentation rate is high in almost all patients.
    10. Serum hyperviscosity is likely in patients with >4 g/dl of IgG or IgA paraproteins or >3 g/dl of IgM paraprotein.
    11. Urinalysis may indicate infection or nephrotic syndrome. The standard dipstick frequently misses the light chains. Bence Jones protein may be detected by

a sulfasalicylic acid screen or urine protein electrophoresis.

- Markers of immunoproliferative disease
  1. Serum protein electrophoresis (SPEP) can detect a paraprotein with a concentration as low as 0.2 g. It is positive in 75% of MM patients and all WM patients.
  2. Urine protein electrophoresis (UPEP) detects light chain proteinuria and albuminuria associated with amyloidosis and other glomerular diseases. It is positive in 65% of MM patients and a small number of those with WM.
  3. Serum and urine immunoelectrophoreses detect the miniscule amounts of protein seen in amyloidosis or "nonsecretory" myelomas. Thus, immunoelectrophoreses are useful when the SPEP and UPEP are negative but there is high clinical suspicion of disease. They also help rule out spurious "pseudo-M-proteins" and identify the subtype of immunoglobulin or light chain. Of the paraproteins:
     a. 50 to 55% are IgG, which are associated with a higher incidence of hypogammaglobulinemia and infection.
     b. 20 to 25% are IgA, which are more likely to be associated with aggressive bony disease, severe hypercalcemia, light chain proteinuria and renal failure, amyloidosis, and hyperviscosity.
     c. 10 to 20% are IgD. Almost all of these have lambda light chains resulting in frequent nephropathy.
     d. Less than 1% are IgE, which is often associated with plasma cell leukemia.
     e. 15 to 25% are light chain only; those with lambda chain disease have frequent nephropathy.

- Features that confirm a malignant gammopathy
  1. Quantitative measurement of immunoglobulin levels detects "immunoparesis" by quantifying the "non-M-spike" gamma globulins. They are low in 80% of MM and 10 to 20% of WM patients.
  2. A skeletal survey (axial skeleton including the skull; ribs, clavicles, and proximal humeri on chest X-ray; and spine and pelvis including proximal femurs) is positive in 80 to 90% of patients.
     a. Of all MM patients, 60 to 70% have lytic lesion, 1 to 2% sclerotic ones, and 5 to 15% have osteopenia only.
     b. In symptomatic patients with nonspecific plain films, CT scans can help separate postmenopausal osteoporotic vertebral fractures from ones associated with MM.
     c. Bone scans are not helpful as they are frequently negative except at sites of secondary fracture.
  3. Bone marrow aspirate and biopsy may detect plasma cell proliferation and dedifferentiation. However, MM involves the marrow in a patchy fashion and biopsies may be negative.

RECOMMENDED DIAGNOSTIC APPROACH

- If the patient has only mild symptoms, with a normal CBC and chemical survey, MGUS or early stage myeloma is most likely. Many of these patients will have been discovered incidentally and the pace of the work-up need not be urgent. It should include SPEP or UPEP, quantitative immunoglobulins, skeletal survey, and, possibly, bone marrow examination.

- In a symptomatic patient, or one who is cytopenic, uremic, or hypercalcemic, the work-up should be done quickly, and treatment initiated promptly:
    1. Rule in myeloma with SPEP or UPEP.
    2. Screen for complications with a chemical survey, CBC, and bone X-rays.
    3. Finish the evaluation with the remainder of the skeletal survey, quantitative immunoglobulins, and bone marrow biopsy to establish stage and prognosis.

Bibliography

Berdmack PA, et al. The POEMS syndrome. Medicine 1980;59:311–320.

Casciato DA, Berenson JH. Immunoproliferative diseases. In: Casciato DA, Lowitz BB, eds. Manual of Clinical Oncology, 2nd ed. Boston, Little, Brown, and Company, 1988.

Cohen HJ. Multiple myeloma in the elderly. Clin Geriat Med 1985;1:827–855.

Cohen HJ. Monoclonal gammopathies and aging. Hosp Pract 1988;23:75–100.

Draedger H, Pruzonski W. Plasma cell neoplasm with peripheral polyneuropathy. Medicine 1980;59:301–310.

Farhargi M, ed. Plasma cell myeloma and the myeloma proteins. Semin Oncol 1986;13(3):259–382.

Kyle R. "Benign gammopathy"—a misnomer? JAMA 1984;251:1849–1854.

Wiernik P, Kyle R, eds. Neoplastic Diseases of the Blood. New York, Churchill Livingstone, 1985.

SECTION VII

ONCOLOGY

48

SPINAL CORD COMPRESSION

CAROLYN COLLINS

The spine is a series of bones running down your back.
You sit on one end and your head sits on the other.

ANONYMOUS

DEFINITION/EPIDEMIOLOGY

- Back pain that develops in a cancer patient should be regarded as a potentially urgent problem.
- Five percent of all patients with disseminated malignancies (Table 48–1) develop an epidural metastasis at some point in their disease. The key to prevention of neurologic compromise is early recognition and institution of treatment prior to the development of neurologic deficits.
- Cord injury occurs when metastases to the vertebral body or pedicle enlarge and compress the underlying cord (Table 48–2) rather than invade the dura.
- It is unusual for epidural disease to develop in the absence of metastases to the vertebral body. This usually develops in patients with lymphoma or myeloma when tumor in the paravertebral space extends through the intravertebral foramen to produce epidural compression.

DIFFERENTIAL DIAGNOSIS (Table 48–3)

While less frequent, metastatic lesions producing intramedullary cord lesions, leptomeningeal lesions or plexopathies must be distinguished from epidural metastases as the approach to treatment is quite different.

CLINICAL FEATURES

- History
  1. The clinical presentation of cord compression is similar regardless of the histology of the malignancy and can be divided into prodromal and compressive phases.
  2. The prodromal phase, characterized by central back pain, occurs in more than 95% of patients.
     a. Epidural lesions typically produce pain, which is gradual in onset and insidiously progressive.

TABLE 48–1. Causes of Spinal Cord Compression by Site of Primary Tumor

Lung carcinoma	16%
Breast carcinoma	12%
Unknown primary	11%
Lymphoma	11%
Myeloma	9%
Sarcoma	8%
Prostate carcinoma	7%
Renal cell carcinoma	6%
Gastrointestinal carcinoma	4%
Miscellaneous	16%

TABLE 48–2. Site of Epidural Metastases

Thoracic spine	59%
Lumbar spine	16%
Cervical spine	15%
Sacral spine	10%

TABLE 48–3. Causes of Low Back Pain

Herniated lumbar disc

Trauma: low back sprain and strain, fracture of spine, pelvis, femur, sciatic, or femoral nerve injury

Tumor: epidural, intramedullary, leptomeningeal, lumbar or sacral plexopathy, spinal metastases, retroperitoneal, pelvic

Infection: herpes zoster, tuberculosis, Guillain-Barré syndrome, discitis, lumbar plexitis, bursitis

Vascular: arterial segmental occlusion, thrombophlebitis

Degenerative: vertebral spondylosis, osteoarthritis, spinal stenosis, hip joint disease

Metabolic: gout, diabetes, osteoporosis

Psychogenic: conversion hysteria, malingering

Miscellaneous: Paget's disease, sciatic nerve entrapment neuropathy

Lhermitte's sign, an electriclike sensation shooting down the back, may occur from an epidural lesion in the cervical spine.

   b. Three types of pain may be present, all of which may be worse at night (increased by recumbency), increased by sudden movements of extreme flexion, extension, rotation of the spine, or Valsalva's maneuver.

      i. Focal bony pain is continuous, aching, and progressive.

      ii. Radicular pain may be lacinating and intermittent. This pain can be mistaken for other disorders such as pleurisy, cholecystitis, pancreatitis, or cardiac ischemia.

      iii. Referred pain is experienced in a site distant from the lesions, but without a radicular component, such as paraspinous discomfort, pain at the midscapular level from cervical disease or pain in the posterior iliac crests from disease at T12 or L1.

3. The compressive phase may produce symptoms suggesting early compromise of neurologic function.

   a. Leg heaviness or clumsiness of gait suggests early motor dysfunction.

   b. Paresthesias may begin in the feet and progress upward as early sensory symptoms.

   c. Constipation and a combination of urinary urgency, frequency, or hesitancy suggest autonomic dysfunction.

   d. Occasionally, impotence may be an early symptom in males.

- Physical Examination
  1. The compressive phase produces a variety of signs on physical examination.

   a. Early in the course, pain can be elicited by percussion over the spine.

   b. The corticospinal tracts, posterior columns, and spinal cerebellar tracts, which are superficially and dorsally located, are the most sensitive to compression by the epidural mass. The neurologic deficit is determined by the level of the involved spinal cord.

  2. Cervical and thoracic cord

   a. Weakness, in a long tract distribution, occurs, causing quadriplegia and paraplegia, respectively, if allowed to progress.

   b. Spasticity and hyperactive reflexes are early signs of myelopathy. Babinski's signs are often present.

   c. Proprioception and vibratory sense may be impaired in the feet.

   d. If affected, the gait may be stiff-legged or ataxic.

   e. A palpable bladder or large postvoid residual may be present. Urinary incontinence is a late sign.

  3. T12 or L1

   a. These lesions may present with sphincter dysfunction as they predominantly affect the conus medullaris.

   b. Sensory loss in the perineum may occur, and there may be absence of an anal wink or bulbocavernosus or cremasteric reflexes.

4. L1 and below
   a. These lesions may affect one or more spinal roots.
   b. A cauda equina syndrome from canal compromise may present with involvement of multiple, and usually bilateral, spinal roots. Motor and sensory loss is often asymmetric. Tone may be reduced or unchanged.
   c. Reflexes are also selectively affected and often diminished, while Babinski's signs are absent.

LABORATORY STUDIES

No laboratory studies help identify spinal cord compression.

RADIOLOGIC IMAGING

- Spinal radiographs
  1. If these are normal at a symptomatic site as defined by focal pain or neurologic dysfunction, there is a 10% chance of epidural disease.
  2. However, epidural disease will be identified in 86% of patients with abnormal radiographs at a symptomatic site and in 43% of asymptomatic patients. The index of suspicion in a patient with vertebral collapse should be very high as 87% will have epidural disease.
  3. Other findings include a paraspinous soft tissue mass and erosion of the vertebral body or the pedicle.
- Radionuclide bone scans
  1. A total body bone scan is a more sensitive test than radiography. However, it is much less specific, and only 69% of patients with an abnormal bone scan at a symptomatic site have epidural disease at that level.
  2. A normal study provides useful evidence against epidural disease, but a positive study is not a good predictor of underlying potential cord compression.
- Myelography. Although long considered to be the preferred procedure to evaluate the spinal canal for epidural disease, it has been largely replaced by magnetic resonance imaging (MRI).
- CT
  1. This provides detailed anatomic definition of vertebral and paravertebral lesions and is more specific than bone scans or plain radiographs in delineating metastatic disease.
  2. Eighty percent of patients with cortical disruption surrounding the epidural space demonstrated on CT scan have tumor extension into the epidural space, as determined by CT myelography.

- MRI
  1. This allows identification of paravertebral tumor extension, additional osseous metastases, and visualization of spinal cord compression occurring between areas of myelographic blocks.
  2. In the detection of spinal cord compression, MRI has been shown, by comparison to surgery, clinical follow-up, and postmortem examinations, to have a specificity of 97%, sensitivity of 93%, and an overall accuracy of 95%.

RECOMMENDED DIAGNOSTIC APPROACH

- The presence of any signs or symptoms other than pain indicates the presence of neural damage. Neurologic deterioration is often quite rapid once signs and symptoms other than pain appear. The best predictor of the outcome of therapy is the pretreatment functional status. Once a neurologic deficit has developed, it is much more likely that treatment will result in stabilization of the symptoms rather than significant improvement.
- An important consideration is the urgency of evaluation in a cancer patient with back pain.
  1. Emergent. Any patient whose history suggests increasing neurologic deficits, or who presents with pain and signs or symptoms of new or progressive spinal cord compression.
  2. Prompt. Patients with back pain with minimal and stable signs of spinal cord compression should be evaluated within the next 24 hours, in the hospital if necessary.
  3. Outpatient evaluation. Patients with back pain only, without evidence of neurologic damage.
- Patients with back pain only without symptoms or signs or neurologic compromise should first have plain radiographs. If these are abnormal, particularly if there is a compression fracture or involvement of a pedicle, then an MRI should be obtained. If radiographs are normal, a radionuclide bone scan would be reasonable to rule out early metastatic bone involvement.
- Patients with back pain with symptoms or signs of neurologic compromise should proceed directly to an MR scan.

Bibliography

Bruckman JE, Bloomer WD. Management of spinal cord compression. Semin Oncol 1978;5:135–140.

Goodkin R, et al. Herniated lumbar disc disease in patients with malignancy. J Clin Oncol 1987;5:667–671.

King CL, Poon PY. Sensitivity and specificity of MRI in detecting malignant spinal cord compression and in distinguishing malignant from benign compression fractures of vertebrae. Magnet Res Imaging 1988;6:547–556.

Portenoy RS, et al. Identification of epidural neoplasm: Radiography and bone scintigraphy in the symptomatic and asymptomatic spine. Cancer 1989;64:2207–2214.

Smoker WR, et al. The role of MR imaging in evaluating metastatic spinal disease. Am J Radiol 1987;149:1241–1248.

Weissman DE, et al. The use of computed tomography of the spine to identify patients at high risk for epidural metastases. J Clin Oncol 1985;3:1541–1543.

Wilson JK, Masaryk TJ. Neurologic emergencies in the cancer patient. Semin Oncol 1989;16:490–503.

49

BREAST NODULES AND CANCER

SUSAN STOVER-DALTON

Deep in her breast lives the silent wound.
VIRGIL, Aeneid IV, 23

DEFINITION

- The breast is comprised of ductal and lobular parenchyma. Breast cancer in these sites may be noninvasive or invasive. The histologic types can be seen in pure forms or combinations, which confounds classification.
- Noninvasive cancers, which account for 10% of cases, include ductal carcinoma in situ (DCIS or intraductal cancer) and lobular carcinoma in situ (LCIS).
  1. Almost half of patients with DCIS present with a palpable breast mass. The usual recurrence of subsequent breast cancer is within the same breast.
  2. LCIS occurs primarily in premenopausal women with a high tendency for multicentric (additional foci within one breast) or bilateral disease. The risk of subsequent invasive disease is increased 10-fold.
- Seventy percent of all breast cancers are infiltrating ductal. These patients can present with a breast mass, sometimes having a characteristic stony hardness to palpation.
- The other histologic variants account for approximately 20% of breast cancer.
  1. Papillary carcinoma is typically multicentric. Mucinous lesions occur primarily in older women with an excellent prognosis.
  2. Infiltrating lobular cancer can present clinically as a vague thickening of the breast and is a slowly growing, less aggressive tumor.
  3. Medullary carcinoma usually is a circumscribed lesion with only low-grade invasiveness, regardless of its size.
  4. Paget's disease of the breast causes nipple discharge or eczematoid skin changes of the nipple. Two-thirds of these patients have an underlying breast cancer.
  5. Inflammatory breast cancer presents with an edematous and erythematous breast and has a high propensity to metastasize.

EPIDEMIOLOGY

Breast cancer is the leading malignancy for American women with the 1989 incidence estimated at 142,000. Breast cancer deaths were 43,000 in 1989, second only to lung cancer. An American women has a 10% lifetime chance of developing breast cancer, with about half dying of the disease.

RISK FACTORS

- Previous breast cancer is associated with 3 times the average risk of a subsequent breast cancer.
- Endocrine. The duration of estrogen stimulation correlates with the incidence of breast cancer. Prolonged estrogen exposure results from early menarche or late menopause and reproduction after age 30 or nulliparity.
- Environment and diet:
  1. The incidence of breast cancer is higher in North America and northern Europe than in Asia. Women of Japanese descent who migrate to the United States have a higher risk than women in Japan.
  2. Women with moderate alcohol consumption (more than 9 drinks per week) have an increased risk of breast cancer.
- Genetic. Women with a family history of breast cancer have twice the normal risk. The risk may be even higher if cancer occurred premenopausally in first-degree relatives (mother, sister, or daughter).
- Age. The incidence of breast cancer increases with age.
- "Benign breast disease." The only subtype of benign breast disease with an increased risk of subsequent breast cancer is atypical hyperplasia. The risk of subsequent breast cancer is increased 4-fold for patients with a prior breast biopsy showing atypical hyperplasia.

DIFFERENTIAL DIAGNOSIS

- Physiologic cyclic hormonal stimulation of breast tissue causes a premenstrual increase in nodularity and size, with a decrease occurring after menstruation. This process occurs variably in different areas of the normal breast, causing further asymmetry. The vast majority of breast nodules result from functional hormonal effects on breast tissue.
  1. Cysts may be the result of physiologic estrogen influences. Other benign proliferation effects can cause fibroadenomas or intraductal papillomas.
  2. Cysts and fibroadenomas are usually smooth with well-defined margins. Fibroadenomas are mobile and are the most common solitary mass in teenagers and women in their twenties.
  3. The density of breast tissue is higher in young women due to more fibroglandular tissue. This has increased texture to palpation when compared to predominantly fatty tissue found in older women.

4. "Fibrocystic disease" includes these proliferative changes. It is perceived by some as a misnomer, since these changes occur as part of a normal continuum.
5. Other palpable abnormalities include abscesses resulting from ductal obstruction or localized hematomas due to trauma.

- The College of American Pathology uses a 3-part classification of benign breast disease:
  1. Nonproliferative
  2. Proliferative without atypia
  3. Atypical hyperplasia

  Only atypical hyperplasia has an increased risk of subsequent breast cancer.

CLINICAL FEATURES

History (see Table 49–1)

- Pain
  1. Cyclic breast pain and nodularity typically resolve after a few months.
  2. The majority of breast cancers are discovered by patients as a painless and hard lump. Breast cancers are only occasionally painful.
  3. Breast pain also commonly occurs due to musculoskeletal strain of the chest wall. Chest wall tenderness is distinguished from breast tenderness by pushing the breast aside and applying direct pressure on the chest wall behind or lateral to the breast.
- Nipple discharge
  1. Nipple discharge is a relatively common finding. Nipple discharge becomes increasingly significant with advancing age. It is rarely associated with cancer in young women.
  2. Bloody discharge results from an intraductal papilloma or an invasive cancer in about one-third of cases.

Examination

- The breast examination.
  1. The optimal time to examine the breast is 1 week postmenstrual.
  2. While the patient is supine, the entire breast is examined with concentric motions.
  3. Breast masses are described by the quadrant in which they are found, with half of breast cancers located in the upper outer quadrant.
  4. Approximately 75% of all breast neoplasms are benign and are usually soft with smooth borders and freely movable. However, some malignant tumors share these characteristics: 40% of cancers have regular borders on palpation and feel soft or cystic, and 60% are freely movable.
  5. Breast cancer is multicentric in up to 13%.

TABLE 49–1. Pertinent Medical History and Physical Examination for the Patient with Breast Cancer

A. History
  1. Breast and axillary symptoms
    a. Breast mass
    b. Breast pain
    c. Nipple discharge
    d. Nipple or skin retraction
    e. Axillary mass or pain
    f. Arm swelling
  2. Medical history of breast disease, including prior biopsies
  3. Reproductive history
    a. Age of menarche
    b. Frequency, duration, and regularity of menstrual periods
    c. Number of pregnancies, children, and abortions
    d. Age at first pregnancy
    e. Age at onset of menopause
    f. History of hormone use, including birth control pills
    g. Breast feeding
  4. Family history: age at diagnosis and death of family members with breast cancer
  5. Review of systems, with particular reference to possible metastatic spread
B. Physical examination
  1. Breast mass
    a. Size
    b. Location (specified by clock position and the distance from edge of the areola)
    c. Shape
    d. Consistency
    e. Fixation to skin, pectoral muscle, or chest wall
  2. Skin changes
    a. Erythema
    b. Edema (note location and extent)
    c. Dimpling
    d. Satellite nodules
  3. Nipple changes
    a. Retraction
    b. Discoloration
    c. Thickening
    d. Reddening
    e. Erosion
  4. Nodal status
    a. Axillary: number, location, size, fixation to other nodes or underlying structures, clinically suspicious or benign
    b. Infraclavicular fullness
    c. Supraclavicular nodes or area swelling

Source: Adapted with permission from Henderson IC, et al. Cancer of the breast. In: DeVita VT, Jr, et al., eds. Cancer: Principles and Practice of Oncology, 3rd ed. Philadelphia, J.B. Lippincott Co., 1989.

6. The nipple should be assessed for discharge, changes in the skin, and the presence of a mass.

• One-half of all patients with breast cancer have metastases, most commonly to the axillary lymph nodes.

LABORATORY STUDIES

• Mammography
  1. Mammography is a low-dose radiography of the breast. It is the only effective imaging modality for detecting asymptomatic or nonpalpable breast cancers and enables further characterization of palpable breast masses.
  2. Mammograms (MGs) are best for the detection of calcifications. Some tumors, such as DCIS, precipitate calcium, and thereby are visualized mammographically. Calcifications can also occur in many benign conditions and in otherwise normal breasts.
  3. MGs are performed prior to breast biopsy to ascertain size of the mass, presence of other masses, and to detect tumor invasion of adjacent skin and chest wall. For masses detected on MGs, a postbiopsy MG confirms removal of the mass.

• Mammographic screening
  1. The goal for breast cancer screening in asymptomatic women is a high sensitivity for early lesions and adequate specificity to avoid the financial and personal costs associated with the work-up of nonmalignant processes.
  2. In one study (see Eddy, 1989), the sensitivity and specificity of MGs were 70% and 99% respectively. Sensitivities are higher in women over 50 due to the greater ability of MGs to detect abnormalities in their predominantly fatty breast tissue.

• Ultrasound (US) is an imaging technique that can determine if a mass is purely cystic (versus mixed or solid) with a sensitivity greater than 90%.

• Fine-needle aspiration (FNA)
  1. For women with a palpable mass, FNA is an office procedure utilizing a 20- to 23-gauge needle.
  2. Fluid aspirated from a cyst is characteristically turbid and straw-colored and is routinely studied to rule out the rarely occurring intracystic cancer. Material from a solid lesion may be studied cytologically.
  3. A combination of mammography plus FNA has a high sensitivity for an early diagnosis of breast cancer, including lesions as small as 2 to 3 mm. For malignant breast cancers, FNA can expedite treatment planning.

• Biopsy
  1. Biopsy is the gold standard for establishing a diagnosis of breast cancer. It is typically a day surgery procedure performed utilizing local anesthesia. Only 10% of women with a positive clinical exam and MG have cancer.

2. Excisional biopsy is preferred with masses smaller than 2 cm, as it removes the entire tumor and allows for pathologic review of the complete specimen. Incisional biopsies are reserved for larger masses.

- Other. Thermography is based on the observation of an increased warmth of the skin overlying breast cancer with a resultant infrared radiation emission. However, clinical use of this modality and also of MRI, CT, and transillumination or diphonography is currently limited.

RECOMMENDED DIAGNOSTIC APPROACH (Figure 49–1)

- An individualized approach to a woman with a breast mass is warranted.
    1. Patients with cyclical nodularity in the absence of other risk factors are usually followed for a few months with subsequent reexamination, and resolution in the majority.
    2. A more expeditious work-up is mandated in the presence of risk factors or clinical features suggestive of malignancy.
- Patients with a mass with "cystic" characteristics (soft, spherical, and well-defined margins) should be referred for FNA for fluid or US to confirm the mass is a cyst.
    1. Patients with a cyst may be followed clinically for a few months. Reaccumulations of fluid may be reaspirated or referred for biopsy.
    2. Ultrasonographic demonstration of mixed or solid-appearing mass indicates proceeding with a FNA or biopsy.
    3. The patient should be referred for biopsy if the FNA result is bloody, nondiagnostic, without fluid, if a residual mass persists after the FNA, or if malignant cells are identified within the cysts.
- For palpable masses without cystic characteristics, patients should have an MG for further characterization, or proceed with FNA or biopsy.
    1. MG-detected abnormalities include densities with microcalcifications, especially if clustered, spiculations, blurred margins or clusters of microcalcifications without a density.
    2. For MGs with abnormal findings, the patient needs referral for FNA or biopsy.
    3. Biopsies or FNAs consistent with cancer necessitate immediate arrangements for staging and commencement of treatment.
    4. For a palpable mass with a negative MG, further evaluation with biopsy or FNA is mandated given the false-negative rate of MG, especially in younger women or those with dense breasts by MG.
- For clinically occult abnormalities detected by screening MG only, further characterization is warranted.

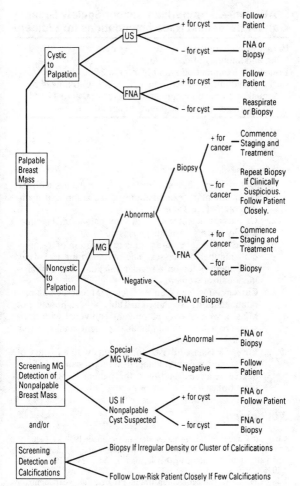

Figure 49–1. Recommended diagnostic approach to breast cancer.

1. For nonpalpable breast masses, the special mammographic views such as cone compression or magnification can be performed. Cone compression of a tumor, including either a fibroadenoma or cancer, does not change its shape, whereas breast parenchyma does alter its shape.
2. An US can be performed if a nonpalpable cyst is suspected.
3. An irregular density or clusters of calcifications should be biopsied as soon as possible. Localization of nonpalpable lesions for biopsy remains a challenge, but is facilitated by the use of guide wires.

TABLE 49–2. American Cancer Society Breast Cancer Screening Recommendations for Women

Breast examination every 1 to 3 years between age 20 and 40, and annually after age 40.

Breast self-examination monthly after age 20.

Baseline mammogram between age 35 and 40, followed by annual or biennial mammograms from ages 40 to 49 and annual mammograms beginning at age 50.

- Screening
  1. Optimal early breast cancer detection occurs with the complementary examinations of palpation and mammography (see Table 49–2).
  2. Of masses detected clinically by palpation, mammography misses or misdiagnoses up to 20%.
  3. Breast self-examination leads to detection of a significant number of masses. The optimal time is 1 week after menses, or on a regular calendar date for postmenopausal women.
  4. Current American Cancer Society MG screening recommendations are shown in Table 49–2. The value of MGs in women over 60 remains equivocal with decisions based on the individual patient and her risk factors.
  5. Earlier MGs are advised for patients with a history of breast cancer or premenopausal breast cancer in first-degree relatives, and/or if the patient is obese with large breasts.

Bibliography

American Cancer Society. Cancer statistics. Cancer 1989;39:3–20.

Azavedo E, et al. Stereotactic fine-needle biopsy in 2,594 mammographically detected non-palpable lesions. Lancet (May 1989):1033–1036.

Baker LH. Breast Cancer Demonstration Project: Five year summary report. Cancer 1982;32:194–225.

Buell P. Changing incidence of breast cancer in Japanese-American women. JNCI 1973;51:1174–1180.

Conont EF, Troupin RH. Ultrasound for breast imaging. Cont Int Med (Jan 1990):34–36.

Devitt JE. False alarms of breast cancer. Lancet (Nov. 1989):1257–1258.

Dupont WD, Page DL. Risk factors for breast cancer in women with proliferative breast disease. N Engl J Med 1985;312:146–151.

Eddy DM. Screening for breast cancer. Ann Intern Med 1989;111:389–399.

Fisher, M, ed. Guide to Preventive Services. Baltimore, Williams and Wilkins, 1989.

Health and Public Policy Committee. The use of diagnostic tests for screening and evaluating breast lesions. Ann Intern Med 1985;103:147–151.

Henderson IC, et al. Cancer of the breast. In: DeVita VT, et al., eds. Cancer: Principles and Practice of Oncology, 3rd ed. Philadelphia, J.B. Lippincott Co., 1989.

Miller AB, et al. Mortality from breast cancer after irradiation during fluoroscopic examinations in patients being treated for tuberculosis. N Engl J Med 1989;321:1285–1289.

Moscowitz M. The predictive value of certain mammographic signs in screening for breast cancer. Cancer 1983;51:1007–1011.

Shapiro S, et al. Ten to fourteen year effect of screening on breast cancer mortality. JNCI 1982;69:349–355.

Venet L, et al. Adequacies and inadequacies of breast examination by physicians in mass screening. Cancer 1971;28:1546–1551.

Willett WC, et al. Moderate alcohol consumption and the risk of breast cancer. N Engl J Med 1987;316:1174–1180.

50

LOCALIZED PROSTATE CARCINOMA

CAROLYN COLLINS

There is a tremendous literature on cancer, but what we know for sure about it can be printed on a calling card.

AUGUST BIER (1861–1949)

DEFINITION

- Prostate carcinoma is the most common tumor in men and is the third leading cause of cancer death in men in the United States. The death rate has reached 30,000 per year.
- In autopsy series, the prevalence rises steadily with age: essentially, all men over 90 years have "histologic" prostate carcinoma. It is uncommon before the age of 40. The prevalence is 60% higher in blacks.
- The presence of circulating male hormones is a necessary condition, as the disease is never seen in castrated males.

DIFFERENTIAL DIAGNOSIS

Causes of palpable abnormalities other than primary cancer include prostatic calculi and infarcts, focal tuberculosis, granulomatous prostatitis, or metastatic extragenital tumors.

CLINICAL FEATURES (Table 50–1)

- Because prostate carcinoma, as opposed to benign prostatic hypertrophy (BPH), arises in the periphery of the gland, obstructive urinary symptoms often occur late in the history of the disease.
- Seventy-five percent of patients clinically diagnosed have disease spread beyond the confines of the prostate gland. Lymphatic spread occurs first to the hypogastric and obturator nodes, followed by the external iliac and presacral drainage. In widespread disease, osteoblastic metastases dominate, although lung, liver, and, infrequently, brain metastases can occur.

TABLE 50-1. American Urologic Society Staging of Prostate Cancer

STAGE	SIGNS, EXTENSIONS	FREQUENCY AT DIAGNOSIS (%)
A1	Not palpable; focal	10
A2	Not palpable: diffuse (Gleason > 4)	
B1	Palpable nodule confined to one lobe, <1.5 cm	15
B2	Palpable nodule >1.5 cm or induration in both lobes	
C	Local extension beyond the prostate	40
D1	Regional nodes involved	35
D2	Distant metastases	<1

HISTORY

- Stage A patients often have symptoms of BPH. Their disease is usually diagnosed following transurethral resection of the prostate (TURP) for obstructive urinary symptoms.

- Stage B patients are often asymptomatic, and their disease is usually discovered during a screening examination.

- Patients with Stage C disease may have a relatively brief history of urinary difficulty when compared with patients with BPH in whom the development of symptoms has been so insidious that the patient may report almost no voiding problems. Occasionally, the presenting symptoms may be the recent onset of impotence. Hematuria is uncommon.

- Stage D disease may present with stiffness, discomfort, or pain due to bony metastases, particularly in the spine or pelvis. Symptoms of prostatic obstruction, radiographic evidence of hydronephrosis, or elevations of prostatic specific antigen (PSA) and/or prostatic acid phosphatase (PAP) may also be present.

SIGNS/PHYSICAL EXAMINATION

- Digital rectal examination (DRE) is the standard against which all other means of prostatic cancer detection have been judged. It should be performed with the patient standing bent over at the waist with his elbows resting on a firm surface. As a screening test, DRE has a sensitivity of 69% and a specificity of 89%.

- In *Stage A,* the prostate gland may be enlarged but no discrete abnormalities are palpable.

- In *Stage B* prostate carcinoma, there is a palpable abnormality of the prostate gland on DRE that appears to be contained within the capsule. A malignant nodule has been said to have the consistency of a button in the middle of a sponge. At biopsy, about half of such palpable nodules are found to be malignant.

- On DRE, *Stage C* carcinoma has invaded the capsule of the gland, extending superiorly into the base of the seminal vesicles, laterally to the pelvic side walls or into the base of the bladder.

- *Stage D* patients may present with variable abnormalities of the prostate gland or findings due to metastasis. On occasion, the only abnormality is an elevated PSA, so-called "stage D-0" disease. These patients have an 80% chance of developing radiologically evident metastatic disease within 2 to 3 years.

LABORATORY STUDIES

- CBC may show evidence of a mild anemia. In advanced disease, there may be cytopenias or a leukoerythroblastic picture reflecting bone marrow involvement.

- Liver function tests may provide a clue to the presence of metastatic disease.

- An abnormal BUN or creatinine suggests tumor that has spread beyond the confines of the gland, resulting in urinary obstruction.

- Alkaline phosphatase may be elevated in patients with bony metastases.

- PAP does not have a high enough sensitivity to be useful as a screening test for prostate carcinoma. In men with advanced disease it can be used as a serum marker for disease activity. Thrombocytosis, hyperthyroidism, myeloma, osteogenic sarcoma, and osteoporosis will also produce elevations in this enzyme.

- PSA
  1. PSA is a protein detected in prostatic tissue (normal, benign hyperplasia, or malignant), seminal fluid, and the sera of patients with prostatic carcinoma.
  2. All patients with invasive carcinoma have serum PSA levels of >2.5 ng/ml. However, cancers may be associated with levels <10 ng/ml.
  3. There is a strong correlation between the pathologic stage and the level of PSA, with a PSA > 40 ng/ml implying stage C or D disease. However, due to substantial overlap, an individual patient's stage cannot be predicted by the PSA level.
  4. The overall sensitivity of PSA in prostatic carcinoma is 96% compared with 63% for PAP. The specificity of PSA and PAP are 97% and 99%, respectively.
  5. Serial determinations of PSA levels may be more sensitive for monitoring therapy, since the PSA titer usually rises before the PAP level and always precedes clinical signs of relapse.
  6. In rare patients with systemic prostatic carcinoma, PSA levels may be normal, probably as a consequence of a poorly differentiated tumor.

IMAGING

- Ultrasonography
  1. The use of high-frequency transrectal ultrasound (TRUS) has established the hypoechoic nature of prostate carcinoma. The accuracy of TRUS in staging prostate cancer is based on the pathologic features that determine the echogenicity.
  2. In a patient with an abnormal DRE or PSA, TRUS is indicated if treatment of early prostate carcinoma is warranted. TRUS adds little if the DRE and PSA are normal.
  3. There is currently no proven role for TRUS in screening for prostate carcinoma.
- Radionuclide scans
  1. All patients with a new diagnosis of prostate carcinoma should undergo a total body bone scan.
  2. Bone scans are more sensitive than plain radiographs in demonstrating bone metastases. However, benign disease such as bone islands, arthritis, and Paget's disease may produce abnormalities on bone scans.
  3. An abnormal bone scan and an elevation of serum PSA and/or PAP levels are very suggestive of unsuspected metastatic disease.
- Radiographic studies
  1. A standard two-view chest X-ray will rule out pulmonary metastases for most patients.
  2. Bone surveys have little value in the evaluation of metastatic disease due to their lower sensitivity. Routine films may demonstrate a benign etiology for abnormal areas on bone scans.
  3. Lymphangiography has an unacceptably high rate of false-negatives (up to 40%) because the standard bipedal study does not image the internal iliac or obturator nodes, which are frequently involved in early nodal dissemination.
  4. CT scans have an accuracy of 65% when compared to a surgical pathologic staging in assessing the extent of primary disease. CT scans cannot demonstrate lymph node metastases unless the nodes are larger than 2 cm; therefore, their accuracy in assessing the presence of nodal metastases is about 70%.
  5. MRI has proved somewhat disappointing in providing further accuracy in staging localized prostate carcinoma. The accuracy in staging early localized carcinoma is about 60%; in advanced local disease it is about 75%.

TISSUE BIOPSY

- There are two putative precancerous lesions of the prostate, prostatic intraepithelial neoplasia (PIN) and atypical adenomatous hyperplasia (AAH).

TABLE 50–2. Pathology of Prostate Carcinoma

Adenocarcinoma (>95%)
Periurethral duct carcinoma
Adenoid cystic carcinoma
Endometroid carcinoma
Carcinosarcoma
Sarcomas
Lymphoma

---

1. PIN is a dysplastic proliferation which has been shown immunohistochemically to progress to invasive carcinoma.
2. AAH is circumscribed proliferation of small glands with an absence of cytologic atypia. The association of AAH with invasive carcinoma is weaker than with PIN.

- Nearly all prostate carcinoma is adenocarcinoma (Table 50–2).

1. Tumor grade, commonly done by the Gleason scores, has prognostic significance in adenocarcinoma. The degree of differentiation of the primary and secondary patterns are each given a score from 1 to 5, the latter being the least differentiated. The primary and secondary pattern scores are added to obtain the total Gleason score.
2. The correlation between the Gleason scores obtained by needle biopsy and the prostatectomy specimen is only 60%.

- The actual diagnosis of prostate carcinoma can only be made by histologic or cytologic evaluation, usually obtained by a needle biopsy.

a. Core biopsies are obtained via a transperineal or transrectal approach. Fine-needle aspiration, which minimizes discomfort and complications, has also been employed.
b. Aspiration and core biopsies are complementary techniques, each of which is limited by relatively small sample sizes. Core biopsy is more specific; aspiration biopsy is more sensitive, allowing larger samples and increasing the probability of detecting multifocal lesions.

TABLE 50–3. Positive Predictive Value of TRUS

DRE RESULT	PSA RESULT	CANCER DETECTION RATE IN PATIENT WITH A POSITIVE TRUS(%)
Abnormal	Abnormal	71
Abnormal	Normal	26
Normal	Abnormal	34
Normal	Normal	5

TABLE 50–4.   Recommended Approach to Diagnosis

DRE Result	PSA Result	
Abnormal	Abnormal	
Abnormal	Normal	→ Proceed to TRUS and biopsy
Normal	Abnormal	
Normal	Normal	→ Consider repeat DRE/PSA in 1 year

RECOMMENDED DIAGNOSTIC APPROACH

- The American Cancer Society recommends that an annual DRE be performed in men over 40.
- The positive predictive values of TRUS for different results of DRE and PSA are shown in Table 50–3.
- Therefore, a reasonable approach to the diagnosis of prostate carcinoma is as shown in Table 50–4. If the biopsy demonstrates PIN/AAH, repeat DRE; PSA and TRUS should be strongly considered in 6 months.

Bibliography

Biondetti PR, et al. Clinical stage B prostate carcinoma: Staging with MR imaging. Radiology 1987;162:325–329.

Boring CC, et al. Cancer statistics, 1991. CA 1991;41:19–51.

Greene DR, Scardino PT. Transrectal ultrasonography for prostate cancer. Principles and Practice of Oncology Updates 1990;4(10): 1–15.

Guinan P, et al. The accuracy of the rectal examination in the diagnosis of prostate carcinoma. New Engl J Med 1980;303:499–503.

Hricak H, et al. Prostatic carcinoma: Staging by clinical assessment, CT, and MR imaging. Radiology 1987;162:331–336.

Lee F, et al. Hypoechoic lesions of the prostate: Clinical relevance of tumor size, digital examination, and prostate specific antigen. Radiology 1989;170:29–32.

Maksem JA, et al. Aspiration biopsy of the prostate. In: Bostwick DG, ed. Pathology of the Prostate, Vol. 15. Contemporary Issues in Surgical Pathology. New York, Churchill Livingstone, 1990, pp. 161–192.

Reflein MD, et al. Comparison of magnetic resonance imaging and ultrasonography in staging early prostate cancer. N Engl J Med 1991;323:621–626.

Ross RK, et al. Serum testosterone levels in healthy young black and white men. JNCI 1986;76:45–48.

Seamonds B, et al. Evaluation of prostate-specific antigen and prostatic acid phosphatase as prostate cancer markers. Urology 1986;28:472–479.

Stamey TA, et al. Prostate-specific antigen as a serum marker for adenocarcinoma of the prostate. N Engl J Med 1987;317:909–916.

51

CANCER OF UNKNOWN PRIMARY SITE

GEORGIANA ELLIS

While there are several chronic diseases more destructive to life than cancer, none are more feared.

CHARLES H. MAYO (1865–1939)

DEFINITION

Cancer of unknown primary site (CUPS) comprises 0.5 to 10% of all malignant diagnoses, and is defined as:

- Unequivocal histologic evidence of malignancy.
- Histology inconsistent with a primary tumor at the biopsy site.
- History (including careful attention to previous malignancies, past biopsies, or excisions), physical exam, chest X-ray, CBC, urinalysis, and stool tests for occult blood fail to indicate a primary site.
- Additional diagnostic studies fail to reveal a primary site. For example, squamous carcinoma presenting in a cervical lymph node is not of unknown primary site until examination by an otolaryngologist with directed biopsies and appropriate scanning fails to reveal a primary site.

DIAGNOSTIC GOALS

- The median survival of patients with CUPS is 3 to 5 months. The plethora of diagnostic studies available to the clinician makes it possible to expend the patient's remaining life expectancy, and possibly financial resources as well, in pursuing a diagnosis, without likely patient benefit.
- Prudent evaluation can be approached by histologic determination of tumor type (adeno- or squamous carcinoma, lymphoma).
- Certain clinical presentations merit special consideration. Evaluation is aimed at identifying those tumors for which effective treatment (cure or palliation) is available (Table 51–1).

TABLE 51–1. Tumors with Effective Therapy

Radiation: head and neck cancer
Surgery: melanoma
Cure possible with systemic (chemo)therapy
  Germ cell tumors
  Hodgkin's disease
  Non-Hodgkin's lymphoma
  Trophoblastic tumors
Control possible with low-morbidity hormonal therapy
  Breast cancer
  Prostate cancer
  Endometrial cancer
Effective chemotherapy (response rate > 50%) available
  Breast cancer
  Ovarian cancer
  Small-cell lung cancer
  Head and neck cancer
  Thyroid cancer

Source: Adapted from Ultmann JE, Phillips TL. Cancer of unknown primary site. In: DeVita VT Jr, et al., eds. Cancer: Principles and Practice of Oncology, 3rd ed. Philadelphia, J.B. Lippincott Company, 1989, pp. 1941–1952; Kirsten F et al., Metastatic adeno- or undifferentiated carcinoma from an unknown primary site: Natural history and guidelines for identification of treatable subsets. Q J Med 1987;62:143–161.

PATHOLOGIC EVALUATION

- The majority of CUPS present as poorly or undifferentiated lesions, suggesting special studies.
- Immunocytochemistry
  1. If rebiopsy is contemplated, appropriate tissue handling (frozen vs. fixed, type of fixative) must be discussed with the pathologist in advance of tissue procurement.
  2. Immunocytochemistry is usually approached via application of a battery of screening antibodies on successive tissue slices, initially to distinguish histologic type (carcinoma vs. sarcoma vs. lymphoma; squamous vs. adenocarcinoma), with subsequent antibody placement as directed by initial results.
     a. Intermediate filament proteins are cytoplasmic components between the small filaments (actin) and larger filaments (myosin and tubulin). There are five classes.
        i. Cytokeratins are characteristic of cells of epithelial origin. The presence of cytokeratin expression indicates carcinoma, while the pattern of expression may differentiate adenocarcinoma from squamous carcinoma, or mesothelioma from adenocarcinoma.
        ii. Vimentin characterizes cells of mesenchymal origin. It is commonly expressed in a number of sarcomas, and is co-expressed by a small

    subset of carcinomas (renal cell, endometrial).

   iii. Desmin is expressed by cells of muscle origin.

   iv. Glial fibrillary acidic protein is expressed by neuroglia cells.

   v. Neurofilament is expressed by neurons.

  b. Antibodies to lymphoid antigens can distinguish poorly differentiated lymphomas. Positive immunostaining with LeuM1 or peanut-agglutinin may suggest Hodgkin's disease.

  c. Antibodies to melanoma-specific antigens (HMB45) may clarify this diagnosis.

  d. Occasional organ-specific antibodies are available, e.g., for prostate (PSA, PAP) or thyroid.

  e. Antibodies for neuroendocrine markers (neuron-specific enolase, chromogranin, synaptophysin) are useful in the diagnosis of small-cell carcinoma, pheochromocytoma, carcinoid, and paraganglioma.

  f. Antibodies to hormone receptors, such as estrogen receptor, may help clarify the diagnosis of breast cancer, but can also be seen in other tumors such as melanoma.

- Electron microscopy is of limited availability because of cost. Many of its previous applications have been supplanted by immunocytochemistry. It may provide information when improper tissue fixation precludes interpretable immunocytochemistry.

- Cytogenetics may support specific diagnoses, such as the presence of an isochromosome of the short arm of chromosome 12 (i12p), seen in a large percentage of germ cell tumors. Cytogenetics, however, are as yet insufficiently delineated to merit the time required for results.

- Clinical correlation. Although improved diagnostic certainty may not confer more certain therapeutic outcome, it may augment the diagnosis of curable or treatable malignancies.

SPECIAL CLINICAL SYNDROMES

A number of clinical presentations of CUPS merit special attention, having a somewhat better prognosis than CUPS in general.

- Cervical lymph nodes

 1. Squamous or undifferentiated carcinoma presenting in cervical lymph nodes without an apparent head and neck primary (after examination by an otolaryngologist and CT or MRI of the head) is found, if the primary later becomes apparent, to be of head and neck origin about 80% of the time.

 2. Median survival may exceed 2 years with aggressive local therapy with or without chemotherapy.

- Axillary lymph nodes, females
  1. Adenocarcinoma presenting in an axillary lymph node in females may represent occult breast carcinoma in up to one-half of such patients in whom a primary site is eventually found.
  2. Median survival may exceed 3 years. There is no survival advantage for one form of local management over another (excision of the axillary node alone vs. subsequent radiation or chemotherapy).
- Malignant ascites, females. Usually due to ovarian carcinoma. CT scan should detect this.
- Melanoma metastatic to lymph node. This should be approached as any stage II melanoma; treatment outcome does not differ from stage II melanomas where the primary was identified.

ADDITIONAL STUDIES

If the above initial evaluation, ancillary studies, and sophisticated tissue review fail to suggest a primary site, and one of the special clinical syndromes is not present, further evaluation should include:
1. CT scans of abdomen and pelvis, which detect a primary site in one-third of patients. The group at Vanderbilt also recommends chest CT to look for midline germ cell tumors.
2. Tumor markers
   a. Alpha-fetoprotein (αFP) and beta-human chorionic gonadotropin (β-HCG) as evidence of extragonadal germ cell tumors.
   b. PAP or PSA as evidence of metastatic prostate cancer.

REMAINING CUPS

- Following the above approach, a variable proportion of cases remain truly unknown. There are 2 broad categories:
  1. Adenocarcinoma of unknown primary. These patients are generally elderly, have multiple visceral metastatic sites (liver, lung, bone), show poor response to "empiric" chemotherapy, and have a median survival of 4 months.
  2. Poorly differentiated carcinoma. These patients are often young, with variable disease sites including the mediastinum, retroperitoneum, and lymph nodes. They comprise 10 to 15% of reported series of adenocarcinoma of unknown primary site. Some appear curable with cisplatin-based chemotherapy, and may have extragonadal germ cell tumors. Poorly differentiated adenocarcinoma is included in this group, and "apparent cures" occur in some patients.

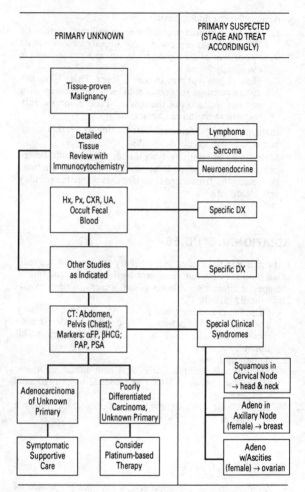

Figure 51–1. Recommended diagnostic approach to carcinoma of unknown primary site.

RECOMMENDED DIAGNOSTIC APPROACH
(see Figure 51–1)

Bibliography

Altman E, Cadman E. An analysis of 1539 patients with cancer of unknown primary site. Cancer 1986;57:120–124.

Bosl GJ, et al. i(12p): A specific karyotypic abnormality in germ cell tumors. Proc Am Soc Clin Oncol 1989;8:131A.

Corwin DJ, Gown AM. Review of selected lineage-directed antibodies useful in routinely processed tissues. Arch Pathol Lab Med 1989;113:645–652.

DeBraud F, et al. Metastatic squamous cell carcinoma of an unknown primary localized to the neck: Advantages of an aggressive treatment. Cancer 1989;64:510–515.

Gatter KC, et al. Clinical importance of analyzing malignant tumors of uncertain origin with immunohistologic techniques. Lancet 1985;1:1302–1305.

Greco FA, et al. Advanced poorly differentiated carcinoma of unknown primary site: Recognition of a treatable syndrome. Ann Intern Med 1986;104:547–553.

Hainsworth JD, Greco FA. Managing carcinoma of unknown primary site. Oncology 1988;2:43–54.

Hamilton CS, Langlands AO. ACUPS (adenocarcinoma of unknown primary site): A clinical and cost benefit analysis. Int J Rad Oncol Biol Phys 1987;13:1497–1503.

Kirsten F, et al. Metastatic adeno- or undifferentiated carcinoma from an unknown primary site: Natural history and guidelines for identification of treatable subsets. Q J Med 1987;62:143–161.

Mackay B, Ordonez NG. Tumors of unknown origin: The role of the pathologist. Advances Oncol 1989;5:13–19.

McMillan JH, et al. Computed tomography in the evaluation of metastatic adenocarcinoma from an unknown primary site: A retrospective study. Radiology 1982;143:143–146.

McNutt MA, et al. Monoclonal antibodies to cytokeratins in diagnostic immunocytochemistry. In: Wick MR, Siegal GP, eds. Monoclonal Antibodies in Diagnostic Immunohistochemistry. New York, Marcel Dekker, 1988, pp. 51–70.

Shah JP. The unknown primary in the head and neck: Evaluation of the patient. In: Chretien PB, et al., eds. Head and Neck Cancer, vol. 1, Philadelphia, BC Dekker Inc., 1985, pp. 283–285.

Ultmann JE, Phillips TL. Cancer of unknown primary site. In: DeVita VT Jr, et al., eds. Cancer: Principles and Practice of Oncology, 3rd ed. Philadelphia, J.B. Lippincott Company, 1989, pp. 1941–1952.

SECTION VIII

ENDOCRINOLOGY

52

HIRSUTISM

DAVID HINDSON

Babies haven't any hair
Old men's heads are just as bare;
Between the cradle and the grave
Lies a haircut and a shave.

SAMUEL HOFFENSTEIN (1890–1947)

DEFINITION AND EPIDEMIOLOGY

1. *Hirsutism* is abnormal hairiness, especially excessive male pattern hair growth in women. *Hypertrichosis* means a generalized (sexual and nonsexual) apparent increase in hair growth. Hirsutism is a common clinical problem. One study found 10% of women to have hirsutism.

2. There are several types of hair (Table 52–1). The gonadal sex steroids have major effects on hair. Hirsutism results from the conversion of vellus to terminal hair under the influence of androgens in sex-dependent areas. The number of hair follicles in these areas does not increase, and the capacity to develop hirsutism under the influence of androgens is quite variable.

DIFFERENTIAL DIAGNOSIS

1. In hypertrichosis (Table 52–2), there is an apparent increase in body hair generally. This occurs because of increased pigmentation and therefore visibility of the vellus hair without actual transformation to terminal hair.

2. Increased androgen effect at sex-dependent hair follicles causes hirsutism.

3. By far the most common causes of hirsutism (Table 52–3) are idiopathic hirsutism (IH) and polycystic ovary syndrome (PCO; Stein-Leventhal syndrome).

4. IH and PCO are related functional disorders probably resulting from any of several interrelated primary perturbations of the hypothalamic-pituitary-ovarian (HPO) axis.

5. By strict definition, IH would include only women with hirsutism without menstrual disorder or virilization, and PCO would require the demonstration of classic polycystic ovaries. In practice, there is a great deal of overlap between IH and PCO, and they are best considered as 2

TABLE 52–1. Types of Hair

Lanugo: fine, short, lightly pigmented, seen in newborn
Vellus: soft (nonmedullated), short (<2 cm), usually
  nonpigmented, unnoticeable, covers most of body in
  adults
Terminal: stiff (medullated), long, pigmented, visible
  Sex-dependent: axilla, pubis, face, chest, abdomen, back
  Sex-independent: eyebrows, eyelashes, corona of scalp
Vibrisae: nares

TABLE 52–2. Causes of Hypertrichosis

Congenital
Central nervous system (postencephalitic, multiple
  sclerosis, trauma)
Malignancy
Starvation (including anorexia nervosa)
Juvenile hypothyroidism
Porphyria cutanea tarda
Drugs (phenytoin, diazoxide, minoxidil, glucocorticoids,
  penicillamine, cyclosporine)

TABLE 52–3. Causes of Hirsutism

Ovarian
  Neoplastic
  Nonneoplastic
    PCO
    IH
    Insulin resistance syndromes
Adrenal
  Neoplastic
  Nonneoplastic
    Cushing's disease
    CAH
    Adrenal causes PCO and IH
Hyperprolactinemia
Drugs: exogenous androgens
Increased hair follicle androgen sensitivity

degrees of severity and clinical expression of the same disorder.

6. In PCO, an altered endocrine milieu (increased androgens, increased estrogens, increased luteinizing hormone (LH)–to–follicle-stimulating hormone (FSH) ratio often without cycling, and decreased progesterone) causes the important clinical consequences:
    a. Hirsutism with occasional virilization
    b. Infertility and menstrual irregularities
    c. Unopposed estrogen stimulation of the uterine endometrium

7. Several types of ovarian neoplasms may secrete testosterone.
    a. These are usually of the sex cord stromal category (Sertoli-Leydig, granulosa stromal, lipoid cell, etc.).
    b. The majority of androgen-producing ovarian tumors are palpable at pelvic examination.

8. All forms of insulin-resistance syndromes are associated with IH or PCO. Insulin increases follicular atresia in the ovary resulting in increased androgen production. Whether mild insulin resistance is a cause or effect in the more common forms of IH or PCO is controversial.

9. Adrenal gland neoplasms (almost always carcinomas) are an uncommon cause of hirsutism and virilization.

10. Cushing's disease (bilateral adrenal hyperplasia due to excessive pituitary ACTH) is associated with moderate increase in androgens along with the increase in glucocorticoids. It is uncommon compared to IH and PCO and is recognized by the many other features of excessive glucocorticoids (Cushing's syndrome).

11. Late onset (or "attenuated") congenital adrenal hyperplasia (CAH) is now increasingly recognized and may mimic IH or PCO. Recent studies found that 1.2 to 6% of patients initially diagnosed with IH have late-onset CAH.

12. Approximately 25% of women with prolactinoma and the amenorrhea/galactorrhea syndrome have IH or PCO. All hirsutism patients with menstrual irregularities or amenorrhea should be examined for galactorrhea, and hyperprolactinemia suspected.

13. The use of exogenous androgens (e.g., among female athletes) may cause hirsutism or virilization.

14. Increased hair follicle sensitivity to androgens with normal androgen levels may comprise a small subset of patients with IH.

CLINICAL FEATURES

1. The clinician has two major tasks:
    a. Distinguish abnormal hirsutism requiring evaluation and treatment from a normal variant needing only reassurance and sometimes cosmetic treatment.
    b. Identify serious underlying disease from clinical features.

TABLE 52–4. Frequency of Terminal Hair Growth in Normal Women

Location	%
Arms and legs	84
Linea alba (''male escutcheon'')	35
Face (mainly upper lip)	26
Chest (mainly periareolar)	17
Lumbosacral area	16
Chin	5
Sternum	3

2. Terminal hair growth is seen in a portion of normal women (Table 52–4).
   a. Older women have increased terminal hair growth on the face, while it is decreased elsewhere.
   b. Normal women do not have terminal hair on the upper back or upper abdomen.
   c. Scoring systems for hirsutism are available (see Ferriman and Gallwey, 1961), and it is important at the initial visit to examine all areas and document the hair growth by description or photography.
3. Hirsutism is one of the earliest signs of excessive androgens.
   a. With more marked elevation of androgen levels, virilization may occur (Table 52–5). Clitoromegaly with a length-time-width index greater than 36 mm^2 is virtually pathognomonic but not always present.
   b. Advanced virilization is unusual in IH or PCO and alerts the clinician to the possibility of more serious underlying disease.
4. IH (Table 52–6) represents the largest group of patients presenting with a complaint of increased hair growth.
   a. By strict definition, this group refers only to women with continued normal ovulatory menses; however, most practitioners include patients with menstrual disorders without demonstrable polycystic ovaries.

TABLE 52–5. Androgen Effects in Women

Mild to moderate
  Hirsutism
  Acne/Oily skin
  Menstrual irregularity
  Increased libido
Virilization (''masculinization'')
  Clitoromegaly
  Male pattern balding
  Deepening of voice
  Increased muscle mass
  Male body habitus

TABLE 52–6. Idiopathic Hirsutism

Onset: peripubertal
Menses: normal or irregular (oligomenorrhea or
  amenorrhea)
Exam: no virilization, often obese
Course: stable

    b.   There is much overlap with PCO on the one end and normal variant on the other.

    c.   The clinical course is stable or slowly progressive hirsutism.

5.   The features of PCO are similar to but more marked than IH (Table 52–7).

    a.   The onset is also at or near the time of puberty.

    b.   Anovulatory menses or amenorrhea and infertility are the rule.

    c.   Obesity is common and the attendant insulin resistance is felt causal by some.

    d.   The classic polycystic ovary is 2 to 5 times normal size and shows multiple follicular and atretic cysts.

6.   Late-onset CAH may mimic IH or PCO but may have an earlier (prepubertal) onset, more rapid or progressive course, more severe virilization, or short stature.

7.   Virilizing tumors of the ovary or adrenal are rare. Generally, virilization accompanies the hirsutism. Most of these tumors in the ovary are palpable on pelvic exam and many of the adrenal tumors are palpable on abdominal exam.

8.   Cushing's syndrome is recognized by the concomitant features of hypercortisolism (hypertension, central obesity, moon facies, striae, proximal muscle weakness, plethora, and bruising).

9.   Clinical features unusual for IH or PCO which should prompt a more thorough search for another etiology include:

    a.   Progressive hirsutism

    b.   Onset before or after the time of puberty

    c.   Virilization or severe hirsutism

    d.   Galactorrhea

    e.   Hypertension

    f.   Signs of Cushing's syndrome

    g.   Pelvic or abdominal mass

TABLE 52–7. Polycystic Ovary Syndrome

Onset: peripubertal
Menses: irregular or amenorrhea (50 to 60%)
Infertility
Exam: hirsutism (70 to 80%), obesity (40 to 50%), mild
  virilization (occasional)
Polycystic ovaries

LABORATORY STUDIES

- Serum testosterone is the measure of the total bound and unbound testosterone in the blood.
    1. In normal women, this level is stable without a pulsatile pattern or circadian rhythm. The normal level in women is 20–70 nanograms (ng)/dl.
    2. In women with IH or PCO, the serum testosterone is often elevated (70 to 80% in PCO; 40 to 70% among all hirsute women; 20 to 30% in hirsute women with regular ovulatory menses). The level in these conditions is generally only mildly to moderately elevated.
    3. A testosterone greater than 200 ng/dl is extremely unusual in IH or PCO and should suggest a testosterone secreting tumor of the ovary or adrenal.
- Dehydroepiandrosterone sulfate (DHEA-S) is virtually completely derived from adrenal glands.
    1. Its serum level has replaced urinary 17-ketosteroids as a measure of adrenal androgen secretion. The normal serum level is less than 450 μg/dl.
    2. The level is elevated in some patients with IH or PCO.
    3. It is markedly elevated in virilizing adrenal carcinoma, and a level greater than 700 μg/dl should prompt a search for an adrenal carcinoma.
    4. Moderate elevations in the range of 450 to 700 μg/dl may be seen in IH/PCO, CAH, and some virilizing adrenal tumors.
    5. The DHEA-S level is not a good screen for late-onset CAH because it is usually normal.
- 17-Hydroxyprogesterone (17-OHP) is the substrate for the 21-hydroxylase enzyme.
    1. In late-onset CAH caused by a deficiency of this enzyme, basal levels of 17-OHP are often elevated.
    2. However, the basal level may be normal, and an ACTH-stimulated 17-OHP level is necessary for the diagnosis. A basal morning 17-OHP is measured, 0.25 mg of synthetic ACTH is given intravenously, and the stimulated 17-OHP level is measured 1 hour later.
    3. The response in late-onset CAH is much greater than in normals or patients heterozygous for the enzyme deficiency, and the test clearly distinguishes late-onset CAH from normal.
- Serum prolactin is usually markedly elevated in prolactinoma and may be mildly elevated (doubled) in IH/PCO.
- Measures of adrenal glucocorticoid secretion are generally normal unless the hirsutism is caused by Cushing's disease.

RECOMMENDED DIAGNOSTIC APPROACH

1. For patients with clinical features of IH or PCO, Figure 52–1 outlines the recommended laboratory evaluation.
2. Serum testosterone and DHEA-S levels are obtained.
    a. A greatly elevated testosterone suggests a tumor of the ovary or adrenal, and further search is necessary.

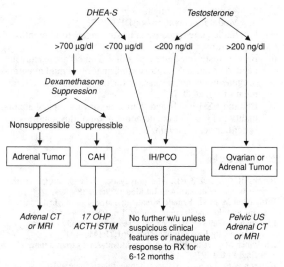

Figure 52–1. Recommended evaluation for hirsutism.

    b. A normal or moderately elevated testosterone is consistent with IH/PCO, and further work-up to identify the exact cause is not necessary and often futile.

3. A greatly increased level of DHEA-S is suggestive of an adrenal carcinoma but may occasionally occur in CAH.

    a. Such a result should be further evaluated with a repeat DHEA-S level after 5 days of dexamethasone suppression (2 mg QID).

    b. Suppression on dexamethasone suggests CAH and appropriate precursor levels should be obtained.

    c. Nonsuppression suggests an adrenocortical carcinoma.

4. A serum prolactin level should be obtained if there is a menstrual disorder or galactorrhea.

    a. Patients with a level more than twice the upper limit of normal should be evaluated for a pituitary tumor.

    b. A lesser degree of elevation is common in IH and PCO.

5. The low prevalence (1 to 6% of hirsute women) and the high rate of false-negatives of the basal 17-OHP levels argue against screening all hirsute women with 17-OHP levels. ACTH stimulation of the 17-OHP level should be measured in the following circumstances:

    a. Hirsutism before puberty

    b. Progressive hirsutism

    c. Hypertension

    d. Virilization

    e. Short stature

    f.   Appropriate family history
    g.   Moderate elevations of DHEA-S
    h.   Inadequate response of hirsutism to 6 to 12 months of therapy

6. Free testosterone and 3 alpha-diol G levels are usually not needed because laboratory confirmation of mild hyperandrogenemia is not necessary for the diagnosis and treatment of IH/PCO.

7. LH and FSH levels and their ratio have a typical abnormality in PCO, but the demonstration of this abnormality is neither necessary nor helpful.

Bibliography

Barnes R, Rosenfeld RL. The polycystic ovary syndrome: Pathogenesis and treatment. Ann Int Med 1989;110:386–399.

Biffignandi P, et al. Female hirsutism: Pathophysiological considerations and therapeutic implications. Endo Rev 1984;5:498–513.

Ferriman D, Gallwey JD. Clinical assessment of body hair growth in women. J Clin Endocrinol Metab 1961;21:1440–1447.

Kirschner MA, et al. Idiopathic hirsutism: An ovarian abnormality. N Engl J Med 1976;294:637–640.

Kuttenn F, et al. Late onset adrenal hyperplasia in hirsutism. N Engl J Med 1985;313:224–231.

Leshin M. Hirsutism. Am J Med Sci 1987;294:369–383.

McKnight E. The prevalence of "hirsutism" in young women. Lancet 1964;1:410–413.

Rittmaster RS, Loriaux DL. Hirsutism. Ann Int Med 1987;106:95–107.

Siegel SF, et al. ACTH stimulation tests and plasma dehydroepiandrosterone sulfate levels in women with hirsutism. N Engl J Med 1990;323:849–854.

Speroff L, et al. Hirsutism. In: Speroff L, et al. eds., Clinical Gynecologic Endocrinology and Infertility, 4th ed. Baltimore, Williams and Wilkins, 1989.

White PH, et al. Congenital adrenal hyperplasia. N Engl J Med 1987;316:1519–1524; 1580–1586.

53

AMENORRHEA

MITCHELL KARTON

In diagnosis, think of the easy first.
MARTIN FISCHER (1879–1962)

DEFINITION

- Primary amenorrhea is present if:
  1. There is an absence of menses at age 14, associated with lack of normal growth or absence of normal secondary sexual development, or both.
  2. There is an absence of menses by age 16, even in the presence of normal growth and normal secondary sexual characteristics.
- Secondary amenorrhea is defined as:
  1. Absence of menstruation for 6 months (or for a duration equal to 3 consecutive cycles) in a woman with a history of regular menses, or absence of menstruation for 12 months in a woman with a history of irregular menses.
  2. Physiologic causes of secondary amenorrhea include pregnancy, puerperal amenorrhea, and normal menopause. Secondary amenorrhea in women of childbearing age should be considered the result of pregnancy until proved otherwise.

DIFFERENTIAL DIAGNOSIS (Table 53–1)

- Primary amenorrhea
  1. This is a rare disorder. Over 95% of normal girls have their first menstrual period by age 15.
  2. Sixty percent of cases of primary amenorrhea are caused by errors in gonadal or genital development:
     a. Gonadal dysgenesis, 30% (including Turner's syndrome)
     b. Müllerian dysgenesis, 20%
     c. Errors in genital development such as male pseudohermaphroditism, 10%
  3. The other 40% of patients have primary amenorrhea caused by:
     a. Hypogonadotropism (10%)
     b. Endocrinopathies
     c. Gonadal resistance syndromes
     d. Outflow tract abnormalities

TABLE 53–1. Causes of Primary and Secondary Amenorrhea

Primary amenorrhea
  A. Fetal errors in genital differentiation
     1. Male pseudohermaphroditism caused by deficient testosterone synthesis
     2. Male pseudohermaphroditism caused by 5-alpha-reductase deficiency
     3. Male pseudohermaphroditism caused by androgen resistance
        a. Complete testicular feminization
        b. Incomplete testicular feminization
        c. Familial incomplete male pseudohermaphroditism (type 1)
     4. Female pseudohermaphroditism with fetal and postnatal androgen excess
  B. Fetal errors in gonadal development
     1. True hermaphroditism
     2. Gonadal dysgenesis with stigmata of Turner's syndrome
     3. Mixed gonadal dysgenesis
  C. Fetal errors in gonaductal development
     1. Müllerian dysgenesis
  D. Ovarian follicles insensitive to gonadotropins
     1. 17-Alpha-hydroxylase deficiency
     2. "Resistant ovary syndrome"
  E. Hypothalamic-pituitary diseases
     1. Familial hypogonadotropic hypogonadism
     2. Pituitary tumors
     3. Idiopathic panhypopituitarism
  F. Unknown
     1. Polycystic ovary disease (chronic anovulation)
     2. Delayed menarche
     3. Systemic diseases
Secondary amenorrhea
  A. Anatomic abnormalities
     1. Intrauterine synechiae (Asherman's syndrome): postsurgical, postinfective, postabortive, posttraumatic, or after IUD use
     2. Müllerian abnormalities or agenesis
     3. Testicular feminization
     4. Hysterectomy
  B. Primary ovarian failure (with high gonadotropin levels)
     1. Congenital: gonadal dysgenesis, gonadotropin resistance
     2. Acquired: premature primary ovarian failure (postinfectious, postoperative, postchemotherapy, postradiation, autoimmune oophoritis, gonadotropin resistance)
  C. Secondary ovarian failure (with low or normal gonadotropins)
     1. Galactorrhea-amenorrhea syndromes with high prolactin

Table continued on following page

TABLE 53–1. Causes of Primary and Secondary Amenorrhea Continued

2. Intrinsic disease of hypothalamus or pituitary: tumors, trauma, postsurgical or postradiation effects, Sheehan's syndrome, empty-sella syndrome
3. Extrinsic disease: psychogenic; from starvation (anorexia nervosa); exercise; after oral contraceptive pill use; excessive estrogen from obesity, age, or thyroid disease; endocrinopathies; intercurrent systemic disease; drug-induced; idiopathic

D. Chronic anovulation with increased ovarian steroid production
1. Ovarian tumors, both feminizing and masculinizing
2. Polycystic ovary syndrome (PCO syndrome, continuous estrus syndrome)

Source: Adapted from Williams R, et al. Textbook of Endocrinology, 7th ed. Philadelphia, W.B. Saunders Company, 1985.

4. Some conditions classically associated with secondary amenorrhea, such as PCO syndrome, may develop early enough to prevent even the first menstrual cycle.

- Secondary amenorrhea
  1. Secondary amenorrhea (excluding pregnancy and menopause) is much more common than primary amenorrhea.
  2. The causes of secondary amenorrhea can be divided into:
     a. Anatomic abnormalities.
     b. Primary ovarian failure with high gonadotropin levels.
     c. Secondary ovarian failure with low gonadotropin levels (owing to either pituitary or hypothalamic disease).
     d. Chronic anovulation with increased ovarian steroid production such as from tumors or polycystic ovary disease. Fifty percent of patients with anovulation are amenorrheic.

HISTORY AND SIGNS AND SYMPTOMS

The clinical findings may be grouped according to the anatomic level of abnormality.

- Outflow tract
  1. Asherman's syndrome
     a. History. Endometritis, surgery (including cesarean section and myomectomy), use of an intrauterine

device, and, rarely, tuberculosis or schistosomiasis are associated with this condition.

  b. Diagnosis is made by hysteroscopy or hystero-
  salpingography.

2. Müllerian dysgenesis

  a. History. There is cyclic abdominal pain and distention from hematocolpos, hematometra, or hemato-
  peritoneum; puberty, growth, and development
  are normal.

  b. Physical examination. Careful pelvic examination
  is used to determine the presence of abnormalities
  including imperforate hymen; the presence of a
  vagina (if present, its patency); and the presence
  and patency of the cervix and uterus.

  c. Laboratory findings. There is a normal female
  karyotype (46XX), which differentiates this disorder from male pseudohermaphroditism.

  d. X-ray. Urinary tract abnormalities (30%) and skeletal malformations (12%) occur.

  e. Ultrasound is used to rule out endometriomas.

3. Male pseudohermaphroditism

  a. History. Puberty is normal or minimally delayed.
  Often there is a positive family history of sexual
  immaturity and infertility and a possible history of
  inguinal hernia.

  b. Physical examination

    i. Examination shows variable virilization due
    to the possibility of some androgen effect,
    but usually there is a normal female pheno-
    type.

    ii. The patient may be tall with a eunuchoidal
    tendency; if there is complete testicular femi-
    nization, the female external genitalia are im-
    mature, and if incomplete, clitoromegaly may
    be present.

    iii. Fifty percent of patients have inguinal hernias
    (cryptorchid testes).

  c. Laboratory findings. There is a normal male
  karyotype (46XY). Testosterone levels are normal
  male or slightly elevated.

• Ovaries

1. Gonadal dysgenesis (Turner's syndrome)

  a. History. There is a history of delayed puberty,
  edema of the extremities in the neonatal period,
  and growth retardation that became evident by the
  third or fourth year of life.

  b. Physical examination shows short stature, webbed
  neck, shield chest, increased carrying angle, and
  immature female external genitalia and secondary
  sex characteristics. Coarctation of the aorta may
  occur.

  c. Laboratory findings. The karyotype is 45XO. Serum gonadotropin levels are elevated.

  d. Chest X-ray may suggest coarctation of the aorta,
  skeletal malformations, or urinary tract abnormalities.

2. Premature ovarian failure
   a. History. The patient should be questioned regarding signs and symptoms of other autoimmune glandular diseases, rheumatoid arthritis, and myasthenia gravis.
   b. Laboratory findings. Laboratory tests should include:
      i. Thyroid function tests, including thyroid-stimulating hormone (TSH) and antithyroid antibodies.
      ii. Morning serum cortisol level.
      iii. Rheumatoid factor, antinuclear antibodies, and antiacetylcholine receptor antibodies.
      iv. Serum gonadotropin levels, which are elevated.

3. PCO syndrome
   a. History. Growth, development, and puberty are normal. This may be associated with diabetes mellitus or dysfunctional uterine bleeding.
   b. Physical examination shows hirsutism, with occasional evidence of virilization. Obesity is common and acanthosis nigricans may occur.
   c. Laboratory findings. There is a normal female karyotype. The LH : FSH ratio may be elevated.

4. Ovarian tumors
   a. History. There are occasional symptoms as a result of thyroid or serotonin excess in benign cystic teratomas.
   b. Physical examination. There are signs of virilization with arrhenoblastoma and hypertension. Diabetes is associated with lipoid cell tumors; many tumors are palpable on pelvic examination.

• Pituitary
   1. Tumors
      a. History
         i. There may be a history of headache, blurred vision, or bitemporal hemianopsia. Hemianopsia is a very late finding with large tumors such as craniopharyngiomas.
         ii. Symptoms of hypothyroidism, adrenal insufficiency, and diabetes insipidus may occur, especially with craniopharyngiomas. Galactorrhea may result from prolactin-secreting micro- and macroadenomas.
      b. Physical examination may reveal visual field defects; occasional evidence of acromegaly; Cushing's syndrome; sexual infantilism (craniopharyngioma); and galactorrhea.
      c. Laboratory findings
         i. There may be alterations in adrenocorticotropic hormone (ACTH), cortisol, growth hormone (GH), TSH, and antidiuretic hormone (ADH) levels.
         ii. Serum prolactin is elevated in 20% of women with secondary amenorrhea and in 50% of patients with galactorrhea-amenorrhea.

      d. X-ray. Skull X-rays may show calcification (craniopharyngioma). If the prolactin level or sella is abnormal, a CT or MR scan should be obtained.

  2. Idiopathic panhypopituitarism

      a. History. There may be a history of previous operations, pituitary radiation, and postpartum hemorrhage (Sheehan's syndrome).

      b. Physical examination. There may be evidence of hypothyroidism, adrenal insufficiency, and loss of axillary and pubic hair.

      c. Laboratory findings. Serum TSH, ACTH, GH, and gonadotropin levels are low.

- Hypothalamus

  1. Anorexia nervosa

      a. History. This condition is usually not associated with other medical problems. Bulimia, self-induced vomiting, lightheadedness, and constipation are common. The onset is usually between 10 and 30 years of age.

      b. Physical examination

         i. Anorexia nervosa is associated with a 25% weight loss or weight 15% below normal for age and height.

         ii. Findings may include hypotension, bradycardia, lanugo, and yellowish palms from hypercarotenemia.

         iii. The mental status examination is notable for denial, rigidity, a distorted body image, and thought content often focused on hoarding or unusual handling of food.

      c. Laboratory findings. The gonadotropin levels are low, cortisol high, and prolactin normal. The TSH and T_4 are normal, T_3 low, and reverse T_3 high.

  2. Anorectic reaction associated with exercise

      a. History. The patient exercises regularly and makes a conscious attempt to lower body weight and percentage of body fat. The patient usually has high stress levels.

      b. Physical examination. The mental status examination is notable for insight into the problem and absence of denial.

      c. Laboratory findings. Exercise is associated with elevated prolactin, ACTH, and GH levels and decreased gonadotropins.

  3. "Postpill" amenorrhea. Amenorrhea may persist after discontinuation of hormonal contraceptives. Evaluation is recommended only after 6 months following discontinuation of oral contraceptive pills or 12 months after the last injection of Depo-Provera.

RECOMMENDED DIAGNOSTIC APPROACH

- Initial steps

  1. History and physical examination (see Figure 53–1). Important clinical features include:

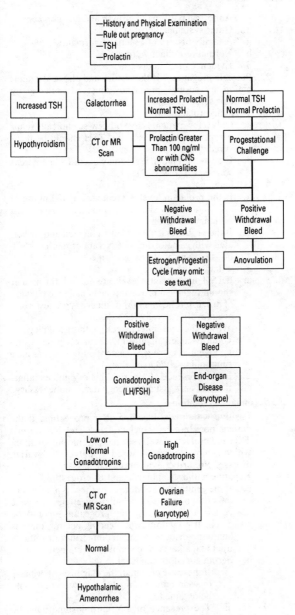

Figure 53–1. Flow diagram for evaluation for amenorrhea.

a. Unusual stress factors
b. Malnutrition
c. Exercise history
d. Medications

      e. Abnormal patterns of growth and development

      f. Other systemic illnesses

      g. A family history of genetic abnormalities

      h. Normal reproductive tracts

      i. Evidence of CNS disease

2. Possible pregnancy. If the history and physical examination are normal, pregnancy must be excluded by urine or serum pregnancy tests.

3. TSH and prolactin level

      a. Only a few patients have otherwise clinically inapparent hypothyroidism, but TSH should be measured.

      b. Elevated prolactin levels may occur for many reasons (see Table 53–2).

4. CT scan

      a. If the prolactin level is greater than 100 ng/ml, a CT or MR scan should be obtained to rule out a pituitary adenoma.

      b. If the prolactin level is mildly elevated and associated with galactorrhea or CNS abnormalities, a CT or MR scan should be performed.

5. Progestational challenge

      a. If TSH and prolactin levels are normal, the patient should receive a progestational challenge (100 mg of progesterone in oil IM or medroxyprogesterone acetate, 10 mg orally for 5 days).

      b. Within the subsequent week, withdrawal bleeding confirms an endometrium adequately primed with endogenous estrogen, a patent outflow tract, and a functioning HPO axis.

      c. In the presence of a normal history and examination, this progestin challenge test is unnecessary.

• Secondary evaluation

1. Positive withdrawal bleeding after progestins. If the patient does not have galactorrhea and has normal TSH and prolactin levels, she has chronic anovulation, which is almost always caused by polycystic ovarian disease. No further evaluation is necessary.

2. Negative withdrawal bleeding after progestins

      a. If the genitalia are abnormal or there is a history of infection or trauma (including curettage), a cyclic course of estrogens and progestins should be given. If no withdrawal bleeding occurs, there is anatomic disease of the endometrium or outflow tract and a karyotype should be obtained.

      b. Serum gonadotropin levels

            i. If these are elevated, the diagnosis of primary ovarian failure is made. A karyotype should be obtained.

            ii. The presence of a Y chromosome must be determined by karyotyping in all cases of elevated gonadotropins in women under the age of 30. The Y chromosome is associated with testicular tissue within the gonad, which indicates a predisposition to virilization and malignant tumor formation (25% of cases).

TABLE 53–2. Prolactin Levels Under Various Abnormal Conditions (Approximate Ranges)

Condition	Range[a] (ng/ml serum)	Comments
Primary hypothyroidism	30–100	Confirm with elevated TSH
Polycystic ovary syndrome	20–50	30–50% of patients have elevation
Anorexia nervosa	10–50	Often mild elevation of GH
Renal failure	10–50	Probably decreased clearance
Chronic high-level exercise	10–50	
Pituitary tumors		
Microadenomas	20–200	Not a firm distinction
Macroadenomas	>200	
Drug use		
Phenothiazines or other neuroleptics	20–200	Usually a dose-related return to normal after discontinuation
Birth control pills or other estrogens	15–50	About 1/3 of patients have mild elevations; if there is no return to normal, evaluate for pituitary tumor
Reserpine, amphetamines, and methyldopa	15–30	Usually mild elevations
Morphine, methadone	10–75	With chronic use, levels tend to be higher

[a] Normal: <23 follicular; 5–40 luteal.

Thirty percent of patients with a Y chromosome show no evidence of virilization.

iii. If the levels are normal or low, the patient should be evaluated for pituitary or hypothalamic tumors. If CT and/or MR scans are normal, the patient has functional hypothalamic amenorrhea.

Bibliography

Kleinberg D, et al. Galactorrhea: A study of 235 cases, including 48 with pituitary tumors. N Engl J Med 1977;296:589–600.

Morris DV, et al. The investigation of female gonadal dysfunction. Clin Endo Metab 1985;14:125.

Muschak A, et al. Clinical and laboratory evaluation of patients with primary amenorrhea. Obstet Gynecol 1981;57:715.

Speroff L, et al. Clinical Gynecologic Endocrinology and Infertility, 4th ed. Baltimore, Williams and Wilkins, 1989.

Williams RH, et al. Textbook of Endocrinology, 7th ed. Philadelphia, W.B. Saunders, 1985.

54

METABOLIC BONE DISEASE

NORMAN R. ROSENTHAL

Thy bones are hollow.

SHAKESPEARE (1564–1616) Measure for Measure

OSTEOPOROSIS

General Comments and Differential Diagnosis

- Primary osteoporosis is most commonly observed in elderly women and men. With the exception of patients treated chronically with steroid medication, secondary causes of osteoporosis remain uncommon (Table 54–1).
- In all causes the underlying disturbance is an increased rate of bone resorption relative to formation with eventual net loss of bone mass. Mineralization of bone remains intact.
- Secondary osteoporosis
  1. Glucocorticoid excess
     a. Chronic treatment with steroids produces severe osteoporosis that is indistinguishable from primary osteoporosis.
     b. Endogenous Cushing's syndrome can cause osteoporosis, but it is a rare finding in the osteoporotic population.
  2. Hyperthyroidism
     a. Clinically apparent bone disease as part of the initial presentation of thyrotoxicosis is rare today. Nonetheless, patients should be screened with thyroid function tests.
     b. Excessive thyroid hormone replacement therapy can promote a reduction in bone density. Whether this results in a higher fracture rate is uncertain.
  3. Hyperparathyroidism
     a. Patients rarely demonstrate classical bone changes of chronic parathyroid hormone (PTH) excess (osteitis fibrosa cystica).
     b. Secondary osteoporosis is the more typical skeletal manifestation of this disease. Attenuated bone mass is often detected by dual photon absorptiometry.
     c. An elevated serum calcium and a low normal serum phosphate indicates the need to exclude hyperparathyroidism.

TABLE 54–1. Classification of Osteoporosis

Primary osteoporosis
  Postmenopausal
  Senile (age-related)
Secondary osteoporosis
  Endocrine abnormality
    Hyperparathyroidism
    Cushing's syndrome
    Hyperthyroidism
    Testosterone deficiency
    Diabetes mellitus
  Drugs
    Corticosteroids
    Heparin
    Alcohol
  Immobilization
  Malignancies
    Multiple myeloma
    Lymphoma
    Leukemia
  Miscellaneous
    Systemic mastocytosis
    Chronic liver disease
    Rheumatoid arthritis

4. Testosterone deficiency
   a. Premature loss of gonadal function can lead to clinically significant reductions in bone mass.
   b. Loss of libido, erectile dysfunction, and change in shaving habits are common associated symptoms.
   c. Men who present with osteopenia before the age of 65 should have serum LH and testosterone levels measured.
5. Diabetes mellitus. Although decreased bone density can be seen in patients with insulin-dependent diabetes, clinically significant osteoporosis is not common.
6. Immobilization. Prolonged periods of bedrest such as occurs with spinal cord diseases can result in profound bone loss due to increased bone resorption and diminished bone formation. Young patients can develop hypercalcemia in addition to hypercalciuria.
7. Malignancies. Multiple myeloma should be considered in the patient complaining of back pain from a vertebral body compression fracture who is found to have an anemia and an elevated ESR.

Clinical Features

- Symptoms/History
  1. General. The typical patient with primary osteoporosis is a light-framed elderly Caucasian woman over the age of 65 years. A positive family history is common (Table 54–2).

TABLE 54–2. Risk Factors for Primary Osteoporosis

Gender: female
Race: Caucasian or Asian
Family History: positive for osteoporosis
Premature menopause: surgical or autoimmune
Body habitus: slim
Lifestyle
sedentary
cigarettes
Gravida status: nulliparous
Dietary factors
low calcium intake
alcohol overuse
? high sodium intake
? high phosphate intake
? high caffeine intake

2. Acute back pain. This is usually located in the lower thoracic and upper lumbar region. It results from vertebral body compression fractures. Lifting, stooping, or coughing are frequent precipitating events. Radicular pain is uncommon.
3. Chronic back pain. This may be due to paravertebral muscle spasm associated with compression fractures.
4. Spinal deformity. Chronic vertebral compression fractures may cause progressive loss of height and dorsal kyphosis ("dowager's hump").
5. Long bone fractures most commonly occur in the femoral neck or distal radius.

- Signs/Examination
  1. Few characteristic features are found on examining the patient with primary osteoporosis. Physical findings indicative of secondary causes of osteoporosis may be present.
  2. Tenderness on palpation over recently fractured vertebrae and spasm of paravertebral muscles commonly occur. Dorsal kyphosis can progressively worsen and create a pronounced downward angulation of the ribs.

Laboratory Findings

- In typical primary osteoporosis, serum calcium, phosphate, and alkaline phosphatase concentrations are normal. The diagnosis is based in part on the exclusion of causes of secondary osteoporosis.
- Imaging studies
  1. The most common feature is radiographic osteopenia. (Table 54–3).
     a. The earliest and best visualized changes occur in the spine, which has predominantly trabecular bone.

TABLE 54–3. Features of Vertebral Osteopenia

Generalized thinning

Loss of transverse trabeculation with the paradoxical appearance of both cortical end-plate region accentuation and vertical striations.

Biconcave compression of cortical end-plates ("codfish deformity")

Anterior wedge compression fractures

    b. Osteoporosis in regions that are predominantly cortical bone such as the skull, phalanges, and long bones is manifest as an overall increase in skeletal translucency.

    c. Routine skeletal radiographs do not show osteopenia until a 30 to 50% reduction of bone mass has occurred.

2. More sensitive techniques for measuring bone density include:

    a. Single photon absorptiometry

    b. Dual photon absorptiometry

    c. Dual energy X-ray absorptiometry

    d. Quantitative computed tomography (QCT)

3. These techniques can detect reduced bone density before it is seen on plain films and can monitor the rate of change of bone mass over time.

    a. Each method is widely available, and their choice in clinical practice reflects differences in accuracy, precision, cost, radiation exposure, patient acceptance, and bone site measurement.

    b. Although preliminary reports attest to the value of bone mass measurement in predicting future fracture rates in disease-free patients, no consensus exists for its use in the screening of unselected asymptomatic persons.

OSTEOMALACIA

General Comments and Differential Diagnosis

- Osteomalacia is due to a disorder of bone mineralization with subsequent accumulation of unmineralized bone matrix. This bone is weaker than normal and subject to deformity (in children) and fracture under normal stresses.

- Disturbances in either vitamin D or phosphate metabolism underlie this syndrome. In contrast to osteoporosis, a patient with osteomalacia has both osteopenia on skeletal films and changes in serum calcium and phosphate homeostasis.

- Vitamin D–related diseases (Table 54–4)

    1. Nutritional deficiency

       a. This problem is rare today but can occur in elderly patients with both deficient dietary intake and limited sunlight exposure.

TABLE 54–4. Classification of Osteomalacia

Vitamin D–related disease
- I. Nutritional deficiency
- II. Malabsorption
  - a. Small intestine disease
  - b. Pancreatic insufficiency
  - c. Bile salt depletion
  - d. Postgastrectomy
- III. Altered Metabolism
  - a. Defective synthesis of 25(OH)-D
    1. Chronic liver disease
    2. Anticonvulsant drug therapy
  - b. Defective synthesis of $1,25(OH)_2$-D
    1. Chronic renal failure
    2. Vitamin D–dependent rickets, Type I
  - c. End organ resistance to $1,25(OH)_2$-D
    1. Vitamin D–dependent rickets, Type II

Phosphate-related disease
- I. Renal phosphate wasting
  - a. Familial hypophosphatemic rickets
  - b. Fanconi's syndrome
  - c. Oncogenic osteomalacia
- II. Malnutrition
- III. Phosphate-binding antacid abuse

Miscellaneous
- I. Bisphosphonates
- II. Systemic acidosis
- III. Total parenteral nutrition

---

   b. Infants who are exclusively breast fed without vitamin supplementation are also at risk.
2. Malabsorption is the most common cause of vitamin D–deficient osteomalacia.
3. Altered vitamin D metabolism
  - a. Severe liver disease rarely causes clinical disorders related to vitamin D metabolism unless associated with obstruction of the biliary tree and subsequent malabsorption.
  - b. Anticonvulsant drugs infrequently cause osteomalacia, but patients at risk indicate a history of poor dietary intake and poor sunlight exposure.
  - c. Chronic renal failure
    - i. Renal damage leading to impaired conversion of 25-hydroxyvitamin D [25(OH)-D] to its active metabolite 1,25-dihydroxyvitamin D [$1,25(OH)_2$-D] is the most common form of osteomalacia due to altered vitamin D metabolism.
    - ii. Renal osteodystrophy covers a spectrum of disorders, but osteomalacia is usually the earliest bone lesion reflecting reduced levels of $1,25(OH)_2$-D and toxic effects of aluminum. Other lesions include:
      - (a). Hyperparathyroidism
      - (b). Osteoporosis

   (c). Osteosclerosis

   (d). Aluminum-induced osteomalacia

  iii. The dominant bone lesion varies among patients, and a given patient might exhibit combinations of histologic abnormalities. A metabolic bone biopsy will clarify this issue.

- Phosphate-related diseases (see Table 54–4)
  1. The most common mechanism for chronic hypophosphatemia is renal phosphate wasting. Inadequate dietary intake and impaired intestinal absorption by phosphate-binding antacids rarely lead to this metabolic disturbance.
  2. Familial hypophosphatemic rickets
     a. This is one of the most common forms of osteomalacia, and is an X-linked dominant disorder that causes bone disease and short stature in children.
     b. These patients demonstrate renal phosphate wasting and inappropriately low levels of $1,25(OH)_2$-D.
     c. An adult form of this disease can occur as either a sporadic or familial condition.
  3. Renal tubular disorders (Fanconi's syndrome)
     a. These cause excessive renal loss of phosphate, amino acids, magnesium bicarbonate, glucose, and uric acid.
     b. This syndrome can be sporadic or inherited or can result from dysproteinemias, Wilson's disease, heavy metal poisoning, tetracycline, or glycogen storage diseases.
  4. Oncogenic osteomalacia
     a. This syndrome occurs when highly vascular, usually benign tumors of mesenchymal origin secrete a circulating factor capable of causing phosphaturia.
     b. The level of $1,25(OH)_2$-D is suppressed.
     c. These tumors can be small and difficult to localize, but excision of the tumor results in complete clinical recovery.
     d. Other tumors reported to cause this syndrome include prostatic cancer, epidermal nevus syndrome, and fibrous dysplasia.
- Miscellaneous causes of osteomalacia
  1. Etidronate, a bisphosphonate used to treat osteoporosis and Paget's disease, inhibits bone mineralization and can result in osteomalacia if administered either at too high doses or for long periods.
  2. Longstanding acidosis of any cause can promote osteomalacia. Distal renal tubular acidosis must be excluded.
  3. Total parenteral nutrition can result in osteomalacia if solution phosphate concentrations are not adequate.

Clinical Features

- Symptoms/History
  1. Adults with mild osteomalacia are often asymptomatic.
  2. Eventually patients complain of bone pain, commonly

in the ribs, pelvis, and/or legs, and proximal muscle weakness. These symptoms are often vague and insidious in onset.
3. Symptoms of hypocalcemia, such as paresthesias or tetany, are also rarely encountered.
- Signs/Examination
1. Proximal muscle weakness and bone tenderness, especially over tibia surfaces, are usually present.
2. Unlike rickets, skeletal deformities are rare. However, children may have short stature, bowing of legs, and skull deformities.

Laboratory Findings

- Biochemical abnormalities of serum calcium and/or phosphate in the presence of osteopenia indicate that osteomalacia, not osteoporosis, is the underlying disorder.
- Pathophysiology
1. In defense against hypocalcemia, PTH release mobilizes calcium directly from bone and kidney, and indirectly from the gut by stimulating the renal production of $1,25(OH)_2$-D, the active vitamin D metabolite.
2. As a consequence of vitamin D deficiency or altered metabolism, hypocalcemia will result in a state of secondary hyperparathyroidism.
3. Chronic hypophosphatemia is usually the result of renal phosphate wasting. Some disorders are associated with other renal transport defects such as excessive urinary excretion of amino acids, glucose, magnesium, bicarbonate, and uric acid. Hypophosphatemia is normally a potent stimulator of $1,25(OH)_2$-D production, but the tubular defect may cause a reduced level of circulating $1,25(OH)_2$-D.
- Typical laboratory findings in vitamin D–related osteomalacia are:
1. Serum calcium: low or low-normal
2. Serum phosphate: low or low-normal
3. Serum alkaline phosphatase: elevated
4. Serum parathyroid hormone: elevated
5. Serum 25(OH)-D: low
6. Serum $1,25(OH)_2$-D: normal
7. Urine calcium: low
- Typical laboratory results in phosphate-related osteomalacia are:
1. Serum calcium: normal
2. Serum phosphate: low
3. Serum PTH: normal
4. Serum alkaline phosphatase: elevated
5. Serum 25(OH)-D: normal
6. Serum $1,25(OH)_2$-D: low or low-normal
- Imaging studies
1. In adults, the most common skeletal X-ray feature is generalized osteopenia that is usually indistinguishable from that seen in osteoporosis.

2. The presence of pseudofractures (Looser's zones or Milkman fractures), which are narrow radiolucencies extending from the cortex partway through the long bones, pelvis, and scapulae is uncommon but pathognomonic of osteomalacia.
3. Patients with secondary hyperparathyroidism have subperiosteal bone resorption; those with osteosclerosis may have a "rugger jersey spine."

RECOMMENDED DIAGNOSTIC APPROACH

- Make the diagnosis of osteopenia by imaging study. Most commonly, this occurs with routine X-rays of an asymptomatic person or during the evaluation of a patient presenting with back pain or a long bone fracture.
- Unselected screening for osteopenia with sensitive bone density measurement techniques is currently not recommended. Clinical situations where it may be useful include:
  1. Patients with equivocal X-ray evidence of osteopenia.
  2. Perimenopausal women considering long-term estrogen therapy.
  3. Patients with disorders such as primary hyperparathyroidism, hyperprolactinemic amenorrhea, or exogenous steroid usage in whom the presence of early secondary osteoporosis might lead to medical or surgical intervention.
  4. Monitoring drug efficacy when treating patients for osteoporosis.
- Once osteopenia is detected, screen for osteomalacia with serum electrolyte, urea nitrogen, creatinine, calcium, phosphate, and alkaline phosphatase determinations. If these are abnormal, characterize the abnormality with PTH and vitamin D determinations.
- Screen for secondary osteoporosis with measurements of serum calcium, protein electrophoresis, thyroid function tests, and serum LH and testosterone levels. Check the CBC and ESR, and, perhaps a urine protein electrophoresis. If clinically indicated, screen the patient for endogenous corticosteroid overproduction.

Bibliography

Health and Public Policy Committee, American College of Physicians. Bone mineral densitometry. Ann Intern Med 1987;107:932–936.

Jackson JA, Kleenekoper M. Osteoporosis in men: Diagnosis, pathophysiology, and prevention. Medicine 1990;69:137–152.

Lukert BP, Raisz LG. Glucocorticoid-induced osteoporosis: Pathogenesis and management. Ann Intern Med 1990;112:352–364.

Melton LJ III, et al. Screening for osteoporosis. Ann Intern Med 1990;112:516–528.

Riggs LB, Melton JL. Clinical heterogeneity of involutional osteoporosis: Implications for preventive therapy. J Clin Endo Metab 1990;70:1229–1232.

Tiegs RD, ed. Metabolic bone disease, parts 1 and 2. Endocrinol Metabol Clin North Amer 1989;18:833–1031 and 1990;19:1–209.

55

THYROID DISEASE

MITCHELL KARTON

> New York, the nation's thyroid gland.
>
> CHRISTOPHER MARLEY (1890–1957)

GENERAL COMMENTS

- Hypo- and hyperthyroidism are functional abnormalities of thyroid metabolism with a number of causes (Tables 55–1 and 55–2).
- The most common abnormality of thyroid structure is the goiter, which is defined as an enlargement of the thyroid gland (Table 55–3). A goiter may be diffuse or nodular. It may be associated with hypo-, hyper-, or euthyroid states.

THYROID FUNCTION TESTS (Table 55–4)

- Serum triiodothyronine (T_3) and total thyroxine (T_4) levels
  1. More than 99% of serum T_3 and T_4 is bound to serum carrier proteins and is inactive. Levels of free (physiologically active) hormone may be measured by radioimmunoassay.
  2. A cheaper and easier approach measures total T_4 (bound and unbound) and uses an indirect measurement of the T_4 free fraction known as the T_3 uptake test (T_3U, previously called T_3 resin uptake). The T_3U measures the degree of saturation of the available T_4 binding sites on the major carrier protein thyroxine-binding globulin (TBG).
  3. If TBG is increased (by medication or other illnesses) and thus produces abnormally high total T_4 measurements, but free T_4 is normal, the T_3U will be low, and the product of total $T_4 \times T_3U$, known as the free thyroid index (FT_4I), falls within the normal range.
  4. If the patient is truly hyperthyroid, the total T_4 and the T_3U are elevated, as is the FT_4I.
  5. The reverse of these situations occurs with a euthyroid patient with lowered TBG and one with hypothyroidism.
- Thyroid-stimulating hormone (TSH)
  1. TSH stimulates all steps in hormone synthesis and secretion. It can be measured by radioimmunoassay.
  2. Hypothyroid patients have a high serum TSH level except for hypothyroidism resulting from intrinsic pituitary or hypothalamic disease (rare).

TABLE 55–1. Classification of Hypothyroidism

Thyroid
- A. Thyroprivic (insufficient functional tissue)
  1. Postablative: surgery or radioactive iodine
  2. Primary idiopathic
  3. Sporadic cretinism (aplasia/dysplasia)
  4. Endemic cretinism (often atrophic)
  5. Congenital TSH resistance
  6. Postradiation (e.g., for lymphoma)
- B. Goitrous
  1. Endemic iodine deficiency with or without goitrous cretinism
  2. Hashimoto's thyroiditis
  3. Defective hormone biosynthesis
     Iodide transport
     Organification defect
     Iodotyrosine coupling defect
     Iodotyrosine dehalogenase defect
     Abnormal iodoprotein secretion
  4. Goitrogens
     Dietary: rutabaga, white turnip, soy, cabbage
     Maternally transmitted: iodides, antithyroid agents
     Drug-induced: lithium, para-aminosalicylic acid, phenylbutazone, iodides, propylthiouracil, methimazole, cobalt, resorcinol

Suprathyroid
- A. Hypothalamic
- B. Pituitary
  1. Tumor
  2. Necrosis (Sheehan's syndrome)
  3. Isolated TSH deficit (extremely rare)

TABLE 55–2. Classification of Thyrotoxicosis

With hyperthyroidism
  Graves' disease
  Toxic multinodular goiter
  Toxic adenoma (uninodular goiter)
  Thyroid carcinoma
  TSH hypersecretion (pituitary adenoma) (rare)
  Trophoblastic disease: hydatidiform mole, choriocarcinoma

Without hyperthyroidism
  Thyroiditis: pyogenic, subacute (de Quervain's), chronic painless with transient thyrotoxicosis
  Ectopic thyroid tissue: struma ovarii
  Thyrotoxicosis factitia
  Jodbasedow phenomenon: iodide-induced

TABLE 55–3. Goiters and Nodules

DISEASE STATUS	GLAND	CLINICAL
Goitrous hypothyroidism	Smooth, diffusely enlarged	Hypothyroid
Hashimoto's disease	Pebbly, diffusely firm, mildly enlarged	Eu- or hypothyroid
Graves' disease	Smooth, diffusely enlarged	Hyperthyroid
Multinodular goiter	Large goiter, irregular with many nodules	Eu- or hyperthyroid
Adenoma	Solitary nodule	Eu- or hyperthyroid
Hemorrhage into preexistent nodule	Acute painful enlargement	Euthyroid
Subacute thyroiditis	Usually tender, finely nodular swelling	Hyperthyroid
Carcinoma	Usually single hard nodule or normal gland with regional adenopathy	Euthyroid

3. TSH levels may help monitor thyroid replacement in hypothyroidism. A normal level implies an adequate dose, but clinical status is the ultimate criterion.
4. Newer "supersensitive" TSH assays may help differentiate between a low serum TSH (thyrotoxicosis or pituitary hypothyroidism) and low-normal levels. Supersensitive TSH assays may become the universal thyroid function test.

- Thyrotropin-releasing hormone (TRH) stimulation test
  1. When a patient has sufficient or increased levels of thyroid hormone, the response of TSH secretion to administration of TRH is greatly diminished. This occurs in thyrotoxicosis, elderly patients, and in euthyroid Graves' disease with ophthalmopathy.
  2. In hypothyroid patients and premenopausal women in the preovulatory phase of the menstrual cycle, the TSH response is increased.
  3. This test is useful in the following situations:
     a. Diagnosis of early or developing hyperthyroidism, when the total T_4 may still be within the normal range: response of TSH to exogenously administered TRH is blunted.
     b. Separation of pituitary from hypothalamic hypothyroidism, when both T_4 and TSH are below normal: if pituitary, the TSH response is "blunted" or

TABLE 55–4. Thyroid Function Tests

CONDITION	T_4 AND T_3	T_3U	FT_4I	TSH	RAIU	TRH STIMULATION
Hypothyroidism	Low	Low	Low	High[a]	Low or normal	Augmented response
Hyperthyroidism	High	High	High	Normal or low	High[b]	Blunted response
Euthyroid "sick" syndrome	Low[c]	High	Low	Normal	Normal	Normal
Pregnancy, estrogens, acute liver disease, acute intermittent porphyria	High	Low	Normal	Normal	Normal	Normal
Androgens, hypoproteinemia, chronic liver disease, glucocorticoid excess	Low	High	Normal	Normal	Normal	Normal

[a] Pituitary or hypothalamic hypothyroidism is associated with a low or normal TSH.
[b] Thyrotoxicosis caused by thyroiditis or exogenous administration of thyroid hormone is associated with a low RAIU.
[c] Reverse T_3 is elevated, except in certain cases of chronic renal disease in which T_3 is elevated and reverse T_3 normal.

absent; if hypothalamic, TSH increases normally after TRH administration, but after an hour's delay, due to the need for synthesis to occur.

c. Diagnosis of euthyroid Graves' disease with ophthalmopathy: if the TSH response is decreased, the test is helpful; a normal response is nondiagnostic.

d. Predicting the adequacy of T_4 suppression in patients with thyroid cancer. Some patients have undetectable basal T_4 levels, but still have a normal TRH stimulation response.

- Radioactive iodine uptake (RAIU)
  1. This test involves giving the patient a dose of iodine-131 (^{131}I) and assessing radioactivity in the gland at selected time intervals (usually after 24 hr).
  2. In a hyperthyroid patient with hormone overproduction there is an increased uptake (usually greater than 30% at 24 hr). If a patient is hypothyroid, the RAIU is often low.
  3. This test helps differentiate between causes of thyrotoxicosis. If the gland is overproducing thyroid hormone (e.g., Graves' disease), the RAIU is increased. If the thyrotoxic state is the result of release of prestored hormone from an inflamed gland (e.g., thyroiditis) or of exogenous thyroid hormone administration, the RAIU is decreased.

- "Euthyroid sick syndrome"
  1. Serious nonthyroidal illnesses, starvation, and the postsurgical state can produce a characteristic pattern of thyroid function abnormalities that must be differentiated from hypothyroidism.
  2. The T_3 is low, T_4 is low to normal, T_3U and reverse T_3 are increased. The TSH level is normal.
  3. Chronic liver disease may cause an elevated T_4, T_3, and TSH. In patients with chronic renal disease, the reverse T_3 may not be elevated.

HYPOTHYROIDISM

- Definition
  1. Hypothyroidism is characterized by insufficient production of thyroid hormone. Hypothyroidism may be primary or secondary (due to intrinsic pituitary or hypothalamic disease).
  2. Myxedema consists of hypothyroidism plus deposition of hydrophilic mucopolysaccharides in the ground substance of the dermis and other tissues.
  3. Congenital hypothyroidism associated with myxedema, mental retardation, and other developmental abnormalities is called cretinism.

- Epidemiology and general comments
  1. Primary hypothyroidism may be goitrous resulting from excessive stimulation of the gland by TSH with inadequate compensatory production of thyroid hor-

mone. Primary hypothyroidism may also be thyroprivic, from the loss of enough thyroid tissue so enough hormone for metabolic needs cannot be produced.

2. Hashimoto's thyroiditis, a chronic lymphocytic infiltration of the gland, is the most common cause of goitrous hypothyroidism in North American adults, especially middle-aged females. It is also the most common cause of sporadic goiter in children. There is a familial predisposition.

3. In areas of the world that have iodine deficiency, endemic goiter and goitrous cretinism may be found more frequently. Congenital hypothyroidism occurs in 1 of 5000 births.

4. The most common cause of thyroprivic hypothyroidism is postablative hypothyroidism, which usually appears after treatment for Graves' disease.

5. Primary idiopathic hypothyroidism may be part of an autoimmune constellation, including pernicious anemia, SLE, rheumatoid arthritis, Sjögren's syndrome, or chronic active hepatitis.

6. Pituitary and hypothalamic insufficiency account for less than 5% of all cases of hypothyroidism.

- Clinical features
  1. Features pertinent to all cases of hypothyroidism include prior thyroid disease and treatment and goitrogenic drugs and foods (see Table 55–1).
  2. The symptoms and signs of hypothyroidism vary with the patient's age:
     a. Infant. Developmental milestones are delayed; cretinous physicality (short stature, a broad nose, widely set eyes, a protruding tongue, and a protuberant abdomen with umbilical hernia); mental retardation.
     b. Children. Signs include mental retardation, short stature, delayed puberty, and poor school performance.
     c. Adult. The onset is nonspecific and insidious. There may be a continuum of the following signs and symptoms:
        i. Lethargy, cold intolerance, constipation, and menorrhagia or amenorrhea
        ii. Slowing of intellectual processes and motor activities, decreased appetite and weight gain, and bradycardia
        iii. Hair that becomes coarse and dry and then falls out, muscular stiffness, voice deepening with hoarseness, and diminished hearing
        iv. Delay in relaxation time of deep tendon reflexes, pale and cool doughy skin, flat expressionless facies, cardiomegaly, possibly with a pericardial effusion, adynamic ileus, and ataxia
        v. Myxedematous coma with hypothermia and respiratory depression
  3. Features relevant to Hashimoto's thyroiditis include a history of other autoimmune disorders and a goiter that

usually has a well-delineated scalloped margin and a rubbery or pebblelike consistency. The goiter is nontender, and the pyramidal lobe may be prominent.

- Laboratory features
  1. Thyroid function tests
     a. The T_4 and FT_4I are low, TSH high, and RAIU low.
     b. In pituitary or hypothalamic hypothyroidism, TSH is normal or low, and the TRH stimulation test differentiates between the causes.
     c. In Hashimoto's disease, the early stages are characterized by a normal T_4/T_3 with high TSH and slightly high RAIU. In later stages, there is low T_4, then low T_3 and very high TSH with low RAIU.
  2. High-titer antibodies directed against various thyroid antigens especially antithyroglobulin antibody and antimicrosomal antibody, are common in Hashimoto's disease. Occasionally, they are present in primary idiopathic hypothyroidism as well.
  3. Other laboratory abnormalities may include elevations of serum cholesterol, creatine phosphokinase, aspartate aminotransferase (AST, SGOT), and LDH levels.
  4. Ten percent of patients with idiopathic primary hypothyroidism have histamine-fast achlorhydria.
  5. The EKG may show bradycardia, low voltage, and inverted T waves.
  6. X-rays may show retarded bone age, epiphyseal dysgenesis, and delayed dental development in infants. Children may have delayed union of epiphyses. Adults may have an enlarged cardiac shadow.

THYROTOXICOSIS

- Thyrotoxicosis is a clinical syndrome resulting from an excess of functioning thyroid hormone. It may result from hyperthyroidism (sustained hyperfunctioning of the thyroid gland), but not all thyrotoxic states are associated with hyperthyroidism (see Table 55–2).
- Important causes of thyrotoxicosis are:
  1. Graves' disease, characterized by hyperthyroidism with diffuse toxic goiter, ophthalmopathy, and dermopathy. These manifestations are independent in appearance and natural history.
  2. Toxic multinodular goiter is an enlarged thyroid gland with more than one region with altered structure and function. No inflammation or neoplasia is present.
  3. Toxic adenomas are well-encapsulated single nodules (occasionally 2 or 3) functioning autonomously in the absence of TSH.
  4. Subacute thyroiditis (de Quervain's) is a temporary inflammation of the thyroid gland that is usually associated with an antecedent viral infection. Transient hyperthyroidism caused by leakage of excess preformed hormone from the gland characterizes both this condi-

tion and chronic painless thyroiditis with transient thyrotoxicosis.

5. Thyroid storm
   a. This syndrome of severe life-threatening thyrotoxicosis is characterized by the abrupt onset of fever, hypotension with volume depletion, tachyarrhythmias, diarrhea, jaundice, and CNS abnormalities. The syndrome may rapidly progress to coma, shock, and death.
   b. Thyroid storm is rare but may occur as a complication of surgery, infection, diabetic ketoacidosis, or trauma in incompletely treated or undiagnosed hyperthyroid patients.
   c. Thyroid storm is diagnosed clinically; laboratory studies cannot differentiate it from chronic thyrotoxicosis.

• Epidemiology and general comments
   1. Graves' disease occurs primarily in the third or fourth decade. It is more common in women and has familial predisposition.
   2. Toxic multinodular goiter is primarily a disease of the elderly. It often arises out of a longstanding simple goiter. Both conditions involve attempted compensation (by TSH-stimulated growth) for decreased efficiency of hormone synthesis.
   3. Toxic adenoma usually occurs in patients in their 30s or 40s. Unlike Graves' disease, there is no ophthalmopathy or dermopathy, and the thyrotoxic symptoms are usually less severe.

• Clinical features
   1. Graves's disease
      a. History
         i. Primary complaints include anxiety, restlessness, excessive sweating, heat intolerance, insomnia, weight loss despite good appetite, and hyperdefecation.
         ii. Premenopausal females may complain of oligomenorrhea or amenorrhea.
         iii. In older patients, cardiac symptoms (palpitations, angina, dyspnea) or myopathic symptoms (weakness, especially proximal) may predominate.
      b. Physical examination
         i. General signs include visible restlessness and "frightened facies." The eyes stare, with widened palpebral fissure and lid lag.
         ii. The skin is warm, moist, and velvety. The hair is silky and fine and alopecia may occur. The nails may be separated from the nail bed.
         iii. Cardiovascular signs include sinus tachycardia or atrial fibrillation, loud S_1, systolic flow murmur, and possible cardiomegaly and CHF.
         iv. Neurologic signs include hyperreflexia, fine tremor of fingers and tongue, and proximal muscle weakness.

    v. There is asymmetric, possibly lobular, diffuse goiter. Bruits may be present over the thyroid gland.

    vi. Graves' ophthalmopathy should be distinguished from the reversible ocular signs of sympathetic overstimulation. There is true exophthalmos with proptosis, ophthalmoplegia, first with loss of superotemporal gaze and eventually all but downward gaze; and chemosis. Conjunctival and periorbital edema may lead to corneal ulceration and optic atrophy.

    vii. Graves' dermopathy may develop during thyrotoxicosis or after treatment. There is pretibial myxedema that is notable for well-demarcated peau d'orange skin, pruritus, and hyperpigmentation over the dorsum of the legs and feet. Occasionally, clubbing of the fingers and toes is present (thyroid acropachy).

2. Toxic multinodular goiter (MNG)
   a. History
      i. Toxic MNG is commonly asymptomatic and an incidental finding on physical examination.
      ii. When symptoms occur, cardiac symptoms predominate.
      iii. Complaints specifically referable to the goiter may include dysphagia, stridor, dyspnea, and hoarseness. If hemorrhage into the gland occurs, acute painful neck enlargement may be the presenting sign.
      iv. If the patient has a history of neck irradiation, malignancy should be considered.
   b. Physical examination
      i. General examination may show signs of apathetic hyperthyroidism in the elderly, such as asthenia, emotional lability, muscle weakness, and wasting.
      ii. In the head and neck there may be evidence of upper airway obstruction, hoarseness, and Horner's syndrome.
      iii. The thyroid is enlarged with multiple nodules of varying consistency. Nodules are palpable when the gland is twice normal size and visible at 3 times normal size.

3. Toxic adenoma
   a. Often there is a long history of a neck lump. Symptoms of thyrotoxicosis usually are present only with nodules larger than 3 cm.
   b. The thyroid has a smooth well-defined mass that moves with the thyroid. There are no bruits over the gland.

4. Thyroiditis
   a. Pyogenic thyroiditis is characterized by swelling, tenderness, erythema, and pain over the gland. Constitutional symptoms and signs of infection are usually present.

b. Subacute thyroiditis often follows an upper respiratory infection. The gland is usually painful and has tender nodularity on examination. Occasionally there is no pain over the gland and referred pain to the ear or jaw and systemic malaise dominate the clinical picture.

c. Chronic thyroiditis with thyrotoxicosis is characterized by a painless firm gland of normal or only slightly enlarged size.

5. Solitary thyroid nodules

a. Approximately 70% of thyroid nodules are "cold" on isotope scan. Only 10% are hyperfunctioning thyrotoxic adenomas which suppress the function of the rest of the gland.

b. "Cold" nodules are typically benign, but 10 to 20% of all "cold" nodules harbor malignancy.

c. Historical and examination features that suggest malignancy are listed in Table 55–5.

- Laboratory features

1. Graves' disease

a. Thyroid function test changes include high T_4/T_3, T_3U, FT_4I, and RAIU. TSH by supersensitive assay should be suppressed.

b. Long-acting thyroid stimulators (LATS) are present in half of patients.

c. Occasionally all are normal except for high T_3 and FT_3I.

d. For confirmation of diagnosis in early thyrotoxicosis (such as euthyroid Graves' disease with ophthalmopathy), the TRH stimulation test should be used.

e. Thyroid scans show diffuse thyromegaly.

2. Toxic MNG

a. Usually all laboratory results are within the normal range. If T_3 is in the upper range or normal,

TABLE 55–5. Thyroid Nodules: Risk Factors for Malignancy

	HIGHER RISK	LOWER RISK
Age	Younger than 30 Older than 65	Middle age
Sex	Male	Female
Consistency	Hard	Soft
Size	Enlarging	Shrinking
Radiation history	Yes	No
Adenopathy	Yes	No
Solitary	Yes	No[a]
Thyroid function tests	Normal	Hyper- or hypothyroid
RAIU	Cold	Hot
Ultrasound	Solid	Cystic

[a] Multinodular glands in patients with a history of neck irradiation are still worrisome.

hyperthyroidism may be present because the T_3 level usually decreases with age.

b. To confirm early disease, the TRH stimulation test should be used.

c. Scans only confirm diagnosis of multinodularity, not thyrotoxicosis.

d. Neck X-rays may show punctate calcifications of medullary carcinoma or concentric calcifications of a benign nodule. Barium swallow may show esophageal or tracheal displacement.

3. Toxic adenoma

   a. Thyroid function tests remain normal until late, when T_4 and T_3 both increase.

   b. The thyroid scan shows a hot nodule with early uptake and no T_3 suppression (although early there may be some function in the rest of the gland).

4. Thyroiditis

   a. In subacute thyroiditis, key laboratory findings are an elevated ESR and a depressed RAIU. Early thyroid function tests may be elevated owing to leakage of hormone, with transiently hypothyroid values later.

   b. In chronic thyroiditis with thyrotoxicosis, laboratory tests show slightly elevated T_4/T_3 with low RAIU, normal or slightly elevated ESR, and absent or low antibody levels.

5. Solitary thyroid nodule. Risk for malignancy may include normal thyroid function tests, a "cold" nodule on scan, and a solid (not cystic) nodule on ultrasound examination. Diagnosis of malignancy must be made by needle aspiration or biopsy, or surgery.

RECOMMENDED DIAGNOSTIC APPROACH

- Hypothyroidism

  1. A normal TSH rules out hypothyroidism (unless there is a pituitary or hypothalamic cause).

  2. An elevated TSH with low T_4 and T_3U rules in hypothyroidism.

     a. The TRH stimulation test is used to differentiate between pituitary and hypothalamic causes when secondary hypothyroidism is suspected.

     b. Antibody titers are used to confirm Hashimoto's thyroiditis. If the diagnosis is unclear, and certainty is necessary, biopsy should be performed.

- Thyrotoxicosis

  1. Thyrotoxicosis is ruled out with a normal T_4 and T_3U, though, occasionally, only T_3 is elevated. The TSH level measured by a supersensitive assay may help distinguish between suppressed and low-normal values.

  2. Thyrotoxicosis is ruled in with an elevated T_4 and T_3U. Occasionally, only T_3 is elevated, and it should be

measured if thyrotoxicosis is strongly suspected but
FT$_4$I is normal.

a. The TRH stimulation test is used to diagnose early
thyrotoxicosis or euthyroid Graves' disease with
ophthalmopathy.

b. RAIU helps to differentiate between hyperthyroidism and thyrotoxicosis without hyperthyroidism (e.g., thyroiditis, thyrotoxicosis factitia).

c. Thyroid scans help to locate functioning ectopic
thyroid tissue.

• Solitary nodules

1. Malignancy is ruled out with a "hot" nodule on thyroid
scan.

2. Malignancy is ruled in with positive biopsy results.

Bibliography

Borst GC, et al. Euthyroid hyperthyroxinemia. Ann Intern Med
1983;98:366–378.

Chopra IJ, et al. Thyroid function in nonthyroidal illnesses. Ann Intern
Med 1983;98:946–957.

DeGroot LJ, et al. Endocrinology, 2nd ed. Philadelphia, W.B. Saunders, 1989.

Ehrmann DA, Sarne DH. Serum thyrotropin and the assessment of
thyroid status. Ann Intern Med 1989;110:179–181.

Hamburger JI. The various presentations of thyroiditis: Diagnostic
considerations. Ann Intern Med 1986;104:219–224.

Helfand M, Crapo LM. Screening for thyroid disease. Ann Intern Med
1990;112:840–849.

Helfand M, Crapo LM. Monitoring therapy in patients taking levothy-
roxine. Ann Intern Med 1990;113:450–454.

Ingbar S, Braverman LH. Werner's The Thyroid, 5th ed. Philadelphia,
J.B. Lippincott, 1986.

Rojeski MI, Gharib H. Nodular thyroid disease. N Engl J Med
1985;313:428–436.

Stanbury JB, Wang C-A. Nontoxic goiter. Thyroid Today 1981;4:3.

56

ADRENAL GLAND DISEASES

WILFRED Y. FUJIMOTO

In treating a patient, let your first thought be to strengthen his natural vitality. New medicine, and new methods of cure, always work miracles for a while.

WILLIAM HEBERDEN (1710–1801)

GLUCOCORTICOID EXCESS (CUSHING'S SYNDROME)

Definitions and General Comments

- Cushing's syndrome results from excess glucocorticoid. An exogenous excess is far more common than an endogenous one.
- Endogenous overproduction of glucocorticoid results from dysfunction of the homeostatic system of cortisol production (hypothalamus, pituitary, or adrenal cortex) or ectopically produced adrenocorticotropic hormone (ACTH).
- Cushing's syndrome refers to all clinical situations in which there is an excess of cortisol. Cushing's disease refers to Cushing's syndrome due to primary ACTH overproduction by the pituitary.

Differential Diagnosis

There are 4 underlying causes of endogenous Cushing's syndrome.

- Pituitary Cushing's syndrome
  1. ACTH overproduction causes bilateral adrenal hyperplasia and overproduction of cortisol and, to a lesser extent, other adrenal steroids. Pituitary ACTH overproduction causes two-thirds of all cases of endogenous hypercortisolism.
  2. Pituitary Cushing's syndrome is usually caused by a pituitary adenoma, most of which are microadenomas.
  3. Pituitary Cushing's syndrome is more common in females. The majority of cases occur in adults.

Adapted, with permission of author and publisher, from Fujimoto WY. Disorders of glucocorticoid homeostasis. In: Metz R, Larson E, eds. Blue Book of Endocrinology. Philadelphia, W.B. Saunders Company, 1986.

- Adrenal adenoma
  1. Cortisol-producing adenomas are usually unilateral and usually produce only cortisol. Thus, the clinical manifestations reflect pure glucocorticoid excess without symptoms of mineralocorticoid or sex steroid overproduction.
  2. Because adrenal sex steroid production may be diminished, the female patients, in contrast to those with pituitary Cushing's syndrome, usually do not have hirsutism or menstrual irregularities.
- Adrenocortical carcinoma
  1. The great majority of adrenocortical cancers produce excessive quantities of all adrenal hormones; in most of them androgens predominate.
  2. In adult males, the effects of excessive adrenal androgen may not be clinically apparent. In females and male children, adrenal cancers produce a Cushing's syndrome with conspicuous evidence of androgen excess usually manifest by rapidly progressive hirsutism.
  3. A few adrenal cancers produce estrogens, causing feminization in males.
  4. In children, adrenal cancer is the most common cause of endogenous Cushing's syndrome.
- Ectopic ACTH production
  1. Almost one-sixth of patients with Cushing's syndrome have ectopic ACTH production.
  2. Ectopic Cushing's syndrome is largely a disease of men and most often occurs in patients with lung cancer, especially small cell carcinomas. Many patients with lung cancer have elevated levels of circulating ACTH, but few show clinical evidence of hypercortisolism, because tumor ACTH may be biologically inert.
  3. Other tumors that may produce clinically apparent Cushing's syndrome include thymoma, bronchial carcinoid, carcinoma of the pancreatic islet, medullary cancer of the thyroid, and pheochromocytoma.
  4. The predominant clinical features are profound weakness, hyperpigmentation, weight loss, and edema. Ectopic Cushing's syndrome usually lacks the somatic features of other Cushing's syndromes (striae, obesity with characteristic fat distribution, plethora, and hirsutism), because the patient does not survive long enough for them to become apparent.
  5. The clinical manifestations of the ectopic Cushing's syndrome may be the first indication of an occult neoplasm, but the underlying tumor is usually obvious.

Clinical Features

The signs and symptoms of Cushing's syndrome are due to excess cortisol production modified by the underlying cause.

- Excess cortisol production (Table 56–1)
  1. The predominant metabolic effect of cortisol is stimulation of gluconeogenesis causing glucose production at the expense of protein anabolism.

TABLE 56–1. Manifestations of Hypercortisolism

Weight gain	Accumulation of adipose tissue, particularly centripetal (face, neck, trunk, limb girdles)
	Hyperphagia
Protein wasting	Thin skin
	Striae
	Capillary fragility (ecchymoses)
	Muscle wasting
	Muscle weakness
	Osteopenia (osteoporosis)
	Poor wound healing
	Growth retardation (children)
Carbohydrate intolerance	Increased glucose production, insulin resistance, impaired glucose utilization, hyperglycemia
Mineralocorticoid effect of cortisol	Hypertension, hypokalemia
Depressed immunity	Increased susceptibility to infections
Other	Downy hirsutism
	Oligomenorrhea
	Plethora
	Erythrocytosis
	Decreased intestinal calcium absorption
	Hypercalciuria
	Personality changes

2. Gluconeogenic action causes glucose intolerance and protein wasting manifest by muscle laxity and wasting (abdominal protuberance, flat buttocks, shrunken thighs), loss of subcutaneous protein (thin skin, striae), loss of bone matrix (osteopenia), poor wound healing, and capillary fragility (ecchymoses).

- Cushing's syndrome

  1. Clinical manifestations vary according to the cause.
  2. In ACTH excess, the patient usually shows the effects of glucocorticoid excess and evidence of androgen overproduction (hirsutism, acne, and occasionally frank virilization).
  3. Duration and extent of cortisol overproduction, age, gender, and the patient's underlying state of health are also important.

Laboratory Features

The diagnostic work-up is directed primarily at 2 questions: 1. Is there overproduction of glucocorticoid? 2. If so, what is the source of that overproduction?

- "Overnight" dexamethasone suppression test
  1. This is the customary first step in the work-up. The patient takes 1 mg of dexamethasone orally at about 11:30 p.m. (before retiring). Plasma cortisol is measured the next morning at 8:00 a.m.
  2. The patient should omit all but essential medications during the day preceding the morning sample and should arrive at the laboratory in a relaxed state.
  3. A plasma cortisol level of ≤ 5 μg/dl essentially excludes the possibility of Cushing's syndrome because the sensitivity exceeds 95%.
  4. False-positive tests (plasma cortisol > 5 μg/dl) may occur in up to one-fourth of hospitalized or chronically ill patients. Other causes include:
     a. Failure to take the dexamethasone at the proper time.
     b. Accelerated metabolism of dexamethasone (caused by drugs such as barbiturates, phenytoin, rifampin, or others that induce hepatic enzymes).
     c. Increased cortisol binding protein due to estrogen administration and obesity (15%).
     d. Depression, anxiety, anorexia nervosa, and uremia.
- Urinary free cortisol
  1. The 24-hour urine collection period should not include the time during which a dexamethasone suppression test is done.
  2. Urinary free cortisol reflects the free (unbound) cortisol concentration in plasma which increases disproportionately when the total plasma cortisol exceeds the level of saturation of corticosteroid binding globulin (about 20 μg/dl).
  3. Urinary free cortisol above 100 μg/day indicates excessive cortisol production. When the urinary free cortisol excretion rate is clearly diagnostic (above 200 μg/day), the presence of hypercortisolism is confirmed.
- "Formal" dexamethasone suppression test
  1. When measurement of urinary free cortisol is equivocal, this test can confirm the diagnosis of hypercortisolism and indicate the cause of the Cushing's syndrome. The test is performed as follows:

Day 1: baseline 24-hour urinary cortisol determination

Day 2: baseline 24-hour urinary cortisol determination

Day 3: administration of low-dose dexamethasone (0.5 mg every 6 hours) while collecting the urine to determine the 24-hour urinary cortisol

Day 4: administration of low-dose dexamethasone again during collection of 24-hour urinary cortisol

Day 5: administration of high-dose dexamethasone (2.0 mg every 6 hours) during collection of 24-hour urinary cortisol

Day 6: administration of high-dose dexamethasone during collection of 24-hour urinary cortisol

2. Urinary cortisol excretion that remains above 25 μg/24 hr after low-dose dexamethasone administration indicates Cushing's syndrome.

3. Failure of the cortisol to be suppressed after high-dose dexamethasone administration usually indicates adrenal Cushing's syndrome or ectopic Cushing's syndrome. Some patients with pituitary Cushing's syndrome fail to show suppression.

4. Suppression of the 24-hour urinary cortisol excretion to about 50% of baseline on the high dose in association with nonsuppression on the low dose indicates pituitary Cushing's syndrome.

5. The urinary dehydroepiandrosterone or 17-ketosteroids should be measured on days 1 and 2. Markedly elevated levels strongly suggest adrenal cancer.

- Imaging techniques (Table 56–2). The plasma ACTH assay and newer imaging techniques frequently obviate the need for the "formal" dexamethasone test.

Recommended Diagnostic Approach (Figure 56–1)

- Confirm a clinical diagnosis of Cushing's syndrome with the overnight dexamethasone suppression test. A positive test should be confirmed with a urinary free cortisol measurement. Occasionally the latter is the initial test of choice (if a false-positive overnight test is likely).

- Measure the plasma ACTH level

1. In Cushing's syndrome due to adrenal adenomas or carcinomas, the level is low.
2. In ectopic Cushing's syndrome, the level is very high.
3. In pituitary Cushing's syndrome the ACTH levels may be moderately elevated or normal.

TABLE 56–2. Anatomic Localization Tests

Pituitary Cushing's syndrome
  Visual fields
  Head CT scan
  Head MR scan
Adrenal Cushing's syndrome
  Abdominal CT scan
  Abdominal MR scan
  Abdominal ultrasound
  Adrenal scintiscan
  Venography
  Adrenal vein cortisol
  Arteriography
Ectopic Cushing's syndrome
  Chest X-ray
  Chest or abdominal CT scan
  Bronchogram
  GI X-ray

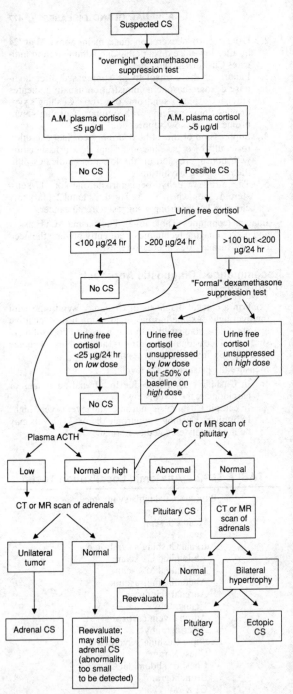

Figure 56–1. Diagnosis of Cushing's syndrome (CS). Exogenous glucocorticoids have been excluded.

- If the ACTH level is low, an abdominal CT or MR scan should be done to evaluate the adrenal glands.
- If ACTH levels are moderately high or normal, a CT or MR scan of the head should be done because of possibility of pituitary Cushing's syndrome. The CT scan shows a pituitary tumor in 80% of cases.
- If ACTH levels are very high and ectopic Cushing's syndrome is suspected, the highest yield procedures to find the responsible tumor are chest X-ray and chest CT scan.
- Occasionally in the search for suspected adrenal adenoma, other procedures, including adrenal scintiscan, venography or arteriography, or sampling of adrenal venous blood for cortisol are necessary.

GLUCOCORTICOID DEFICIENCY

Definitions and General Comments

- Glucocorticoid deficiency may be caused by adrenocortical destruction, a defect in cortisol biosynthesis, or deficient pituitary ACTH secretion.
- Addison's disease or primary adrenocortical insufficiency is glucocorticoid deficiency caused by adrenocortical destruction. Its incidence is the same in men and women and may occur at any age.
- Secondary adrenocortical insufficiency is caused by ACTH deficiency. It may be isolated or associated with deficiency of other pituitary hormones (hypopituitarism).

Differential Diagnosis

- Primary adrenocortical insufficiency
  1. This condition is now most often caused by idiopathic adrenal atrophy and may be caused by autoimmune adrenalitis. Sixty percent of patients have antiadrenal antibodies in the sera.
  2. Patients with idiopathic adrenal failure also have an increased risk of developing primary hypothyroidism, diabetes mellitus, idiopathic hypoparathyroidism, primary gonadal failure, or pernicious anemia as a result of autoimmune destruction of these other tissues.
  3. Infectious destruction of the adrenal glands by tuberculosis, previously the most common cause of primary adrenocortical insufficiency, now accounts for 20% of all cases.
  4. Other causes of primary adrenocortical failure are systemic fungal diseases, metastatic tumor to the adrenals, amyloidosis, adrenal hemorrhage (from anticoagulant therapy, sepsis, or trauma), and adrenalectomy.
- Secondary adrenocortical insufficiency. This is caused by deficient ACTH production by the pituitary. The most common cause is suppression of ACTH secretion by chronic glucocorticoid therapy for nonendocrine disease. ACTH deficiency may also arise from a primary pituitary or hypothalamic disorder.

Clinical Features

- Origin of glucocorticoid deficiency
  1. In primary adrenocortical insufficiency there is combined glucocorticoid and mineralocorticoid deficiency (Table 56–3), while in secondary adrenocortical insufficiency, mineralocorticoid production is unimpaired.
  2. In secondary adrenocortical insufficiency there may be clinical signs of deficiency of pituitary hormones in addition to ACTH.
- Primary adrenocortical insufficiency. In most cases primary adrenocortical insufficiency has a gradual onset. Compensatory increases in ACTH and renin enable the adrenal glands to secrete enough cortisol and aldosterone in the absence of stress. When more than 90% of the adrenal cortex has been destroyed, or stress occurs, compensation is inadequate.
- Acute adrenal insufficiency (Addisonian crisis). This condition is marked by nausea, vomiting, hypotension, abdominal pain, extreme muscle weakness, confusion, and, ultimately shock.
- Chronic adrenal insufficiency. The degree of insufficiency ranges from complete failure to a minor impairment of adrenal reserve capacity.
  1. Symptoms may be nonspecific and include weakness, weight loss, anorexia, and hypotension. If any of these

TABLE 56–3. Manifestations of Primary Adrenocortical Insufficiency

Cortisol deficiency

    Gastrointestinal: anorexia, nausea, vomiting, diarrhea, abdominal pain, weight loss, hypochlorhydria

    Mental: enervation, confusion, psychosis

    Metabolism: impaired fat mobilization and utilization, decreased gluconeogenesis, liver glycogen depletion, hypoglycemia

    Cardiovascular: impaired pressor response to catecholamines, hypotension

    Renal: impaired "free water" clearance

    Pituitary: increased ACTH secretion, hyperpigmentation

    Muscular: asthenia

    Other: eosinophilia, mild anemia

Aldosterone deficiency

    Inability to conserve sodium: decreased extracellular fluid and blood volume, weight loss, decreased cardiac size and output, prerenal azotemia, increased renin production, weakness, hypotension, postural syncope, shock

    Impaired renal secretion of potassium and hydrogen: hyperkalemia, mild acidosis

4 features are absent, the patient probably does not have Addison's disease.

2. A major complaint is asthenia, both mental and physical. Patients lose weight but may not do so until adrenal failure is well advanced.

3. Anorexia, nausea, and constipation alternating with diarrhea are increasingly frequent complaints as the disease progresses.

4. Skin pigmentation
   a. This often leads to suspicion of primary adrenal insufficiency. It is caused by increased melanin in the skin, particularly in regions normally pigmented and exposed to sunlight or pressure.
   b. Skin creases and scars acquired after the onset of adrenal insufficiency tend to be pigmented, while scars present before onset of primary adrenal failure remain unpigmented.
   c. Mucosal pigmentation of the mouth, conjunctiva, and vagina may also occur.
   d. Pigmentation may precede other features of hypoadrenalism by many years and may be first appreciated by the patient as a better suntan that lasts longer than usual.
   e. Vitiligo occurs in 10 to 20% of patients with primary adrenal failure.

5. Loss of body hair, reflecting loss of adrenal androgen production, may occur in women.

Laboratory Features

Since there is impaired tolerance to stress when cortisol is deficient, these manifestations typically become more pronounced during times of stress.

- Since one of the predominant metabolic effects of glucocorticoids is to stimulate gluconeogenesis, deficiency of cortisol results in fasting hypoglycemia.

- Glucocorticoids have cardiovascular and renal effects, and deficiency of cortisol results in impaired ability for free water excretion (causing hyponatremia). Hyperkalemia and azotemia may occur.

- Glucocorticoids stimulate hematopoiesis, gastric acid production, and reduction of blood eosinophils. Mild anemia, hypochlorhydria, and eosinophilia may occur in deficiency.

- Short ACTH stimulation test
  1. This is the customary first step in evaluation of a patient thought to have primary or secondary adrenocortical insufficiency.
  2. A blood sample is obtained for measurement of basal plasma level of cortisol. A portion of the sample is also set aside in case measurement of plasma ACTH concentration or aldosterone concentration is indicated after the results of this screening test are known.
  3. Cosyntropin (synthetic alpha [1-24]-ACTH), 0.25 mg, is then administered to the patient IM or IV, and blood

samples are withdrawn at 30 and 60 minutes for measurement of plasma cortisol. An additional sample is saved for possible determination of plasma aldosterone levels at a later time.

4. A normal response is marked by a basal plasma cortisol level $\geq 5\ \mu g/dl$, an increment $> 7\ \mu g/dl$, and a maximal value $> 18 \mu g/dl$.

5. If the patient is suspected of being in Addisonian crisis and immediate administration of glucocorticoid is deemed essential, dexamethasone should be used. The ACTH test can be done while dexamethasone is being given, since the latter does not interfere with subsequent measurements of plasma cortisol.

6. If a low level of cortisol is present, plasma ACTH should be measured in the sample that was set aside previously.

   a. Low plasma cortisol levels with elevated plasma ACTH levels are found with primary adrenocortical insufficiency.

   b. In fully developed secondary adrenocortical failure, ACTH is low.

   c. Since ACTH has a very short plasma half-life, if a patient is given glucocorticoids, the ACTH level will fall to the normal range within 15 to 30 minutes, even if it was initially elevated.

7. Plasma aldosterone levels may also be measured.

   a. The plasma aldosterone increment following ACTH stimulation is normally at least 5 ng/dl greater than baseline.

   b. With primary adrenocortical failure, aldosterone also fails to show the normal increase after ACTH stimulation, whereas in secondary adrenal failure, aldosterone has a normal increase.

- Metyrapone test

1. In cases in which adrenocortical insufficiency is unlikely but should be excluded, the metyrapone test may be performed. When the diagnosis of adrenocortical insufficiency is strongly suspected, the ACTH stimulation test (Figure 56–2) should be used. The metyrapone test is used much less frequently than the ACTH stimulation test.

2. Metyrapone is a competitive inhibitor of 11-beta-hydroxylase and thus inhibits the conversion of 11-deoxycortisol to cortisol.

3. The normal response to a block in cortisol biosynthesis is an increase in ACTH secretion with a consequent increase in steroid synthesis and a rise in the intermediate proximal to the block (11-deoxycortisol).

4. Metyrapone is given as a single dose of 30 mg/kg between 11 p.m. and midnight. The plasma deoxycortisol and cortisol are measured the following day at 8 a.m.

5. The 8 a.m. plasma 11-deoxycortisol level rises from baseline levels of $< 3\ \mu g/dl$ to $> 7\ \mu g/dl$ in normal subjects (with a concomitant fall in plasma cortisol to $< 6\ \mu g/dl$).

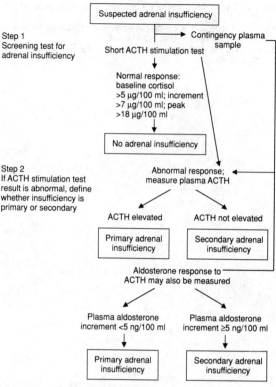

Figure 56–2. Diagnosis of adrenocortical insufficiency.

Recommended Diagnostic Approach

If the clinical picture suggests adrenocortical insufficiency, the following questions must be answered:

1. Is there inadequate production of glucocorticoid?
2. Is endogenous ACTH low or high?

The recommended diagnostic approach is shown in Figure 56–2.

Bibliography

Bayliss RIS. Adrenal cortex. Clin Endocrinol Metab 1980;9:477–486.

Burke CW. Adrenocortical insufficiency. Clin Endocrinol Metab 1985;14:947–976.

Carpenter PC. Diagnostic evaluation of Cushing's syndrome. Clin Endocrinol Metab 1988;17:445–472.

Howlett TA, et al. Cushing's syndrome. Clin Endocrinol Metab 1985;14:911–945.

Kaye TB, Crapo L. The Cushing syndrome: An update on diagnostic tests. Ann Intern Med 1990;112:434–444.

Kreiger DT. Physiopathology of Cushing's disease. Endocrinol Rev 1983;4:22–43.

57

PHEOCHROMOCYTOMA

DAVID HINDSON

Disease is very old, and nothing about it has changed. It is we who change, as we learn to recognize that which was formerly imperceptible.

JEAN MARTIN CHARCOT (1825–1893)

DEFINITION AND EPIDEMIOLOGY

1. Pheochromocytoma (pheo) is a tumor of the adrenal medullary or chromaffin cells. The tumor cells synthesize and secrete catecholamines (epinephrine, norepinephrine, and dopamine), often in bursts, and these secretory products are responsible for the many symptoms and signs of pheo.
2. The prevalence among hypertensive patients is estimated at 1 per 1000.
3. Ninety percent of these tumors are sporadic and 10% are familial.
4. The tumor is solitary in 90% of patients. It is located within the adrenal in 90% (usually 2 to 10 cm in size). Ten percent of pheos are extraadrenal (intraabdominal in 99%).

CLINICAL FEATURES

1. The hallmark of pheo is the presence of hypertension and "spells" (Table 57–1). Hypertension is the most consistent finding, present in more than 90% of patients. There is only a weak correlation between serum catecholamine levels and the blood pressure.
2. Most patients with pheo are symptomatic and suffer paroxysmal attacks (Table 57–2). Although usually discrete and of short duration, attacks may last a few hours.
3. Common symptoms during a spell include headache, palpitations, and sweating (see Table 57–1).
   a. Weakness and exhaustion are often prominent symptoms.
   b. Glucose intolerance is frequent, but overt diabetes is not common.
   c. Constipation and occasional pseudo-obstruction may occur.
   d. Arrhythmias may occur during a paroxysm.
   e. Postural hypotension is often present related to hypovolemia.

TABLE 57-1. Clinical Features of Pheochromocytoma

Hypertension (>90%)
    Sustained
    Sustained with labile character
Paroxysmal attacks ("spells")
    Headache (common)
    Palpitations (common)
    Sweating (common)
    Abdominal or chest pain
    Anxiety
    Tremor
    Pallor
    Nausea and/or vomiting
Postural hypotension
Weakness and exhaustion
Glucose intolerance, diabetes mellitus
Constipation
Hypermetabolism with heat intolerance, weight loss
Cholelithiasis

    f. Left ventricular hypertrophy and failure may result from the hypertension.

DIFFERENTIAL DIAGNOSIS

1. The symptoms and signs of pheo may suggest a number of alternative diagnoses (Table 57–3).
2. The proper patient selection for screening for pheo is controversial. Table 57–4 lists some of the widely accepted circumstances that should prompt further diagnostic testing.

TABLE 57-2. Pheochromocytoma Paroxysms

Symptoms (see Table 57–1)
Frequency: several per day to weekly
Duration: minutes to hours (usually <1 hr)
Usually stereotypic in a patient
Precipitants
    Usually unidentified
    Stress
    Anesthesia
    Exercise
    Pressure on tumor
    Sexual intercourse
    Drugs
    Radiographic contrast

TABLE 57–3. Differential Diagnosis

Hypertension: essential or secondary
Chronic anxiety or panic disorder; hyperventilation
Migraine
Thyrotoxicosis
Drug withdrawal or adverse effect
Autonomic dysreflexia
Angina pectoris
Factitious

LABORATORY STUDIES

1. Routine laboratory studies are generally unrevealing.
2. Biochemical testing for pheo includes either measurement of catecholamines in serum or urine or their metabolites in urine (Table 57–5).
   a. All tests are best performed in a drug-free patient; however, it is often difficult or dangerous to discontinue all medications.
3. Total catecholamines in the serum must be measured under rigorous conditions because of the effects of physiologic stimuli (e.g., upright posture, stress) on their level.
   a. The patient should be supine in a quiet room with blood drawn from an indwelling venous catheter in place for 30 min.
   b. Values less than 700 pg/ml are considered normal; values greater than 2000 pg/ml are usually diagnostic; values between 700 and 2000 are equivocal.
4. Urine vanillylmandelic acid (VMA) or metanephrines may be measured by a 24-hr urine collection or a timed 2-hr collection expressed as a ratio to creatinine.
   a. Values of urinary VMA greater than 11 mg/24 hr or metanephrines greater than 1.8 mg/24 hr are abnormal.
   b. Most often, all of the tests are markedly abnormal in patients with pheo, but false-negative or equivocal results do occur.
   c. For hypertensive patients with spells of headache, palpitation, and sweating, the predictive value of a

TABLE 57–4. Indications to Screen for Pheochromocytoma

Multiple endocrine neoplasia (MEN) II or III kindred
Phakomatoses
Incidentally discovered adrenal mass
Malignant hypertension
Paroxysmal or markedly labile hypertension
Hypertension with paroxysms of suggestive symptoms

TABLE 57–5. Diagnostic Tests for Pheochromocytoma

	SENSITIVITY (%)	SPECIFICITY (%)
Plasma catecholamines (>700 pg/ml)	60–95	80–95
Urinary metanephrines (>1.8 mg/24 hr)	60–95	80–95
Urinary VMA (>11 mg/24 hr)	50–90	80–95

single negative test is 98% and the predictive value of a positive test is 30 to 50%.

    d. Thus, any of these tests is adequate to rule out pheo, but a firm biochemical diagnosis requires either markedly abnormal test results or confirmatory diagnostic tests.

5. For patients in whom biochemical testing yields equivocal results, the clonidine suppression test is an excellent confirmatory test.

    a. Clonidine, 0.3 mg, is given orally to a supine patient through an indwelling venous catheter, and plasma catecholamines are measured after 3 hr.

    b. Patients with essential hypertension or other diagnoses will have catecholamine levels suppressed to less than 500 pg/ml. Patients with pheo do not show a significant decrease.

    c. Both groups generally have a significant fall in blood pressure.

6. Provocative tests have largely been abandoned because of their danger.

7. Localization studies should only be undertaken after a clinical and biochemical diagnosis has been established.

    a. Unless biochemical confirmation is obtained, an incidental adrenal mass will confound the clinical situation.

    b. Scanning with ^{131}I-metaiodobenzylguanidine (MIBG), a substance preferentially localized to adrenergic tissue, gives functional information about the tumor and is extremely helpful in locating extraadrenal pheos.

    c. CT and MRI studies are both excellent at identifying tumors within the adrenal.

    d. If the clinical situation suggests extraadrenal tumor is likely, an MIBG scan should be performed first and used as a guide for CT or MRI.

RECOMMENDED DIAGNOSTIC APPROACH

1. Figure 57–1 shows the approach for patients with low or moderate clinical suspicion for pheo.

    a. A single negative biochemical test excludes the diagnosis, and further testing is unnecessary.

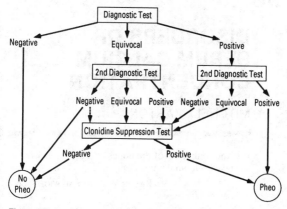

Figure 57–1. Low or moderate suspicion of pheochromocytoma.

    b. Two different clearly positive tests are likely diagnostic.

    c. For patients with a positive and negative test, a positive and equivocal test, or 2 equivocal results, a clonidine suppression test should be performed.

2. When there is strong clinical suspicion of pheo, it is necessary to confirm both negative and positive results.

Bibliography

Benowitz NL. Pheochromocytoma: Recent advances in diagnosis and treatment. West J Med 1988;148:561–567.

Bravo EL, Gifford RW. Pheochromocytoma: Diagnosis, localization, and management. N Engl J Med 1984;311:1298–1303.

Cryer PE. Pheochromocytoma. Clin Endocrinol Metab 1985;14:203–220.

Greene JP, Guay AT. New perspectives in pheochromocytoma. Urol Clin North Amer 1989;16:487–503.

Shapiro B, Fig LM: Management of pheochromocytoma. Endocrinol Metab Clin North Am 1989;18:443–481.

Velchik MG, et al. Localization of pheochromocytoma: MIBG, CT, and MRI correlation. J Nuc Med 1989;30:328–336.

Young MJ, et al. Biochemical tests for pheochromocytoma: Strategies in hypertensive patients. J Gen Intern Med 1989;4:273–276.

58

DISORDERS OF SERUM CALCIUM CONCENTRATION

MITCHELL KARTON

It is the soundness of the bones that ultimates itself in the peach-bloom complexion.

RALPH WALDO EMERSON (1860)

HYPERCALCEMIA

Definition and General Comments

- The normal total serum calcium (Ca) is between 8.9 and 11 mg/dl (4.4 and 5.5 mEq/L).
- Approximately 40% of total Ca is bound to serum proteins.
  1. Between 80 and 90% of the protein-bound Ca is bound to albumin. The protein-bound fraction is in equilibrium with the ultrafilterable Ca, which consists of ionized (50% of serum) and complexed (10% of serum) components.
  2. The ionized fraction (normal values 4.4 to 5.1 mg/dl [2.2 to 2.6 mEq/L]) is the biologically active form of Ca.
- Variations in serum proteins alter measurements of total serum Ca. For each decrease of 1 g/dl of serum albumin, the serum calcium drops by 0.8 mg/dl.
- Changes in pH affect the protein binding of Ca. Each decrease/increase of 0.1 in pH decreases or increases the protein-bound Ca by 0.12 mg/dl (i.e., acidosis increases the ionized fraction of Ca and alkalosis decreases it).

Clinical Features

- The clinical features of hypercalcemia include specific findings of the underlying disease and effects of hypercalcemia in the organ systems.
- Some patients with serum Ca concentrations as high as 14 mg/dl may lack symptoms altogether. Hypomagnesemia and hyperkalemia accentuate the neurologic and cardiovascular effects of hypercalcemia.
- Signs and symptoms include:
  1. Gastrointestinal. Anorexia, constipation, nausea, vomiting, peptic ulcer pain, and acute pancreatitis.

2. Genitourinary. Polyuria, polydipsia, renal insufficiency, calculi, and nephrocalcinosis.
3. Neurologic. Fatigue, muscle weakness, depressed tendon reflexes, disorientation, stupor, coma, and death.
4. Psychiatric. Apathy, depression, or psychotic behavior.
5. Metastatic calcification. Ocular keratopathy, nephrocalcinosis, chondrocalcinosis, vascular calcification, and periarticular calcification.

Differential Diagnosis (See Table 58–1)

- Hyperparathyroidism (HPT)
  1. Primary HPT accounts for half of cases of hypercalcemia.
     a. Its incidence has increased 10-fold, partly due to earlier detection by automated biochemical testing.
     b. There are 35,000 to 85,000 new cases in the United States each year. Postmenopausal females are at the greatest risk, with an incidence greater than 1 case per 1000 population. At all ages, women with HPT outnumber men by 3 : 1.

TABLE 58–1. Causes of Hypercalcemia

Common
  Primary hyperparathyroidism (50% of cases)
  Secondary hyperparathyroidism
  Malignancy (35% of cases)
    Without metastases: lung, kidney, or gastrointestinal
    With metastases: breast, lung, kidney, thyroid,
      prostate, ovary, head, and neck
  Multiple myeloma
  Sarcoidosis
  Hyperthyroidism
  Acute adrenal insufficiency
  Thiazides
Uncommon
  Hypervitaminosis D
  Hypervitaminosis A
  Milk-alkali (Burnett's) syndrome
  Leukemia and lymphoma
  Hypothyroidism
  Immobilization: in the young with rapid growth and in the
    old with Paget's disease
  Diuretic phase of acute renal failure
  Acromegaly
  Pheochromocytoma
  Berylliosis
  Vasoactive intestinal peptide (VIP)–producing tumor
  Pulmonary granulomatous disease (e.g., tuberculosis,
    coccidioidomycosis)
  Hypophosphatemia
  Hypercalcemia of infancy
  Iatrogenic causes: estrogens, antiestrogens, lithium

2. The triad of nephrolithiasis, metabolic bone disease, and hypercalcemia characterize HPT. Serum Ca is usually high, and serum phosphate (P_i) is usually low but may be normal, especially if renal failure is present.
3. Serum chloride
   a. The level is usually above 103 mEq/L in primary HPT and less than 98 mEq/L with hypercalcemia of malignancy.
   b. Patients with primary HPT have impaired HCO_3 reabsorption in the proximal tubule with resulting HCO_3 loss and renal tubular acidosis.
4. Serum chloride–phosphate ratio
   a. If the ratio is greater than 33 (i.e., due to acidosis and phosphate wasting), HPT is suggested. If the ratio is less than 30, the hypercalcemia is probably not due to HPT.
   b. The sensitivity of the chloride-phosphate ratio is greater than 90%. However, the large variance of phosphate values impedes its usefulness and reliability.
5. Corticosteroid suppression test
   a. Patients with primary HPT have no hypocalcemic response to 10 days of glucocorticoid administration.
   b. Patients with myeloma, sarcoidosis, vitamin D intoxication, and some tumors may respond with a lowering of the serum Ca level.
6. Thiazide provocation test
   a. This may produce sustained hypercalcemia in patients with primary HPT and a borderline elevation of serum Ca. Some patients with vitamin D intoxication and metabolic bone disease may also have sustained increase in serum Ca.
7. Serum immunoreactive parathyroid hormone (iPTH) levels.
   a. Definitive diagnosis depends upon simultaneous demonstration of hypercalcemia and inappropriately elevated serum iPTH levels.
   b. Most patients with primary HPT and serum Ca above 12 mg/dl have unequivocally elevated iPTH, whereas most patients with hypercalcemia related to neoplasia have normal or undetectable iPTH levels.
   c. In mild cases of HPT, this may be equivocal. Patients with known malignancies, high serum Ca, and elevated levels of iPTH are very likely to have coexistent primary HPT.
8. Despite the availability of diagnostic tests, primary HPT is commonly diagnosed clinically because it is a chronic disease with evidence of the clinical triad noted above. Therefore, if isolated hypercalcemia is a recent discovery, without any historical symptoms, a thorough search for causes other than primary HPT must be made.
- Malignancy
  1. The annual incidence of hypercalcemia associated with

malignancy is 150 patients per 1 million population per year.

    a. Squamous cell lung cancer appears with hypercalcemia in 10 to 15% of cases (small-cell carcinoma is almost never associated with high Ca).

    b. One-third of patients with advanced breast cancer develop hypercalcemia at some stage during the course of the disease.

    c. Other solid tumors include squamous cell tumors of the head and neck, thyroid gland, ovary, hypernephroma, and prostate.

    d. Myeloproliferative causes include myeloma, leukemia, lymphoma, and Hodgkin's disease.

2. No single test can differentiate between hypercalcemia caused by primary HPT and that caused by malignancy.

    a. Hypercalcemia of malignancy may be associated with a PTH-related protein, related to local bony involvement, or associated with hematologic malignancies.

    b. An elevated excretion of nephrogenous cyclic adenosine monophosphate (n-cAMP) is usually present in primary HPT and in patients with hypercalcemia due to PTH-related protein.

    c. The new generation of two-site assays for intact PTH measures only biologically active PTH and does not cross-react with PTH-related protein. Thus, a normal or elevated iPTH level in a hypercalcemic cancer patient strongly suggests concomitant primary HPT.

- Sarcoidosis. Mild hypercalcemia is present in 10% of cases. It indicates widespread disease, usually with pulmonary involvement.

- Thyrotoxicosis. Hypercalcemia with a normal iPTH is seen in approximately 25% of hyperthyroid patients. The symptoms leading to medical evaluation are usually those of hyperthyroidism, not of hypercalcemia.

- Adrenal insufficiency. The elevated Ca returns to normal with adrenal replacement therapy.

- Vitamin D intoxication. Vitamin D intoxication requires months of ingestion of greater than 100,000 units of D_2 or D_3 and is rare.

- Milk-alkali syndrome. This syndrome has been rare since the introduction of nonabsorbable antacids.

- Medications. Hypercalcemia may be found in patients taking thiazide diuretics. Many such patients also have HPT, but they should be evaluated after stopping the medication.

Recommended Diagnostic Approach

- Clinical evaluation
  1. Determine the acuteness of symptoms. Review medications and symptoms that suggest a disease associated with hypercalcemia.

   2. Physical examination may reveal findings due to hypercalcemia or to its cause.
- Laboratory findings
  1. General. These include serum Ca, P_i, chloride, alkaline phosphatase, and iPTH levels if necessary. The N-terminal PTH assay should be used in patients with renal insufficiency if a 2-site assay is not available.
  2. ESR may be helpful for myeloma, malignancy, and tuberculosis.
  3. Serum and urine protein electrophoreses or immunoelectrophoreses may indicate myeloma.
  4. Other tests may include thyroid function tests, acid phosphatase for prostatic disease, liver function tests for metastatic disease, morning cortisol for Addison's disease, and PFTs, skin tests, and sputum cultures as needed.
- Other diagnostic procedures. Tests that may help diagnose the cause of hypercalcemia include:
  1. Hand X-rays for subperiosteal resorption, demineralization, and cysts
  2. Chest X-ray
  3. IV pyelogram for renal stones
  4. Mammography
  5. Skull films for lytic lesions
  6. Bone scans for metastases
  7. Bone marrow aspirate (for myeloma or tuberculosis)
  8. Biopsy material (for malignancy or sarcoidosis)

HYPOCALCEMIA

Definition

Hypocalcemia is defined as a total serum Ca concentration below 8.9 mg/dl.

Clinical Features

Hypocalcemia causes 5 categories of signs and symptoms.
- Tetany
  1. There is a range of symptoms from circumoral paresthesias to stiff hands and feet to frank carpopedal spasm.
  2. Chvostek's sign consists of a twitch of the facial muscles elicited by a sharp tap over the facial nerve in front of the ear. The sign may be positive in 10% of normal adults.
  3. Trousseau's sign is the induction of latent carpopedal spasm by reducing the circulation in the arm with a blood pressure cuff. It is rarely positive in normal adults.
- Other neurologic signs include diminished or absent deep tendon reflexes, occasional papilledema, and seizures.
- Mental status disturbances include irritability, confusion,

memory loss, depression, delusions or hallucinations, seeming mental retardation, and mental instability.

- Skin abnormalities. There may be dryness of skin and hair, alopecia, and brittle nails. Subcapsular cataracts are often visible with the naked eye.
- Gastrointestinal. The patient may complain of vague crampy abdominal pain with episodic vomiting and diarrhea.

Differential Diagnosis and Laboratory Features (See Table 58–2)

- Hypoalbuminemia. Hypoalbuminemia causes a decreased total serum Ca level. A normal serum ionized Ca level precludes symptoms of hypocalcemia.
- Idiopathic hypoparathyroidism
  1. This rare disease should be considered in patients with symptomatic hypocalcemia, hyperphosphatemia, and

TABLE 58–2. Causes of Hypocalcemia

Hypoalbuminemia
Hypoparathyroidism
Pseudohypoparathyroidism
Vitamin D deficiency
Nutritional calcium deficiency
Malabsorption
   Postsurgical
   Sprue
   Chronic pancreatitis
   Obstructive jaundice
   Biliary cirrhosis
   Cathartic ingestion
Abnormal metabolism of vitamin D
   Renal disease
   Vitamin D–dependent rickets
   Hepatic dysfunction
Hyperphosphatemia: administered phosphate, renal disease, cytotoxic drugs
Acute pancreatitis
Hypomagnesemia
Postoperative: after thyroidectomy, after parathyroidectomy
Renal tubular acidosis
Medullary carcinoma of the thyroid causing excess calcitonin
Toxic shock syndrome
Medications
   Binders: EDTA, citrate, phytate
   Anticonvulsants
   Gentamicin
   Mithramycin
   Magnesium sulfate (IV)
   Fluoride intoxication
   Calcitonin

normal renal function. Most cases are sporadic and present before early adolescence.
   2. Diagnosis is based on:
      a. Decreased or absent iPTH levels
      b. Low urinary cAMP excretion which increases 10- to 20-fold after PTH administration)
   3. Hypoparathyroidism may coexist with other autoimmune diseases such as Addison's disease, Hashimoto's thyroiditis, diabetes mellitus, and pernicious anemia. Parathyroid antibodies may exist in one-third of cases.

- Pseudohypoparathyroidism
   1. Signs and symptoms are the same as for hypoparathyroidism. In addition, skeletal abnormalities (short fourth and fifth metacarpals and metatarsals), short stature, mental retardation, and moon facies are found in patient or siblings. There is a female-to-male patient ratio of 2 : 1.
   2. The iPTH levels are normal or increased.
   3. The basal levels of nephrogenous cAMP or total cAMP excretion are low, with little or no response of urinary cAMP to PTH.

- Malabsorption
   1. Incidence of this is increased in patients with small bowel disease or obstructive jaundice, and after small bowel surgery.
   2. There is increased PTH with decreased vitamin D levels. There may be other signs of malabsorption.

- Renal failure
   1. Abnormalities in this setting include hyperphosphatemia, chronic acidosis, and elevated BUN and serum creatinine levels.
   2. Ectopic soft-tissue calcification due to hyperphosphatemia may occur.

- Acute pancreatitis. Hypocalcemia is transient, occurring within the first 30 hr and improving after the acute episode.

- Hypomagnesemia
   1. The primary mechanism is impairment of PTH secretion, but peripheral resistance to PTH also occurs.
   2. Hypomagnesemia is most common in alcoholics and others with chronically poor nutrition.

- Postsurgical hypocalcemia
   1. This occurs in less than 5% of postthyroidectomy patients, usually within 24 hr and especially after removal of a large goiter.
   2. After parathyroidectomy, the serum Ca concentration depends on the amount of remaining functional parathyroid tissue and preexisting clinical bone disease which is associated with recalcification tetany, or the "hungry bones" syndrome.

- Medication-related hypocalcemia
   1. Patients receiving large amounts of blood by transfusion are vulnerable to citrate-induced complexing of Ca.

2. Patients treated with chronic anticonvulsant therapy may be susceptible if they are not treated with supplemental vitamins D_2 and D_3.
3. Gentamicin, amphotericin B, and cisplatin may cause hypomagnesemia with subsequent hypocalcemia.

Recommended Diagnostic Approach

- Clinical features
    1. The dietary history is important with special reference to symptoms of malabsorption. Other pertinent features include alcohol history, medications, and family history (stature, skeletal abnormalities, and autoimmune polyglandular syndromes).
    2. Physical examination may reveal abnormalities as noted above.
- Laboratory findings
    1. The following studies should be obtained routinely:
        a. Serum calcium, phosphate, magnesium, urea nitrogen, and creatinine
        b. Serum albumin and total protein
        c. Serum iPTH and vitamin D levels
    2. Clinical findings may indicate a serum amylase level and evaluation for malabsorption
    3. Measurement of urinary cAMP may be necessary.
    4. Hands and feet should be X-rayed. Ultrasound may be used to assess the pancreas.

Bibliography

Lufkin EG, et al. Parathyroid hormone radioimmunoassay in the differential diagnosis of hypercalcemia due to primary hyperparathyroidism or malignancy. Ann Intern Med 1987;106:559–563.

Mundy R, et al. The hypercalcemia of cancer: Clinical implications and pathogenetic mechanisms. N Engl J Med 1984;310:1718–1727.

Nusynowitz RL, et al. The spectrum of hypoparathyroid states: A classification based on physiologic principles. Medicine 1979;55:109.

Ralston SH, et al. Relative contribution of humoral and metastatic factors to the pathogenesis of hypercalcemia in malignancy. Br Med J 1984;288:1405–1411.

Strewler GJ, Nissenson RA. Nonparathyroid hypercalcemia. Adv Intern Med 1987;33:235–258.

59

DIABETES MELLITUS

MICKEY EISENBERG

Man may be captain of his fate, but he is also the victim of his blood sugar.

WILFRED G. OAKLEY (1905–   )

DEFINITION

Diabetes is a heterogeneous group of diseases with glucose intolerance in common (Table 59–1).

- Diabetes mellitus (DM) is defined by abnormally high plasma glucose levels. It is a chronic disorder characterized by abnormal metabolism of carbohydrate, protein, fat and is accompanied, after some time, by specific microvascular, macrovascular, and neuropathic complications. There are 3 clinical subclasses of DM.

  1. Type I. Patients with type I DM have severe insulinopenia and are prone to development of ketoacidosis. They are dependent on exogenous insulin to prevent ketoacidosis and death. Ten percent of all cases of DM are type I. Although it may occur at any age, the major peak of onset occurs at about 11 or 12 years, and nearly all patients diagnosed before age 20 are of this type. They are usually lean and often have recent significant weight loss, polyuria, and polydipsia.

  2. Type II
     a. Patients with type II DM may be asymptomatic at diagnosis. Although the symptomatology of type II DM is less obvious than type I, this type of diabetes is also accompanied by vascular and neuropathic complications.
     b. In patients with type II DM, insulin resistance (decreased tissue sensitivity or responsiveness to exogenous and endogenous insulin) is usually present, and insulin levels may be low, normal, or high.
     c. Patients are not prone to develop ketoacidosis except during periods of stress, such as infections, trauma, or surgery.
     d. Type II diabetes can occur at any age but is usually diagnosed after age 30.

Adapted with permission from Physicians Guide to Insulin-Dependent (Type I) Diabetes: Diagnosis and Treatment. Alexandria, VA, American Diabetes Association, 1988.

e. About 75% of patients are obese or have a history of obesity at the time of diagnosis, but type II DM can occur in nonobese individuals as well, especially in the elderly.

f. Although patients with type II DM are not dependent on exogenous insulin for survival, many patients require insulin for adequate glycemic control, especially at times of metabolic stress.

3. Other types. This category, which is numerically the smallest, includes DM associated with certain diseases or conditions (see Table 59-1).

- Impaired glucose tolerance (IGT)

1. Patients with IGT have plasma glucose levels that are lower than those considered diagnostic for DM.

2. Twenty-five percent of patients with IGT eventually develop DM.

3. Although patients with IGT do not appear to have an increased risk for the microvascular complications seen with DM, they may have a greater than normal risk for atherosclerotic disease.

- Gestational diabetes mellitus (GDM)

1. GDM refers to glucose intolerance with onset or first detection during pregnancy. Women with known DM before conception are not part of this class.

2. GDM occurs in 2% of pregnant women, usually during the second or third trimester.

3. Fetal morbidity and mortality are increased by the presence of GDM. Thus, all pregnant women should be screened for GDM between the 24th and 28th weeks of pregnancy.

4. After parturition, patients with gestational diabetes should be reclassified on the basis of plasma glucose testing as having DM, IGT, or a previous abnormality of glucose tolerance (see below). In most cases, glucose tolerance in women with gestational diabetes returns to normal after delivery. Within 5 to 10 years of parturition, however, one-third of women with GDM develop overt DM (usually type II).

EPIDEMIOLOGY AND GENERAL COMMENTS

- Type I DM

1. Type I DM results from immunologic destruction of the beta cells. It is a heterogeneous disorder in terms of precipitating events.

2. Genetic factors are probably important. However, twin studies indicate that only 50% of identical twins of type I patients develop the disease.

3. The majority of patients have circulating islet cell antibodies at the time of diagnosis. In some patients acute physiological stress, e.g., viral infections, may precipitate the clinical syndrome.

4. Type I DM accounts for 3% of all new cases of diabetes diagnosed in the United States. Although it is much

TABLE 59–1. Types of Diabetes Mellitus and Other Categories of Glucose Intolerance

CLINICAL CLASS	DISTINGUISHING CHARACTERISTICS
I Insulin-dependent diabetes mellitus (IDDM); Type I	Patients may be of any age, are usually thin, and usually have abrupt onset of signs and symptoms with insulinopenia before age 30. These patients often have strongly positive urine ketone tests.
II Non–insulin-dependent diabetes mellitus (NIDDM); Type II (obese or nonobese)	Patients usually are older than 30 years at diagnosis, obese, and have relatively few classic symptoms. They are not prone to ketoacidosis except during periods of stress.
III Other types of DM	Patients with other types of DM have certain associated conditions or syndromes.
A. Secondary to: Pancreatic disease	Examples: pancreatectomy, hemochromatosis, cystic fibrosis, chronic pancreatitis

Endocrinopathies   Examples: acromegaly, pheochromocytoma, Cushing's syndrome, primary hyperaldosteronism, glucagonoma

Drugs and chemical agents   Examples: certain antihypertensive drugs, thiazide diuretics, glucocorticoids, estrogen-containing preparations, psychoactive agents, catecholamines, nicotinic acid

B. Associated with:
Insulin-receptor abnormalities   Examples: acanthosis nigricans
Genetic syndromes   Examples: hyperlipidemia, muscular dystrophies, Huntington's chorea

Miscellaneous conditions   Examples: malnutrition ("tropical diabetes")

Other categories of impaired glucose tolerance:
Impaired glucose tolerance (IGT: obese or nonobese)   Patients with IGT have plasma glucose levels higher than normal but not diagnostic for DM.

Gestational diabetes mellitus (GDM)   Patients with GDM have the discovery of glucose intolerance during pregnancy.

501

less common in the general population than type II diabetes, type I DM is not rare among children and young adults.

5. The annual incidence among people under age 20 years is 15 per 100,000 (1 new case/7000 children/yr) and makes type I diabetes 3- to 4-fold more common than chronic childhood diseases such as cystic fibrosis, peptic ulcer, juvenile rheumatoid arthritis, or leukemia, and nearly 10-fold more common than nephrotic syndrome, muscular dystrophy, or lymphoma. After age 20 the yearly incidence decreases to 5 per 100,000.

6. The incidence is similar in men and women, lower in blacks than whites, and markedly less common in Hispanics, Asian Americans, and native Americans. Two to five percent of siblings of individuals with type I diabetes develop the disorder.

- Type II DM
  1. Type II DM accounts for approximately 90% of the diabetic patients in the United States. The prevalence of diagnosed type II DM in the United States is about 6 million people or 2.5%. There is probably an equal number of undiagnosed cases.

  2. The prevalence of type II DM is markedly increased among American Indians, blacks, and Hispanics. It increases with age and obesity. The annual incidence is increasing.

  3. The etiology of type II DM remains unknown. Genetic and environmental factors seem important. Although type II DM is not associated with specific HLA tissue types, there is 90 to 100% concordance in identical twins. There are families in which type II DM is present in children, adolescents, and adults and in which an autosomal dominant inheritance has been established. This form of diabetes was formerly referred to as maturity-onset diabetes of the young (MODY).

  4. Unlike type I DM, circulating islet cell antibodies are rarely present. Intake of excessive calories leading to weight gain and obesity is probably an important factor in the pathogenesis of type II DM.

  5. Obesity is a powerful risk factor and even small weight losses are associated with return of plasma glucose levels toward normal in many patients.

HISTORY

- Clinical presentation of type I diabetes
  1. The presentation of type I diabetes covers a broad range from mild nonspecific symptoms to frank coma.
  2. In children, correct diagnosis is often delayed because polyuria is incorrectly attributed to urinary tract infection or enuresis; anorexia rather than polyphagia may occur; and fatigue, irritability, weight loss, deterioration of school performance, and enuresis are ascribed to emotional problems. In some cases, failure to thrive

may be an overlooked indication of diabetes in a young child.

3. Fewer patients present with severe metabolic decompensation today than in the past, and more than 70% of cases are diagnosed within 1 month of onset of symptoms. Nevertheless, delayed diagnosis continues to be a serious and sometimes fatal problem, especially among younger children.

4. The frequency of coma as a presenting feature in children less than 2 years old is approximately 40% compared to less than 10% in those older than 15 years. In children, coma remains an important cause of death; approximately 5% of children presenting in coma die during the acute phase of the disease.

5. The frequency of various clinical and laboratory characteristics in type I diabetes is shown in Figure 59–1.

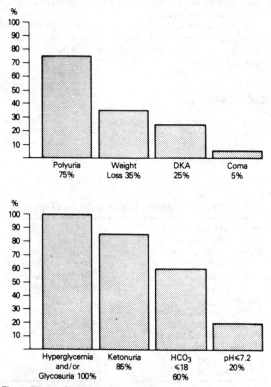

Figure 59–1. Clinical (top) and laboratory (bottom) presentations of type I diabetes. DKA = diabetic ketoacidosis. *Data from* MS Eberhardt, unpublished observations.

In young adults, the presentation is often less acute, although an absolute requirement for insulin becomes evident with time.

LABORATORY STUDIES

- Indications and criteria for screening tests. Screening tests for DM should be limited to the following individuals:
  1. People with a strong family history of DM
  2. Women with a morbid obstetrical history or a history of babies over 9 lb at birth
  3. All pregnant women between 24 and 28 weeks of pregnancy
  4. Patients with a history of recurrent skin, genital, or urinary tract infections
- It is particularly important to screen all pregnant women for GDM. Nearly 100,000 women with GDM give birth each year. GDM is associated with increased perinatal morbidity.
- The recommended screening test for nonpregnant adults and children is a fasting plasma glucose level. In pregnant women a 50-g oral glucose load is recommended for screening. All women with a history of IGT or GDM should be screened before planned conception. Tables 59–2 and 59–3 contain normal glucose levels and criteria for positive screening tests.

DIAGNOSIS

- Indications for definitive diagnostic testing. Diagnostic testing should be done only when there are definite indications, such as
  1. Positive screening test results

TABLE 59–2. Normal Plasma Glucose Values

Nonpregnant adults	
Fasting plasma glucose	<115 mg/dl
Plasma glucose values	30 min < 200 mg/dl
after 75-g oral	60 min < 200 mg/dl
glucose dose	90 min < 200 mg/dl
	120 min < 140 mg/dl
Children	
Fasting plasma glucose	<130 mg/dl
Plasma glucose value	120 min < 140 mg/dl
after glucose dose of	
1.75 g/kg ideal body	
weight up to	
maximum of 75 g	

Note: Glucose values above these concentrations but below criteria for diabetes mellitus or impaired glucose tolerance should be considered nondiagnostic.

TABLE 59–3. Criteria for Screening Tests

Nonpregnant adults. A fasting plasma glucose
determination should be used for screening. Fasting
plasma glucose level of 115 mg/dl or greater is considered
an indication for diagnostic testing (see Table 59–4).

Children. A fasting plasma glucose determination should be
used for screening. Fasting plasma glucose level of 130
mg/dl or greater is considered an indication for diagnostic
testing (see Table 59–4).

Pregnant women. An oral glucose tolerance test with 50-g
glucose load is recommended for screening. Fasting
plasma glucose level above 105 mg/dl or plasma glucose
level of 140 mg/dl or greater 1 hr later is considered an
indication for diagnostic testing (see Table 59–4).

---

2. The presence of obvious signs and symptoms of diabetes mellitus (polydipsia, polyuria, polyphagia,
   weight loss)
3. An inconclusive clinical picture such as glycosuria or
   equivocal elevation of a random plasma glucose level

- Diagnostic tests for DM
  1. When diagnostic testing for DM is indicated, a firm
     diagnosis should be made on the basis of plasma glu-
     cose levels. Although glycosuria is strongly suggestive
     of diabetes in symptomatic patients, it does not make
     the diagnosis of DM.
  2. There are currently insufficient data to support the use
     of glycosylated hemoglobin measurements for the di-
     agnosis of diabetes. The choice of diagnostic tests and
     their interpretation are different for nonpregnant
     adults, children, and pregnant women (Table 59–4).
  3. Tests for DM should not be done in the presence of
     factors that impair glucose tolerance, such as certain
     drugs (Table 59–5), stress, marked restriction of carbo-
     hydrate intake, or prolonged physical inactivity. Fur-
     thermore drugs and chemicals that may cause lower
     than normal plasma glucose (e.g., monoamine oxidase
     inhibitors, propranolol, alcohol, and large quantities of
     salicylates) as well as those that may elevate plasma
     glucose levels (see Table 59–5) should be discontinued
     when possible before testing.
        As noted above, the standard oral glucose tolerance
     test (OGTT) is usually unnecessary for diagnosis of
     DM. When it is indicated, the OGTT is useful only if
     done with strict adherence to proper methods (Table
     59–6).

EVALUATION AND CLASSIFICATION OF PATIENTS BEFORE TREATMENT

Before therapy is initiated to treat DM or IGT, the patient
should have a complete medical evaluation and be classified
appropriately. Diagnostic criteria are shown in Table 59–4.

TABLE 59–4. Diagnostic Criteria for Diabetes Mellitus, Impaired Glucose Tolerance, and Gestational Diabetes

Nonpregnant adults

Criteria for DM. Diagnosis of DM in nonpregnant adults should be restricted to those who have *one* of the following:

Random plasma glucose level of 200 mg/dl or greater *plus* classic signs and symptoms of DM including polydipsia, polyuria, polyphagia, and weight loss

Fasting plasma glucose level of 140 mg/dl or greater on at least 2 occasions

Fasting plasma glucose level less than 140 mg/dl *plus* sustained elevated plasma glucose levels during at least 2 OGTTs. The 2-hr sample and at least one other between 0 and 2 hr after 75-g glucose dose should be 200 mg/dl or greater. OGTT is not necessary if patient has fasting plasma glucose level of 140 mg/dl or greater.

Criteria for IGT. Diagnosis of IGT in nonpregnant adults should be restricted to those who have *all* of the following:

Fasting plasma glucose of less than 140 mg/dl

2-hr OGTT plasma glucose level of between 140 and 200 mg/dl

Intervening OGTT plasma glucose level of 200 mg/dl or greater

Pregnant women

Criteria for GDM. After an oral glucose load of 100 g, diagnosis of GDM may be made if 2 plasma glucose values equal or exceed (in mg/dl)

Fasting	1 hr	2 hr	3 hr
105	190	165	145

Children

Criteria for DM. Diagnosis of DM in children should be restricted to those who have *one* of the following:

Random plasma glucose level of 200 mg/dl or greater *plus* classic signs and symptoms of diabetes mellitus, including polyuria, polydipsia, ketonuria, and rapid weight loss

Fasting plasma glucose level of 140 mg/dl or greater on at least 2 occasions *and* sustained elevated plasma glucose levels during at least 2 OGTTs. Both the 2-hr plasma glucose and at least one other between 0 and 2 hr after glucose dose (1.75 g/kg ideal body weight up to 75 g) should be 200 mg/dl or greater.

Criteria for IGT. Diagnosis of IGT in children should be restricted to those who have *both* of the following:

Fasting plasma glucose concentration of less than 140 mg/dl

2-hr OGTT plasma glucose level of greater than 140 mg/dl

TABLE 59–5. Drugs Associated with Abnormal Glucose Tolerance or Diabetes Mellitus

Hormones and related agents
 ACTH
 Catecholamines (epinephrine, isoproterenol, levodopa)
 Dextrothyroxine
 Estrogens (oral contraceptives)
 Glucocorticoids (cortisone and derivatives)
 Thyroxine and triiodothyronine (toxic doses)
Diuretics and antihypertensive drugs
 Chlorthalidone (Hygroton, Combipres, Regroton)
 Clonidine (Catapres, Combipres)
 Ethacrynic acid (Edecrin)
 Furosemide (Lasix)
 Thiazides (Diuril, Hydrodiuril, etc.)
Psychoactive agents
 Chlorprothixene (Taractan)
 Haloperidol (Haldol)
 Lithium (Lithane, Eskalith)
 Phenothiazines (Thorazine, Trilafon, Etrafon, Triavil, etc.)
 Tricyclic antidepressants
  Amitriptyline (Elavil, Endep, Triavil, etc.)
  Desipramine (Norpramin, Pertofrane)
  Doxepin (Adapin, Sinequan)
  Imipramine (Presamine, Tofranil)
  Nortriptyline (Aventyl)
Miscellaneous
 Antineoplastic drugs (L-asparaginase, streptozotocin)
 Indomethacin
 Isoniazid (INH)
 Nicotinic acid

Source: Reprinted with permission from Barker LR, et al., eds. Principles of Ambulatory Medicine, 2nd ed. Baltimore, Williams & Wilkins, 1988, p. 957.

- Evaluation and classification of the patient helps the physician to determine the presence of underlying diseases that need further study and detect complications frequently associated with DM.

    Generally, initial assignment of the patient can be made on the basis of diagnostic test results, a complete personal and family history, and complete physical evaluation. Patients should not be classified on the basis of age alone or on the basis of selected therapy.

- Special problems in classification
    1. IGT vs. DM
        a. IGT does not constitute a definitive diagnosis of DM. The label of IGT itself may cause problems for the patient with employers and insurance companies.
        b. Because the finding of IGT may identify a person with higher than normal risk of developing DM and

TABLE 59-6. Oral Glucose Tolerance Test

Patient Selection

Certain patients should be excluded from OGTT because their responses will be difficult to interpret. Examples include patients that have chronic malnutrition, restricted CHO intake (<150 g/day for >3 days), or bedrest for 2–3 days. Test results are invalid in patients experiencing acute medical or surgical stress: such patients probably should not be tested until several months after recovery.

Patient preparation

The patient should discontinue medication 3 days before testing when possible and should also eat and drink nothing except water for 10 to 14 hr before the test. If the patient's diet contains 150 g CHO/day, a preparatory diet high in carbohydrates is not necessary.

Test method

Schedule the test in the morning to exclude diurinal influence on test results. Instruct the patient to refrain from smoking and from drinking coffee just before and during the test. Draw a blood sample for determination for fasting plasma glucose. Give the patient a standard glucose solution (75 g for nonpregnant adults, 100 g for pregnant women, and 1.75 g/kg ideal body weight up to 75 g for children). Ask the patient to remain quiet for the duration of the test (2 hr for children and nonpregnant adults, 3 hr for pregnant women). Start timing when the patient begins to drink the solution, and obtain samples at appropriate intervals. In nonpregnant adults and children, obtain blood samples every 30 min for 2 hr. In pregnant women, obtain blood samples every hr for 3 hr.

---

atherosclerotic heart disease, most physicians continue to regularly observe the patient.

    c. If the patient with IGT is obese, attention should be given to weight control and to modification of vascular risk factors.

2. Type I vs. type II DM

    a. It may be difficult to assign the patient to a particular subclass of DM. The thin, type II patient who has been taking insulin often looks like a type I patient.

    b. A newly diagnosed child or adolescent who is a member of a family with an autosomal dominant form of inheritance of diabetes usually has type II diabetes and should not be classified as type I on the basis of age alone.

    c. There are patients with characteristics of type II diabetes who may require insulin therapy for glycemic control but are not dependent on it to prevent ketoacidosis or sustain life. These patients should not be classified as type I simply on the basis of insulin therapy. They are "insulin treated," not "insulin dependent."

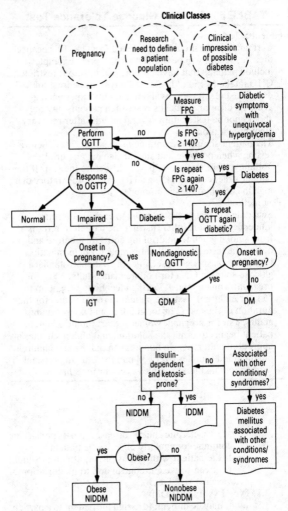

Figure 59–2. Procedure for classifying adult patients with diabetes mellitus. (FBS = fasting blood sugar) (From Eisenberg MS. Diabetes mellitus. In Cummins RO, Eisenberg MS, eds. Blue Book of Medical Diagnosis. Philadelphia, W.B. Saunders, 1986, p. 402.)

d. Currently, it is not necessary for clinicians to measure islet cell antibodies or the degree of insulin secretion. In research studies, measurement of plasma C-peptide after an oral stimulus is often used as an index of insulin secretion; however, it is not a useful classification tool.

e. A history of ketoacidosis or the detection of moderate to strong urine ketones in the presence of hyperglycemia in an unstressed patient strongly supports a diagnosis of type I DM. The absence of urinary ketones is of no diagnostic value.

f. Generally, if the patient is less than 30 years old, not obese, and has signs and symptoms of DM and an elevated fasting blood glucose, the physician should assume type I diabetes and treat with insulin.

- Reclassification of the patient. After therapy is initiated, the patient should be reevaluated periodically and reclassified accordingly. In this regard, it is important to reemphasize that the specific therapy used to treat a patient is not the determining factor in classification.

RECOMMENDED DIAGNOSTIC APPROACH

Figure 59–2 is a flow diagram illustrating the set of measurements and decisions needed to classify an individual case. The presence of such obvious diabetic symptoms as polyuria, polydipsia, ketonuria, and rapid weight loss, together with ketonuria or gross and unequivocal elevation of plasma glucose, is usually sufficient to make the diagnosis of diabetes. In the absence of these signs and symptoms, however, quantitative measurements of glucose under carefully standardized conditions are the prescribed methods for making a clinical diagnosis of diabetes.

60

HYPERLIPIDEMIA

DAVID K. LEE

A feast of fat things, a feast of wines on the lees.

ISAIAH 25:6

DEFINITION

- Hyperlipidemia is an abnormally high level of circulating fatty substances in the blood. Since fats are insoluble in blood, they are bound to specialized lipoproteins. Circulating fats of greatest clinical importance are cholesterol (C) and triglycerides (TGs).
- Measured C and TG levels in any population assume a normal distribution, so designation of any given level as "abnormal" is somewhat arbitrary, and has changed dramatically in recent years. In the United States, the National Cholesterol Education Program (NCEP) has recommended the following levels for adults:

	Normal	Borderline	Abnormal
Serum C (mg/dl)	<200	200–239	>240

- Lipid levels are strongly influenced by metabolic, genetic, and dietary factors.

ETIOLOGY

- Lipid disorders can be primary or secondary. Secondary causes of high C include hypothyroidism, nephrotic syndrome, obstructive liver disease, porphyria, and dietary excess of saturated fat and C.
- Elevated TGs are seen in obesity, uncontrolled DM, renal failure, excessive alcohol intake, glycogen storage diseases, and lipodystrophy.
- Lipid values can also be altered by medications, including oral contraceptives, estrogens, beta blockers, thiazides, and glucocorticoids.
- Primary hyperlipidemias may be classified by numerical types (Table 60–1) or descriptively (Table 60–2).

TABLE 60-1. Classification of Hyperlipidemia

Type	Lipid Involved	Mechanism
I	Chylomicron TG	Lipoprotein lipase not activated
IIa	C	Genetic lack of LDL receptors
IIb	C and TG	IIa plus elevated VLDL
III	C and TG	Large VLDL remnants cannot be cleared from the circulation
IV	TG	Overproduction of VLDL
V	Chylomicron TG	Genetic predisposition plus aggravating secondary factor (e.g., diabetes mellitus)

HISTORY

1. The clinical history is often important for the conditions that can trigger a secondary hyperlipidemia. A careful medication history should be taken.
2. For familial or genetic hyperlipidemias, a careful family history is critical.
   a. The patient may be unaware of his kindred's lipid history, so a background of coronary artery disease (especially before age 55) should be sought.
   b. Hypertriglyceridemia of any cause can trigger pancreatitis when levels are greater than 1000 mg/dl.
3. Treatment decisions of hyperlipidemia to prevent atherosclerosis may hinge on the presence of other risk factors, since there is a dynamic interplay between these factors. The NCEP noted 7, in addition to already established atherosclerotic disease (Table 60-3).

TABLE 60-2. Genetic Classification of Hyperlipidemia

Familial hypercholesterolemia: Genetically mediated lack of LDL receptors with common clinical characteristics

Polygenic (severe primary) hypercholesterolemia: Elevated C values, usually over 300 mg/dl, in a familial pattern but not mediated by other mechanisms listed

Familial combined hyperlipidemia: Multiple lipoprotein patterns in a single family, usually types IV, IIa, IIb, or V (Table 60-1)

Familial dysbetalipoproteinemia: Same as type III (Table 60-1)

Familial hypertriglyceridemia: Overproduction of VLDL coupled with mild defect in lipolysis, often aggravated by obesity or excess alcohol intake. Usually accompanied by low HDL-C levels.

Familial type I and familial type V: Same as types I and V (Table 60-1) but in a demonstrated familial pattern

TABLE 60-3. Other Coronary Heart Disease Risk Factors

Male gender
Family history (definite MI or sudden death in a parent or sibling before the age of 55)
Cigarettes: currently smoking more than 10 cigarettes per day
Hypertension
HDL-C < 35 mg/dl
Diabetes mellitus
Severe obesity (>30% over ideal body weight)

Source: Adapted from Expert Panel. Report of the National Cholesterol Education Program Expert Panel on detection, evaluation, and treatment of high blood cholesterol in adults. Arch Intern Med 1988;148:36–69.

PHYSICAL EXAMINATION

1. Most patients with hyperlipidemia have no physical signs.
2. Xanthomas may be tendonous, tuberous, or eruptive.
   a. Tendonous xanthomas can be palpated or may be visible as nodularities in extensor tendons, especially the Achilles tendon. They are seen most commonly with types II and III hyperlipidemia.
   b. Tuberous xanthomas occur on the elbows, hands, or other soft tissue areas and are most common in type III hyperlipidemia. Early tuberous xanthomas can be flat and seen in the palmar creases.
   c. Eruptive xanthomas are small papular clusters of lesions with a yellow center and red halo, seen in types I and V hyperlipidemias, which have very high TG levels in the chylomicron fraction.
3. Examination of the eyes
   a. Corneal arcus, a white ring around the cornea, often presents in older people and blacks without signifying hyperlipidemia. In younger patients and in whites, it has greater significance.
   b. Xanthelasma are flat plaques on the eyelids or near the eye. About half the patients with xanthelasma have significantly elevated low-density lipoprotein-C (LDL-C) levels.
   c. Lipemia retinalis results from TG levels >1200 mg/dl seen in types I and V. Blood in the retinal vessels assumes a "cream of tomato soup" appearance.

LABORATORY STUDIES

- For screening purposes, the total C is acceptable and patients need not be fasting.
- If the total C value is elevated or the TG and high-density lipoprotein-C (HDL-C) levels are important, they should be obtained after a 12- to 14-hr fast.

- Total C is largely composed of LDL-C, HDL-C, and very low-density lipoprotein-C (VLDL-C).
  1. HDL-C values can be determined directly without an ultracentrifuge.
  2. The VLDL-C is approximated by TG/5 for TG levels below 450 mg/dl.
  3. Thus, the atherogenic LDL-C value can be estimated using the formula below.

$$\text{LDL-C} = \text{Total C} - \text{TG/5} - \text{HDL-C}$$

- The NCEP makes treatment recommendations based on this calculation, where:

	Normal	Borderline	High
LDL-C (mg/dl)	<130	130–159	>160

- The NCEP keys its recommendations around LDL-C levels and treats a low HDL-C as an independent risk. The ratio of total C/HDL-C is occasionally used with a ratio of <3.3 being low risk, 4.5 average risk, and >6.0 high risk.
- Measurement of the constituent apolipoproteins of LDL and HDL is commercially available. Although these may be useful in specialized cases, in general, they are currently beyond the need of most clinical practice.

RECOMMENDED DIAGNOSTIC APPROACH

1. Screen all adults (or at least those with increased risk of coronary artery disease) with a random total serum C level.
2. If that value is elevated, redetermine a fasting total C along with TG and HDL-C. Then calculate the LDL-C fraction. Two such measurements should be made 1 to 8 weeks apart. This is especially important if treatment decisions depend on the values.
3. As part of the evaluation, take a careful history with attention to diet, family history (of lipids or coronary artery disease), medications, other coronary risk factors, and conditions that might cause a secondary hyperlipidemia.
4. Consider electrophoresis or ultracentrifugation if physical findings or family history suggest type III dysbetalipoproteinemia.

Bibliography

Basinski A, et al. Detection and management of asymptomatic hypercholesterolemia, a policy document by the Toronto working group on cholesterol policy. Toronto, Ontario Ministry of Health, 1989.

Expert Panel: Report of the National Cholesterol Education Program expert panel on detection, evaluation, and treatment of high blood cholesterol in adults. Arch Int Med 1988;148:36–69.

Keys A, ed. Coronary heart disease in seven countries. Circulation 1970;41(suppl 1):I1–I211.

Martin MJ, et al. Serum cholesterol, blood pressure, and mortality: Implications from a cohort of 361,622 men. Lancet 1986;2:933–936.

Pearson TA, Becker DM, eds. The Johns Hopkins Lipid Education Program, Segment 2, Screening Strategies for Lipid Disorders. Baltimore, Johns Hopkins University, 1985, pp. 8–9.

Schaefer EJ, Levy RI. Pathogenesis and management of lipoprotein disorders. N Engl J Med 1985;312:1300–1310.

Stamler J. Population studies. In: Levy RI, et al., eds. Nutrition, Lipids, and Coronary Diseases: A Global View. New York, Raven Press, 1979, pp. 25–88.

SECTION IX

NUTRITION

61

NUTRITION ASSESSMENT

JEAN M. STERN, *and*
    SAUNDRA N. AKER

Power of nutrient reaches to bone and to all the parts of
bone, to sinew, to vein, to artery, to muscle, to membrane, to flesh, fat, blood, phlegm, marrow, brain, spinal marrow, the intestines and all their parts, it reaches
also to heat, breath, and moisture.

HIPPOCRATES

NUTRIENT REQUIREMENTS

- Requirements for calories, protein, and fluids vary with
  age, body composition, activity, and stress.
  1. The basal energy expenditure (BEE) is a calculated
     estimate of the calorie requirement for a fasting, non-
     stressed person at rest.
  2. Modifications of the BEE are required for activity,
     growth, fever, trauma, or other stresses.
- Calories
  1. Basal calorie requirement
     a. Adults: The Harris-Benedict equation provides
        the daily BEE in kcal for adults at or near ideal
        body weight (IBW) (Table 61–1).

  Men: BEE (kcal) = 66 + (13.7 × actual weight in
  kg) + (5 × height in cm) − (6.8 × age in years)

  Women: BEE (kcal) = 655 + (9.6 × actual weight
  in kg) + (1.7 × height in cm) − (4.7 × age in years)

  For obese patients, the corrected IBW, which accounts for increased lean body mass to support
  extra weight, should be used in place of the actual
  weight:

  Corrected IBW = [(actual
  weight − IBW) × 0.25] + IBW

Preparation of this chapter was supported in part by grant numbers
CA18029, CA38552, HL36444, and DK35816 from the National Cancer
Institute, National Heart Lung and Blood Institute, and the Clinical
Nutrition Research Unit, Department of Health and Human Services.

TABLE 61–1. Ideal Body Weights for Adults

HEIGHT (CM)	WEIGHT (KG)	
	Women	Men
152	50.0 ± 4	
156	51.3 ± 4	
160	53.6 ± 4	
164	56.6 ± 5	62.4 ± 5
168	59.0 ± 5	64.7 ± 5
172	61.4 ± 5	68.0 ± 5
176	64.4 ± 5	70.8 ± 6
180	67.2 ± 5	73.6 ± 6
184	69.6 ± 5	76.8 ± 7
188		80.0 ± 7
192		82.4 ± 7

Weights were measured without shoes or clothing. The ± refers to the weight range between the 25th and 75th percentile of each height category.

Source: Modified from Hathaway ML and Foard ED. Heights and Weights of Adults in the U.S. Washington DC USDA, ARS, Home Economics Research Report Number 10, Table 80, 1960.

    b.   Children and adolescents (less than 45 kg and 3 to 16 years old):

$$\text{Males: BEE (kcal)} = 859 + [18.7 \times (\text{weight in kg} - 15)]$$

$$\text{Females: BEE (kcal)} = 800 + [19.7 \times (\text{weight in kg} - 15)]$$

  2. Total energy expenditure. Energy requirement = BEE × activity factor (AF) × injury factor (IF) × other factors as applicable (use all multipliers that apply) (Table 61–2).

- Protein
  1. Protein is required for tissue anabolism, enzyme and hormone synthesis, immune function, and maintenance of acid-base and fluid balances.
  2. Protein requirements vary with age, body size, organ function, illness, and catabolic drug therapy.
  3. During high stress such as wound healing, sepsis, and trauma, nutrition support should provide 16 to 24 non-protein calories per gram of protein (100 to 150 non-protein calories/g nitrogen).

Age	Baseline daily protein requirement (g/kg of IBW)	Stress daily protein requirement (g/kg of IBW)
Adult	0.8–1.0	1.5 (during sepsis, may be 2.0–2.5)
15–18	0.9	1.8
11–14	1.0	2.0
7–10	1.0	2.0–2.4
4–6	1.2	2.4–3.0

TABLE 61–2. Energy Expenditure Factors

CLINICAL CONDITION	CORRECTION FACTOR
Activity	
Confined to bed	1.1—1.2
Light activity	1.3
Moderate activity	1.5
Heavy activity	1.75
Injury state	
Fever	1.0 + 0.13 per degree C over 37.0
Elective surgery	1.0–1.2
Peritonitis	1.2–1.5
Multiple fractures	1.2–1.35
Major sepsis	1.4–1.8
Thermal injury	
0–20%	1.0–1.5
20–40%	1.5–1.85
40–100%	1.85–2.1
Starvation	1.7
Growth (children, adolescents)	1.1

- Fluid
  1. For persons over 20 kg, maintenance fluid requirements are based on the body surface area (Figure 61–1). Maintenance fluid requirements are:

     Adults and children > 20 kg: 1500 ml/square meter
     Children ≤10 kg: 100 ml/kg
     Children 10–20 kg: 1000 ml + 50 ml/kg over 10 kg

  2. The fluid requirements may decrease during hepatic, renal, or cardiac dysfunction. Additional fluid is required during the following:
     a. Increased respiratory rate
     b. Fever (13% increase for each degree above 37.0°C)
     c. GI losses
     d. Hemorrhage
     e. Hot, dry environment
     f. Polyuria
     g. Vomiting
- Nutrient absorption. Nutrient deficiencies may occur in persons with dysfunctional or surgically removed intestinal segments (Table 61–3). Biochemical monitoring may aid diagnosis.

CLINICAL ASSESSMENT

- Early nutrition assessment and support can decrease morbidity and mortality in the hospitalized patient. Historical or examination features that suggest nutritional deficiency include:
  1. Unintentional weight loss in the prior 3 months:
     a. To less than 90% of usual body weight for adults

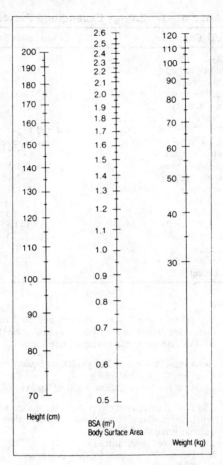

Figure 61–1. Body surface area nomogram. The body surface area (BSA) is indicated where a straight line connecting the height and weight levels intersects the surface area column. Adapted from Behrman RE, et al. Nelson's Textbook of Pediatrics, 12th ed. Philadelphia, WB Saunders Company, 1983, p. 1814.

    b. To less than 95% of usual body weight for children
2. Potential sources of nutrient loss (e.g., diarrhea).
3. Nothing by mouth for greater than 3 days or significantly low oral intake for greater than 7 days (e.g., anorexia, vomiting, esophagitis, or mucositis).
4. Elevated metabolic requirements (see above).
5. Medical diagnoses with higher risk of malnutrition: acquired immunodeficiency syndrome, cancer, decubiti, diabetes, GI disease or surgery, hepatic disease, hyperemesis gravidarum, renal failure, respiratory failure, sepsis, wounds.

TABLE 61–3. Nutrient Absorption

SITE	NUTRIENTS ABSORBED
Duodenum	Monosaccharides, amino acids, iron, calcium, magnesium, chloride, sodium
Proximal jejunum	Monosaccharides, amino acids, peptides, fatty acids, monoglycerides, glycerol, cholesterol; vitamins A, C, E, K; water-soluble vitamins: folate, riboflavin, niacin, pyridoxine, thiamin; copper, zinc, sodium, phosphorus
Distal jejunum	Majority of nutrients are absorbed in first 3 feet of jejunum. Distal segment assumes absorption after resection or disease.
Ileum	Vitamins B_{12}, C; bile salts, cholesterol, water, electrolytes
Colon	Water, electrolytes

6. Weight abnormality: less than 80% or greater than 120% of IBW. In determining this, the patient's actual height and weight must be measured, as patient reports of these are often inaccurate.

- Diet history. Pertinent features of the dietary history include:
  1. Current diet including food and fluid intake records
  2. Recent diet modifications
  3. Physical problems interfering with oral intake
     a. Dentures or poor dentition
     b. Oral lesions
     c. Chewing or swallowing difficulties
     d. Limited use of arms and hands
  4. Use or abuse of vitamin, mineral, or other nutrition supplements
  5. Eating habits
  6. Activity prior to hospitalization

- Medications may alter nutrient absorption or utilization (Table 61–4).

- Laboratory evaluation may be useful, but values may be altered by nonnutritional factors and may not be sensitive to early nutritional deficiencies.
  1. Immunologic function tests aid assessment of nutrition status only in conjunction with other biochemical parameters. Examples include the WBC and lymphocyte counts and the delayed cutaneous hypersensitivity reactions.
  2. Biochemical assays of nutrition status
     a. Nitrogen balance may be estimated using the formula below. A value less than 1 indicates a cata-

Text continued on page 530

TABLE 61–4. Drug and Nutrient Interactions

DRUG	NUTRIENTS WITH POTENTIALLY INCREASED LOSSES OR ELEVATED REQUIREMENTS[A]
Analgesics	
Alcohol	Vitamins B_{12}, A, C; folate; pyridoxine; thiamin; Ca^{2+}; Mg^{2+}; Zn
Aspirin	Vitamins C, K; folate; iron
Colchicine	Vitamins A, B_{12}; folate; K^+; Mg^{2+}; carotene; lactose; fat; nitrogen
Indomethacin	Iron; protein
Antacids	
AlOH/MgOH	Vitamin A; thiamin; Ca^{2+}; PO_4
Bicarbonate	Folate; iron
Antiarrhythmics	
Digitalis	K^+
Antiarthritics, chelating agents	
Penicillamine	Pyridoxine; Cu; Zn
Anticonvulsants	Vitamins C, D; folate; Ca^{2+}
Phenytoin	
Primidone	
Phenobarbital	
Antifungals	
Amphotericin B	K^+; Mg^{2+}; nitrogen
Antidepressants	
Amitriptyline	Riboflavin
Imipramine	Riboflavin

Antihyperlipemics	
Cholestyramine	Vitamins B_{12}, A, D, K; folate; Ca^{2+}; Fe; carotene; fat; medium chain triglycerides; glucose; cholesterol
Clofibrate	Vitamins B_{12}; E; iron; carotene; medium chain triglycerides; glucose
Antihypertensives	
Hydralazine	Pyridoxine
Antimicrobials	
Cephalosporin	Vitamin K
Gentamicin	K^+; Mg^{2+}
Neomycin	Vitamins B_{12}, A, D, K; Ca^{2+}; K^+; Mg^{2+}; Na^+; iron; lactose; fat; protein; sucrose
Pentamidine	Folate, K^+
Purimethamine	Folate
Tetracycline	Vitamins C, K; riboflavin; Ca^{2+}; Mg^{2+}; iron; Zn
Tobramycin	K^+
Trimethoprim-sulfamethoxazole	Vitamin K (with long use); folate
Antineoplastics	
Actinomycin-D	Vitamin B_{12}; Ca^{2+}; iron; fat
5-Fluorouracil	Thiamin
Methotrexate	Vitamin B_{12}; folate; carotene; fat; lactose; cholesterol
Antiparkinsons	
L-Dopa	Vitamin C; pyridoxine
Antituberculars	
Cycloserine	Vitamin B_{12}; folate; pyridoxine; Ca^{2+}; Mg^{2+}
Isoniazid (INH)	Vitamin B_{12}; E; folate; niacin; pyridoxine; Ca^{2+}; Mg^{2+}
Para-amino salicylate	Vitamins B_{12}; K; folate; fat
Cathartics	
Phenolphthalein	Vitamins C, D; Ca^{2+}; K^+

Table continued on following page

TABLE 61–4. Drug and Nutrient Interactions Continued

DRUG	NUTRIENTS WITH POTENTIALLY INCREASED LOSSES OR ELEVATED REQUIREMENTS[a]
Corticosteroids	Vitamin D; Ca^{2+}; K^+; PO_4; Zn; protein
Diuretics	
Chlorthalidone	K^+; Mg^{2+}
Ethacrynic acid	Ca^{2+}; K^+; Mg^{2+}
Furosemide	Ca^{2+}; K^+; Mg^{2+}; Zn
Hydrochlorothiazide	Riboflavin; K^+; Mg^{2+}; Zn
Spironolactone	Ca^{2+}; Mg^{2+}
Triamterene	Folate; Ca^{2+}
Hormones	
Oral contraceptives	Vitamin C; folate; pyridoxine; Zn
Hypnotics/Sedatives	
Glutethimide	Vitamin D; Ca^{2+}
Immunosuppressants	
Cyclosporine	Mg^{2+}
Laxatives	
Mineral Oil	Vitamins A, D, E, K; Ca^{2+}; PO_4; carotene
Other	
Diphosphonates	Vitamin D; Ca^{2+}
H_2 receptor antagonists	Vitamin B_{12}
para-Aminobenzoic acid	Vitamin D
Potassium chloride	Vitamin B_{12}
Sulfasalazine	Folate, Fe

[a] Most of these are clinically significant only with prolonged use.

TABLE 61–5. Implications of Visceral Proteins on Nutrition Status

VISCERAL PROTEINS	HALF-LIFE	NUTRITION-RELATED ALTERATIONS	NON-NUTRITION ALTERATIONS
Albumin	18–20 days	Decreased: chronic protein deficiency, malabsorption, protein-losing enteropathy	Decreased: serious infections, trauma, nephrotic syndrome, liver disease, preeclampsia, blood loss, overhydration Increased: exogenous albumin, blood or plasma support
Prealbumin (Transthyretin)	2 days	Decreased: calorie, protein deficiency	Decreased: liver disease, inflammatory diseases, trauma, chronic illness
Retinol binding protein	8–12 hours	Decreased: calorie, protein deficiency	Decreased: liver disease, inflammatory diseases, trauma, chronic illness Increased: renal disease
Transferrin	7–8 days	Decreased: calorie, protein deficiency Increased: iron deficiency	Decreased: multiple transfusions Unreliable in acute phase of illness or injury

TABLE 61–6. Clinical Signs of Nutrient Deficiencies

CLINICAL FINDING	POSSIBLE DEFICIENCY
Skin	
Xerosis	Essential fatty acid
Subcutaneous fat loss, fine wrinkling	Protein; energy
Purpura, increased bruising	Vitamins C, K
Pressure sores, poor wound healing	Protein; energy; vitamin C; pyridoxine; riboflavin; Zn; essential fatty acids
Oral Cavity	
Cheilosis (at corners of mouth, especially)	Protein; niacin; pyridoxine; riboflavin
Ageusia, dysgeusia	Zn
Magenta tongue	Riboflavin
Glossitis	Vitamin B_{12}; folate; pyridoxine; iron
Fiery red tongue	Vitamin B_{12}; folate
Glands	
Goiter	Iodine
Hypogonadism, delayed puberty	Zn

528

Heart	
Cardiac arrhythmias	Mg^{2+}; K^+
Cardiac dysfunction	PO_4
Cardiomyopathy	Selenium
Bone	
Bone pain	Vitamins C, D; Ca^{2+}; PO_4; minimal sunlight exposure
Bone deformities	Vitamin D; minimal sunlight exposure
Muscle	
Myalgia	Biotin; thiamin; selenium
Muscular weakness	Na^+; K^+
Muscle cramps	Cl^-; Na^+
Neurologic	
Disorientation	Thiamin; Na^+; water
Other	
Anemia	Vitamins B_{12}, E; biotin; folate; pyridoxine, iron; copper
Growth retardation	Protein; energy; vitamin D; Ca^{2+}; Mg^{2+}; Zn
Glucose intolerance	Chromium

bolic state while a value greater than 5 indicates an anabolic state. The factor 4 accounts for nitrogen losses not measured by the UUN, including stool, skin, and nonurea nitrogen:

$$\text{Nitrogen balance} = \text{Dietary nitrogen (g)} - \text{UUN} - 4$$

where dietary nitrogen (g) = dietary protein (g)/6.25; UUN = urinary urea nitrogen, obtained from a 24-hr urine collection

    b.   Serum visceral proteins (Table 61–5)
  3.   Clinical findings (Table 61–6)

Bibliography

Anderson CF, et al. The sensitivity and specificity of nutrition-related variables in relationship to duration of hospital stay and rate of complications. Mayo Clin Proc 1984;59:477–483.

Hathaway ML, and Foard ED. Heights and Weights of Adults in the U.S., Washington DC, USDA, ARS, Home Economics Research Report Number 10, 1960.

Krause MV, Mahan LK. Food, Nutrition, and Diet Therapy, 8th ed. Philadelphia, W.B. Saunders, 1990.

Linn BS, Robinson DS. The possible impact of DRGs on nutritional status of patients having surgery for cancer of the head and neck. JAMA 1988;22:514–518.

Long CL, et al. Metabolic response to injury and illness: Estimation of energy and protein needs from indirect calorimetry and nitrogen balance. J Paren Ent Nutr 1979;3:452–456.

Powers DE, Moore AO. Food Medication Interactions, 6th ed. Phoenix, AZ, F-M I Publishing, 1988.

SECTION X

**INFECTIOUS
DISEASES**

62

FEVER OF UNKNOWN ORIGIN

DAVID C. DUGDALE

Perhaps a fever (which the Gods forefend) may bring
your youth to some untimely end.

DRYDEN

DEFINITION

- Fever is a cardinal sign of disease.
  1. Most febrile illnesses due to viral or bacterial infections last 2 weeks or less and resolve without specific treatment.
  2. The definition of fever of unknown origin (FUO) used in patient series is:
     a. Presence of fever for at least 3 weeks.
     b. A documented temperature of at least 38.3°C (101°F) on several occasions.
     c. Failure to make the diagnosis after at least 1 week of study in the hospital.
- Evolution of medical care has changed the diseases that cause FUO. In practice, "FUO" refers to a febrile illness lasting more than 3 weeks, and the requirement of hospitalization is not stringent; this change of definition does not change the diagnostic approach to the syndrome.

DIFFERENTIAL DIAGNOSIS (Table 62–1)

- The axioms of evaluation of FUO patients are:
  1. Clinical clues are of critical importance in formulating the diagnostic approach.
  2. FUO is usually due to an atypical presentation of a relatively common disease.
  3. No "routine" evaluation is universally recommended. In general, with the exception of serologic and microbiologic studies, blood tests evaluate the degree of illness, while clinical findings and imaging studies provide direction for making a tissue diagnosis.
- Differences in frequencies of categories from various series are partially related to the study population.
  1. Increased use of prosthetic devices has led to their involvement as causes of FUO.
  2. HIV infections may cause prolonged fever or contribute to the atypical presentation of infectious diseases.

TABLE 62–1. Percentage of Cases by Diagnosis

	1952–1957 SERIES (YALE)	1970–1980 SERIES (UNIV. OF WASH.)	1986 SERIES (SOUTHWESTERN)
Infection	36	31	50
Abdominal abscess	11	10	4
Mycobacteria	11	5	5
Cytomegalovirus (CMV)	0	4	4
Urinary tract infection	3	3	9
Sinusitis/Dental	0	2	1
Osteomyelitis	0	2	4
Endocarditis	5	0	5
Vascular graft/catheter	0	2	4
Other (fungal, Epstein-Barr Virus (EBV) and others)	6	3	14
Neoplasm	19	31	15
Lymphoma	6	16	3

Leukemia	2	5	0
Solid tumors	9	10	12
Other	2	0	0
Collagen vascular disease	15	9	2
Still's disease	2	4	0
SLE	5	0	0
Polyarteritis nodosa	0	2	0
Giant cell arteritis	2	1	0
Rheumatic fever	6	1	0
Other	0	1	2
Granulomatous disease (sarcoidosis, Crohn's disease, granulomatous hepatitis)	4	7	2
Miscellaneous (hematomas, pulmonary emboli, familial Mediterranean fever, drug fever, alcoholic hepatitis, atrial myxoma)	16	7	22
Factitious fever	3	3	0
Undiagnosed	7	12	9

3. Difficulty with interpretation of pathologic material often delays the diagnosis of lymphomas.
4. Among solid tumors, renal, hepatic, colon, and adrenal carcinomas, and tumors metastatic to the liver have been implicated in causing FUO.
5. Patients who remain undiagnosed have a good prognosis (83% resolution at 1 year and 4% mortality).

CLINICAL FEATURES

- History. Historical information is critical to directing the evaluation of FUO patients.
  1. Specific dysfunctional organs (abdominal or flank pain, cough)
  2. Travel history (malaria after incomplete prophylaxis, amebic liver abscess, babesiosis, or Lyme disease after visits to Mexico, Cape Cod, or tick-infested areas of the United States)
  3. Familial illness (familial Mediterranean fever)
  4. Medications (rash and eosinophilia are not usual: alphamethyldopa, quinidine, procainamide, penicillins, isoniazid, phenytoin, cephalothin, sulfonamides, antihistamines, and iodide are common causes of drug fever)
  5. Medical history (subphrenic abscess in a patient post-abdominal surgery, hematomas after trauma or percutaneous diagnostic procedures, vascular access devices, prosthetic joints)
  6. Animal contact (psittacosis, brucellosis, leptospirosis, or trichinosis)
  7. Psychiatric history (factitious illness more common in female health-care workers or those with borderline personality disorder)
- Examination. Clinical signs are rarely pathognomonic but help guide further diagnostic studies and biopsies.
  1. Fever should be documented to exclude factitious fever by supervised temperatures or simultaneous oral and rectal temperatures. Fever pattern is rarely helpful (Table 62–2).
  2. Lymphadenopathy, hepatosplenomegaly, and pathologic masses must be detected to optimize biopsy site selection.
  3. Cutaneous manifestations may suggest the diagnosis. Factitious illness with true fever may have skin lesions due to self-inoculation.
  4. Cardiac murmurs suggest endocarditis or atrial myxoma.
  5. Bony tenderness may result from osteomyelitis or metastatic malignancy.
  6. Arthritis is frequent with collagen vascular diseases. Temporal artery tenderness suggests giant cell arteritis.
  7. Dental percussion tenderness suggests apical abscess.
  8. Rectal examination may suggest a neoplasm.
  9. Serial physical examinations may reveal new clinical clues or ones whose significance was underestimated.

TABLE 62–2. Causes of Prolonged Fever

Colon carcinoma
Fabry's disease
Granulomatous hepatitis
Malaria
Osteomyelitis
Regional enteritis
Renal cell carcinoma
Subphrenic abscess
Vasculitis
   Polyarteritis nodosa
   Polymyalgia rheumatica
   Still's disease
Whipple's disease

Source: Adapted from Wolff SM, et al. Unusual etiologies of fever and their evaluation. Ann Rev Med 1975;26:277–281.

LABORATORY STUDIES

- Useful tests include:
  1. Review of all previous studies. A review of reports is not adequate as "fresh looks" at data may reveal findings that were overlooked (e.g., bone lesions on IV pyelogram (IVP) films).
  2. Cultures of blood, urine, sputum, and other body fluids should be routinely collected for bacterial, fungal, viral, and mycobacterial pathogens.
     a. Unless obtained during antibiotic therapy, more than 4 blood cultures are unnecessary.
     b. Prolonged incubation to detect fastidious organisms is important (Table 62–3).
  3. CBC and blood film examination may find infections (malaria, babesiosis, or *Borrelia recurrentis*) or indicate a bone marrow biopsy (pancytopenia, myelophthisis).
  4. Tuberculin skin tests (5-tuberculin unit PPD) with controls. In FUO patients, TB is extrapulmonary.
  5. Urinalysis may demonstrate persistent bacterial infection, sterile pyuria (TB), hematuria (hypernephroma), or proteinuria (vasculitis).
  6. Hepatic enzymes are essential clues to granulomatous hepatitis and neoplasms.

TABLE 62–3. Fastidious Organisms That Cause Endocarditis

Hemophilus parainfluenza
Hemophilus aphrophilus
Actinobacillus actinomycetemcomitans
Eikenella corrodens
Cardiobacterium hominis
Kingella kingae

TABLE 62–4. Diagnostic Yield of Biopsies

Bone marrow	14%
Liver	13%
Lymph node	35%
Other	38%
All biopsies	22%
Laparotomy	48%

Source: Adapted from Larson EB, et al. Fever of undetermined origin: Diagnosis and follow-up of 105 cases, 1970–1980. Medicine 1982;61:269–292.

7. Serologic studies may detect some infections:
   a. HIV, CMV, EBV, or heterophile antibody
   b. Rapid plasma reagin (RPR) and confirmatory tests for syphilis
   c. Amebic hemagglutination (not complement fixation, which is insensitive)
   d. Q-fever, Brucella, Lyme disease

- Radiographic examination. X-rays should generally be used to study symptomatic sites.
  1. Chest X-rays should be universal.
  2. Bone X-rays should be done of symptomatic sites.
  3. Sinus X-rays should be done if a nasogastric tube has been used. CT scans are more sensitive for sinusitis than are X-rays.
  4. Dental X-rays should be considered in all patients as symptoms of apical abscesses are subtle.
  5. Barium studies should be reserved for those with GI symptoms or possible inflammatory bowel disease.
  6. Abdominal ultrasound detects hepatobiliary tract disease and intrarenal or perirenal infections but lacks sensitivity for intraabdominal abscesses.
  7. CT of the abdomen has replaced the lymphangiogram and nearly replaced the IVP and liver-spleen scan. Its sensitivity and specificity in detecting intraabdominal and intrahepatic abscesses is 90–95%. It is useful to image major vascular structures. CT improves the

TABLE 62–5. Method of Final Diagnosis

Nonlaparotomy tissue biopsy	36%
Laparotomy	21%
Clinical course	13%
Radiographic studies or scans	11%
Autopsy	10%
Nontissue culture	5%
Serology	5%
Other	1%

In 3 cases, 2 separate sources of information were critical to making the diagnosis.
Source: Adapted from Larson EB, et al. Fever of undetermined origin: Diagnosis and follow-up of 105 cases, 1970–1980. Medicine 1982;61:269–292.

TABLE 62–6. Work-up of the Patient with FUO

Basic procedures for evaluation of FUO
  History, physical, and review of medication
  Review of previously done studies; consider repeating
    those of questionable quality or with direct clinical
    relevance
  Blood cultures
  CBC with differential white cell count
  Erythrocyte sedimentation rate
  Urinalysis
  RPR and HIV
  Renal and thyroid function tests, liver and muscle
    enzymes, albumin, globulin
  Tuberculin skin tests with controls
  Stool for occult blood
  Antinuclear antibody and rheumatoid factor
  Serum sample to be saved for future use (frozen)
  Chest X-ray
  Biopsy of tissue as clinically indicated
    Bone marrow (abnormal CBC, disseminated infection
      or tumor)
    Liver (abnormal liver enzymes, disseminated infection
      or tumor)
    Temporal artery
    Abnormal lymph node or pathologic mass
    Muscle (polyarteritis nodosa)
Second-level procedures for evaluation of FUO
  Abdominal CT
  Dental X-ray
  Lumbar spine X-ray
  Sinus X-ray or CT
  Viral, amebic, bacterial serologies
  "Blind" (i.e., independent of clinical findings) bone
    marrow biopsy
Third-level procedures for evaluation of FUO
  Abdominal ultrasound
  Echocardiogram
  Indium-111–labeled leukocyte scan
  Barium studies of the GI tract
  Small bowel and/or rectal biopsy
  Muscle biopsy
  Temporal artery biopsy
  Laparoscopy or laparotomy
  Therapeutic trial

      yield of tissue biopsies and laparotomies, but does not
      obviate them.
   8. MRI as currently practiced is not superior to CT in
      detection of intraabdominal abscesses.
- Radionuclide scans. Use of these should be judicious due
  to excessive false-positive studies.
   1. Liver-spleen scans have, unless a functional as-
      sessment is needed, been replaced by ultrasound and
      CT.

2. Bone scans are the most sensitive test for osteomyelitis, but most patients with FUO due to osteomyelitis have plain film abnormalities.
3. Gallium scans done in the absence of localizing clinical clues are not helpful.
4. Indium-111–labelled leukocyte scans are very sensitive to infectious causes of FUO but have a high rate of false positive and borderline results. Use with a radionuclide bone scan may help diagnose prosthesis-associated osteomyelitis.

- Tissue biopsy or laparotomy. These have the highest yield in cases with localized findings (Table 62–4).
  1. A bone marrow biopsy should be considered in most patients.
  2. The absence of clinical signs pointing to the abdomen or a normal abdominal CT scan make a positive laparotomy unlikely.
- Therapeutic trials
  1. As a rule, therapeutic trials add confusion to the clinical picture.
  2. The trial should be directed toward a single disease.
  3. Naproxen has been advocated in the differential diagnosis of patients with known malignancy and FUO (i.e., fever that resolved with naproxen was neoplastic), but its use has not been proven in the broad spectrum of FUO patients.

RECOMMENDED DIAGNOSTIC APPROACH

The best results are obtained by following clinical clues and positive studies to a tissue diagnosis. The method of final diagnosis in patients with FUO is dominated by biopsy, laparotomy, and clinical course (Table 62–5). Not all studies listed in Table 62–6 are applicable to all patients.

Bibliography

Barbado FJ, et al. Fever of unknown origin: A survey on 133 patients. J Med 1984;15:185–192.

Chang JC, Gross HM. Utility of naproxen in the differential diagnosis of fever of undetermined origin in patients with cancer. Am J Med 1984;76:597–603.

Gleckman R, et al. Fever of unknown origin: A view from the community hospital. Am J Med Sci 1977;274:21–25.

Kerttula Y, et al. Fever of unknown origin: A follow-up investigation of 34 patients. Scand J Infect Dis 1983;15:185–187.

Larson EB, et al. Fever of undetermined origin: Diagnosis and follow-up of 105 cases, 1970–1980. Medicine 1982;61:269–292.

Mackowiak PA, LeMaistre CF. Drug fever: A critical appraisal of conventional concepts. Ann Int Med 1987;106:728–733.

Petersdorf RG, Beeson PB. Fever of unexplained origin: Report of 100 cases. Medicine 1961;40:1–30.

Rowland MD, DelBene VE. Use of body computed tomography to evaluate fever of unknown origin. J Infect Dis 1987;156:408–409.

Schmidt KG, et al. Indium-111-granulocyte scintigraphy in the evaluation of patients with fever of undetermined origin. Scand J Infect Dis 1987;19:339–345.

Smith JW. Southwestern medical conference: Fever of undetermined origin: Not what it used to be. Am J Med Sci 1986;292:56–64.

Weinstein L. Clinically benign fever of unknown origin: A personal retrospective. Rev Infect Dis 1985;7:692–699.

63

FEVER IN THE IMMUNO-COMPROMISED HOST

OLIVER W. PRESS

Behold, the bush burned with fire, and the bush was not consumed.

EXODUS 3:2

DEFINITIONS

- Fever is defined as an oral temperature $\geq$ 100.2°F (37.8°C) or a rectal temperature of $\geq$ 101.2°F (38.4°C).
- Immunocompromised hosts may have any of the following immune deficits (Table 63–1):
  1. Neutropenia (a neutrophil count $\leq$ 500 cells/mm^3) is the greatest risk factor for bacterial and fungal infections.
  2. Defective neutrophil function.
  3. Cellular immune dysfunction results from deficiencies in the numbers or activity of T lymphocytes and macrophages.
  4. Humoral immune dysfunction results from defective immunoglobulin production (e.g., B-lymphocyte and plasma cell disorders).
  5. Obstruction of body luminal structures promotes stasis of body fluids and overgrowth of microorganisms.
  6. Disruption of mucocutaneous barriers
  7. Splenic dysfunction causes defective production of antibodies against encapsulated organisms and impaired phagocytosis of microbes.

DIFFERENTIAL DIAGNOSIS OF FEVER IN THE IMMUNOCOMPROMISED HOST

- Infection with bacterial, viral, fungal, or parasitic organisms can be demonstrated by culture or serology in 65% of febrile immunocompromised patients (Table 63–2).
- The underlying disease may be responsible for fever in patients with malignant ("tumor fever") or collagen vascular disease. This diagnosis is always one of exclusion. The neoplasms most commonly associated with intrinsic fever include lymphomas, leukemias, renal cell and adrenal carcinomas, hepatomas, and tumors metastatic to the liver.

- Drug fever typically appears idiosyncratically 7 to 10 days after exposure to an offending drug (e.g., penicillins, cephalosporins, sulfonamides, thiazides) and may occur in association with a pruritic, maculopapular rash or eosinophilia. Some medications predictably produce fever within hours of drug exposure (amphotericin, bleomycin, high dose cytosine arabinoside, and antithymocyte globulin).
- Transfusions commonly cause febrile reactions as a result of alloimmunization to leukocyte antigens.
- Hematomas can produce prolonged fever even if they are uninfected. Concealed hematomas are most commonly located in the retroperitoneum.
- Pulmonary emboli are associated with fever in 50% of cases.
- Splenic infarcts should be suspected in patients with left-sided abdominal pain and fever.
- Graft vs host disease (GVHD) occurs in 30 to 60% of patients receiving allogeneic bone marrow transplants, and may also occur rarely in immunocompromised patients transfused with unirradiated blood products. The disease generally appears with fever, rash, diarrhea, and liver dysfunction.
- Miscellaneous causes of cryptic fever include adrenal insufficiency, catheter infections, mycobacterial disease (the patient may be anergic), abdominal abscesses, and systemic viral infections, including cytomegalovirus, Epstein-Barr virus, and anicteric hepatitis (A, B, or C).

CLINICAL FEATURES OF FEVER IN THE COMPROMISED HOST: HISTORY AND PHYSICAL EXAMINATION

- A careful review of the patient's medical history is mandatory.
- A history of recent travel and exposure to pets and infection should be carefully elicited.
- Localizing symptoms are of paramount importance.
- The medication list should be scrutinized and unnecessary drugs discontinued.
- Careful and repeated physical examinations should be performed in a search for signs of local inflammation, catheter infection, mental status changes, nuchal rigidity, lesions in the fundi and on the skin, periodontal infections, lymphadenopathy, pulmonary consolidation, hepatosplenomegaly, abdominal tenderness, or perirectal cellulitis. The physical examination reveals no source of infection in 55% of patients with documented bacteremia.
- The cardinal symptoms and signs of infection may be absent in immunocompromised patients. Neutropenic patients may not generate pus, sputum, or signs of local inflammation. Meningitis with opportunistic pathogens occurs without meningismus in 63% of cases. Only 8% of neutropenic patients with pneumonia have purulent spu-

TABLE 63-1. Infections in Immunocompromised Hosts

Defective Defense Mechanism	Typical Disease Setting	Typical Infecting Organisms	Types of Infection
Neutropenia	Leukemia Bone marrow transplantation	Gram-negative rods[a] *S. epidermidis* *S. aureus* *Candida* *Aspergillus*	Septicemia, pneumonia, typhlitis, meningitis
Defective neutrophil function	Uremia Alcoholism Diabetes mellitus Chronic granulomatous disease	*S. aureus* *Candida*	Recurrent abscesses, septicemia
Cellular immune dysfunction	AIDS Hodgkin's disease Kidney transplants	*Pneumocystis carinii* *Cryptococcus* Mycobacteria Cytomegalovirus Herpes simplex *Cryptosporidium* *Toxoplasma* *Strongyloides*	Pneumonia, meningitis, cutaneous lesions, diarrhea, septicemia

Humoral immune dysfunction	Multiple myeloma, Chronic lymphocytic leukemia, Agammaglobulinemia	*Listeria* *Salmonella* *S. pneumoniae,* *Hemophilus influenzae* *Neisseria meningitidis* Gram-negative rods[a]	Septicemia, pneumonia, meningitis
Obstruction of lumina	Cancer	Gram-negative rods[a] *Bacteroides* *Enterococcus*	Septicemia
Disruption of mucocutaneous barriers	Burns, Cancer chemotherapy	*S. epidermidis* *S. aureus* Gram-negative rods[a] (esp. *Pseudomonas*)	Local infections, septicemia
Splenic dysfunction	Sickle cell anemia, Splenectomy	*S. pneumoniae* *Hemophilus influenzae* *Neisseria meningitidis*	Septicemia

[a] The most common pathogenic gram-negative rods in immunocompromised hosts include *Escherichia coli,* *Enterobacter cloacae,* *Klebsiella,* and *Pseudomonas aeruginosa.*

545

TABLE 63–2. Frequency of Various Types of Infections in Immunocompromised Patients[a]

PATHOGEN	MULTIPLE MYELOMA (%)	RENAL TRANSPLANTS (%)	MARROW TRANSPLANTS (%)	AIDS (%)
Bacteria (overall)	(78)	(16)	(35–40)	(25–50)
Enteric gram-negative rods				
Escherichia coli	26	1	2	<1
Klebsiella	8	<1	3	<1
Enterobacter	0	<1	2	<1
Pseudomonas	12	3	2	<1
Other	—	0	1	<1
Salmonella	<1	<1	0	2
Staphylococcus epidermidis	—	1	12	2
S. aureus	20	1	3	3
Streptococcus pneumoniae	52	<1	5–10	1
Enterococcus	0	<1	1	<1
Bacteroides	0	<1	0	<1
Hemophilus influenzae	10	1	0	<1
Mycobacterium	4	<1	0	25–50[b]

Other	0	4	5	1
Viruses (overall)	(2)	(24)	(40–70)	(>90)
Cytomegalovirus	0	21	45	73
Herpes zoster	2	2	30–40	NA
Herpes simplex	0	NA	40–50	28
Fungi (overall)	(0)	(4)	(22)	(90)c
Aspergillus	0	2	4–10	<1
Candida	0	2	10–15	80–90c
Cryptococcus	0	<1	1	9–13
Protozoa (overall)	(0)	(<1)	(6)	(80)
Pneumocystis	0	0	6	60–80
Toxoplasma	0	0	<1	3–11
Strongyloides	0	0	<1	3
Cryptosporidium	0	0	0	11

a Percentage of patients acquiring infection with the stated pathogen. Many patients had more than one infection, hence totals do not equal the sum of the individual infection incidences.

b 90% of mycobacterial infections in AIDS are *M. avium-intracellulare*; 10% are *M. tuberculosis*.

c The majority of candidal infections in AIDS are oral (thrush). About 25% have invasive candidiasis at autopsy.

NA = data not available

547

tum, and 38% have a normal chest X-ray. Only 11% of neutropenic patients with urinary tract infections have pyuria.

- Factors that favor a microbial origin rather than an underlying disease as the cause of fever include appearance of skin lesions, mental deterioration, hypotension, hyperventilation, disseminated intravascular coagulation, hemolysis, metabolic acidosis, localized pain, and oliguria.

CLINICAL APPROACH TO FEVER IN THE IMMUNOCOMPROMISED HOST: LABORATORY STUDIES

- General laboratory studies
  1. A CBC, smear, white cell differential, and platelet count should be done.
  2. Routine serum chemistries (electrolytes, BUN, creatinine, transaminases, bilirubin) should be done to assess metabolic acidosis and renal insufficiency due to septic shock or liver function abnormalities from hepatitis or hepatic metastases.
  3. Gram's stains of sputum, urine, CSF, pus, and other body fluids (e.g., pleural effusions or ascites) should be performed. Special stains (Ziehl-Neelsen for mycobacteria, India ink of CSF for cryptococcus, immunofluorescent stains for CMV, *Legionella,* and *Pneumocystis*) should be performed when the diagnosis eludes initial evaluation.
  4. Cultures of the pharynx, perirectal area, stool, urine, sputum, blood, skin vesicles, and other body fluids (pleural effusions and ascites) should be obtained for routine microbiologic studies for bacteria, fungi, viruses, and mycobacteria. Anaerobic cultures should be performed on blood and other body fluids, and blood cultures should be incubated for prolonged periods (4 weeks) to allow growth of fastidious organisms. Antibiotic removal devices may be useful when patients are receiving antibiotics, and the "DuPont isolator" will enhance recovery of mycobacteria and *Candida* from blood cultures (especially in AIDS patients).
  5. Microscopic evaluation of fresh stool specimens may demonstrate *Strongyloides stercoralis* larvae or *Cryptosporidium.*
  6. Serologic testing should be performed for *Legionella pneumophila,* cryptococcal antigen, HIV, hepatitis A and B, cytomegalovirus, Epstein-Barr virus, and toxoplasmosis.
  7. Coagulation studies may detect disseminated intravascular coagulation.
- Radiographic studies and special tests
  1. An initial chest X-ray should be done for all patients. Serial chest radiographs are useful for monitoring evolving pneumonias (such as in cytomegalovirus infection or *Pneumocystis*).

2. Localizing signs should be investigated with appropriate studies.
3. Sinus X-rays or a limited sinus CT scan may reveal occult sinusitis.
4. Radionuclide scans of bone, lung, and liver/spleen are useful in cases of suspected osteomyelitis, pulmonary embolism, and splenic infarction, respectively.
5. The usefulness of gallium-scans and indium-labeled white cell scans is controversial. Although many cases of occult infection have been diagnosed with the aid of these techniques, the frequency of false-positive and false-negative results (14 and 4%, respectively for gallium) limits their utility. In addition, these methods are technically difficult in neutropenic patients.

- Invasive procedures
  1. Biopsy of skin lesions should be performed for pathology and culture (bacterial, fungal, and viral) to detect leukemia cutis, ecthyma gangrenosum (due to *Pseudomonas aeruginosa*), or disseminated candidiasis.
  2. Bone marrow or lymph node biopsy may reveal histologic or microbiologic evidence of tuberculous, fungal, or *Salmonella* infection or tumor (lymphoma, Kaposi's sarcoma). In patients with AIDS and fever of unknown source, Bishburg, et al. found that bone marrow biopsy yielded diagnoses of infection in 42% of the patients. It had a sensitivity of 94% for *Mycobacterium avium–intracellulare* and 31% for *Cryptococcus neoformans*.
  3. Liver biopsy should be considered for patients with hepatic dysfunction.
  4. Peripheral venous and routine subclavian catheters should be removed, culture samples should be taken, and new catheters should be inserted. Right atrial Hickman and Broviac catheters need not be removed unless there is evidence of persistent catheter infection after administration of appropriate antibiotics.
  5. Special tests for patients with pulmonary infiltrates:
     a. Gram's stain and culture of sputum should be routinely ordered but usually are nondiagnostic.
     b. Bronchoscopy with bronchoalveolar lavage and/or transbronchoscopic biopsy is now the procedure of choice for diagnosing pulmonary infections in immunocompromised hosts.
        i. Bronchoalveolar lavage is particularly effective in AIDS patients: for PCP the sensitivities of lavage and transbronchoscopic biopsy are 86 and 87%, respectively, and that of both techniques together, 98%.
        ii. The risk of pneumothorax with transbronchial biopsy is 9% (5.9% require tube thoracostomy).
     c. Open lung biopsy has the highest diagnostic yield of any diagnostic pulmonary procedure, but is associated with considerable morbidity. Empiric normal antibiotic coverage with combination regimens is advocated by many clinicians rather than proceeding to open lung biopsy if suspected pneumonia eludes diagnosis with bronchoscopy.

6. Diagnostic procedures for patients with headache, stiff neck, or mental status changes:
   a. CT of the head can rule out a brain abscess or hemorrhage.
   b. Lumbar puncture should be performed even with minimal CNS symptoms as long as there is no evidence of increased intracranial pressure or severe thrombocytopenia (<50,000 mm^3). The common pathogens producing meningitis in compromised patients do not cause prominent meningeal symptoms. CSF should be analyzed for cell count, protein, glucose, Gram's and acid-fast stain, India ink examination, cryptococcal antigen determination, and bacterial, mycobacterial, and fungal cultures.

RECOMMENDED DIAGNOSTIC APPROACH

- Initial evaluation
  1. Perform detailed history and physical examination.
  2. Obtain routine laboratory tests: CBC, with differential, chemistry panel, and urinalysis.
  3. Draw 2 blood cultures 15 min apart. In patients with central venous catheters: 1 culture should be drawn through each lumen of the catheter and 1 through a peripheral vein.
  4. Obtain Gram's stain and culture of other sites: pharynx, sputum, urine, skin lesions, ascites, pleural effusions.
  5. If diarrhea is present, obtain stool for fecal leukocyte stain, ova and parasite examination, *Clostridium difficile* toxin assay, and culture.
  6. Perform a chest X-ray.
  7. If a specific anatomic site is implicated by symptoms or signs, specific imaging studies should be ordered:
     a. For abdominal pain: obtain upright and supine abdominal radiographs.
     b. For CNS complaints (headache, drowsiness, stiff neck): a head CT scan and lumbar puncture should be performed.
  8. Empiric antibiotic administration must be initiated in all febrile neutropenic patients while awaiting culture results.
- Further evaluation. If the patient remains febrile more than 48 hr after institution of empiric antibiotic therapy, and initial tests have not delineated an etiology, the following studies should be considered:
  1. Review of medication list with discontinuation of any unnecessary drugs.
  2. Daily blood cultures while febrile and neutropenic.
  3. Repeat cultures of other suspicious sites.
  4. Culture and immunofluorescent stain of any mucocutaneous lesions for Herpes simplex and zoster.
  5. Serologic tests for *Legionella,* toxoplasmosis, CMV.
  6. Bronchoscopy and bronchoalveolar lavage if pulmo-

nary infiltrates are present. Specimens should be analyzed with Gram's, fungal, and acid-fast stains, bacterial, fungal, and mycobacterial culture, immunofluorescent staining for CMV, *Pneumocystis,* and *Legionella,* and centrifugation cultures for CMV.
7. Biopsy skin lesions, lymph nodes, liver, and bone marrow for histologic examination and culture.
8. Sinus radiographs to look for occult sinusitis.
9. Abdominal CT scan to look for occult abscesses.

Bibliography

Armstrong D. Opportunistic infections in the acquired immune deficiency syndrome. Sem Oncol 1987;14:40–47.

Bishburg E, et al. Yield of bone marrow culture in the diagnosis of infectious diseases in patients with acquired immunodeficiency syndrome. J Clin Micro 1986;24:312–314.

Bodey GP. Infection in cancer patients. Am J Med 1986;81:11–26.

Crawford SW, et al. Rapid detection of cytomegalovirus pulmonary infection by bronchoalveolar lavage and centrifugation culture. Ann Int Med 1988;108:180–185.

Lazarus HM, et al. Infectious emergencies in oncology patients. Sem Oncol 1989;16:543–560.

Meyers JD. Infection in bone marrow transplant recipients. Am J Med 1986;81:27–38.

Peterson PK, et al. Infectious diseases in hospitalized renal transplant recipients. Medicine 1982;61:360–372.

Rubin RH. Empiric antibacterial therapy in granulocytopenia induced by cancer chemotherapy. Ann Int Med 1988;108:134–136.

Whimbey E, et al. Bacteremia and fungemia in patients with the acquired immunodeficiency syndrome. Ann Int Med 1986;104:511–514.

Wong B. Parasitic diseases in immunocompromised hosts. Am J Med 1984;76:479–486.

64

OTITIS, PHARYNGITIS, AND SINUSITIS

PAUL G. RAMSEY, *and* DOUGLAS S. PAAUW

The ears should be kept perfectly clean; but it must never be done in company. It should never be done with a pin, and still less with the fingers, but always with an ear-picker.

St. Jean Baptiste de la Salle (1651–1719)

OTITIS

Definition

- Acute otitis media is a suppurative process that is related to eustachian tube blockage with subsequent accumulation of fluid in the middle ear. Bacteria may gain access to the middle ear by reflux up the eustachian tube, although other pathogenic mechanisms such as hematogenous spread of bacteria occur.
- Noninfected secretory middle ear effusions are called serous otitis media.
- Otitis externa refers to infection of the external ear, often related to trauma.

Epidemiology

- Otitis media and serous otitis are common problems among children less than 6 years of age but are uncommon in adults.
- Otitis externa is a common problem in adults and children. Predisposing factors include trauma, heat, humidity, excessive contact with water, and skin disorders such as psoriasis or seborrhea.
- Viral infection is an important predisposing factor for otitis media, though viruses are infrequently isolated from middle ear effusions. In children, infection with respiratory syncytial virus and adenovirus, and in adults, infection with influenza virus often precede otitis media.

Etiology and Clinical Manifestations

- Otitis media
    1. Onset is associated with pain in the ear and fever in 40 to 60% of cases, and occasionally is associated with nausea, vomiting, vertigo, or hearing loss.

2. Otoscopic examination of the color, contour, translucence, and mobility of the tympanic membrane help distinguish otitis media from serous otitis.
3. The most common causative organisms are *Streptococcus pneumoniae* and nontypable strains of *Hemophilus influenzae*. *Moraxella catarrhalis* (formerly called *Branhamella catarrhalis*), *Streptococcus pyogenes*, and staphylococcal species are found in small numbers of patients.
4. *S. pneumoniae* and *H. influenzae* cause most cases of bullous myringitis. *Mycoplasma pneumoniae* is rarely isolated from the middle ear.
5. In the neonate and in immunosuppressed adults, gram-negative bacteria and *S. aureus* may cause otitis.

• Otitis externa
1. Patients with otitis externa usually have pain in the affected ear but rarely have fever.
2. Examination reveals erythema, serosanguinous or purulent discharge, and granulation tissue in the external auditory canal.
3. *Pseudomonas aeruginosa* and *S. pyrogenes* are common causes of otitis externa in children and adults. Otitis externa is relatively common in HIV-infected patients, and may involve atypical organisms (*Pneumocystis carinii*).

• Complications of otitis include:
1. Mastoiditis and temporal bone osteomyelitis.
2. Invasive otitis externa due to infection with *P. aeruginosa*, which usually occurs in elderly diabetic patients. The infection spreads in the soft tissue to the base of the skull and may be associated with cranial nerve palsies.

Laboratory Evaluation

• Myringotomy. Diagnosis of otitis media may be made most specifically by myringotomy, but this procedure is rarely indicated. Myringotomy may be considered in the following situations:
1. For patients with severe systemic toxicity
2. For immunosuppressed patients
3. For patients who have not responded to prior antibiotic therapy
4. For patients with signs of spread of infection beyond the middle ear (mastoiditis or temporal bone osteomyelitis)

• Tympanometry. This objective test of tympanic membrane compliance may be useful to examine individuals with chronic otitis.
• X-rays or CT. These studies evaluate for spread of infection beyond the ear.

Recommended Diagnostic Approach

• Otitis is usually diagnosed on the basis of clinical findings. Treatment is usually empiric based on epidemiologic features, but a specific microbiologic diagnosis should be made in some cases (see above).

- Complications of otitis may be suspected by clinical findings and confirmed by radiographic or CT examinations.

PHARYNGITIS

Definition

Pharyngitis is an infection of the oropharynx. Most infections are self-limited, but a variety of complications may occur, including:

1. Otitis media and sinusitis.
2. Epiglottitis.
3. Peritonsillar abscess (quinsy): This is a complication of streptococcal pharyngitis.
4. Nonsuppurative sequelae of *S. pyogenes* infection: acute rheumatic fever, glomerulonephritis, and scarlet fever.
5. Diphtheria is a rare complication of *Corynebacterium diphtheriae* infection.

Epidemiology

Viruses cause most cases of pharyngitis, but bacteria (primarily *S. pyogenes*) may cause as many as 25% of cases in epidemic situations.

- Age
  1. Pharyngitis in children is commonly caused by viruses, including respiratory syncytial virus, adenovirus, parainfluenza virus, rhinovirus, and enteroviruses.
  2. In adults, parainfluenza and influenza viruses, adenovirus, and enteroviruses also cause pharyngitis, but Epstein-Barr virus and herpes simplex virus should also be considered.
  3. *S. pyogenes* infections occur most frequently in school-age children, and *M. pneumoniae* causes pharyngitis in individuals of ages 10 to 25. *Chlamydia pneumoniae* (TWAR) may also cause pharyngitis in this age group.
- Clinical setting. In crowded living conditions (schools and military settings) adenovirus is the most important cause of pharyngitis. *S. pyogenes* infections also occur frequently in these settings, with the highest incidence in the winter.

Clinical Manifestations and Microbiology

- Symptoms
  1. Sore throat, the hallmark symptom of pharyngitis, usually develops acutely.
  2. General malaise, myalgia, fever, and upper respiratory tract symptoms including coryza, cough, and laryngitis may be present.
- Physical findings

1. Physical findings do not allow diagnosis of a specific etiology.
2. Exudative pharyngitis. This is not a specific finding for streptococcal infection. It can be seen with Epstein-Barr virus, adenovirus, herpes simplex virus, and other viral infections. Many patients with Epstein-Barr virus infection may also have beta-hemolytic streptococci isolated from the pharynx.
3. Tender cervical lymphadenopathy with an exudative pharyngitis and leukocytosis (WBC > 15,000/mm³) suggests streptococcal infection.
4. Findings of scarlet fever. A bright erythematous rash with a sandpaper feel involving the trunk and face and skin folds (Pastia's lines) also suggests streptococcal infection. The rash usually spares the palms and soles and desquamates in the resolving phase.
5. Peritonsillar abscess (quinsy)
   a. Adults in the second or third decade of life may develop peritonsillar abscesses due to infection with beta-hemolytic streptococci and rarely with *S. aureus*.
   b. The superior pole of the tonsil is the common location for abscess formation. Symptoms include sore throat, dysphagia, and impaired palatal motion. Trismus may result from irritation of the internal pterygoid muscle.
   c. Physical examination reveals a fluctuant mass, and the uvula is often displaced from the midline.
6. An adherent gray-black membrane, with edema of the fauces, suggests diphtheria. The onset of this infection is abrupt with rapid spread of the tonsillar exudate. Symptoms and signs include severe lethargy, stridor, cranial and peripheral nerve palsies, and airway obstruction.
7. Epiglottitis
   a. Dysphagia out of proportion to the signs of pharyngitis suggests epiglottitis.
   b. Patients appear anxious and sit leaning forward. Respiratory stridor may be present. Secretions can be seen in the back of the oral cavity, and epiglottitis can be confirmed by the presence of an erythematous epiglottis projecting over the tongue.
   c. If epiglottitis is suspected, examination, which may precipitate airway obstruction, should be performed only if personnel and equipment are available for emergency endotracheal intubation or tracheostomy.

Diagnostic Tests and Differential Diagnosis

It is important to distinguish self-limited benign infections (viral and *Mycoplasma* infections) from infections associated with morbidity and potential mortality.

- Throat cultures are necessary to diagnose group A streptococcal pharyngitis. Throat swabs should be cultured also for *N. gonorrhoeae* if the clinical setting suggests this diagnosis.

- Rapid Strep antigen: Rapid streptococcal antigen tests may be processed within 10 min. The sensitivity is 75 to 90%, with specificity over 95%.
- Lateral neck X-rays
  1. Recognition of the complications of pharyngitis depends primarily on the history and physical examination.
  2. Lateral neck X-rays are important for diagnosing epiglottitis and may demonstrate an enlarged epiglottis.

Recommended Diagnostic Approach

- If the patient presents with severe pharyngitis, then use a rapid Strep antigen test with treatment if the result is positive. If the result is negative, throat culture for Strep should be done.
- Consider other diagnostic tests based on epidemiologic or clinical clues: Monospot, diphtheria culture, *N. gonorrhoeae* culture.
- If clinical suspicion is very high (fever, exudate present, headache, adenopathy), then treatment with no culture or rapid Strep antigen test is an acceptable option.
- If pharyngitis is mild, then use of throat culture alone is sufficient. There is no danger in withholding treatment until culture results are available.

SINUSITIS

Definition

- Bacterial, viral, and occasionally fungal infections of the paranasal sinuses may cause acute or chronic sinusitis.
  1. *H. influenzae, S. pneumoniae,* and other streptococci are the primary pathogens causing acute sinusitis. Anaerobic organisms are primarily implicated in cases of chronic disease.
  2. It is often difficult to distinguish infectious sinusitis from noninfectious allergic conditions.
- Maxillary sinusitis is extremely common (1% of viral upper respiratory infections are complicated by acute maxillary sinusitis). Complications related to maxillary sinusitis are rare.
- Frontal sinusitis is unusual but may be complicated by potentially life-threatening infections such as cranial osteomyelitis, brain abscess, frontal subperiosteal abscess, epidural abscess, or subdural abscess.
- Bacterial infection of the ethmoid sinus is a common cause of orbital cellulitis.
- Sphenoid sinusitis is rare, but the relationship of the sphenoid sinus to the pituitary gland, optic canals, dura mater, and cavernous sinus may lead to severe complications.

Epidemiology and Predisposing Factors

- Associated infections. Most cases follow viral upper respiratory tract infection. Symptoms of viral infection that persist longer than 7 days should raise the question of sinusitis.

- Mechanical problems. A deviated nasal septum, facial trauma, and nasal polyps disrupt the normal sinus drainage pattern, predisposing patients to sinusitis.

- Allergies. Allergic rhinosinusitis is an important predisposing condition for infectious sinusitis.

- Extension of odontogenic infections. This may lead to complicated bacterial sinusitis.

- Cystic fibrosis. Most patients with cystic fibrosis develop bacterial sinusitis.

- Immunosuppressed patients. Immunosuppressed patients may develop complications of sinusitis due to unusual organisms.
    1. Rhinocerebral mucormycosis is most commonly seen in patients with diabetic ketoacidosis.
    2. Invasive aspergillosis usually occurs in the setting of neutropenia.

- AIDS. Sinusitis is extremely common in AIDS patients. The most common organisms are *H. influenzae* and *S. pneumoniae*. Occasionally, fungal pathogens may be present.

- "Nosocomial sinusitis." Sinusitis should be considered in all patients with fever in association with prolonged nasotracheal or nasogastric intubation.

Clinical Features

- Maxillary sinusitis
    1. This form is associated with facial pain, purulent nasal discharge, and altered facial sensation. Facial pain may be aggravated by stooping. Headache and fever occur in a minority of patients.
    2. Sinus transillumination is helpful in diagnosing cases of acute maxillary sinusitis but is less helpful in the setting of chronic disease. The finding of opaque sinuses correlates with active purulent infection.

- Frontal sinusitis
    1. Patients with acute frontal sinusitis often have symptoms of pain and tenderness over the frontal sinus.
    2. Fever, purulent nasal discharge, and signs of involvement of the maxillary sinuses may be seen.
    3. Pitting edema over the forehead suggests a possible diagnosis of a subperiosteal abscess ("Pott's puffy tumor").

- Ethmoiditis. Ethmoiditis may be associated with orbital complications.
    1. Edema or cellulitis of the eyelid.
    2. "Orbital cellulitis" characterized by tenderness of the eye, ophthalmoplegia, chemosis, proptosis, and ery-

thema and edema of the lids. Orbital or subperiosteal abscess may occur.

3. Other complications include meningitis, epidural abscess, or cavernous sinus thrombosis.

- Sphenoid sinusitis

1. Headache is the most common initial symptom in patients with sphenoid sinusitis. Pain is often unilateral and may involve the frontal, temporal, or occipital regions. Patients may have unexplained tenderness over the vertex of the skull or over the mastoid.

2. Fever is frequently present in patients with acute sphenoiditis but may be absent in patients with chronic infection.

3. Extension of infection from the sphenoid sinus may lead to cavernous sinus thrombosis, pituitary insufficiency, bitemporal hemianopsia, and meningitis. Clinical features of septic cavernous sinus thrombosis include abrupt onset of photophobia, headache, ophthalmoplegia, chemosis, and proptosis.

4. *S. aureus* is the most frequent cause of septic cavernous sinus thrombosis, but gram-negative organisms and anaerobes have also been implicated.

Recommended Diagnostic Approach

- Most cases of acute maxillary sinusitis can be diagnosed by sinus transillumination.
- Radiologic examination is the most sensitive and specific test.

1. The Water's view provides the best examinations of the maxillary sinuses. Findings of opacity or air fluid level or mucosal thickening greater than 8 mm correlate with purulent sinusitis.

2. X-ray examination is essential for diagnosing frontal, ethmoid, and sphenoid sinusitis.

- CT examinations may be needed for diagnosis of sphenoid sinus infection.
- Direct sinus aspiration is the only procedure that can provide accurate information concerning etiology. Nasal swab cultures do not correlate with cultures of material obtained by direct sinus aspiration.

Bibliography

Berg O, et al. Discrimination of purulent from nonpurulent maxillary sinusitis: A clinical and radiographic diagnosis. Ann Otolaryngol 1981;90:272–275.

Doroghazi RM, et al. Invasive external otitis: Report of 21 cases and review of the literature. Am J Med 1981;71:603–614.

Kohan D, et al. Otologic disease in patients with acquired immune deficiency syndrome. Ann Otol Rhino Laryngol 1988;97:636–640.

Levy ML, et al. Infections of the upper respiratory tract. Med Clin North Am 1983;67:153–171.

Lew D, et al. Sphenoid sinusitis: A review of 30 cases. N Engl J Med 1983;309:1149–1153.

Mayosmith MF, et al. Acute epiglottitis in adults. N Engl J Med 1986;314:1133–1139.

Pelton Si, Klein JO. The draining ear: Otitis media and extrena. Infect Dis Clin N Am 1988:2:117–129.

Todd JK. The sore throat: Pharyngitis and epiglottitis. Infect Dis Clin N Am 1988:2:149–162.

65

BRONCHITIS AND PNEUMONIA

KEITH LEYDEN

As has been belch'd on by infected lungs.

SHAKESPEARE (1564–1616) Pericles, IV, vi

ACUTE BRONCHITIS

Definition and General Comments

- Definition
  1. Acute bronchitis is an inflammatory condition of the tracheobrochial tree that does not involve the alveoli.
  2. Chronic bronchitis is a noninfectious disease that occurs in patients with a history of chronic exposure to inhaled toxins, usually tobacco smoke.
- Epidemiology. Specific risk factors for acute bronchitis include young age, old age with chronic respiratory illness, asthma, exposure to air pollutants (especially nitrogen oxides, sulfur dioxide, and cigarette smoke), and exposure to cold, damp environments.
- Etiology (Table 65–1)
  1. Viruses cause over 95% of acute bronchitis cases. *Mycoplasma pneumoniae* is the most common nonviral cause.
  2. Throat cultures taken at the time of illness often demonstrate *Streptococcus pneumoniae, Staphylococcus aureus,* or *Hemophilus influenzae;* however, the etiologic roles for these organisms remain unclear.
  3. In normal individuals the bronchi are sterile. In 82% of patients with chronic obstructive pulmonary disease (COPD), pathogenic bacteria chronically colonize the bronchi. In these individuals, a bacterial etiology of acute bronchitis is more common.

Differential Diagnosis (Table 65–2)

The differential diagnosis of acute bronchitis includes any acute process which presents with cough. The diagnosis of bronchitis is one of exclusion.

Clinical Features

- History
  1. The clinical hallmark of acute bronchitis is the presence of cough. Important historical information

TABLE 65–1. Causes of Acute Bronchitis

Viral	Bacterial
Influenza	*Bordetella pertussis*
Adenovirus	*Streptococcus*
Rhinovirus	*pneumoniae*
Coronavirus	*Hemophilus influenzae*
Parainfluenza virus	*Staphylococcus aureus*
Respiratory syncytial	Bacterialike
virus	*Mycoplasma pneumonia*
Rubeola	*Chlamydia psittaci*
Rubella	(TWAR)

      includes associated symptoms such as fever, sinus pain or discharge, dyspnea, wheezing, chest pain, unilateral or bilateral lower extremity edema; exposure to environmental toxins and smoking; difficulty swallowing or history of foreign body aspiration.

2. Acute bronchitis is nearly always preceded by an upper respiratory tract infection manifested by malaise, coryza, sore throat, rhinorrhea, and lethargy.

3. The onset of cough in acute bronchitis occurs concurrently with nasal and pharyngeal complaints in 30 to 50% of patients. While these upper respiratory complaints often subside within 3 to 4 days, 45% of patients with acute bronchitis are still coughing at 2 weeks, and 25% at 3 weeks.

4. In patients with chronic bronchitis, preceding URI symptoms are often absent. Sputum production is usually increased and is notably thickened and purulent.

- Physical exam
  1. In otherwise healthy patients with bronchitis, physical exam findings are minimal or absent.
  2. Fever is unusual in bronchitis caused by rhinovirus or coronavirus. Influenza virus, adenovirus, and *M. pneumoniae* typically have temperature elevations up to 39°C.
  3. In patients with an exacerbation of chronic bronchitis, hypoxemia and acidemia that may develop can lead to

TABLE 65–2. Differential Diagnosis of Patients Presenting with Cough

Pharyngitis
Laryngitis
Diphtheric laryngitis
Pneumonia
Aspiration of foreign body
Sinusitis
Lung cancer
Asthma
Reflux esophagitis
Pulmonary embolus
Congestive heart failure

abnormalities including tachypnea, tachycardia, cyanosis, lethargy, bronchospasm with acute right-sided heart failure (cor pulmonale), and lower extremity edema.

Laboratory Evaluation

- Sputum cultures. With the exception of patients with COPD in whom a bacterial etiology for bronchitis is more likely, sputum cultures are of little use. In the COPD patient, results of a properly obtained sputum may be helpful in guiding therapy.
- Radiologic examination. The chest X-ray is normal in bronchitis.

Recommended Diagnostic Approach

- In otherwise healthy patients without historical features consistent with congestive heart failure, pneumonia, allergy, asthma, or foreign body, and a normal exam, no further evaluation is necessary.
- In patients with COPD, obtain a WBC count, sputum Gram's stain, and chest X-ray to rule out pneumonia.

PNEUMONIA

Definition and General Comments

- Definition
  1. Pneumonia is an inflammatory process involving the lung parenchyma. Except in immunocompromised patients, an infiltrate must be present on a chest radiograph to make the diagnosis.
  2. Community-acquired pneumonia refers to any pneumonia contracted outside of the hospital.
  3. Atypical pneumonia refers to a community-acquired pneumonia caused by a nonpyogenic organism.
  4. Aspiration pneumonia refers to the aspiration of large quantities of oropharyngeal contents, primarily in patients with impaired consciousness or altered swallowing.
  5. Nosocomial pneumonia is one that is acquired in the hospital setting.
- Epidemiology
  1. The estimated incidence of pneumonia is 1.5 cases per 100 persons per year.
  2. The overall mortality for all age groups is 24 per 100,000. It is much higher for patients over the age of 65. Of those elderly requiring hospitalization, the fatality rate is 12%. Pneumonia is the sixth most common cause of death in the United States and the most common cause of infection-related death.
- Pathogenesis. Microorganisms gain entry to the lung through one of three mechanisms:

1. Aspiration of oropharyngeal or nasopharyngeal microbes (e.g., pneumococcus)
2. Inhalation of airborne microbes (e.g., *Legionella*)
3. Hematogenous spread from distant sites of infection (e.g., *S. aureus* in intravenous drug users)

· Etiology: (Tables 65–3 and 65–4).

Clinical Features (See Specific Common Pathogens)

· History. The most common symptoms of pneumonia are cough, fever, dyspnea, and chest pain.
   1. A *cough* is almost always reported in patients with pneumonia. The 2 major exceptions are elderly and immunocompromised individuals. Bacterial pneumonias most commonly are associated with purulent, rust-colored, or bloody sputum. *M. pneumoniae, Pneumocystis carinii, Legionella* (initially), and viral pneumonias most commonly have nonproductive coughs.
   2. Chest pain, usually pleuritic, is a frequent but not invariable complaint.
· Physical exam
   1. Fever is usually present. The major exceptions include

TABLE 65–3. Etiologic Agents of Acute Pneumonia in Adults

Bacterial	Rickettsial
Streptococcus pneumonia	*Coxiella burnettii*
Staphylococcus aureus	Bacterialike agents
Hemophilus influenzae	*Mycoplasma pneumoniae*
Mixed anaerobic bacteria	*Chlamydia pneumoniae*
Escherichia coli	(TWAR)
Klebsiella pneumoniae	*Chlamydia trachomatis*
Enterobacter cloacae	Mycobacterial
Serratia marsescens	*Mycobacterium*
Pseudomonas aeruginosa	*tuberculosis*
Legionella pneumophilia	Parasitic
Viral	*Pneumocystis carinii*
Influenza A virus	
Influenza B virus	
Adenovirus types	
Cytomegalovirus	
Fungal	
Aspergillus spp.	
Candida spp.	
Coccidioides immitis	
Cryptococcus neoformans	
Histoplasma capsulatum	

Source: Adapted from Donowitz GR, Mandell GL. Acute pneumonia. In: Mandell GL, Douglas RG, Bennett JE, eds. Principles and Practice of Infectious Diseases, 3rd ed. New York, Churchill Livingstone, 1990, p. 541.

TABLE 65–4. Etiologies of Community-Acquired Pneumonias

PATHOGEN	ESTIMATED PERCENTAGE
Streptococcus pneumoniae	25–40
Hemophilus influenzae	4–15
Mycoplasma pneumoniae	3–14
Staphylococcus aureus	2–10
Legionella species	1–22
Virus (esp. influenza A)	1–10
Pneumocystis carinii	1–6
Other gram-negative bacilli	2–8
Other (fungi, mycobacteria)	<1
Mouth anaerobes	unknown
No pathogen identified	3–40

elderly and debilitated patients with overwhelming infection.

2. Tachycardia is a natural response to fever. A pulse temperature deficit (relative bradycardia) suggests infection with influenza virus, *Mycoplasma, Legionella, Chlamydia,* or *Francisella tularensis.*
3. Tachypnea is common. Cyanosis strongly suggests hypoxia.
4. Examination of the chest
   a. Early in pneumonia, auscultation of the chest may reveal only decreased breath sounds. As the infection progresses, rales may be heard. Frequently the chest X-ray still shows no infiltrate at this stage.
   b. Evidence of consolidation (dullness to percussion, bronchial breath sounds, egophony ["E to A changes"], and tactile fremitus) is highly suggestive of a bacterial process, though dullness to percussion may also signify pleural effusion.
   c. Patients with influenza virus, *Mycoplasma, Chlamydia* (TWAR and *C. psittaci*), and *Coxiella burnetii* (Q fever) demonstrate few if any abnormalities on chest exam, despite the presence of impressive infiltrates on chest film.
5. The presence of a splenectomy scar suggests the possibility of infection with encapsulated organisms (pneumococcus, *H. influenzae*).
6. Mental status changes can result from hypoxia and/or concurrent meningitis from the infecting organism. This may be the only sign of infection in elderly patients.

Laboratory Evaluation (See Specific Common Pathogens)

• The WBC count is usually elevated in bacterial pneumonia. It may be normal in the atypical pneumonias (mycoplasma, virus, chlamydiae).

- Sputum. The gross and microscopic evaluation of properly collected sputum is the most important test in the microbiologic diagnosis of pneumonia. In 60% of cases, it leads to a presumptive diagnosis.
  1. Appearance
     a. Color. A yellow-green color indicates purulence and is the most common sputum color in patients with bacterial pneumonia. "Rusty" sputum is most commonly (although not solely) associated with pneumococcus. "Currant jelly" sputum is found in *Klebsiella pneumoniae* infections.
     b. Amount. In a majority of bacterial infections, there is copious production. In atypical pneumonias and dehydrated patients, sputum may be scant.
     c. Consistency. Most bacterial pneumonias cause purulent sputum. Watery samples are seen in patients with *Mycoplasma* infection.
     d. Odor. Feculent sputum suggests anaerobic organisms.
  2. Microscopic evaluation
     a. Gram's stain
        i. To assure minimal oropharyngeal contamination, the sample should have ≥25 neutrophils and ≤10 epithelial cells per low-power field (100×).
        ii. Physician evaluation of gram stains is most reliable for the diagnosis of *S. pneumoniae* (gram-positive, lancet-shaped diplococci), and least reliable for the diagnosis of *H. influenzae* (small gram-negative coccobacilli).
        iii. The presence of WBCs without bacteria suggests *Mycoplasma,* virus, or *Legionella.*
     b. Direct fluorescent antibody stain (see below.)
     c. Giemsa or Gomori's methenamine silver stain. In HIV-positive patients, the sensitivity of this stain for *P. carinii* is 50 to 80%.
     d. Acid-fast stain is used to detect *M. tuberculosis.*
     e. Fungal stains may be indicated in selected patients.
- Cultures
  1. Sputum
     a. Sputum cultures are clinically less useful than gram's stains in making a causative diagnosis.
     b. Cultures are negative in 45 to 50% of patients with bacteremic pneumococcal and *H. influenzae* pneumonias. Many organisms (e.g., *Legionella*) require special culture techniques.
     c. Sputum cultures are probably most useful in the diagnosis of tuberculosis.
  2. Blood. Blood cultures have a low sensitivity (10 to 20%), but they are highly specific.
- Serologic studies. A variety of serologic tests are used to confirm a clinically suspected etiology. Organisms include: *Legionella* spp., *M. pneumoniae, Coxiella burnetii, Chlamydia* spp., and influenza.

- DNA hybridization probes provide rapid detection of specific organisms.
- Invasive testing (Table 65–5). In selected individuals (immunocompromised hosts, patients with overwhelming pneumonia, patients with a high suspicion for tuberculosis, or patients who fail to respond to therapy or have recurrent pneumonias), a microbiologic diagnosis is needed.
- Radiologic evaluation (see also specific common pathogens)
  1. Lobar consolidation, although suggestive of bacterial pneumonia in general, is seen routinely with pneumococcus.
  2. Bilateral diffuse infiltrates imply *P. carinii* or viral etiology.
  3. *M. tuberculosis* and *Klebsiella pneumoniae* have a predilection for upper lobe involvement. In addition, *K. pneumoniae* is classically associated with bulging or sagging of the major fissure.
  4. Infiltrates in the superior or basilar segments of lower lobes or posterior segments of upper lobes suggest aspiration.
  5. Cavitation suggests infection with *S. aureus*, Gram-negative bacilli, and *M. tuberculosis*.
  6. A perihilar distribution of infiltrates is frequently noted in early *M. pneumoniae* or influenza infection.

Specific Common Pathogens

- *Streptococcus pneumoniae.* Pneumococcus is the most common cause of community-acquired pneumonia.
  1. Clinical presentation. Abrupt onset with a single shaking chill (80% of cases).
  2. Physical exam. Patients are ill-appearing and febrile, frequently to 40°C. Tachycardia and tachypnea are present. Pleural effusions are present in 20% of cases.
  3. Laboratory findings (Table 65–6). Leukocytosis is typical.
  4. Radiographic findings. Lobar or sublobar consolidation is classic.
- *Haemophilus influenzae*
  1. Clinical presentation. Fever, chills, cough, and dyspnea are the most common complaints.

TABLE 65–5. Invasive Diagnostic Tests

Type of Invasive Test	Diagnostic Yield (%) (Range)[a]	Complication Rate (%)
Percutaneous needle aspirate	23 (8–35)	13
Transbronchial biopsy	43 (5–76)	13
Open lung biospy	68 (46–95)	10–18

[a] In immunocompromised patients.

TABLE 65–6. Diagnostic Tests for
Streptococcus Pneumoniae

Test	Sensitivity (%)	Specificity (%)	Positive Predictive Value (%)
Gram's stain (lancet-shaped diplococci in any field)	85	85	78
Gram's stain (>10 lancet-shaped diplococci per oil immersion field [1000×])	62	85	90
Sputum culture	24	90	—
Blood culture	25	100	100

2. Physical exam. There may be minimal temperature, pulse, and respiratory rate elevations. Rales are found on exam but evidence of lobar consolidation is often lacking.
3. Laboratory findings. Gram's stain of the sputum shows numerous polymorphonuclear leukocytes amid small pleomorphic gram-negative coccobacilli. Bacteremia occurs in 33% of cases.
4. Radiographic findings. Bronchopneumonia is the most common pattern seen with *H. influenzae,* but lobar consolidation can occur.

- *Mycoplasma pneumoniae* is the most common cause of community-acquired pneumonia in young adults without underlying risk factors. Infections increase in frequency in the fall and early winter.
  1. Clinical presentation (Table 65–7). The onset of the disease is insidious in 60% of patients. Patients do not appear ill. A variety of rashes may be seen, including macular, maculopapular, vesicular, urticarial, and erythema multiforme.
  2. Extrapulmonary manifestations
     a. Cold agglutinins (33 to 72%)
     b. Autoimmune hemolytic anemia (24%)
     c. Meningitis and meningoencephalitis (4%)
     d. Myopericarditis (4%)
  3. Laboratory findings (Table 65–8)
     a. WBC is 10,000 or less in 75% of cases.
     b. Gram's stain of sputum reveals polymorphonuclear leukocytes with no predominant organism.
     c. A 4-fold rise in complement fixation titers in acute and convalescent sera (2 to 3 weeks apart) confirms a clinical diagnosis. A single titer of 1:64 on acute sera is presumptive evidence of infection.
  4. Radiographic findings. Chest X-ray findings vary. Patterns correspond to clinical presentation.

TABLE 65–7. Signs and Symptoms of *M. pneumoniae*

SYMPTOMS	% OF PATIENTS
Cough	95
Malaise	75
Headache	72
Chills	68
Sore throat	51
Purulent sputum	20
Pleuritic chest pain	30
Rhinorrhea	32
Myalgias/arthralgias	32
Earache	24
Nausea/vomiting	29
Diarrhea	13
SIGNS	
Fever (39°C)	82
Rales	80
Pharyngitis	41
Rash	20
Lymphadenopathy	21
Bullous myringitis	12

a. Patchy bronchopneumonia (40%)—insidious onset and nonspecific symptoms.
b. Lobar or segmental consolidation (40%)—acute onset suggestive of bacterial pneumonia.
c. Interstitial (20%)—longer duration of symptoms with less fever and more dyspnea.
d. Pleural effusions are seen in 20% of patients.

TABLE 65–8. Diagnostic Tests for *Mycoplasma pneumoniae*

TEST	SENSITIVITY (%)	SPECIFICITY (%)	POSITIVE PREDICTIVE VALUE (%)	COMMENTS
Cold agglutinins (serum)	56	96	65	
Complement fixation titer (serum)	68	100	100	Requires 2–3 wks
DNA probe (sputum)	90	97		Rapid. Expensive
Culture (sputum)	100	unknown		Current gold standard Requires 2 wks

- *Staphylococcus aureus* causes a destructive necrotizing process occurring commonly in immunocompromised hosts (specifically those with humoral defects and chronic disease) and in healthy adults as a complication of influenza A.

  1. Clinical presentation. Aerogenic *S. aureus* pneumonia has an abrupt onset with hectic fevers, multiple chills, productive cough, and pleuritic chest pain. In hematogenously spread pneumonia, the onset of illness is less dramatic.

  2. Physical exam. In aerogenic pneumonia patients usually appear toxic, and have tachycardia and temperature elevation >40°C. Lung findings are variable. In the hematogenous form, evidence of endocarditis such as a new heart murmur, splinter hemorrhages and Roth's spots, should be sought.

  3. Laboratory findings. The WBC is usually above 15,000/mm³. Gram's stain reveals large gram-positive cocci in clusters and polymorphonuclear leukocytes. Positive blood cultures occur in 20%.

  4. Radiographic findings. Bilateral lower lobe bronchopneumonia is characteristic. Abscess, pleural effusions, and empyema are common complications. The radiographic appearance of single or multiple small round infiltrates is characteristic of hematogenously acquired *S. aureus* pneumonia.

- *Legionella pneumophila*

  1. The organism is spread via drinking water, and infection follows direct inhalation of the organism from aerosols of contaminated water.

  2. Clinical features. *Legionella* may present in either an insidious or abrupt fashion. Anorexia, weakness, and malaise occur in 100% of cases. Ninety-five percent of patients note fever. Cough, present in 90%, is usually not a major complaint. It is initially dry but may become productive or bloody.

  3. Physical exam. Nonremitting temperature elevation in excess of 39°C is seen in >80%. Relative bradycardia is noted in 60%. Tachypnea, rales, and evidence of consolidation are present.

  4. Laboratory findings (Table 65–9). Leukocytosis of 10,000/mm³ or greater is typical. Alkaline phosphatase, bilirubin, and transaminase levels are often elevated. Hyponatremia and hypophosphatemia are common.

  5. Gram's stain of sputum shows few to moderate polymorphonuclear cells and rarely, faintly staining gram-negative rods.

  6. Radiographic findings
     a. Initially, the chest radiograph may show a patchy alveolar infiltrate in a single lobe. This usually progresses to consolidation of the involved lobe. Lower lobes are more often affected.
     b. Small pleural effusions are noted in 50% of patients.
     c. In 25% of patients, macroscopic abscesses are seen, often small and multiple.

TABLE 65–9. Diagnostic Tests for
Legionella pneumophila

TEST	SENSITIVITY (%)	SPECIFICITY (%)	COMMENTS
Serum indirect fluor. antibody	75	90–95	Rapid
Direct immunofluor. antibody (sputum)	60–90	99	
Culture (charcoal yeast extract agar; sputum)	80–100	100	Requires selective media and 3 to 5 days
DNA probe (sputum)	57	99	Expensive; may not be as specific as originally thought

- Influenza. Influenza A is the most common viral cause of pneumonia in the adult civilian population. The peak incidence of influenza occurs in winter. Bacterial superinfection complicates 1% of influenza A pneumonias (*S. pneumoniae, S. aureus,* and *H. influenzae*).
  1. Clinical presentation. Near the end of a typical influenza illness, which consists of fever, headache, sore throat, myalgia, and malaise, the patient suddenly worsens. Cough, initially productive of scant watery sputum then progressing to mucoid or blood tinged, becomes a prominent feature. Pleuritic chest pain is present in 50% of patients.
  2. Physical exam. Temperature is elevated to 38 to 39°C. Chest findings include rales. Without bacterial superinfection, signs of lobar consolidation are absent.
  3. Laboratory findings
     a. The WBC ranges from normal to moderately elevated (15,000/mm³).
     b. A Gram's stain shows few leukocytes and no predominant organism.
     c. Virus isolation can be obtained via tissue culture. Specimens are obtained from nasopharyngeal swabs, sputum, throat washings, transtracheal aspirates, or lung biopsy. Culture requires 7 days and is only 60% sensitive.
  4. Radiographic findings. In primary influenzal pneumonia, perihilar infiltrates are present. If superinfection is present, the infiltrates may be lobar.

Recommended Diagnostic Approach

- Establishing the presence of pneumonia
  1. Obtain a history and perform a physical examination.
  2. Draw a CBC. The absence of a leukocytosis does not

TABLE 65–10. Important Environmental Factors in Pneumonia

PNEUMONIA ASSOCIATED WITH	ENVIRONMENTAL HISTORY
Anthrax	Exposure to cattle, swine, horses, goat hair, wool, hides
Brucellosis	Exposure to cattle, goats, pigs; employment as abattoir worker or veterinarian
Melioidosis	Travel to W. Indies, Australia, Guam, Southeast Asia, South and Central America
Plague	Exposure to ground squirrels, chipmunks, rabbits, prairie dogs, rats
Tularemia	Exposure to tissue or body fluids of infected animals (rabbits, hares, foxes, squirrels) or to bites of an infected arthropod (flies, ticks) Handling or ingesting poorly cooked meat from an infected animal
Psittacosis	Exposure to birds (parrots, budgerigars, cockatoos, pigeons, turkeys)
Leptospirosis	Exposure to wild rodents, dogs, cats, pigs, cattle, horses, or exposure to water contaminated with animal urine
Coccidioidomycosis	Travel to San Joaquin Valley, S. California, S.W. Texas, S. Arizona, New Mexico
Histoplasmosis	Exposure to bat droppings or dust from soil enriched with bird droppings
Q fever	Exposure to infected goats, cattle, sheep and their secretions (milk, amniotic fluid, placenta, feces)
Legionnaires' disease	Exposure to contaminated aerosols (e.g., air coolers, hospital water supplies)

Source: Donowitz GR, Mandell GL. Acute pneumonia. In: Mandell GL, et al., eds., Principles and Practice of Infectious Diseases, 3rd ed. New York, Churchill Livingstone, 1990, p. 542.

    rule out pneumonia, and in fact may be a poor prognostic sign.

3. Obtain a good quality sputum for Gram's stain and possibly culture. The lack of purulent sputum can be an etiologic clue, or mean that the patient is dehydrated.

4. Obtain a chest radiograph. With the exception of immunocompromised patients or severely volume-

TABLE 65–11. Epidemiologic Categories of Pneumonia

CATEGORY	ORGANISMS TO CONSIDER
Community-acquired pneumonia	Pneumococci, *Mycoplasma, Hemophilus influenzae* viruses, *Legionella*
Community-acquired aspiration	Pneumococci, anaerobic bacteria (mouth flora)
Postinfluenzal pneumonia	Pneumococci, *Hemophilus influenzae, Staphylococcus aureus*
Alcoholism	Pneumococci, *Klebsiella pneumoniae, Hemophilus influenzae, Mycobacterium tuberculosis*
Intravenous drug use	Pneumococci, *Staphylococcus aureus*
HIV-positive patient	*Pneumocystis carinii,* pneumococci, *Hemophilus influenzae*
Immunocompromised patient	Bacteria, viruses, fungi, parasites
Nosocomial pneumonia/ aspiration	Gram-negative bacilli, staphylococci, *Legionella*
Nursing home patient	Pneumococci, *Klebsiella pneumoniae, Hemophilus influenzae, Staphylococcus aureus, Mycobacterium tuberculosis,* influenzae
Cystic fibrosis patients	*Pseudomonas aeruginosa, Staphylococcus aureus*

depleted patients, an infiltrate must be present on the radiograph to make the diagnosis of pneumonia.

5. Blood cultures should be drawn on any ill-appearing patient with an infiltrate on chest X-ray.

6. An arterial blood gas should be considered on patients who are tachypneic or cyanotic.

- Ascertaining a "likely" etiology. Even with aggressive investigation, a specific etiology is established in only 50 to 60% of patients.

1. Based on historical considerations, assign the patient to a clinical and epidemiologic category (Tables 65–10, 65–11, and 65–12).

2. Examine the sputum Gram stain for predominance of a single organism.

3. In a patient with an atypical presentation, consider obtaining serologic studies for eventual confirmation of the clinical diagnosis.

4. DNA probe studies should be considered in patients with a history consistent with *Legionella*. This test is rarely indicated for suspected *Mycoplasma* infections

TABLE 65–12. Etiology of Acute Pneumonia Based Upon Differences in Presentation

FEATURE	CLASSICAL PRESENTATION	ATYPICAL PRESENTATION
Onset	Abrupt	Gradual
Fever > 39°C	Common	Less common
Chills	Common	Uncommon
Pleuritic pain	Common	Uncommon
Tachycardia > 130/min	Frequent	Rare
Consolidation	More common	Less common
Pleural effusion	More common	Less common
Sputum volume	Abundant	Minimal
Sputum character	Thick, purulent	Thin, mucoid
Sputum Gram's stain	"Single predominant organism." Many polys[a]	No polys[a]; some monos[b]. Scattered normal flora
Leading causes	*S. pneumonia* *H. influenzae* *Klebsiella pneumonia* *S. aureus*	*Mycoplasma* Viruses *Legionella* *Chlamydia* (TWAR)

[a] poly = polymorphonuclear leukocytes.
[b] mono = mononuclear cells.

given the expense of the test and the low mortality rate of this pathogen.

5. In HIV-positive patients always consider the possibility of *Pneumocystis* and other unusual organisms.

Bibliography

Edelstein PH, Meyer RD. Legionaires' disease: A review. Chest 1984:85:114–120.

Fine MJ, et al. Prognosis of patients hospitalized with community-acquired pneumonia. Am J Med 1990;88:1–7.

Garibaldi RA. Epidemiology of community-acquired respiratory tract infections in adults: Incidence, etiology and impact. Am J Med 1985;78:32–37.

Grayston JT, et al. A new *Chlamydia psittaci* strain, TWAR, isolated in acute respiratory tract infections. N Engl J Med 1986:315: 161–168.

Levy M, et al. Community-acquired pneumonia: Importance of initial noninvasive bacteriologic and radiographic investigations. Chest 1988;92:43–48.

Mansel JK, et al. *Mycoplasma pneumoniae* pneumonia. Chest 1989;95:639–646.

66

TUBERCULOSIS

RICHARD ALBERT

Consumption catch thee!

SHAKESPEARE (1564–1616)
Timon of Athens, IV, iii, 201

DEFINITIONS

- Tuberculosis (TB) is an acute or chronic infection caused by *Mycobacterium tuberculosis*.
  1. Tuberculous infection means that the tubercle bacillus has become established but there are no symptoms or evidence of active disease, and bacteriologic studies are negative.
  2. Tuberculosis implies that an infected person has a disease process involving one or more organs, and bacteriologic studies are positive.
- Acquisition of disease
  1. Patients with pulmonary tuberculosis generate organisms in small particles (droplet nuclei), 1 to 4 μm in diameter, whenever they cough or speak. When inhaled by susceptible hosts, the bacteria multiply without initial resistance. Subsequently, the organisms become engulfed by phagocytes but may remain viable within the intracellular environment. During the initial infection, the bacilli spread through lymphatics to regional lymph nodes and hematogenously throughout the body. In about 5% of patients, initial control is inadequate and progressive disease results. Usually the cell-mediated immunity that develops is able to limit further multiplication of the organisms, the infection is controlled, and the patient remains asymptomatic with the only evidence of disease being conversion of the tuberculin (PPD) test result to positive.
  2. In 5 to 15% of patients who acquire asymptomatic disease, active tuberculosis develops after a variable interval (2 yr to decades). Factors favoring reactivation include old age, immunosuppressive therapy, alcoholism, and undernutrition. The most common location for recurrent disease is the upper lung zones. However, other areas of the lung may be involved, as may other nonpulmonary foci.
- Definitive diagnosis usually requires demonstration of *M. tuberculosis* in tissues by histologic examination or in secretions or body fluids by stains and culture. The need for definitive diagnosis, particularly by culture, cannot be overemphasized.

574

- Other mycobacterial disease. Disease similar to that caused by *M. tuberculosis* can be caused by other myco-bacteria such as *M. kansasii* and *M. avium-intracellulare*. The transmission and pathogenesis of infection with these organisms is poorly understood.

EPIDEMIOLOGY

In 1989, 21,520 cases of tuberculosis were reported to the CDC. The rate of decrease in annual cases has fallen off in the last several years due to a high incidence of tuberculosis in HIV-positive patients (frequently with extrapulmonary mani-festations), in HIV-negative IV drug users, elderly nursing home residents, and other population segments. Over 10 mil-lion people are infected with *M. tuberculosis* in the United States, and these people have a lifelong risk of developing the disease.

HISTORY

The history usually does not contribute to the diagnosis unless contact with a patient having active tuberculosis can be estab-lished. Many patients with active disease come to medical attention only through case-finding activities (investigation of contacts of patients with active disease) or by further investi-gation of patients who convert their tuberculin skin tests.

SIGNS AND SYMPTOMS

- Although active disease may be found in asymptomatic individuals, symptoms of disease are usually present. Symptoms may have an insidious onset. Common symptoms include fatigue, anorexia, and weight loss, which may have been present for weeks to months. Pa-tients may have an acute febrile illness resembling influ-enza or they may have a low-grade fever. Some have a fever of undetermined origin. Other findings depend on the organ system involved.
- Pulmonary tuberculosis. Cough with mucoid or mucopu-rulent sputum is the most common manifestation of pulmo-nary tuberculosis (except in children, in whom cough is unusual). Hemoptysis is rare. When it is observed in pa-tients with chest roentgenographic evidence of posttuber-culous scarring, the possibility of an aspergilloma should be considered.
- Meningeal tuberculosis. Tuberculous meningitis usually causes fever, a change in mental status, headaches, or seizures. Cranial nerve abnormalities (especially III and VI) are common. Pulmonary or miliary disease is usually present, and the purified protein derivative (PPD) test is usually positive.
- Abdominal tuberculosis. Ascites, fever, and abdominal pain are characteristic of peritoneal disease. Half of pa-

tients have no evidence of pulmonary disease, but pleural effusions may be present. PPD is positive in more than 80% of the patients. Peritoneal tuberculosis is often misdiagnosed as Crohn's disease, appendicitis, or carcinoma. Patients with anal or rectal tuberculosis present with fistulae or abscesses and usually have concurrent pulmonary disease.

- Genitourinary tuberculosis. Genitourinary tuberculosis should be considered whenever patients have dysuria, pyuria without bacteriuria, unexplained hematuria or proteinuria, a beaded vas deferens on palpation, or epididymitis. Women may have menorrhagia, oligomenorrhea, amenorrhea, pelvic inflammatory disease, or infertility. The IV pyelogram may be abnormal.

- Lymph node tuberculosis. Any lymph node may have tuberculous infection. Hilar or mediastinal adenopathy may be present during the initial pulmonary infection, particularly in children and in patients with HIV infection. Cervical and supraclavicular adenopathy is common and usually occurs in patients without roentgenographic evidence of pulmonary involvement. Nodes in these areas may drain spontaneously. In adults, *M. tuberculosis* is almost always the causative organism. In children, other mycobacteria may be responsible.

- Bone and joint tuberculosis. The skeleton (most commonly the lower spine and weight-bearing joints) is affected in approximately 1% of patients with tuberculosis. Half of these have no evidence of pulmonary involvement.

- Pericardial tuberculosis. Most patients with tuberculous pericarditis are dyspneic and have extensive pulmonary involvement. Constriction with impaired right ventricular filling may result.

- Laryngeal tuberculosis. Patients with laryngeal tuberculosis have hoarseness or a sore throat. Extensive pulmonary involvement is usually seen. Sputum smears are markedly positive.

- Miliary tuberculosis. Patients may have acute onset of fever and shortness of breath or may only describe nonspecific generalized symptoms. Miliary tuberculosis may precede the development of the miliary pattern seen on chest X-rays. Patients may have hepatomegaly, splenomegaly, generalized lymphadenopathy, or meningitis.

- Other organs. Tuberculosis rarely may cause adrenal insufficiency, chronic otitis media, mastoiditis, and perirectal abscesses or fistulae.

LABORATORY AND X-RAY STUDIES

- Chest X-ray. Pulmonary tuberculosis is often first suspected on the basis of chest X-ray findings. Patients with inactive disease may have a hilar node and peripheral calcification (Ghon complex) and/or apical lung scarring. Active disease may cause an apical lesion (often mottled in appearance), which may go on to cavitate. Virtually any chest roentgenographic abnormality can be caused by tuberculosis, and patients with active disease may have normal chest X-rays.

- Sputum. Specific instructions regarding sputum collection are needed. Three good-quality early morning specimens are sufficient. Sputum production can be induced by inhalation of hypertonic saline solution (3 to 10%) or collected by nasotracheal suction or bronchoscopy. Brushings can be obtained for culture during this procedure. Tissue can be obtained by transbronchial biopsy for histologic examination as well as for culture.

- Gastric fluid. Aspiration of gastric fluid after an 8- to 10-hr fast can be cultured for tuberculosis.

- Urine. The first specimen voided in the morning is preferred. Several collections are required. Broad-spectrum antibiotics in the urine may result in negative cultures.

- Other specimens. Pleural, cerebrospinal, peritoneal, and pericardial fluids should be analyzed for cell counts, protein, and glucose. A high protein level (greater than 3 g/dl), lymphocytosis, and low glucose levels are usually found in patients with tuberculous infections. To increase diagnostic yield, biopsy of pleural and peritoneal tissues should be performed at the time of thoracentesis or paracentesis. Specimens should also be acquired from the lung, pericardium, lymph nodes, bones, joints, bowel, salpinges, and epididymis when noninvasive techniques fail to establish the diagnosis. In cases in which hematogenous or miliary disease is possible, bone marrow, lung, or liver biopsy for histologic examination and culture should be considered.

- Tuberculin skin testing. The cell-mediated immune response to infection with mycobacteria produces delayed hypersensitivity to culture extracts. Not all reactive patients are infected with *M. tuberculosis* since cross-reactivity to nontuberculous mycobacteria can occur. The larger the reaction, the more likely it is that it is caused by *M. tuberculosis*.

   The area of induration should be determined 48 to 72 hr after intradermal injection of 0.1 ml of Tween-stabilized PPD containing 5 tuberculin units (also known as intermediate-strength PPD). Finding an area of induration greater than 10 mm in diameter indicates infection; it does not imply the presence of active disease. The infection may have occurred as recently as 2 weeks previously, or in the far distant past. In evaluation of close contacts of patients with active disease or in patients infected with the HIV, a reaction of 5 mm is considered positive. A negative test does not exclude infection, even in the absence of anergy. First- (1 tuberculin unit) and second-strength (250 tuberculin units) tuberculin tests have limited, if any, diagnostic use.

- Staining and culture techniques for tuberculosis. Water-soluble dyes are taken up through the wall of the tubercle bacillus and cannot be eliminated by an acid wash. "Acid-fastness" is not a property exclusive to *M. tuberculosis*.

Nontuberculous mycobacteria and nocardia are also acid-fast. Culturing is considerably more sensitive than the acid-fast smear to detect mycobacteria. Culturing is essential to distinguish *M. tuberculosis* from other mycobacteria, as well as to test for drug susceptibility.

RECOMMENDED DIAGNOSTIC APPROACH

The diagnostic approach must be customized to the patient's clinical findings and type of tuberculosis suspected. Diagnosis rests on culture or histologic evidence of tuberculous bacilli. In children with hilar adenopathy and contact with a known TB case, bacteriologic proof may not be required.

- Low suspicion of pulmonary TB. A chest X-ray is an adequate initial procedure. Three early morning sputum specimens for staining and culture are indicated when the chest X-ray is suggestive of TB.

- High suspicion of pulmonary TB. Chest X-ray and collection of three early morning sputum specimens for staining and culture are initial diagnostic steps. If tuberculosis is not proved, the next diagnostic steps should be based on the availability of specimens (e.g., pleural fluid, pleural tissue), and the signs, symptoms, and seriousness of the illness. It is useful to culture for tuberculosis when the urinalysis is abnormal without explanation or if intravenous pyelography suggests tuberculosis.

Bibliography

Bailey WC, et al. (American Thoracic Society and Centers for Disease Control). Treatment of tuberculosis and other mycobacterial diseases. Am Rev Respir Dis 1983;127:790–796.

Centers for Disease Control. Screening for tuberculosis and tuberculosis infection in high-risk populations. MMWR 1990;39:1–12.

Chaissors RE, Slutkin G. Tuberculosis and human immunodeficiency virus infection. J Infect Dis 1989;159:96–100.

Farer LS, et al. Control of tuberculosis. Am Rev Respir Dis 1983;128:336–342.

Jukubonski A, et al. Clinical features of abdominal tuberculosis. J Infect Dis 1988;158:687–692.

Weg JG, et al. (American Thoracic Society and Centers for Disease Control). Diagnostic standards and classification of tuberculosis and other mycobacterial diseases. Am Rev Respir Dis 1981;123:343–358.

67

INFECTIVE ENDOCARDITIS

C. SCOTT SMITH

Pathologists have long known . . . that rheumatic fever "licks at the joints, but bites at the heart".

QUOTED by ALVAN FEINSTEIN (1964)

DEFINITION

Infective endocarditis (IE) is a microbial infection of a platelet-fibrin vegetation on a cardiac valve or, less commonly, on the mural endocardium. Most infections are caused by bacteria and are associated with continuous bacteremia.

EPIDEMIOLOGY AND CLASSIFICATION

- Clinical Classification
  1. Native valve endocarditis (Figures 67–1 and 67–2). In approximately 30% of infections, the patient's heart has no underlying structural abnormality. The underlying cardiac lesions in the remaining 70% have changed markedly over time as rheumatic disease has become less frequent. The major categories of lesions currently are:
     a. Mitral valve prolapse (30%). These patients almost uniformly have regurgitant murmurs and redundant myxomatous valvular tissue on echocardiogram, and not just simple systolic clicks.
     b. Degenerative lesions of the aortic or mitral valves (20%).
     c. Congenital heart disease (13%). Includes bicuspid aortic valve, ventricular septal defect, and pulmonary stenosis.
     d. Rheumatic heart disease (6%).
     e. Hypertrophic cardiomyopathy (5%).
  2. Intravenous drug use–associated endocarditis (IVDU) (Figures 67–3 and 67–4). There is no grossly evident underlying structural abnormality in 70% of these cases. However, the tricuspid valve may suffer microinjury from particulate matter injected intravenously (e.g., contaminants of the drugs).
  3. Prosthetic valve endocarditis occurs in 3% of patients at 1 yr and 4 to 6% of patients at 4 yr after valve placement. It remains a risk as long as the valve is in

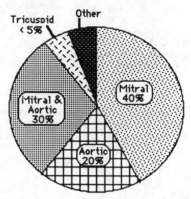

Figure 67–1. Valves affected in native valve endocarditis.

place. There is no difference in risk between mechanical and bioprosthetic valves, nor is there a difference between valve sites. The disease is commonly divided into early prosthetic valve endocarditis (EPVE), which occurs within 2 months of placement, and late prosthetic valve endocarditis (LPVE) after 2 months.

EPVE (Figure 67–5) is usually a consequence of perioperative contamination. It is rapidly progressive, and fever, valvular insufficiency, or CHF are strongly suggestive of the diagnosis.

LPVE (Figure 67–6) is more commonly associated with incidental bacteremia (tooth extraction, genitourinary procedures, IV catheter infection). Clinically, it behaves more like subacute native valve endocarditis with insidious onset and more prominent systemic symptoms.

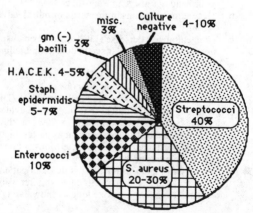

Figure 67–2. Etiology of native valve endocarditis.

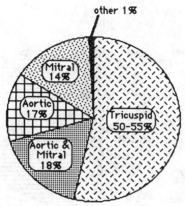

Figure 67–3. Valves affected in IVDU-associated endocarditis.

- Acute and subacute classification. IE has been divided into acute and subacute forms depending on whether untreated patients could be expected to survive for more than or less than 8 weeks.
  1. Subacute bacterial endocarditis (SBE) most commonly involves the left side of the heart and particularly affects previously damaged valves. It is frequently insidious in onset and often results in fatigue, malaise, arthralgias, and weight loss. SBE often involves less virulent pathogens (*S. viridans,* enterococci).
  2. Acute bacterial endocarditis (ABE) has a more rapid and fulminant course. Different organisms have different valvular predilections. *Staphylococcus aureus* often infects the tricuspid valve, *Candida* species favor left-sided valves, and *Pseudomonas* infections are of-

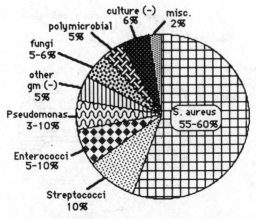

Figure 67–4. Etiology of IVDU-associated endocarditis.

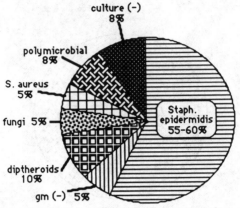

Figure 67–5. Etiology of early prosthetic valve endocarditis.

ten biventricular and multivalvular. Persons with ABE are more likely to have rigors, sweats, chills, meningismus, leukocytosis, and elevation of the erythrocyte sedimentation rate. The organisms are generally more virulent and include *S. aureus, S. pneumoniae, S. pyogenes, N. meningitidis,* and *H. influenzae.*

- Classification by etiologic agent
  1. Penicillin-sensitive streptococci. Penicillin-sensitive streptococci (minimal inhibitory concentration for penicillin < 0.1 μg/ml) are the most common causes of IE and are isolated from more than 45% of all cases of endocarditis. Species in this category include viridans streptococci (*S. sanguis, S. mutans, S. mitior*); group D streptococci (*S. bovis, S. equinas*); *S. pyogenes;* and *S. pneumoniae* (in which IE may present as meningi-

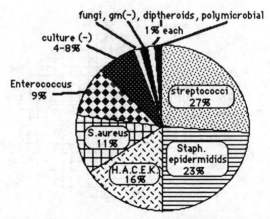

Figure 67–6. Etiology in late prosthetic valve endocarditis.

tis). *S. bovis* in the elderly is often associated with carcinoma or atypical polyps of the colon.

2. Enterococci. Enterococci, a subset of group D streptococci, are less sensitive to penicillin and cause approximately 10% of all IE. Among enterococci, *S. faecalis* is the most common offender. The usual predisposing situation to this infection is in elderly men after genitourinary manipulation. Patients usually have preexisting cardiac lesions or artificial valves and a subacute presentation.

3. Staphylococci. IE due to staphylococci may follow a fulminant acute course with multiple complications (congestive heart failure, renal failure, metastatic infection, emboli) and high mortality. Among IVDUs, IE is usually right-sided, and in non-IVDUs, usually left-sided. Among non-IVDUs approximately 50% of staphylococcal IE has no identifiable portal of entry.

   Staphylococcal bacteremia is 5 times as common as IE, so positive blood cultures do not necessarily mean IE (Table 67–1).

4. HACEK organisms. The "HACEK" organisms are fastidious, slow-growing gram-negative coccobacillary bacteria that prefer incubation in a CO_2-enhanced atmosphere and are penicillin-sensitive. They may present as "culture-negative" subacute endocarditis, especially in late prosthetic valve endocarditis or native valve endocarditis. The group name derives from the causative organisms: <u>H</u>aemophilus species (*aphrophilus, parainfluenza, paraphrophilus*); <u>A</u>ctinobacillus actinomycetemcomitans; <u>C</u>ardiobacterium hominis; <u>E</u>ikenella corrodens; and <u>K</u>ingella kingii.

TABLE 67–1. Factors That Distinguish *S. Aureus* Endocarditis from Bacteremia

Diagnostic of endocarditis	Supportive of endocarditis
1. New pathologic or changing heart murmur	1. Rheumatic valvular heart murmur
2. Major embolic event(s)	2. Community-acquired bacteremia, delayed treatment, no primary site of infection
3. New splenomegaly (rare)	
4. Peripheral microembolic signs (rare)	
Characteristic of endocarditis	Suggestive of bacteremia
1. Intravenous drug use	1. Hospital-acquired bacteremia
2. Prosthetic valve	2. Promptly treated bacteremia related to wounds or use of intravenous devices
3. Meningitis *(de novo)*	
4. Severe renal failure, microscopic hematuria (especially casts)	
5. Cardiac conduction defects, pericarditis, congestive heart failure	
6. Teichoic acid antibodies (substantial titer)	

5. Other gram-negative bacteria. Gram-negative IE is uncommon but the incidence has increased as a result of IV drug use, cardiac valve replacement, immunosuppressive therapy, and widespread use of antibiotics.

6. Fungi. Infection with fungi is uncommon but there is increasing incidence with prosthetic valves, IVDU-associated endocarditis, and IV hyperalimentation. Among non-IVDUs, fungal species include *Candida albicans* and *Aspergillus* species. In IVDUs, the chief fungi are *C. parapsilosis, C. tropicalis,* and *C. stellatoidea.*

Fungal IE characteristically produces bulky left-sided vegetations on the valve. Major emboli are common. Tissue invasion is also common.

7. Culture-negative endocarditis. The blood cultures are persistently negative in 4–10% of endocarditis cases. Advances in microbiologic techniques are offset by the increased use of preculture outpatient antibiotics and by the occurrence of nonbacterial IE.

DIFFERENTIAL DIAGNOSIS (Table 67–2)

CLINICAL FEATURES

History (Table 67–3)

The constellation of symptoms in any given patient is quite variable, and some authorities estimate that the reliance on the classic diagnostic criteria would result in failure to suspect IE in up to 90% of cases. Elderly patients have fewer symptoms and diminished febrile response to IE.

Physical Exam (Table 67–4)

- Skin
  1. Splinter hemorrhages are linear, subungual hemorrhages in the middle of the nail bed (their most common cause is trauma). Proximal and transverse splinters are more specific for SBE than distal and longitudinal ones.
  2. Petechiae may continue to occur for a few weeks despite adequate antibiotic coverage and do not portend

TABLE 67–2. Differential Diagnosis of Infective Endocarditis

Acute rheumatic fever with carditis
Collagen vascular disease (especially SLE)
Atrial myxoma
Nonbacterial thrombotic endocarditis
Paraneoplastic disease (especially hypernephroma)
S. aureus bacteremia without endocarditis

TABLE 67–3. Symptoms of Infective Endocarditis

SYMPTOMS	PERCENT
Fever	80–90
Chills	40
Weakness	40
Dyspnea	40
Sweats	25
Anorexia	25
Weight loss	25
Malaise	25
Cough	25
Skin lesions	20
Stroke	20
Nausea and vomiting	20
Headache	15
Myalgia and arthralgia	15
Edema	15
Chest pain	15
Delirium and coma	10
Hemoptysis	10
Back pain	10
Abdominal pain	10–15

treatment failure. They are normal in the conjunctive and mucous membranes after heart/lung bypass associated with valve replacement and do not indicate early prosthetic valve endocarditis.
3. Osler's nodes are tender reddish-purple subcutaneous

TABLE 67–4. Physical Findings in Infective Endocarditis

FINDINGS	PERCENT
Fever	90
Heart murmur	85
Changing murmur	5–10
New murmur	3–5
Embolic phenomena	>50
Skin manifestations	50
Osler's nodes	10–23
Splinter hemorrhages	15
Petechiae	20–40
Janeway's lesions	<10
Splenomegaly	20–57
Septic complications (pneumonia, meningitis, etc.)	20
Mycotic aneurysms	20
Clubbing	12–52
Retinal lesions	5–10
Signs of renal failure	10–15

nodules. They generally develop in the tuft of the finger and can be the result of microemboli.

4. Janeway lesions are more widespread on the palms or soles than Osler's nodes and are further distinguished by being painless. They are generally more hemorrhagic than nodular.

- Funduscopic
  1. Petechiae or flame hemorrhages
  2. Cotton wool exudates
  3. Roth's spots are oval pale areas of the retina with a surrounding zone of hemorrhage.

LABORATORY STUDIES

- Blood cultures. Blood culture remains the principal diagnostic test for IE. Success of pathogen recovery depends primarily on the volume of blood; however, other factors include the number of cultures, processing techniques, type of pathogen involved, and preculture use of antibiotics. Not significant in IE are the timing of cultures or the site.

  1. Number of blood cultures. Current recommendations are for 3 sets of blood cultures in the first 24 hr.
  2. Volume of blood. This is the most important factor in successful diagnosis. Ten ml is the minimum essential volume per culture.
  3. Preculture antibiotics. There is a decrease in bacterial yield with preculture antibiotics. Treatment does not halt the disease or prevent the ultimate positivity of the culture.
  4. Timing of blood cultures. Because the bacteremia is continuous, there is no advantage from cultures obtained with temperature spikes or over specified intervals.
  5. Site of blood culture. There are measurable but not significantly greater numbers of bacteria in arterial versus venous blood. In practice, arterial cultures show no advantage over venous cultures.
  6. Special considerations (Table 67–5). Several organ-

TABLE 67–5. Causes of Apparent Culture-Negative Endocarditis

Prior antimicrobial treatment (most common cause)
HACEK organisms
Q fever
Fungi
Acid-fast bacilli
Chlamydia
Noninfective endocarditis
? L forms of bacteria
? Virus
Brucellosis
Legionella

isms are slow growing (HACEK organisms, *Candida* species, diphtheroids) and cultures that are not initially positive should be kept 14 to 21 days.

While no consensus exists as to how far to look for a microbiologic diagnosis before declaring the case culture-negative, the Mayo Clinic recommends:

 a. Reviewing history of previous antibiotic use, IVDU, exposure to gonococcus, brucellosis, psittacosis, nongonococcal urethritis or cervicitis, Q fever, and recent dental or dermatologic manipulation
 b. Gram's stain, biopsy, and culture any cutaneous lesion
 c. Obtaining blood culture results from the referring hospital
 d. Using nutritional supplements in the culture (CO_2 enhanced for HACEK, charcoal-yeast for *Legionella*, etc.) and continuous incubation for 3 to 4 weeks with blind subcultures and Gram's stains
 e. Obtaining 2 blood cultures each for *Brucella, Neisseria,* and fungi
 f. Repeat 2 sets of routine blood cultures
 g. Obtain serologies for the organisms listed above
 h. Echocardiography
 i. Bone marrow biopsy and culture

- Immunologic testing. A normal ESR is extremely rare in IE (Table 67–6).
- Echocardiography. Some bacteremic patients without clinical findings of IE in fact have vegetations that can be demonstrated by echocardiography (less than 10%). Echocardiography, however, is not routinely useful. The sensitivity of M-mode echocardiography in one series was 37%, specificity 96%, predictive value of positive test 76%, and predictive value of a negative test 80% (Come et al, 1982). A study by Buda et al. (1986) found that when a vegetation was visualized, there was a significantly worse clinical outcome. In general, echocardiography is useful for confirming the diagnosis of IE when it is suspected clinically.
- Electrocardiogram (ECG). The ECG is useful for detecting

TABLE 67–6. Mediators of the Immune Response in IE

	PERCENT OF CASES WITH ABNORMAL RESULT
Anemia	70–90
Erythrocyte sedimentation rate (mean 57)	90–100
Rheumatoid factor	40–50
Hypergammaglobulinemia	20–30
Hypocomplementemia	5–15
Proteinuria	50–65
Microscopic hematuria	30–50
Red blood cell casts	12

abnormalities resulting from myocardial abscesses (partial or complete heart blocks, premature ventricular contractions) or MI secondary to emboli.

- Cardiac catheterization. Indications for catheterization include preoperative hemodynamic assessment in patients with congestive heart failure, persistent sepsis, or recurrent embolism. Cardiac catheterization is also useful for evaluation of ruptured sinus of Valsalva aneurysms, valve ring abscesses, mycotic aneurysms, and for quantitative culture on both sides of tricuspid and pulmonary valves in right heart IE with negative echocardiographic results.

RECOMMENDED DIAGNOSTIC APPROACH

- History (high index of suspicion required). Important factors include:
  1. Malaise, anorexia, weight loss, low-grade fever
  2. Underlying heart disease (rheumatic, valvular, or congenital)
  3. IVDU
  4. Recent procedures (dental, urologic, gynecologic, or GI manipulations)
  5. Prior antibiotic use
  6. History of prosthetic valve
- Physical examination. This should especially cover vital signs, cardiac findings, and peripheral stigmata of disease (see Table 67–4)
- Laboratory tests
  1. Blood culture (3 times)
  2. CBC and ESR
  3. Urinalysis (presence of RBC or red cell casts)
  4. Chest X-ray
  5. Serum creatinine
  6. ECG
- Presumptive treatment. Patients with significant fever who do not have an obvious source and who have a high clinical suspicion for IE (i.e., IVDU, peripheral stigmata of IE, new or changed heart murmur, etc.) should be treated presumptively after cultures are obtained.

Bibliography

Baddour LM, Bisno AL. Infective endocarditis complicating mitral valve prolapse: Epidemiologic, clinical, and microbiologic aspects. Rev Inf Dis 1986;8(1):117–137.

Buda AJ, et al. Prognostic significance of vegetations detected by two-dimensional echocardiography in infective endocarditis. Am Heart J 1986;112(6):1291–1296.

Calderwood SB, et al. Prosthetic valve endocarditis. Analysis of factors affecting outcome of therapy. J Thorac Cardiovasc Surg 1986;92:776–783.

Come PC, et al. Diagnostic accuracy of M-mode echo in active Infective Endocarditis and prognostic implication of ultrasound detectable vegetations. Am Heart J 1982;103:839.

Douglas A, et al. Fever during treatment of endocarditis. Lancet June 1986;8494:1341–1343.

McKinsey DS, et al. Underlying cardiac lesions in adults with infective endocarditis. The changing spectrum. Am J Med 1987;82:681–688.

Terpenning MS, et al. Infective endocarditis: Clinical features in young and elderly patients. Am J Med 1987;83:626–634.

68

SKIN INFECTIONS

PAUL G. RAMSEY, *and*
DOUGLAS S. PAAUW

When you are skinning your customers, you should leave some skin on to grow so that you can skin them again.

NIKITA KHRUSHCHEV

DEFINITION

Most primary skin infections are caused by bacteria and fungi. Primary cutaneous infections are classified according to their appearance. Trauma such as surgery, puncture wounds, burns, and bites often provide the site of entry for infectious agents, although in many patients no entry site is apparent.

- Cellulitis is a spreading superficial erythematous lesion that is warm to the touch.
- Impetigo appears as a confluent group of vesicles or pustules with a characteristic superficial crust.
- Folliculitis is a purulent infection of hair follicles and appears as small pustular lesions in the distribution of body hair.
- Furuncles or common boils are cutaneous abscesses related to obstructed hair follicles or sebaceous glands. Carbuncles are large furuncles.
- Ulcerative lesions are deep erosions with dermal destruction. A crust of necrotic material may cover the base of an ulcer.
- Cutaneous mycoses may cause a variety of clinical findings (see section on clinical features).

EPIDEMIOLOGY

- Young children are more likely than adults to develop facial cellulitis and frequently acquire and spread impetigo.
- Adults with venous insufficiency, peripheral vascular disease, superficial mycoses, and primary skin diseases are likely to develop cellulitis of the extremities.
- Risk of surgical wound infection is related to type and length of surgery as well as to the skill of the personnel.
- Prolonged bed rest predisposes patients to ischemic necrosis of the skin surface and decubitus ulcers.
- Animal exposure is an important risk factor for unusual bacterial infections such as tularemia or anthrax.

- Infection by unusual bacteria may be related to occupation.
- Puncture wounds are associated with a risk of anaerobic infections (tetanus) and the acquisition of unusual organisms (*Pseudomonas aeruginosa* infection of the feet).
- IVDUs have a high rate of superficial and deep skin infections. Unusual organisms including mouth flora (*Eikenella corrodens*) can occur due to the practice of licking needles.

CLINICAL FEATURES

- Cellulitis: Microbiology and types of infection
    1. Staphylococci and streptococci
        a. *S. aureus* and beta-hemolytic streptococci (usually group A but occasionally groups B, C, D, F, and G) are the most common causative agents of cellulitis. Beta-hemolytic streptococci and *S. aureus* may be present together.
        b. Typical skin findings include erythematous warm spreading lesions with indistinct borders. Bullous lesions suggest *S. aureus* infection. A primary skin lesion (due to trauma, superficial mycoses, or ischemic disease) is often present. Lymphangitic spread and regional adenopathy may occur.
    2. Erysipelas is an erythematous indurated inflammatory lesion that often has a shiny appearance. Its sharply demarcated raised border is a distinguishing feature. Erysipelas may involve the face or the lower extremities. Group A beta-hemolytic streptococci probably cause most cases of erysipelas.
    3. *Haemophilus influenzae* is a common cause of a purplish cellulitis in children, often involving the face. The margins are not sharply demarcated, differentiating this cellulitis from erysipelas.
    4. Gram-negative bacteria including *E. coli, Pseudomonas, Klebsiella,* and *Enterobacter* species may cause cellulitis in patients with venous stasis, ischemia, diabetes mellitus, after surgery, or in IVDUs. Gas may form in the soft tissues.
    5. Synergistic cellulitis, caused by combinations of anaerobic bacteria and gram-negative organisms, may occur in the settings described above. Gas formation is characteristic.
    6. Cellulitis due to animal bites. A gram-negative species, *Pasteurella multocida,* frequently causes cellulitis in the setting of dog and cat bites and scratches.
    7. Cellulitis due to water-related injuries
        a. *Aeromonas hydrophilia* is an aquatic organism that can cause cellulitis after water-related injuries.
        b. *Vibrio* species can infect wounds contaminated by seawater. Cellulitis due to *Vibrio vulnificus* can be rapidly spreading and progress to septicemia.
- Impetigo
    1. Impetigo is caused by group A streptococci or *S. aureus.* Breaks in the skin may be obvious in pa-

tients with staphylococcus disease but absent with streptococci.

2. The vesiculopustular lesions of impetigo are usually perioral but may involve the extremities.

- Erysipeloid is a distinctive type of purplish cellulitis with raised well-defined borders that occurs on the hands or fingers of fishermen or meat handlers. It is caused by *Erysipelothrix rhusiopathiae*.

- Most episodes of folliculitis are caused by *S. aureus* or *Candida* species. *Pseudomonas aeruginosa* acquired from bathing in hot tubs and spas causes a severe form of folliculitis ("hot tub folliculitis") that is associated with fever and systemic symptoms.

- Erythrasma is an infection of intertriginous skin that is characterized by red or brownish patches and caused by *Corynebacterium* species.

- Furuncles caused by *S. aureus* commonly occur in the axilla, the groin, and around the nose and lips. Some individuals are prone to chronic staphylococcal carriage and recurrent furunculosis. Furuncles usually are not associated with systemic findings.

- Ulceronodular skin lesions are often associated with fever and regional lymphadenopathy.

  1. Tularemia is associated with animal (especially rabbit) or tick exposure. The primary skin lesion is a pruritic red papule. An ulcer with sharply defined edges and a depressed center appears 4 days after inoculation.

  2. Anthrax is associated with exposure to hairs, hides, animal products, fertilizer, and herbivores. A "malignant" pustule appears 2 to 5 days after inoculation. The characteristic skin lesion begins as a red papule, which vesiculates and forms a black eschar surrounded by a rim of nonpitting, painless brawny edema.

  3. Swimming pool granuloma. This lesion is caused by *Mycobacterium marinum* and is acquired from fish tanks or swimming pools. The incubation period is uncertain. Skin lesions consist of groups of papules on an extremity, which progress to ulceration and scab formation.

  4. Sporotrichosis may be acquired from exposure to plants (including decaying vegetation). After an incubation period ranging from 1 to 12 weeks, papular skin lesions appear. These lesions often ulcerate and are usually arranged in a "lymphocutaneous" distribution extending from the hand up the forearm.

- *Trichophyton* and *Microsporum* species. These fungal infections of epidermal tissues occur anywhere on the body with keratinized tissues (skin, hair, and nails). In general, these specialized fungi are not capable of invading deeper tissues.

RECOMMENDED DIAGNOSTIC APPROACH

The clinical appearance of skin infections and epidemiologic factors should allow the clinician to make a diagnosis in many patients without the use of other diagnostic tests. It is important to be aware of systemic sequelae of primary skin infections such as sepsis (from *S. aureus, H. influenzae, Vibrio vulnificus*), glomerulonephritis (*Streptococcus pyogenes*), and deep tissue invasion (myonecrosis or fasciitis).

- Blood cultures should be performed if a patient has signs of systemic toxicity, especially in the setting of possible *H. influenzae* cellulitis or staphylococcal abscesses.
- Culture of purulent material
    1. In patients with folliculitis, cutaneous abscesses, or ulcerative lesions, this method should be considered if the patient is acutely ill or immunosuppressed.
    2. In patients with impetigo, cultures are generally not needed. If performed, specimens should be collected by swabbing the base of the vesiculopustular lesions after removing the crust.
- Needle aspiration
    1. The yield of culture of needle aspirate of the advancing edge of cellulitis is low.
    2. A skin biopsy improves the yield but should be reserved for patients at risk for unusual organisms (diabetics) or with unusual clinical features.
- Serologic tests such as streptozyme are not useful in the clinical management of primary skin infections.
- Wood's light examination may assist in making the diagnosis of erythrasma (a coral red fluorescence is seen) and infections with *Microsporum* species (blue-green fluorescence is seen).
- Potassium hydroxide (KOH) preparation is useful in the diagnosis of superficial mycoses.
- Special cultures, serology, or fluorescent antibody stains may be indicated in selected circumstances, e.g., tularemia, anthrax, sporotrichosis, or swimming pool granuloma.
- X-ray or CT examinations may be indicated if gas-forming organisms or underlying osteomyelitis are suspected.

Bibliography

Dellinger EP. Severe necrotizing soft-tissue infections: Multiple disease entities requiring a common approach. JAMA 1981;246:1717.

Fierer J, et al. The fetid foot: Lower-extremity infections in patients with diabetes mellitus. Rev Infect Dis 1979;1:210.

Fleisher G, et al. Cellulitis: Bacterial etiology, clinical features, and laboratory findings. J Pediatr 1980;97:591.

Hill MK, Sanders CV. Localized and systemic infection due to vibrio species. Inf Dis Clin NA 1987;3:687.

Hook EW, et al. Microbiologic evaluation of cutaneous cellulitis in adults. Arch Intern Med 1986;146:295.

Steinberg DG, Stollerman GH. Dangerous pyogenic skin infections. Hospital Pract 1989;24:95.

69

SEXUALLY TRANSMITTED DISEASES

MICKEY EISENBERG

Two minutes with Venus, two years with mercury.

APHORISM

GENERAL COMMENTS

Diagnosis of sexually transmitted diseases (STDs) is complicated by several factors.

1. Symptoms resulting from STDs overlap considerably, thus making it difficult to determine the pathogenic organism on the basis of symptoms alone.
2. Laboratory tests to identify all pathogenic organisms are not readily available. Thus, sometimes it is a practical necessity to make a presumptive diagnosis without laboratory confirmation.
3. Patients may be infected with more than one pathogen (Table 69–1).

DIAGNOSIS OF STD

Criteria for presumptive and definitive diagnosis are presented. A presumptive diagnosis is sufficient grounds for initiation of therapy.

- **Gonorrhea**
    1. Etiology. *Neisseria gonorrhoeae,* a gram-negative diplococcus.
    2. Epidemiology. One million cases are reported annually in the United States. Actual incidence is probably 2 to 3 times higher.
    3. Typical clinical presentation
        a. Men usually have dysuria, frequent urination, and purulent urethral discharge; however, they may be asymptomatic.

Portions of this chapter are adapted from material generously supplied by Walter Stamm, M.D., and Hunter Handsfield, M.D., and the Seattle Sexually Transmitted Disease Training Program, Harborview Medical Center, Seattle, Washington, and Centers for Disease Control, Case Definitions for Public Health Surveillance. MMWR 1991;39:1–42.

TABLE 69–1. Classification of STDs

Bacteria	Viruses
Neisseria gonorrhoeae	Herpes simplex virus
Treponema pallidum	HIV
Chlamydia trachomatis	*Molluscum contagiosum*
Mycoplasma hominis	Hepatitis A
Ureaplasma urealyticum	Hepatitis B
Hemophilus ducreyi	Cytomegalovirus
Calmmatobacterium	Genital warts
granulomatis	Protozoa
Shigella species	*Trichomonas vaginalis*
Campylobacter fetus	*Entamoeba histolytica*
Gardnerella vaginalis[a]	*Giardia lamblia*
Streptococcus, group B[a]	Others
	Phthirus pubic (crab louse)
	Sarcoptes scabiei (scabies mites)

[a] May not be associated with sexual transmission.

    b. Women may have abnormal vaginal discharge, abnormal menses, dysuria, or may be asymptomatic.
    c. Anorectal and pharyngeal infections are common in homosexual men and heterosexual women. Often these are asymptomatic, but proctitis generally produces mild rectal pain or discharge.
  4. Diagnosis (Table 69–2)

PRESUMPTIVE	DEFINITIVE
Microscopic identification of typical gram-negative intracellular diplococci on smear of urethral or rectal exudate (men) or endocervical material (women)	Growth on selective medium with confirmatory laboratory testing
Sensitivity of Gram's stain: male urethritis (98%), female cervix (50%), rectal (20%)	A definitive diagnosis is required if the specimen is extragenital, from a child, or medicolegally significant

- **Chlamydia**
  1. Etiology. *Chlamydia trachomatis*.
  2. Epidemiology. Up to several million cases annually.
  3. Typical clinical presentations. Infection with *Chlamydia trachomatis* may cause urethritis, epididymitis, cervicitis, acute salpingitis, or other syndromes when sexually transmitted. Perinatal infections may result in inclusion conjunctivitis or pneumonia among newborns. Other syndromes caused by *C. trachomatis* include lymphogranuloma venerum.
  4. Diagnosis requires laboratory confirmation by isolation of *C. trachomatis* by culture or demonstration of

TABLE 69–2. Sampling Sites for Culture of Gonococci

PATIENT CATEGORY	PRIMARY SAMPLING SITE	ADDITIONAL SITES
Men		
Heterosexual	Urethra	Oropharynx if practicing cunnilingus
		Urethral secretion after prostatic massage
Homosexual/bisexual	Urethra	Urethral secretion after prostatic massage
	Anal canal (rectum)	
	Oropharynx	
Women	Cervical os	Urethra and anal canal. (Anal canal is the only positive site in 5% of patients.) Oropharynx if practicing fellatio. Bartholin's glands if bartholinitis
Men and women with disseminated gonococcal infection (DGI)	As above	Blood
		Joint fluid (if present)
		Skin lesions
Newborns with ophthalmia	Conjunctivae	Mother: cervix, urethra, and anal canal

Source: Reprinted with permission from Holmes KK et al. Sexually Transmitted Diseases, 2nd ed., New York, McGraw-Hill, 1990 p. 904.

C. trachomatis in a clinical specimen by antigen detection methods.

- **Pelvic inflammatory disease (PID)**
  1. Etiology. PID is caused by one or more of *N. gonorrhoeae, Chlamydia trachomatis, Mycoplasma hominis,* and anaerobic bacteria.
  2. Epidemiology. Between 600,000 and 1 million cases of PID are estimated to occur in the United States each year. PID causes the most important sequelae of STDs in women: involuntary infertility and ectopic pregnancy.
  3. Typical clinical presentation. There are no generally accepted diagnostic clinical criteria for the diagnosis of PID. The patient may have pain and tenderness involving the lower abdomen, cervix, uterus, and adnexae, often with fever, chills, and elevated WBC count and ESR. The diagnosis is more likely if the patient has multiple sexual partners.
  4. Diagnosis

Presumptive	Definitive
Unilateral or bilateral adnexal tenderness on examination in association with evidence of lower genital tract infection and without associated evidence of other diagnosis (ectopic pregnancy, appendicitis). Positive cervical cultures for *N. gonorrhoeae* and/or *Chlamydia trachomatis* support the diagnosis.	Direct visualization of inflamed (edema, hyperemia, or tubal exudate) fallopian tube(s) at laproscopy or laparotomy makes the diagnosis of PID definite. A culture of the tubal exudate establishes the cause.

- **Syphilis**
  1. Etiology. *Treponema pallidum.*
  2. Epidemiology. There are 30,000 cases annually in the United States. Most new cases occur in homosexual or bisexual men.
  3. Typical clinical presentation
     a. Primary. The classic chancre is single, painless, indurated, and located at the site of exposure. Many are rectal.
     b. Secondary. Patients may have a highly variable skin rash, mucosal patches, condylomata lata, or diffuse lymphadenopathy.
     c. Latent. Patients have no specific clinical signs.
  4. Diagnosis

Presumptive	Definitive
Primary: Patients have typical lesion(s) and	Primary and secondary syphilis definitively

either a newly positive serologic test for syphilis (STS) or an STS titer that is at least 4-fold greater than the last, or there has been syphilis exposure within 90 days of lesion onset.

Secondary: Patients have the typical clinical presentation and a strongly reactive STS.

Latent: Patients have serologic evidence of untreated syphilis without clinical signs.

diagnosed by demonstrating *T. pallidum* with darkfield microscopy or fluorescent antibody techniques in material from a chancre, regional lymph node, or other lesion. A definitive diagnosis of latent syphilis cannot be made under usual circumstances.

- **Nongonococcal urethritis (NGU)**
  1. Etiology. The primary agent is *Ureaplasma urealyticum*. Less common causes are herpes simplex virus and *Trichomonas vaginalis* (Table 69–3).
  2. Epidemiology. This is a relatively common cause of urethritis in men.
  3. Clinical presentation. Men usually have dysuria, frequent urination, and mucoid to purulent urethral discharge. Some infected men are asymptomatic.
  4. Diagnosis

PRESUMPTIVE	DEFINITIVE
Men with typical clinical symptoms, and at least 5 WBC per oil immersion field on an intraurethral smear are presumed to have NGU when the urethral Gram's stain and culture is negative for gonorrhea and chlamydial culture is negative.	Nongonococcal urethritis (NGU) is a clinical diagnosis of exclusion.

- **Mucopurulent cervicitis (also known as endocervicitis)**
  1. Etiology. Cervicitis is present without chlamydial or gonococcal infection. Ulcerative cervicitis is often caused by herpes virus. Often the cause is obscure.
  2. Epidemiology. Cases of mucopurulent cervicitis are similar to urethritis in men.
  3. Clinical presentation. There is a mucopurulent secretion from the endocervix.
  4. Diagnosis. The cervical discharge has increased polymorphonuclear leukocytes seen on Gram's stain. The presence of 5 or more polymorphonuclear neutrophils per oil immersion microscopic field suggests cervicitis. Cervical ectopy is a common sign of mucopurulent cervicitis caused by *C. trachomatis*. Cultures

TABLE 69–3. Etiology of Sexually Transmitted Urethritis in Males

Neisseria gonorrhoeae, 20–30%
Chlamydia trachomatis, 30–50%
Ureaplasma urealyticum, 5–20%
Other, 10–15%
Trichomonas vaginalis, rare
Yeasts, rare
Herpes simplex virus, rare
Adenoviruses, rare
Hemophilus spp., rare
Bacteroides ureaolyticus?
Mycoplasma genitalium?
Other bacterial?

Source: Reprinted with permission from Holmes KK et al. Sexually Transmitted Diseases, 2nd ed., New York, McGraw-Hill, 1990 p. 627.

for *Neisseria gonorrhoeae* and *Chlamydia* should be obtained. Mucopurulent cervicitis (MPC) is a clinical diagnosis of exclusion.

· **Vaginitis**

1. Etiology. Common causes are *Trichomonas vaginalis, Candida albicans,* and *Gardnerella vaginalis* (with anaerobic bacteria). Other infectious, chemical, allergenic, and physical agents may cause vaginitis.

2. Epidemiology. This is an exceedingly common infection in young women. It is not always sexually transmitted.

3. Typical clinical presentation. Clinical findings vary from no signs or symptoms to erythema, edema, and pruritus of the external genitalia. Excessive or malodorous vaginal discharge is a common finding. "External" dysuria and dyspareunia may be prominent.

4. Diagnosis (Table 69–4)

PRESUMPTIVE	DEFINITIVE
Trichomoniasis: Profuse grayish discharge with odor	Trichomoniasis: Typical motile trichomonads are identified in a saline wet mount of vaginal discharge, or a vaginal culture is positive for T. vaginalis.
Bacterial vaginosis: A presumptive diagnosis of bacterial vaginosis is made if three out of the following four criteria are present: grayish-white vaginal exudate, vaginal pH >4.5, clue cells (epithelial cells with adherent bacteria), and amine odor present with 10 percent potassium hydroxide.	Bacterial vaginosis: None. Candidiasis: Microscopic identification of yeast forms (budding cells or hyphae) in Gram's stain or potassium hydroxide wet mount preparations of vaginal discharge.

TABLE 69-4. Symptoms and Laboratory Features of Vaginitis

	NORMAL	TRICHOMONIASIS	BACTERIAL VAGINOSIS	CANDIDIASIS
Symptoms	None	Vulvar pruritus, profuse discharge	Slightly increased discharge, malodorous	Vulvar pruritus, increased discharge
Appearance of discharge	Clear or whitish-grey, nonhomogenous	Grayish-white, homogenous; may be frothy	Grayish-white, homogenous	White, clumped, cottage cheese–like
Amount of discharge	None	Large	Moderate	Scant to moderate
pH of discharge	<4.5	>5.0	>4.5	<4.5
Amine (fishy odor) with 10% KOH	Negative	May be present	Positive	Negative
Microscopy with saline and 10% KOH preparations	Epithelial cells	Motile trichomonad	Clue cells[a]	Leukocytes + yeast and pseudomycelia

[a] Clue cells are epithelial cells with a ragged and refractile appearance that is caused by a large number of adherent bacteria. Up to 10% of Clue cells among epithelial cells may be seen normally.

Source: Reprinted with permission from Holmes, KK, et al. Sexually Transmitted Diseases, 2nd ed., New York, McGraw-Hill, 1990, p. 542.

Candidiasis: The presumptive criteria are typical clinical symptoms of vulvovaginitis (marked itching).

- **Granuloma inguinale (donovanosis)** (Table 69–5)
  1. Etiology. *Calymmatobacterium granulomatis.*
  2. Epidemiology. This condition is exceedingly rare in the United States (fewer than 50 cases per year) and usually occurs in people from Asia, Africa, or the tropics.
  3. Diagnosis

PRESUMPTIVE	DEFINITIVE
Typical clinical presentation is sufficient to suggest diagnosis. Resolution of lesions, following specific antibiotic therapy, supports diagnosis. A history of travel to the tropics (particularly India or Papua New Guinea) among patients or their partners helps to substantiate the clinical impression.	Scrapings or biopsy specimens from the ulcer margin reveal the pathognomonic Donovan bodies on microscopic examination. These appear as gram-negative bacteria in vacuolar compartments within white blood or plasma cells.

- **Lymphogranuloma venereum (LGV)**
  1. Etiology. *C. trachomatis* (LGV serotype).
  2. Epidemiology. LGV is rare in the United States.
  3. Typical clinical presentation
     a. The primary lesion of LGV is a 2 to 3 mm painless vesicle or nonindurated ulcer at the site of inoculation. Patients commonly fail to notice this primary lesion.
     b. Regional adenopathy follows within 1 to 4 weeks and is the most common clinical observation. A sensation of stiffness and aching in the groin, followed by swelling of the inguinal region, is the first symptom for most patients, which may subside spontaneously or proceed to the formation of abscesses that rupture to produce draining sinuses.
  4. Diagnosis

PRESUMPTIVE	DEFINITIVE
Eighty percent of cases have LGV complement fixation titers of 1 : 16 or higher. Since the sequelae of LGV are serious and	Isolation of *C. trachomatis,* serotype L1, L2, or L3, from clinical specimen. Demonstration of inclusion bodies by immunofluorescence in

TABLE 69–5. Clinical Features of Genital Ulcers

	SYPHILIS	HERPES	CHANCROID	LYMPHOGRANULOMA VENEREUM	DONOVANOSIS
Incubation period	2–4 weeks (1–12 weeks)	2–7 days	1–14 days	3 days–6 weeks	1–4 weeks up to 6 months
Primary lesion	Papule	Vesicle	Papule or pustule	Papule, pustule, or vesicle	Papule
Number of lesions	Usually one	Multiple, may coalesce	Usually multiple, may coalesce	Usually one	Variable
Diameter, mm	5–15	1–2	2–20	2–10	Variable
Edges	Sharply demarcated, elevated, round, or oval	Erythematous	Undermined, ragged, irregular	Elevated, round, or oval	Elevated, irregular
Depth	Superficial or deep	Superficial	Excavated	Superficial or deep	Elevated
Base	Smooth, nonpurulent	Serous, erythematous	Purulent	Variable	Red and rough ("beefy")
Induration	Firm	None	Soft	Occasionally firm	Firm
Pain	Unusual	Common	Usually very tender	Variable	Uncommon
Lymphadenopathy	Firm, nontender, bilateral	Firm, tender, often bilateral	Tender, may suppurate, usually unilateral	Tender, may suppurate, loculated, usually unilateral	Pseudoadenopathy

Source: Reprinted with permission from Holmes, KK, et al. Sexually Transmitted Diseases, 2nd ed., New York, McGraw-Hill, 1990, p. 712.

preventable, treatment should not be withheld pending laboratory confirmation.

leukocytes of an inguinal lymph node (bubo) aspirate. Positive microimmunofluorescent serologic test for a lymphogranuloma venereum strain of *C. trachomatis* (in a clinically compatible case).

- **Molluscum contagiosum**
  1. Etiology. Molluscum contagiosum virus.
  2. Epidemiology. Epidemiology is poorly defined.
  3. Typical clinical presentation. The lesions are 1 to 5 mm, smooth, rounded, shiny, firm, flesh-colored to pearly white papules with characteristically umbilicated centers. They are most commonly seen on the trunk and anogenital region and are generally asymptomatic.
  4. Diagnosis

PRESUMPTIVE	DEFINITIVE
Usually on the basis of the typical clinical presentation.	Microscopic examination of lesions or lesion material reveals the pathognomonic molluscum inclusion bodies.

- **Condylomata acuminata**
  1. Etiology. Human papilloma virus.
  2. Epidemiology. Epidemiology is poorly defined.
  3. Typical clinical presentation. Condylomata acuminata appears as single or multiple soft, fleshy, papillary or sessile painless growths around the anus, vulvovaginal area, penis, urethra, or perineum.
  4. Diagnosis

PRESUMPTIVE	DEFINITIVE
A diagnosis may be made on the basis of the typical clinical observations. The possible diagnosis of condylomata lata is excluded by obtaining a test for syphilis.	A biopsy is required to make a definitive diagnosis. Biopsy should be done before initiation of therapy for very atypical lesions for which neoplasia is a consideration.

- **Herpes genitalis**
  1. Etiology. Herpes simplex virus (HSV) types 1 and 2.
  2. Epidemiology. There are an estimated 400,000 to

600,000 primary infections annually and 2 to 3 million recurrent episodes annually.

3. Typical clinical presentation. Multiple vesicles appear anywhere on the genitalia. They spontaneously rupture to form painful shallow ulcers, and resolve spontaneously without scarring. The first occurrence ("initial infection") has a mean duration of 12 days and is often associated with local pain, fever, dysuria, and lymphadenopathy. Subsequent, usually milder, occurrences are termed recurrent infections (mean duration 4 to 5 days).

4. Diagnosis

PRESUMPTIVE	DEFINITIVE
When typical genital lesions are present or a pattern of recurrence has developed, herpes infection is likely. Presumptive diagnosis is further supported by direct identification of multinucleated giant cells with intranuclear inclusions in a clinical specimen prepared by Papanicolaou's or other histochemical stain.	An HSV virus tissue culture demonstrates the characteristic cytopathogenic effect (CPE) following inoculation of a specimen from the cervix, the urethra, or the base of a genital lesion.

- **Chancroid**
  1. Etiology. *Hemophilus ducreyi.*
  2. Epidemiology. Chancroid is rare in the United States but has occurred in epidemics or clusters of cases in the last few years; otherwise, it appears in travelers to the tropics, Southeast Asia, and Africa.
  3. Typical clinical presentation (see Table 69–5). Ulcers usually occur on the coronal sulcus, glans, or shaft. Females are usually asymptomatic. A characteristic inguinal bubo that may rupture occurs in 25 to 60% of cases.
  4. Diagnosis

PRESUMPTIVE	DEFINITIVE
When the only organisms seen in an aspirate from a bubo are arranged in chains or clumps along strands of mucus and are morphologically similar to *H. ducreyi,* the diagnosis is highly likely. A clinical picture consistent with chancroid involving the genitalia or a unilateral	The diagnosis is definitive when *H. ducreyi* is recovered by culture. Biopsy may be diagnostic but is not usually performed.

bubo, or both, is
suggestive. Gram's stain
of the ulcer is not
diagnostic.

- **Pediculosis pubis**
  1. Etiology. The condition is caused by an infestation with *Phthirus pubis* (pubic or crab louse), an ecto-parasite 1 to 4 mm long with segmented tarsi and claws for clinging to hairs.
  2. Epidemiology. Epidemiology is poorly defined.
  3. Typical clinical presentation. Symptoms range from slight discomfort to intolerable itching. Erythematous papules, nits, or adult lice clinging to pubic, perineal, or perianal hairs are present and often are noticed by patients.
  4. Diagnosis

PRESUMPTIVE	DEFINITIVE
A history of recent exposure to pubic lice in a patient with pruritic erythematous macules, papules, or secondary excoriations in the genital region.	Finding of lice or nits attached to genital hairs.

- **Scabies**
  1. Etiology. This is caused by *Sarcoptes scabiei,* the itch mite. The female mite is 0.3 to 0.4 mm long and the male is somewhat smaller. The female burrows under the skin to deposit eggs.
  2. Epidemiology. Epidemiology is poorly defined.
  3. Typical clinical presentation. Symptoms include itching, which is often worse at night, and the presence of erythematous papular eruptions. Excoriations and secondary infections are common. Reddish-brown nodules are caused by hypersensitivity and may de-velop 1 or more months after infection has occurred. The primary lesion is the burrow, and when not obliter-ated by excoriations, it is most often seen on the fingers and interdigital web spaces, penis, and wrists.
  4. Diagnosis

PRESUMPTIVE	DEFINITIVE
The diagnosis is often made on clinical grounds alone. A history of recent exposure to pubic lice in a patient with scabies within the previous 2 months supports the diagnosis.	Definitive diagnosis is made by microscopic identification of the mite or its eggs, larvae, or feces in scrapings from an elevated papule or burrow.

RECOMMENDED DIAGNOSTIC APPROACH

- **Urethritis in men**
  1. Urethritis in men is customarily divided in gonococcal, chlamydial, and nongonococcal urethritis (see Table 69–3).
  2. The urethral Gram's stain is the quickest means of distinguishing gonococcal from nongonococcal urethritis (Figure 69–1).

- **Ulcerative genital lesions** (Figure 69–2 and Table 69–5)
  1. Most ulcerative genital lesions are caused by herpes virus infection. Ten to fifteen percent of genital ulcers are traumatic in origin.
  2. Genital herpes is supported by a history of vesicular lesions becoming ulcerative over several days or by recurrences in the same area. Lymphadenopathy is common but does not help identify etiology.
  3. Darkfield examination should be performed on all ulcerative lesions, regardless of the presence of pain, unless genital herpes seems quite likely.

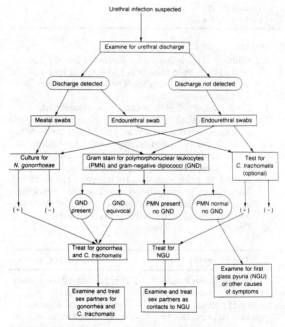

Figure 69–1. Initial diagnosis and management in men with suspected urethritis. (Reprinted with permission from Holmes K, et al. Sexually Transmitted Diseases, 2nd ed. New York, McGraw-Hill, 1990 p. 633.)

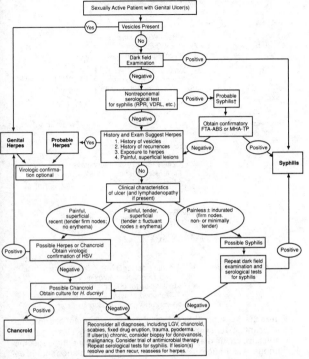

Figure 69–2. Algorithm for the diagnosis of genital ulcer-inguinal adenopathy syndromes in sexually active patients. (Reprinted with permission from Holmes K, et al. Sexually Transmitted Diseases, 2nd ed. New York, McGraw-Hill, 1990 p. 714.)

- **Vaginitis**
  1. Findings on physical and microscopic examination of the discharge usually allow characterization of the vaginitis (see Table 69–4).
  2. There is often considerable overlap of symptoms among vaginitis, urethritis, cervicitis, and salpingitis. Hence, other causes of vaginal discharge and dysuria should be considered if the suspected vaginitis does not respond to therapy.

- **Cervicitis**
  1. Major causes of cervicitis are *C. trachomatis, N. gonorrhoeae,* herpes simplex virus, *Candida albicans,* and *Trichomonas vaginalis.*
  2. Cervicitis may occur alone or in combination with vaginitis. *Candida* and *Trichomonas* are common causes of cervicitis combined with vaginitis. *N. gonorrhoeae* and *Chlamydia* usually cause nonerosive cervicitis without vaginitis. Herpes virus as a cause of cervicitis

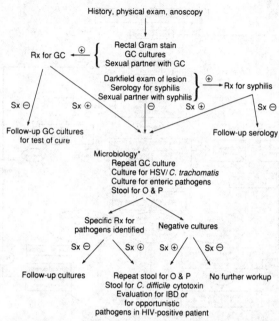

Figure 69–3. Algorithm A: Evaluation and treatment of anorectal and/or intestinal symptoms in homosexual men. This algorithm emphasizes a full diagnostic evaluation and treatment for specific pathogens identified. Ideally, microbiological evaluation should be based on presenting symptoms and sigmoidoscopy findings. Rx = treatment, Sx = symptoms, GC = *N. gonorrhoeae*, O & P = ova and parasites, IBD = inflammatory bowel disease. (Reprinted with permission from Holmes K, et al. Sexually Transmitted Diseases, 2nd ed. New York, McGraw-Hill, 1990 p. 678.)

     produces ulcerative necrotic lesions that are easily seen on pelvic examination.

3. Cultures for gonococcus and chlamydia should be obtained. If risk for STD is high, empiric treatment is usually justified with cultures pending.

· **PID**

1. PID is conveniently categorized into gonococcal and nongonococcal forms. Nongonoccocal PID is caused by *C. trachomatis* (sexually transmitted) and by *Bacteroides fragilis* and anaerobic gram-positive cocci (nonsexually transmitted).

2. PID should be considered in all women with lower abdominal pain. The pain is usually bilateral. Vaginal discharge, menometrorrhagia, dysuria, onset of pain associated with menses, and fever are common symptoms.

· **Infectious proctitis in homosexual men**

1. Major infectious causes of infectious proctitis, primarily occurring among homosexual men, are *N. gon-*

orrhoeae and herpes virus. Other sexually transmitted microorganisms include enteric pathogens (*Shigella, Salmonella, Giardia lamblia* and *Entamoeba histolytica*).

2. Anoscopy is a key diagnostic procedure in defining the cause of proctitis and is necessary to obtain adequate cultures (Figure 69–3).

Bibliography

Centers for Disease Control: Sexually Transmitted Diseases Summary. Centers for Disease Control, Atlanta, GA, 1990.

Eschenbach DA, Hiller SL. Advances in diagnostic testing for vaginitis and cervicitis. J Reprod Med 1989;34(8 Suppl):555–564.

Hanssen PW, et al. Clinical manifestations of vaginal trichomoniasis. JAMA 1989;261:571–576.

Hemsell DL. Acute pelvic inflammatory disease. Etiologic and therapeutic considerations. J Reprod Med 1988;33(1 suppl):119–123.

Holmes K, et al., eds. Sexually Transmitted Diseases, 2nd ed. New York, McGraw-Hill, 1990.

Larsen SA, Syphilis. Clin Lab Med 1989;9:545–557.

Martens MG. Office diagnosis of sexually transmitted diseases. Obstet Gynecol Clin North Am 1989;16:659–677.

McCue JD. Evaluation and management of vaginitis. Arch Intern Med, 1989;149:565–568.

70

URINARY TRACT INFECTIONS

MICKEY EISENBERG

One must agree with Hippocrates, Galen, and many others, ancient and modern, that there is no surer way to determine the temperaments and constitutions of people of either sex than to look at the urine.

DAVACH DE LA RIVIERE (18th century)

DEFINITION

Infections of the urinary tract range in severity from asymptomatic bacteriuria to life-threatening bacteremic pyelonephrtis. "Complicated" urinary tract infections refer to infections resulting from anatomic or physiologic obstruction (renal calculi, anatomic anomalies, indwelling urinary catheters, or urologic manipulation), resistant organisms, or infection in "compromised" patients.

- Asymptomatic bacteriuria
  1. Asymptomatic bacteriuria is defined as the presence of bacteria in the urine without symptoms of infection (urine is normally sterile). It occurs in 1 to 2% of children, 2 to 5% of women of child-bearing age, and in 5 to 15% of older women.
  2. Two to ten percent of pregnant women have asymptomatic bacteriuria. Of pregnant women with first-trimester asymptomatic bacteriuria, 20 to 40% develop pyelonephritis during pregnancy if the bacteriuria is not eradicated.
  3. Asymptomatic bacteriuria is common in elderly men, but does not generally require treatment.
- Acute uncomplicated cystitis
  1. This is an infection of the bladder and/or urethra. It is also known as lower urinary tract infection. Acute cystitis typically occurs in otherwise healthy young women.
  2. *Escherichia coli*, other enterobacteriaciae, *Staphylococcus saprophyticus*, or enterococci account for 90% of cases.
- Acute pyelonephritis
  1. This is an infection of renal parenchyma and is also known as upper urinary tract infection. The usual pathogen is *E. coli*.
  2. One-third of patients with characteristic signs and

symptoms of acute cystitis also have unrecognized infection of the upper urinary tract. (Table 70–1)

- Complicated infections (see Table 70–1)
  1. Pathogens associated with renal calculi include *Proteus* spp., *Klebsiella* spp., enterococci, and *Staphylococcus aureus*.
  2. Pathogens associated with urologic manipulation, ob-

TABLE 70–1. Risk Factors for Occult Renal Infection, Antimicrobial Resistant Pathogen, or "Complicated Urinary Tract Infection"

RISK FACTOR	OCCULT RENAL INFECTION	RENAL PATIENT "COMPLICATED URINARY TRACT INFECTION"
Demographic		
Urban emergency department	Yes	
Lower socioeconomic status	Yes	
Hospital-acquired infection		Yes
Pregnancy	Yes	Yes
Urologic		
Indwelling catheter		Yes
Recent urinary tract instrumentation		Yes
Known urinary tract abnormality or stone	Yes	Yes
Medical		
Previous relapse after therapy for urinary tract infection	Yes	
Previous urinary tract infection before age 12	Yes	
Acute pyelonephritis or more than three urinary tract infections in past year	Yes	
Symptoms for more than 7 days before therapy	Yes	
Recent antibiotic use		Yes
Diabetes	Yes	Yes
Other immuno-suppressing conditions	Yes	Yes

Source: Reprinted with permission from Johnson JR, Stamm WE. Uinary tract infections in women: Diagnosis and treatment. Ann Intern Med 1989; 111:906–917.

struction, indwelling urinary catheter, and nosocomial infections include *Proteus* spp., *Klebsiella* spp., *Enterobacter* spp., *Serratia* spp., *Pseudomonas* spp., *Staphylococcus aureus,* enterococci, and fungi, including *Candida albicans.*

EPIDEMIOLOGY

- In the United States, UTIs account for 5.2 million visits to physicians' offices and 100,000 hospitalizations annually.
- UTIs are very common in women and affect 10% to 20% at some time in their lives. Pregnancy is a risk factor for both asymptomatic and symptomatic infections.
- UTIs in men are almost always associated with functional or anatomic urologic abnormalities. Prostatic hypertrophy and genitourinary instrumentation are the major predispositions to infection.
- Forty percent of nosocomial infections are UTIs. Of nosocomial UTIs, 75% are associated with indwelling urinary catheters and the remainder result from urologic manipulation.

DIFFERENTIAL DIAGNOSIS

Evaluation of patients with symptoms of dysuria should include consideration of:

- Urethritis. This may be caused by *Neisseria gonorrhoeae* or *Chlamydia trachomatis.*
- Vaginitis. This may be caused by vaginal anaerobes (bacterial vaginosis), *Trichomonas vaginalis,* or *C. albicans.*
- Genital herpes infection

CLINICAL FEATURES

There are overlaps in signs and symptoms between patients with upper tract and lower tract infection, but typical clinical pictures are:

- Acute uncomplicated cystitis: urgency, frequent urination, dysuria, and suprapubic discomfort in the absence of fever, flank pain, or systemic symptoms are common.
- Acute pyelonephritis: fever, flank (costovertebral angle) pain, rigors, nausea, vomiting, and myalgia are typical. Urgency, frequent urination, dysuria, and suprapubic pain are often absent in patients with pyelonephritis. Other symptoms include headache, abdominal pain, malaise, and sweats. Patients may have septic shock from gram-negative bacteremic pyelonephritis.

LABORATORY FEATURES

- Pyuria
  1. Determination of the presence or absence of pyuria is essential to the diagnosis of UTI. Patients with pyuria almost always have infected urine.
  2. Hemacytometer use
     a. Fresh, uncentrifuged urine is examined in a hemacytometer chamber.
     b. Fewer than 8 WBCs/ml usually correlates with sterile urine in asymptomatic women.
     c. More than 8 WBCs/ml are present in most patients with acute cystitis (most patients have more than 60 cells/mm^3 according to this technique).
  3. A positive leukocyte esterase test on urinalysis indicates presence of WBCs in the urine, which are a presumptive indicator of infection. The test measures esterase in polymorphic nucleated WBCs only and does not indicate the presence of lymphocytes or epithelial cells; thus for infected urine which has been at room temperature for a while with resulting "disappearance" of WBCs, the test will remain positive. The test may be falsely positive if many vaginal cells contaminate the specimen. Generally the test is reported as negative, trace, or positive. Only the positive should be considered indicative of infection.
- WBC casts are common in pyelonephritis and are not seen in patients with lower tract disease.
- Hematuria may be present in both cystitis (50%) and pyelonephritis.
- There may be bacteriuria; the presence of 1 bacterium per high-power field of uncentrifuged urine correlated with 100,000 bacterial colonies per ml when the urine is cultured.
- Urine culture
  1. An unequivocal diagnosis of UTI requires demonstration of uropathogenic bacteria.
  2. One hundred thousand bacterial colonies per ml is not an absolute requirement for the diagnosis of bacterial infection of the urinary tract. One-third of women with lower UTIs have colony counts in midstream urine of less than 100,000/ml.
  3. Colony counts of 100 to 10,000 bacteria/ml in patients with pyuria and a compatible clinical picture can be of diagnostic importance. In general, significant bacteriuria in acutely symptomatic women is defined as more than 100 colonies/ml of a known uropathogen.
- Nitrite test
  1. The nitrite test is a dipstick test which measures the presence of nitrites in the urine produced by gram-negative organisms.
  2. Nitrites can only be produced by bacteria at body temperature and thus the test (if a UTI is present) is more likely to be positive on urine that has been in the blad-

der for a while. Freshly produced urine may be falsely negative.
- Bladder washout and antibody-coated bacteria tests. These procedures are not routinely done but may be of value in localization of infection in selected cases.
- Rapid diagnostic techniques. These tests generally achieve a sensitivity of 95 to 98% and a negative predictive value of over 99% compared to routine cultures when bacteriuria is defined as 100,000 colonies/ml. However, such a definition will falsely miss patients with low colony count infections.

RECOMMENDED DIAGNOSTIC APPROACH

- Suspected cystitis
  1. Urinalysis. If urinalysis shows the presence of pyuria (as seen using the hemacytometer or as indicated by a positive leukocyte esterase test), or hematuria (present in approximately 50% of patients), or bacteriuria (the nitrite test is a good screening test for the presence of bacteria), there is presumptive evidence of cystitis and empiric treatment can begin without a culture.
  2. Gram's stain for uncomplicated urinary infections is generally not warranted.
  3. For uncomplicated infections urine culture is not warranted as presumptive therapy can begin based on clinical findings. If the patient does not respond to therapy, further evaluation is indicated including a culture. A urine culture should be obtained on all patients with complicated infections.
- Pyelonephritis
  1. Urinalysis. With the exception of WBC casts (which may not be present), the findings are identical to those seen in cystitis.
  2. Urine culture. A culture should be obtained whenever the possibility of pyelonephritis is considered.
  3. Ill patient and/or complicated pyelonephritis
     a. Blood cultures should be done.
     b. WBC count with differential count should be determined.

Bibliography

Johnson JR, Stamm WE. Urinary tract infections in women: Diagnosis and treatment. Ann Intern Med 1989;111:906–917.

Latham RH, et al. Urinary tract infections in adult women caused by *Staphylococcus saprophyticus*. JAMA 1983;250:3063–3066.

Lipsky BA. Urinary tract infections in men. Epidemiology, pathophysiology, diagnosis, and treatment. Ann Intern Med 1989;110:138–150.

Pezzlo M. Detection of urinary tract infections by rapid methods. Clin Microbiol Rev 1988;1:268–280.

Stamm WE. Protocol for diagnosis of urinary tract infection: Reconsidering the criterion for significant bacteriuria. Urology 1988;32(2 Suppl):6–12.

Stamm WE, et al. Diagnosis of coliform infection in acutely dysuric women. N Engl J Med 1982;307:463–468.

71

INFECTIOUS DIARRHEA

PAUL G. RAMSEY, *and*
DOUGLAS S. PAAUW

There is death in the pot.
KINGS II 4:40

DEFINITION

It is helpful to characterize infections of the GI tract by their
pathogenesis:

- Mucosal ulceration. Some microorganisms invade the intestinal wall and cause mucosal ulceration. These infections occur in the large intestine and are defined clinically
  by the finding of blood or polymorphonuclear leukocytes
  (PMNs) in the stool.
- Enterotoxin
  1. Other organisms cause GI symptoms via an entero-
     toxin. Blood and PMNs are usually absent from the
     stool of these patients.
  2. In some cases disease is acquired by ingestion of pre-
     formed toxin (as with *Staphylococcus aureus* and
     Clostridium botulinum); in other cases the toxin is
     formed after ingestion of the organism.

EPIDEMIOLOGY

Important historical factors include:

- Travel history. There are differences in geographic distribution of the organisms causing GI infections. For example, amebiasis should be considered in an individual who
  has traveled to an endemic area such as Mexico.
- Foodborne infections (Table 71–1). Such infections remain
  an important cause of infectious diarrhea in this country.
  Large outbreaks of *Salmonella* infection may be traced to
  restaurants or picnics. Uncooked food is more likely to
  transmit a foodborne infection.
- Water is an important source for infection with *Giardia
  lamblia* and a variety of bacteria.
- Animal contact. Chickens, cats, or dogs may be a source of
  Campylobacter fetus.
- Host factors. Decreased gastric acidity predisposes patients to infection with *E. coli* and *Shigella* species, as well
  as *Giardia*.

TABLE 71–1. Causes of Foodborne Disease

	BACTERIAL	VIRAL
Common	*Salmonella*	Hepatitis A
	Shigella	Norwalk virus
	Clostridium perfringens	
	Staphylococcus	
	Bacillus cereus	
	E. coli 0157:H7	
	Campylobacter fetus	
Rare	Streptococcus groups A & D	Echovirus
	Yersinia enterocolitica	
	Vibrio parahaemolyticus	
	Clostridium botulinum	
	Listeria monocytogenes	

- Prior antibiotic therapy raises the possibility of *Clostridium difficile* infection.
- Person-to-person contact is a major source of transmission of viral infections. In child day-care centers, many bacteria and parasites may be passed.
- Male homosexual activity introduces a large differential diagnosis (*Campylobacter fetus,* gonorrhea, *Chlamydia,* amebiasis, herpes simplex virus) for proctitis.
- Immunosuppressed patients
  1. Such patients may develop severe upper GI (esophageal, gastric, and small intestinal) infections with herpes simplex virus, *Candida* spp., and cytomegalovirus.
  2. Diarrhea is particularly common in HIV-infected patients, with the most frequent infectious causes being CMV, cryptosporidia, salmonella, and *Giardia.*

CLINICAL FEATURES

- History. Important points in the history include:
  1. Upper GI symptoms (nausea and vomiting) versus lower GI symptoms (diarrhea)
  2. Duration of symptoms and incubation period
  3. Character of the diarrhea (volume, watery consistency, blood, or mucus)
  4. Presence of associated findings (fever, flatulence, epigastric bloating, severe abdominal pain)
  5. Renal abnormalities (which suggest *E. coli* 0157 : H7)
  6. Health of family and close associates
  7. Epidemiologic factors (see Epidemiology)
- Initial differential diagnosis based on stool examination
  1. The absence of blood or PMNs in the stool suggests the differential diagnosis listed in Table 71–2.
  2. The finding of blood or PMNs (see Table 71–3) implicates a number of infectious agents, which should be treated with antimicrobial therapy (except for

TABLE 71-2. Infectious Agents Not Associated with Blood or Pus in the Stool

| ORGANISM | INCUBATION PERIOD | UPPER GI SYMPTOMS[a] | | | | ASSOCIATED FINDINGS |
		N	V	C	D	
Viral (in adults)	<7 days	1+	1+	2+	3+	Exposure to children or family members; mild fever and myalgia are often present
S. aureus	1–6 hr	4+	4+	4+	2+	None
C. perfringens	9–18 hr	1+	1+	1+	3+	None
Cholera	1–4 days	1+	1+	0	4+	Lower abdominal cramps and voluminous watery diarrhea
B. cereus	3–12 hr	2+	2+	2+	2+	May appear like staphylococcal or C. perfringens food poisoning
E. coli (enterotoxic)	1–2 days	1+	1+	1+	3+	Fever and myalgia often present
Giardia	7–21 days	2+	0	3+	2+	Midepigastric bloating, flatulence, and diarrhea may be chronic

[a] Symptoms are rated on a scale of 0 to 4+, ranging from absent to most prominent. N = nausea; V = vomiting; C = cramps; D = diarrhea.

TABLE 71–3. Infectious Agents Associated with Blood or Pus in the Stool

| ORGANISM | INCUBATION PERIOD | UPPER GI SYMPTOMS^A | | | | ASSOCIATED FINDINGS |
		N	V	C	D	
Campylobacter fetus	1–5 days	1+	1+	2+	4+	"Sheets" of PMNs in stool
Salmonella spp.	12–48 hr	1+	1+	1+	3+	Fever, myalgia often present
Shigella spp.	1–5 days	1+	1+	2+	4+	Fever, myalgia, many PMNs in stool
E. coli (enterohemorrhagic)	7–8 days	2+	1+	3+	2+	Hemolytic uremic syndrome in up to 10% of cases. Abdominal pain and tenderness can be marked
E. coli (enteroinvasive)	>24 hr	1+	1+	1+	3+	Fever, myalgia

	Incubation	N	V	C	D	Comments
Amebiasis	1–3 weeks	1+	1+	1+	3+	Mild fever
Yersinia enterocolitica	Unknown	0	0	1+	2+	Mesenteric lymphadenitis, reactive polyarthritis
C. difficile	Unknown	1+	1+	2+	3+	History of recent antibiotic use
Vibrio parahemolyticus	1–3 days	1+	1+	2+	3+	Associated with eating raw shellfish, fever, headache. Microscopic exam reveals red and white cells but stools rarely grossly bloody
Aeromonas hydrophila	Unknown	0	0	1+	3+	Watery or bloody diarrhea, symptoms may be prolonged

[a] Symptoms are rated on a scale of 0 to 4+ ranging from absent to most prominent. N = nausea; V = vomiting; C = cramps; D = diarrhea.

Salmonella gastroenteritis). However, the absence of blood and pus does not rule out the possibility of these organisms.

- Laboratory
  1. Examination of stool for PMNs can be done using a Gram's stain or methylene blue technique. Gram's stain also may be useful for diagnosing *Campylobacter fetus* infection.
  2. Stool culture
     a. Stool culture should be performed when there are signs of invasive disease (blood or pus in the stool), or systemic toxicity, or if symptoms persist for more than 24 hr.
     b. Stool cultures are not necessary in all patients, especially if clinical features suggest a benign non-invasive disease.
     c. Culture techniques
        i. Standard culture for "enteric pathogens" (*Salmonella* and *Shigella*).
        ii. Special culture media and temperature conditions for *Campylobacter fetus* are now included in many laboratories as part of the standard culture.
        iii. Special enrichment techniques are necessary to culture for *Yersinia enterocolitica* and *Vibrio* species.
        iv. Some laboratories rapidly identify *Clostridium difficile* by gas-liquid chromatography.
  3. Blood cultures should be performed if a patient has fever or systemic toxicity in association with diarrhea. Bone marrow cultures may be especially useful in the diagnosis of typhoid fever.
  4. Toxin assay for *Clostridium difficile* should be considered in addition to stool culture when this infection is suspected.
  5. Sigmoidoscopy may be useful for identifying the findings associated with *C. difficile* infection (pseudomembranous enterocolitis). Intestinal ulcerations found by sigmoidoscopy may suggest *Entamoeba histolytica* infection.
  6. Serologic techniques are available for amebiasis and salmonellosis.
     a. Indirect hemagglutination serology to identify *E. histolytica* infection is 95% sensitive for extra-intestinal amebiasis and 80% sensitive for intestinal infection.
     b. *Salmonella* titers rise after 1 week of infection in 50% of patients and peak by 4 to 6 weeks in 90 to 95% of patients. *Salmonella* titers are most useful in patients with typhoid or paratyphoid fever.
  7. Stool for ova and parasite examination. This examination should be performed if travel or sexual history suggests ambiasis or if symptoms and epidemiologic findings suggest giardiasis.

RECOMMENDED DIAGNOSTIC APPROACH

- The diagnostic approach is determined by the duration of symptoms, signs, and epidemiologic considerations.
- Patients with symptoms of less than 24 hr (unless febrile or toxic appearing) do not require extensive laboratory tests.
- Patients with symptoms longer than 24 hr and those who are febrile or appear toxic should have a stool Gram's stain and culture.
- Patients who have traveled to areas where amebiasis and giardia are common should have a stool examination for ova and parasites.
- Patients who have recently received antibiotics or been hospitalized should have stool evaluation for the presence of *C. difficile*.

Bibliography

Blaser MJ, Reller LB. *Campylobacter* enteritis. N Engl J Med 1981;305:1444.

Carter AO, et al. A severe outbreak of *Escherichia coli* 0157:H7–Associated hemorrhagic colitis in a nursing home. N Engl J Med 1987;317:1496.

Ho DD, et al. *Campylobacter* enteritis—early diagnosis with Gram's stain. Arch Intern Med 1982;142:1858.

Holmberg S. Vibrios and aeromonas. Inf Dis Clin North Am 1988; 2:655.

MacDonald KC, et al. *Escherichia coli* 0157:H7, an emerging GI pathogen. JAMA 1988;259:3567.

Recommendations for collection of laboratory specimens associated with outbreaks of gastroenteritis. MMWR 1990;39(RR-14):1.

Thorn GM. Diagnosis of infectious diarrheal diseases. Inf Dis Clin North Am 1988;2:747.

72

SEPTIC ARTHRITIS
AND OSTEOMYELITIS

PAUL G. RAMSEY, *and*
DOUGLAS S. PAAUW

Bone of my bones and flesh of my flesh.

GENESIS 2:23

DEFINITION

- Septic arthritis is an infection involving the joint space.
  1. Although polyarticular involvement can occur, a single joint is involved in most cases.
  2. Septic arthritis may mimic noninfectious inflammatory joint diseases and should be distinguished also from septic bursitis, which involves the olecranon or prepatellar bursa.
- Osteomyelitis is an infection of the bone and marrow.
  1. Route of infection
     a. Hematogenous. The infection is hematogenous in 19% of adult cases, most commonly involving the long bones in children and the thoracic vertebrae in adults.
     b. Contiguous spread occurs in 47% of adult cases and is common in the pelvis, skull, and mandible.
     c. Vascular insufficiency accounts for 34% of cases in adults, often in diabetics. The feet are most commonly involved.
  2. Acute versus chronic. Cases are classified as acute during the first occurrence of osteomyelitis. Cases of patients who have a history of prior osteomyelitis are classified as chronic.
  3. Clinical settings. Several special clinical settings of osteomyelitis are recognized: vertebral osteomyelitis, IV drug use, sickle cell anemia, artificial joints, hemophiliacs, osteitis pubis, and puncture wounds.

EPIDEMIOLOGY

- Septic arthritis
  1. Age. Gonococcal infection is the most common cause of septic arthritis in the 15- to 40-year age group.
  2. Inflammatory joint disease. Rheumatoid arthritis, trauma, and gout are predisposing factors for infection and make the diagnosis of septic arthritis more difficult.

3. Infection of a prosthetic device. This condition is difficult to diagnose, since fever is often absent. Joint tenderness may be the only clue to an infected prosthesis.
4. Sexual history. Sexual history is important because of the risk of gonococcal infection.
5. Concurrent infections are common in patients with septic arthritis.
6. IV drug use is a risk factor.

- Septic bursitis. Most patients with septic bursitis involving the olecranon or prepatellar bursa are young to middle-age men with a history of trauma to the site. Some patients may have a history of other diseases involving the bursa, and a few patients have developed infection after intrabursal corticosteroid injection.

- Osteomyelitis

1. Age. There are 2 age peaks: childhood (85% of cases) and the elderly. Bone involvement depends on age: long bones are affected in children; vertebrae in adults.
2. Predisposing conditions for hematogenous infections include IV drug use and hemoglobinopathies. Precipitating factors for osteomyelitis secondary to a contiguous focus of infection include postoperative infections (60% of cases), soft tissue infections, infected teeth, paranasal sinus infections, and radiation therapy.
3. Most patients with osteomyelitis related to vascular insufficiency are diabetic and older than 50.

CLINICAL FEATURES

- Septic arthritis

1. *Neisseria gonorrhoeae*
   a. *N. gonorrhoeae* accounts for 90% of cases in patients ages 15 to 40.
   b. Gonococcal arthritis is one manifestation of disseminated gonococcal infections (DGI). Patients usually have fever; pustular, papular, or petechial skin lesions (fewer than 30 in number); and joint involvement of the wrist, fingers, knees, or ankles. Tenosynovitis is an early finding.
   c. Septic arthritis usually follows with monoarticular involvement of the knees, ankles, or wrists.
   d. In women, disseminated gonococcal infections occur in association with menstruation.
2. *Staphylococcus aureus*
   a. *S. aureus* accounts for approximately 70% of cases of nongonococcal bacterial septic arthritis in adults.
   b. In elderly adults with rheumatoid arthritis, *S. aureus* accounts for more than 90% of cases. Fever is often absent.
3. Beta-hemolytic streptococci (Groups A and B). These organisms may cause mono- or polyarticular septic arthritis, especially in association with bacteremia.
4. Gram-negative bacteria

    a. These bacteria account for 10% of cases of septic arthritis in recent years.

    b. Patients with host-defense abnormalities, chronic diseases, IV drug use, and other noninfectious inflammatory joint disease have an increased risk of developing gram-negative infections.

    c. *Hemophilus influenzae* is a common cause of septic arthritis in children but is uncommon in adults.

  5. Fungal and mycobacterial septic arthritis. Fungal (in immunosuppressed patients and IV drug users) and mycobacterial (in patients with underlying inflammatory joint disease) septic arthritis occur infrequently.

- Septic bursitis
  1. Swelling (100% of cases) and pain (95%) of the prepatellar or olecranon bursa suggest this diagnosis. Fever and chills are common.
  2. Cellulitis is seen in 75% of cases, but joint motion is nearly normal. *S. aureus* and, rarely, beta-hemolytic streptococci cause septic bursitis.

- Osteomyelitis. The clinical features and microbiology vary greatly with age, route of infection, and predisposing illness.
  1. Hematogenous infection
     a. *S. aureus* is responsible for 80% of childhood and 50% of adult cases of hematogenous infection.
     b. Streptococci (10% of cases), enteric gram-negative rods (8%), and *Salmonella* (2%) are other pathogens.
     c. Clinical findings include signs and symptoms localized to the involved bone. Fever, chills, and general malaise are found in less than half of the patients. Some patients have symptoms present for several months before examination.
     d. Vertebral osteomyelitis accounts for 2% of adult hematogenous osteomyelitis. Ninety percent of patients have localized continuous pain lasting longer than 3 months. In bacterial osteomyelitis, the adjacent vertebrae are frequently involved. The spine is a common location for tuberculous osteomyelitis (Pott's disease).
     e. Hematogenous osteomyelitis related to IV drug use often involves the vertebrae (including the cervical vertebrae), sternoclavicular joint, sacroiliac joint, or the os pubis. These infections are often due to gram-negatives (*Pseudomonas aeruginosa* in 60%), and only 15% are caused by *S. aureus*. Patients usually have localized pain without systemic symptoms.
     f. In patients with sickle cell anemia, it is difficult to distinguish bone infarction associated with crisis from osteomyelitis. *Salmonella* species or *S. aureus* osteomyelitis should be suspected in patients with sickle cell disease or other hemoglobinopathies.
  2. Contiguous focus of infection

    a. Osteomyelitis due to a contiguous focus of infection is more common in older patients.

    b. *S. aureus* is the most common bacterial isolate (50% of cases). *S. epidermidis* should be considered a pathogen when it is isolated from bone, especially in the setting of a prosthetic device.

    c. Anaerobic osteomyelitis may be seen in relation to decubitus ulcers, bites, trauma to the head, and intraabdominal infections.

    d. Wounds and draining sinuses are important clues to osteomyelitis due to a contiguous focus of infection. Local inflammatory signs usually are present, although fever often is absent.

3. Vascular insufficiency. Osteomyelitis related to vascular insufficiency is associated with local pain and inflammatory findings, including cellulitis. Most infections are polymicrobial.

4. Prosthetic device infections. Fever and inflammatory signs are often absent, and symptoms of local pain appear in an indolent fashion. *S. epidermidis* is an important pathogen in this setting.

5. Puncture wounds. Osteomyelitis can be an infrequent complication of puncture wounds (usually involving the foot). Most cases are caused by *Pseudomonas aeruginosa*.

LABORATORY STUDIES

• Confirmation of the infectious process

1. Joint aspiration

    a. In diagnosing septic arthritis, joint aspiration is mandatory (Table 72–1).

    b. Radiographic examination may be helpful for demonstrating concomitant osteomyelitis, the presence of joint effusion (especially helpful in cases of hip infections), and loosening of a prosthetic device.

    c. Technetium-99m scanning can be used to define an inflammatory process in a deep-seated joint such as the sacroiliac joint.

2. Aspiration of bursal fluid is necessary to make the diagnosis of septic bursitis. The findings are variable, ranging from serous material to thick pus.

3. Radiologic findings

    a. Osteomyelitis can be suggested by X-ray findings but abnormalities apparent on X-ray examination are delayed at least 10 days after initial symptoms. Early abnormalities include periosteal elevation and soft tissue swelling. After 1 month, areas of sclerotic bone appear. The sensitivity of X-rays in the first few weeks of osteomyelitis is 30%, with a specificity of 89%.

    b. CT scanning can be helpful, especially early in vertebral osteomyelitis, when it can show bony erosion much earlier than plain films.

TABLE 72-1. Characteristics of Arthrocentesis Fluid

Condition	Appearance	Viscosity	Leukocytes (per ml)	Glucose (mg/dl)	Comments
Normal Noninflammatory diseases: osteoarthritis, traumatic arthritis	Clear, straw-colored Clear	High High	75 (15% PMNs) 1000 (15-25% PMNs)	Nearly equal to blood Nearly equal to blood	Acute trauma often causes grossly bloody fluid with RBCs on microscopy
Inflammatory diseases Rheumatoid arthritis	Translucent-opaque, light yellow	Low	2000 (60-75% PMNs)	>25 mg/dl, lower than blood	"Rice bodies" seen
Gout, pseudogout	Translucent-opaque, white	Poor	10-75,000 (60-75% PMNs)	>25 mg/dl, lower than blood	Gout: Needlelike negative birefringent crystals. Pseudogout: Rhomboid weakly positive birefringent crystals.
Infectious diseases Bacterial septic arthritis	Opaque, gray-yellow	Varies	100,000 (>75% PMNs) but lower with partial treatment, low-virulence organisms	<25 mg/dl, lower than blood	

PMN = polymorphonuclear leukocyte.
RBC = red blood cell.
Source: Reprinted with permission of author and publisher from Eisenberg M, Copass M. Emergency Medical Therapy, 3rd ed. Philadelphia. W. B. Saunders Company, 1988, p. 275.

    c. Technetium-99m bone scans may suggest osteomyelitis within 48 hr of symptom onset and, with hematogenous osteomyelitis in children, the sensitivity and specificity are 90%. Specificity may be less in adults with osteomyelitis related to contiguous infections.

    d. Indium-111–labeled white cell scans may be useful in the diagnosis of osteomyelitis when a contiguous infection or inflammatory state is present. Sensitivity for this method approaches 100% with a specificity of 80 to 90%.

- Microbiologic diagnosis
  1. Joint fluid analysis
     a. Gram's stains of synovial fluid are positive in two-thirds of cases.
     b. Aerobic and anaerobic cultures should be performed on all joint fluid aspirates, with particular attention paid to cultures for *gonococci* in the appropriate age groups.
     c. In selected patients with underlying chronic joint disease and indolent symptoms, mycobacterial cultures of the synovial fluid should be performed. However, cultures of synovial tissue have a higher yield. Acid-fast smears of synovial fluid have a 20% yield for tuberculosis.
  2. Blood cultures and cultures from other sites of infection should be performed in patients with septic arthritis.
  3. Culture of bursal fluid
     a. In patients with septic bursitis, culture of the bursal fluid is necessary for microbiologic diagnosis. Gram's stain of fluid is often negative, and culture may grow only a few colonies of *S. aureus*.
     b. Blood cultures are rarely positive in patients with septic bursitis.
  3. Bone biopsies
     a. Bone biopsies are the "gold standard" for defining the cause of osteomyelitis.
     b. Sinus tract cultures often do not predict the findings of bone biopsy culture. If *S. aureus* is isolated as a single organism from a sinus tract, it can be found in 78% of bone biopsy cultures.

RECOMMENDED DIAGNOSTIC APPROACH

- Septic arthritis/septic bursitis
  1. Joint aspiration/bursal aspiration. The fluid should be sent for immediate Gram's stain and bacterial culture. If the patient is at risk for tuberculous disease or has a subacute or chronic presentation, acid-fast smears and mycobacterial cultures should be performed on the joint fluid.
  2. Blood cultures should be done in patients with septic arthritis.

- Osteomyelitis
  1. X-ray. Periosteal elevation and soft tissue swelling are early changes of osteomyelitis with cortical irregularity and sequestrum formation occurring later. A normal X-ray does not rule out osteomyelitis.
  2. Blood cultures may reveal the organism in up to 50% of cases.
  3. Technetium-99m bone scan is not necessary if bony changes are present on X-ray.
  4. Bone biopsy should be done if blood cultures are negative.

Bibliography

Abbey DM, Hosea SW. Diagnosis of vertebral osteomyelitis in a community hospital using computed tomography. Arch Intern Med 1989;149:2029.

Graham BS, Gregory DW. *Pseudomonas aeruginosa* causing osteomyelitis after puncture wounds of the foot. South Med J 1984;77:1228.

Ho G, Jr., et al. Septic bursitis in the prepatellar and olecranon bursae: An analysis of 25 cases. Ann Intern Med 1978;89:21.

McCarthy K., et al. Indium-111-labeled white blood cells in the detection of osteomyelitis complicated by a pre-existing condition. J Nucl Med 1988;29:1015.

Pichichero ME, Friesen HA. Polymicrobial osteomyelitis: Report of three cases and a review of the literature. Rev Infect Dis 1982;4:86.

Sapico FL, Montgomerie JA. Vertebral osteomyelitis in intravenous drug abusers: Report of three cases and review of the literature. Rev Infect Dis 1980;2:196.

Silverthorn KG, Gillespie WJ. Pyogenic spinal osteomyelitis: A review of 61 cases. NZ Med J 1986;99:62.

Waldvogel FA, Vasaey H. Osteomyelitis: The past decade. N Engl J Med 1980;303:360.

Wheat J. Diagnostic strategies in osteomyelitis. Am J Med 1985;78(suppl 6B):218.

73

MENINGITIS AND ENCEPHALITIS

CHRISTINA M. MARRA

MIND, n. A mysterious form of matter secreted by the brain. Its chief activity consists in the endeavor to ascertain its own nature, the futility of the attempt being due to the fact that it has nothing but itself to know itself with.

AMBROSE BIERCE (1842–1914?)

MENINGITIS

Definition

- Meningitis is an infection of the linings of the brain and ventricles. The syndrome consists of fever and stiffness of the neck or back muscles (meningismus), usually with nausea and vomiting and sometimes with photophobia. The very young, very old, and immunocompromised may have minimal signs and symptoms.
- Seizures and mild changes in mental status may be a feature of meningitis and reflect cortical irritation. Focal neurologic abnormalities indicate a complication of meningitis or that the patient has some other disorder.

Clinical and Laboratory Features

- Bacterial meningitis
    1. Epidemiology. Twenty to twenty-five thousand cases of bacterial meningitis are diagnosed in the United States per year, and 80% occur in children <15 years old. Eighty percent are caused by *Haemophilus influenzae, Streptococcus pneumoniae,* and *Neisseria meningitidis.* Age is the most important determinant of etiology (see Table 73–1).
    2. Diagnosis (see Table 73–2)
        a. In bacterial meningitis, the CSF generally shows a neutrophilic pleocytosis with >2000 WBCs/mm^3.
        b. Gram's stain and culture of CSF are usually positive unless the patient has been treated with antibiotics.
        c. Latex agglutination tests on CSF can detect antigens of pneumococci, meningococci, *H. influenzae,* and group B streptococci.
        d. Blood cultures are positive in 30 to 80% of cases.

TABLE 73–1. Age and Etiology of Bacterial Meningitis

First month of life: Escherichia coli, group B streptococci, *Listeria monocytogenes.* One case in four of sepsis is accompanied by meningitis.

1-3 months: E. coli (and occasionally other gram-negatives), group B streptococci, *L. monocytogenes, Streptococcus pneumoniae.*

3 months-18 years: Haemophilus influenzae, Neisseria meningitidis, Streptococcus pneumoniae.

Adults <50 years: S. pneumoniae and *N. meningitis* cause 85% of cases of meningitis in otherwise healthy adults. *Staphylococcus aureus* is seen in the setting of endocarditis.

>50 years: S. pneumoniae, N. meningitidis, L. monocytogenes, gram-negative bacilli.

Cultures of the nose and throat are not useful in the diagnosis of bacterial meningitis. Needle aspiration of middle ear fluid for gram stain may help identify the organism if the CSF smear is equivocal. Urine cultures may be of value in children <1 year of age.

3. Etiology. Specific pathogens
   a. *S. pneumoniae* (pneumococcus)
      i. This is the most frequent cause of meningitis in adults.
      ii. About one-half of cases are associated with a focus of infection in the lungs, middle ear, heart, or paranasal sinuses. Predisposing factors for pneumococcal meningitis include old or recent head trauma, CSF leak, splenectomy, sickle cell disease, bone marrow transplant, and alcoholism.
      iii. In comparison to other common causes of bacterial meningitis, pneumococcal meningitis is more often associated with intracerebral vasculitis, leading to ischemia, infarction, and higher morbidity.
   b. *N. meningitidis* (meningococcus)
      i. Meningococcal meningitis is most commonly seen in patients 5 to 40 years old, but adults of any age can be affected. It is most common in winter and spring.
      ii. Complement deficiency and SLE are associated with recurrences.
   c. *H. influenzae* type b
      i. This organism is the most common cause of bacterial meningitis in the United States, and most commonly occurs in children under 6 years of age.
      ii. It frequently occurs in association with a primary source of infection in this age group, such as pneumonia, otitis media, sinusitis, and cellulitis.

TABLE 73–2. CSF Parameters in Meningitis

Laboratory Parameter	Bacterial Meningitis (Untreated)	Bacterial Meningitis[a] (Partially Treated)	Viral Meningitis	Fungal Meningitis	Tuberculous Meningitis	Carcinomatous Meningitis	Endocarditis
White cell count	↑ (> 1000)[f]	↑ (> 1000)	↑ (< 1000)[c]	↑ (< 500)	↑ (< 1000)	0–500	↑ (< 500)
Polys	↑ (> 60% PMN)	↑ (> 60% PMN)	↑ (10% of Pts.)[a]		↑[a]	0–95%	↑ (28% of patients)
Lymphs			↑	↑			↑ (25% of patients)
Red blood cells	0	0	Variable	0	0	Variable	Occasionally ↑
Glucose	↓ (< 45)[b]	↓ (< 45)	Normal[d]	Normal; slight ↓	↓ (< 45)	↓; Normal	Normal; ↓
Protein	↑ (> 80)	↑ (Variable)	Normal; slight ↑[d]	↑ (> 60)	↑ (> 100)	Usually ↑	Normal; ↑
Gram stain	+ (80%)	+ (60%)	Negative	Negative	+ AFB Stain (80%)	Negative	Unknown
Bacterial culture	+ (> 90%)	+ (65%)	Negative	Negative	+ AFB (85%)	Negative	+ (16%)

a See text for discussion: if polymorphonuclear leukocytes (PMN) > 90% on serial exams, viral etiology is not likely, especially with low (< 500) white cell count (WBC); an average of 13% of patients with TB meningitis will have PMN predominance.

b Or 50%–66% of blood glucose. As many as 40%–50% of patients with bacterial meningitis may have normal CSF glucose.

c 85% < 1000; rare > 2800.

d See text for discussion of major exceptions.

e High percentage is smear positive if 10 cc of CSF is centrifuged and examined for 30–90 min.

f If > 50,000, brain abscess with rupture should be considered.

Source: Modified from Reese RE, Douglas RG, Jr. A Practical Approach to Infectious Diseases. Boston, Little Brown & Co, 1986, p. 125.

      iii. In adults, *H. influenzae* meningitis is uncommon and is associated with otitis media and other parameningeal foci of infection, as well as CSF leaks, immunodeficiency, and alcoholism.

    d. *Listeria monocytogenes*

      i. This organism may be mistaken for skin contaminants (diphtheroids) on gram stain.

      ii. *L. monocytogenes* is a common cause of bacterial meningitis in the compromised host, especially those with T-cell dysfunction. It is also seen in neonates, the aged, alcoholics, in pregnancy, and in normal adults, especially men >45 years of age. Peak incidence is in spring and summer.

      iii. The majority of CSF WBCs can be mononuclear, but this occurs in only 25% of cases. The CSF is frequently sterile, but blood cultures are usually positive.

    e. Gram-negative bacilli. Gram-negative meningitis is seen in neonates, in adults with dural disruption (head trauma, after neurosurgical procedures), and in association with gram-negative sepsis. The most common organisms are *Escherichia coli* and *Klebsiella pneumoniae,* but other organisms such as *Pseudomonas* may be involved.

    f. *Staphylococcus aureus* is an uncommon cause of meningitis and occurs most frequently in the setting of CNS trauma or surgery, or with underlying infections such as endocarditis or parameningeal abscess.

    g. Coagulase-negative *Staphylococcus*. These organisms are common pathogens in ventricular shunt–associated meningitis.

- Aseptic meningitis

  1. Aseptic meningitis is a term used to describe meningitis in the absence of an easily detectable bacterial pathogen in CSF. With more extensive evaluation, an infectious etiology is often identified, such as viral meningitis, partially treated bacterial meningitis, and meningitis due to difficult-to-grow organisms such as mycoplasma, mycobacteria, spirochetes, parasites, and fungi (see Table 73–3).

  2. In viral meningitis, CSF WBC counts range from 10 to 1000/mm^3. Neutrophils can be seen within the first 6 to 24 hr, but lymphocytes usually predominate (see Table 73–2).

  3. Specific viral pathogens

    a. Enterovirus

      i. Enteroviruses include Coxsackie, echo, and polio viruses. Infection is spread by the fecal-oral route and is most common in late summer and fall. Enteroviral meningitis accounts for 80% of identified cases of viral meningitis.

      ii. It is most common in children <14 years of age but can affect any age and is 2 to 3 times

TABLE 73-3. Causes of Aseptic Meningitis

Infectious

Partially treated bacterial meningitis

Parameningeal infection: otitis media, sinusitis, epidural abscess, subdural empyema, brain abscess, cranial osteomyelitis

Infectious processes not contiguous with CSF: endocarditis

Mycoplasma

Mycobacteria

Spirochetes: leptospirosis, syphilis, Lyme disease.

Fungi: *Cryptococcus neoformans, Candida albicans, Coccidioides immitis*

Rickettsia: Rocky mountain spotted fever

Protozoa: *Toxoplasma gondii,* amoebae, malaria

Cestodes: cysticercosis

Viruses: enteroviruses, lymphocytic choriomeningitis, Epstein-Barr, arboviruses, HSV-2, HIV

Noninfectious

Drugs: nonsteroidal anti-inflammatory agents, isoniazid, trimethoprim/sulfamethoxazole

Collagen-vascular diseases: SLE, Sjögren's syndrome

Sarcoidosis

Primary CNS vasculitis

Carcinomatous or lymphomatous meningitis

Stroke

Migraine

Chemical: after neurosurgical procedures, intrathecal injections, subarachnoid hemorrhage

---

    more common than bacterial meningitis in infants.

 iii. The CSF may show a neutrophilic pleocytosis and hypoglycorrhachia. The diagnosis can be made by isolation of virus from CSF, throat, or stool.

 b. Lymphocytic choriomeningitis virus (LCM)

  i. LCM infection causes 1 to 10% of all cases of viral meningitis and mild encephalitis. Infection is acquired through contact with an infected rodent. Person-to-person transmission is not significant. Infection is most common in winter.

  ii. The illness is often biphasic with a flulike prodrome followed by meningitis. The CSF can show a high lymphocyte count and low glucose. The diagnosis is made by isolation of virus from blood, urine, or CSF, or by serology.

 c. Herpes simplex virus type 2 (HSV-2)

  i. HSV-2 is responsible for 0.5 to 5% of all culture-proven cases of viral meningitis. Meningitis usually occurs during primary genital infection.

ii. The diagnosis is made by culture of the CSF or genital lesions.

- Diagnosis of bacterial vs. viral meningitis Table 73–2 and 73–4) Normal CSF cell counts can be seen in bacterial meningitis, and neutrophilic pleocytosis can be seen in viral as well as bacterial meningitis. Of the viral meningitides, LCM, HSV-2, and enteroviral infections are more likely to be associated with low CSF glucose and polymorphonuclear pleocytosis.

Recommended Diagnostic Approach to a Patient with Suspected Meningitis

- Physical examination. In the setting of an acute onset of symptoms, this should be brief and directed.
- Draw blood cultures.
- If examination reveals focal neurologic signs or papilledema, a head CT scan with and without contrast should be performed prior to lumbar puncture to rule out a space-occupying lesion. Empiric antibiotics should be given prior to CT.
- Perform lumbar puncture (LP). If the patient is neurologically normal, evaluate the CSF cell count with differential and Gram's stain, and initiate appropriate therapy based upon results. If the patient is not neurologically normal, treat empirically for bacterial meningitis prior to examination of CSF. The CSF must be examined within 60 to 90 min of collection because the WBC rapidly disintegrate at room temperature.

TABLE 73–4. Historical and Physical Exam Data Suggesting Specific Etiologies of Meningitis

Physical exam
  Petechiae, rashes: meningococci, enteroviruses, *S. aureus,* leptospirosis
  Vesicular skin lesions: herpesviruses
  Parotitis: Coxsackie, LCM, and Epstein-Barr viruses
Underlying conditions
  Diabetes: pneumococci, gram-negative bacilli, staphylococci, *Cryptococcus,* mucormycosis
  Steroid therapy: *Cryptococcus, Mycobacterium tuberculosis*
  Neutropenia: gram-negative bacilli, *S. aureus,* fungi
  T-cell and monocyte dysfunction: *L. monocytogenes,* pneumococcus
  Disruption of dura: pneumococcus, *S. aureus,* coagulase-negative staphylococci, diphtheroids, gram-negative bacilli
Epidemiology
  Sibling with meningitis: Meningococci, *H. influenzae*
  Swimming in fresh water: amoebae
  Summer and fall: enteroviruses, leptospirosis

- If no organisms are seen on Gram's stain, and the patient appears relatively well, some advocate withholding therapy and repeating the LP in 8 hr. This approach is not appropriate if the patient was pretreated with antibiotics, is younger than 1 year of age, is clinically unstable, or deteriorates during the observation period.

ENCEPHALITIS

Definition

Encephalitis refers to infection of brain tissue. Clinically, patients present acutely or subacutely with headache, fever, and signs of parenchymal involvement such as coma, seizures, change in mental status, and focal neurologic findings. They may not have meningismus.

Clinical and Laboratory Features

- Encephalitis is often considered as an etiology in the evaluation of a patient with fever and changes in mental status, but other causes should also be considered (Table 73–5).
- Viral etiologies of encephalitis
    1. Arboviruses (Table 73–6)
        a. There are 450 "strains" of arboviruses. Japanese encephalitis virus is the most important internationally. Nearly all cases in the United States are due to St. Louis, LaCrosse, Eastern equine, and

TABLE 73–5. Differential Diagnosis of Encephalitis

Infectious
Arboviruses: Japanese encephalitis, St. Louis, La Crosse, Eastern Equine, Western Equine viruses
Herpesviruses: HSV-1 and HSV-2, Varicella zoster
Mycobacteria
Mycoplasma
Rickettsia
Spirochetes
Fungi
Protozoa: *Toxoplasma gondii*
Endocarditis: cerebral emboli, ischemic or hemorrhagic stroke
Atypical presentation of bacterial meningitis: *L. monocytogenes*
Parameningeal infection
Bacterial brain abscess
Noninfectious
Metabolic and toxic encephalopathies
Tumors
Stroke
Collagen-vascular disease
CNS vasculitis

TABLE 73–6. Characteristics of Selected Mosquitoborne American Arbovirus Encephalitides Found in the United States[a]

CHARACTERISTIC	WESTERN EQUINE	EASTERN EQUINE	VENEZUELAN	ST. LOUIS	LACROSSE
Geographical distribution	West, Midwest	East, Gulf Coast, South	South	Central, West, South	Central, East
Age group affected	Infants and adults >50 yr old	Children	Adults	Adults > 50 yr old	Children
Mortality (%)	5–15	50–75	1	2–20	<1
Sequelae	Moderate in infants; low in others	80% of survivors	Rare	20% of survivors	Low
Symptoms	Headache, altered consciousness, seizures	Headache, altered consciousness, seizures[a]	Headache, myalgia, pharyngitis	Headache, nausea, vomiting, disorientation, stupor, irritability	Seizures, paralysis, focal weakness

[a] Symptoms are fulminant.

Source: Whitley RJ. Viral encephalitis. New Engl J Med 1990; 323:242–250.

Western equine encephalitis viruses. Disease is transmitted to man by mosquitoes.

b. Most people infected with arboviruses have mild or inapparent infection, but in a few persons, the virus enters the brain. The CSF may be normal, but more commonly shows 5 to several hundred white cells/mm^3 with mostly lymphocytes, although neutrophils may transiently predominate. Protein is normal to mildly elevated, and glucose is usually normal.

c. The diagnosis of arboviral encephalitis is made retrospectively by serology.

d. St. Louis encephalitis is a common cause of epidemic encephalitis in the United States. Asymptomatic or mild infection is common during epidemics, especially in children. The usual clinical presentation includes fever, headache, nausea, and vomiting. Dysuria, pyuria, and the syndrome of inappropriate antidiuretic hormone secretion are sometimes seen.

e. The LaCrosse subtype is the most prevalent and most virulent of the California encephalitis group. Infection is endemic in the eastern United States, with most cases occurring in the upper Mississippi valley. In adults, the virus can also cause inapparent infection, a benign febrile illness, or aseptic meningitis.

f. Eastern equine encephalitis is rare. Small outbreaks occur sporadically along the Atlantic and Gulf coasts. In the absence of equine vaccination programs, epizootics in horses precede disease in humans by a few weeks. The ratio of subclinical to clinical infection is low. The onset of illness is often abrupt and the course is fulminant. Patients frequently have focal abnormalities and may have purulent CSF.

g. Western equine encephalitis causes sporadic infections in the rural western United States. Mild and inapparent infection is common.

2. Herpes simplex virus type 1 (HSV-1)

a. HSV-1 encephalitis is the most common encephalitis in the United States and accounts for the most deaths. Several hundred to several thousand cases are reported each year, compared to 108 cases of arbovirus infection reported in the United States in 1989.

b. The history is nonspecific, and includes fever, headache, and change in the level of consciousness. A prior history of HSV skin lesions does not increase the likelihood of encephalitis.

c. HSV-1 infection frequently involves the frontal and temporal lobes, and focal neurologic findings and focal seizures are present in 85% of patients.

d. The CSF usually shows a lymphocytic pleocytosis with 50 to 1000 WBCs/μl. Neutrophils can be seen early in the illness. Hypoglycorrhachia is seen in 5 to 25% of samples, and protein is usually elevated.

e. Viral culture of CSF is positive in only 4% of those with biopsy-proven infection, and 3% of cases have normal CSF findings.

f. The electroencephalogram (EEG) is the most sensitive test for detecting structural abnormalities and is abnormal in 80% of proven cases.

g. CT is usually normal early in the course of the disease, but CT or brain scan or both are abnormal in about 50% of cases.

h. Diagnosis can only be proven by biopsy, but patients are commonly treated empirically.

Recommended Diagnostic Approach to the Patient with Suspected Viral Encephalitis

- Like viral meningitis, it is not possible to diagnose the etiology of viral encephalitis clinically.
- A detailed history and physical examination, including history of travel, exposure to animals or insects, and skin examination
- CT or MR scan of head with and without contrast
- CSF examination
- EEG. Ancillary procedures such as sinus X-rays, serologic tests, and brain biopsy are indicated in individual cases

Bibliography

Arboviral infections of the central nervous system—United States, 1989. MMWR 1990;39:407: 413–417.

Behrman RE, et al. Central nervous system infections in the elderly. Arch Intern Med 1989;149:1596–1599.

Kim JH, et al. *Staphylococcus aureus* meningitis: Review of 28 cases. Rev Infect Dis 1989;11:698–706.

Pruitt AA, et al. Neurologic complications of bacterial endocarditis. Medicine 1978;57:329–343.

Ratzan KR. Viral meningitis. Med Clin North Am 1985;69:399–413.

Reik L, Jr. Disorders that mimic CNS infections. Neurol Clin 1986;4:223–248

Tunkel AR, et al. Bacterial meningitis: Recent advances in pathophysiology and treatment. Ann Intern Med 1990;112:610–623.

Whitley RJ. Viral encephalitis. N Engl J Med, 1990;323:242–250.

Whitley RJ, et al. Diseases that mimic herpes simplex encephalitis. Diagnosis, presentation, and outcome. NIAID Collaborative Antiviral Study Group. JAMA 1989;262:234–239.

74

ACQUIRED IMMUNODEFICIENCY SYNDROME

DOUGLAS S. PAAUW

As it takes two to make a quarrel, so it takes two to make a disease, the microbe and its host.

CHARLES V. CHAPIN (1856–1941)
The Principles of Epidemiology

DEFINITION

- The Centers for Disease Control have defined a case of acquired immunodeficiency syndrome (AIDS) as an illness characterized by one or more "indicator diseases," depending on the status of laboratory evidence of HIV infection (see Table 74–1). A history of an underlying immunosuppressive disorder in the absence of laboratory evidence of HIV infection precludes the diagnosis of AIDS.
- CDC staging system for HIV-associated illness:
  1. Class I. Acute infection: mononucleosislike syndrome with or without aseptic meningitis, associated with seroconversion to HIV antibody positivity.
  2. Class II. Asymptomatic infection: absence of signs or symptoms of infection.
  3. Class III. Persistent generalized lymphadenopathy: lymph node enlargement greater than 1 cm at 2 or more extrainguinal sites persisting for more than 3 months.
  4. Class IV. Other diseases
     a. Constitutional disease
        i. Fevers > 1 month
        ii. Involuntary weight loss > 10%
        iii. Diarrhea persisting > 1 month
     b. Neurologic disease
        i. Dementia
        ii. Peripheral neuropathy
        iii. Myelopathy
     c. Secondary infectious diseases (Table 74–1)
     d. Secondary cancers
        i. Kaposi's sarcoma
        ii. Non-Hodgkin's lymphoma
        iii. Primary lymphoma of the brain
     e. Other conditions. Presence of clinical findings not classified by other classes or subgroups, including HIV-related thrombocytopenia and lymphoid interstitial pneumonitis.

TABLE 74–1. Indicator Diseases for AIDS

Laboratory evidence of HIV infection not required
  Esophageal or pulmonary candidiasis
  Extrapulmonary cryptococcosis
  Chronic symptomatic cryptosporidiosis
  Kaposi's sarcoma or primary central nervous system
    (CNS) lymphoma in patients < 60 years old
  Disseminated cytomegalovirus infection
  Pulmonary, esophageal, or chronic mucocutaneous
    herpes simplex infection
  Lymphocytic interstitial pneumonitis in patients < 13
    years old
  Disseminated *Mycobacterial avium-intracellulare* or *M.*
    kansasii infection
  Pneumocystis carinii pneumonia (PCP)
  Progressive multifocal leukoencephalopathy
  Toxoplasmosis of the central nervous system
Laboratory evidence of HIV infection required
  Recurrent serious bacterial infections in patients <13
    years old
  Disseminated histoplasmosis or coccidioidomycosis
  HIV encephalopathy
  HIV wasting syndrome ("slim disease")
  Recurrent *Salmonella* bacteremia
  Disseminated mycobacterial infections including *M.*
    tuberculosis
  Kaposi's sarcoma or CNS lymphoma in patients >60
    years
  Small, noncleaved B-cell lymphoma or immunoblastic
    sarcoma

EPIDEMIOLOGY

- High-risk groups for AIDS and HIV infection include (with percentage of diagnosed AIDS cases):
  1. Homosexual/bisexual men (62% of cases)
  2. IV drug user (20% of cases)
  3. Homosexual and IV drug user (7% of cases)
  4. Hemophiliacs (1% of cases)
  5. Transfusion recipients (3% of cases—far greater risk for blood products received between 1978 and March, 1985)
  6. Sexual partners and children of high-risk mothers (4% of cases)
  7. Three percent of AIDS cases do not fit into these categories.

- Progression of HIV infection
  1. Within 8 yr of HIV infection, 30 to 50% of patients develop AIDS.
  2. With the exception of neonates, a younger age at the time of seroconversion is associated with a longer incubation period for AIDS.

LABORATORY PROCEDURES

- ELISA
  1. Screening serologic testing for the HIV virus is done with an enzyme-linked immunosorbent assay (ELISA).
  2. In high-risk groups, it has 98 to 99% specificity. In low-risk groups, the specificity is much lower.
  3. A strongly positive ELISA test in a low-risk population is more likely to be a true positive (87%) than a weakly reactive test (2%).
- Western blot
  1. The Western blot test is more specific for HIV infection than the ELISA. It is used as a confirmatory test for all positive ELISA tests.
  2. It is interpreted by looking for binding of anti-HIV immunoglobulins to specific antigenic bands from disrupted purified whole virus. A Western blot is positive if specific bands are present. The Western blot is negative if no bands are present, and reported as indeterminate if some but not all the diagnostic bands are present.
- T-cell subsets. In HIV disease there is a marked decline in CD_4 lymphocytes (T_4 or T-helper cells) with no change or a slight increase in CD_8 lymphocytes (T_8 or T-suppressor cells). A CD_4 count of $<200/mm^3$ is associated with increased risk of progression to AIDS over the next several years.
- p 24 antigen. p 24 antigen is a component of the HIV. It is a marker of viral replication and when present, a predictor for the development of AIDS.
- Beta-2-microglobulin. This is a protein that is part of the Class I major histocompatibility antigens. Serum levels of this protein reflect lymphocyte turnover. Increased serum levels of beta-2-microglobulin correlate with an increased risk of progression to AIDS.

INITIAL EVALUATION OF THE HIV-POSITIVE PATIENT

Symptoms/History

- A thorough review of systems is important to uncover minor symptoms which may indicate significant disease.
- Visual complaints should be aggressively pursued as cytomegalovirus (CMV) retinitis is vision-threatening. Early intervention can save vision.
- Systemic symptoms include anorexia, fevers, and weight loss.
- Pulmonary symptoms include chronic cough and dyspnea which may indicate PCP or tuberculosis.
- Neurologic symptoms include memory loss and headache. Both are frequent with HIV infection.

- Dysphagia may be due to *Candida* or CMV esophagitis. *Candida* infection, either thrush or esophagitis, occurs in 95% of AIDS patients.

Signs/Examination

- Oral cavity
  1. Oral thrush is a common finding and may be asymptomatic.
  2. Hairy leukoplakia appears as a white thickening with vertical folds, usually found on the lateral aspect of the tongue. It is specific for HIV infection.
  3. HIV-associated gingivitis brings progressive gingival loss and destruction of supporting bone.
- Skin
  1. Seborrheic dermatitis is extremely common. Molluscum contagiosum is seen and can rapidly increase in numbers.
  2. Kaposi's sarcoma (KS) is asymptomatic initially, presenting as a red to purple macule. Older KS lesions may become nodular.
  3. Warts are very common and may be large.
- Eyes. Funduscopic exam is important to evaluate for early CMV retinitis. The typical appearance is one of perivascular exudates and hemorrhage. Early in CMV retinitis these lesions are primarily at the periphery.
- Lymphadenopathy can occur due to acute HIV infection or part of persistent generalized lymphadenopathy (PGL).

Recommended Diagnostic Approach

- Thorough history and physical exam. Oral candidiasis and hairy leukoplakia are associated with progression of HIV disease.
- T-cell subsets should be checked initially.
  1. If the CD_4 count (T_4) is above 600/mm^3, it should be repeated every 6 months.
  2. As the count approaches 500 or as it approaches 200, testing should be every 3 months as pneumocystis prophylaxis and zidovudine (AZT) treatment are based on these cell counts.
- CBC with platelet count.
- Tuberculin skin testing with controls. There is a 4% incidence of TB in HIV-infected patients. Earlier in the course of HIV infection, patients are more likely to react to tuberculin skin tests. Only 10% of HIV-infected patients with CD_4 counts greater than 500 have cutaneous anergy.
- VDRL (serologic test for syphilis). There is a high incidence of syphilis infection among HIV-seropositive populations.

EVALUATION OF DIARRHEA IN THE HIV-POSITIVE PATIENT

Differential Diagnosis

INFECTIOUS

- Bacterial
  1. *Salmonella* causes both diarrhea and recurrent bacteremia in HIV-infected patients.
  2. *Shigella* is a common organism found in homosexual males.
  3. *Campylobacter*—A patient with HIV infection can have severe and prolonged proctocolitis.
  4. *Neisseria gonorrhoeae*
  5. *Treponema pallidum*
  6. *Clostridium difficile* is associated with frequent broad-spectrum antibiotic use.
  7. Mycobacteria—*Mycobacterium avium-intracellulare* complex is a cause of diarrhea late in the course of AIDS.

- Protozoa
  1. *Giardia lamblia* is the most common cause of enteritis in the homosexual male.
  2. *Entamoeba histolytica* is a common cause of acute diarrhea in AIDS patients.
  3. *Cryptosporidia* is a small noninvasive coccidial parasite which commonly causes diarrhea in animals. It was not widely seen as a human pathogen until the AIDS epidemic.
  4. *Isospora belli*—This coccidial parasite appears to be most prevalent in tropical and subtropical climates. It is a common cause of diarrhea in AIDS patients in Africa and Haiti but is uncommon in the United States.

- Viruses
  1. CMV—The majority of patients with HIV infection have evidence of past CMV infection. CMV may cause ulcerations of the esophagus or bowel.
  2. Herpes simplex

NONINFECTIOUS

- KS. GI tract involvement with KS occurs in up to 50% of patients with skin lesions.
- AIDS-associated enteropathy. This entity has been described in a group of patients with persistent diarrhea and no identifiable intestinal pathogens. Biopsies of intestinal mucosa show villous atrophy.
- Lymphoma. Lymphomatous (non-Hodgkin's) involvement of the GI tract is a rare cause of diarrhea.

Clinical Features

SYMPTOMS/HISTORY

1. The presence of predominantly rectal symptoms suggests proctocolitis due to *Neisseria,* herpes simplex, syphilis, *Chlamydia,* or *Campylobacter.*
2. Watery diarrhea without blood is suggestive of *Giardia,* cryptosporidia, or HIV enteropathy.
3. Bloody diarrhea, usually associated with cramping, suggests *Shigella* or *Campylobacter.* Frank hemorrhage can be seen with CMV colitis.

PHYSICAL EXAM

The presence of cutaneous KS can suggest GI involvement. Examination of the anus and rectum should be done including anoscopy to examine for evidence of proctitis.

Recommended Diagnostic Approach

- Examination of the stool for polymorphonuclear leukocytes. Leukocytes on stool Gram's stain or methylene blue exam suggests *Campylobacter, Shigella, Salmonella,* and *Entamoeba histolytica.*
- Stool culture for enteric pathogens including *Campylobacter* and, perhaps, *C. difficile* should be done. If proctitis or proctocolitis is present, rectal swabs for *Neisseria gonorrhoeae, Chlamydia,* and herpes simplex should be sent for culture.
- Stool for ova and parasites. Potential pathogens include *Giardia lamblia, Cryptosporidia, Entamoeba histolytica,* and *Isospora belli.* These organisms should be specified, as special techniques may be involved (e.g., sugar flotation technique or acid-fast stain for *Cryptosporidia*).
- Blood cultures should be performed in patients with fever or protracted diarrhea. *Salmonella* and *Mycobacterium avium-intracellulare* (MAI) are frequent causes of bacteremia.
- Sigmoidoscopy/Colonoscopy may be necessary in patients with hemorrhage or persistent symptoms. This allows for biopsy of focal ulcers (e.g., due to CMV, *E. histolytica*).
- Upper endoscopy with small bowel biopsy should be considered in refractory cases of watery diarrhea with no identified cause. Possible diagnoses include KS, lymphoma, MAI or *Giardia* infection, and AIDS-associated enteropathy.

EVALUATION OF FEVER IN THE HIV-POSITIVE PATIENT

History/Symptoms

- Head and neck. The prevalence of sinus disease in AIDS patients is high.

- Oral cavity. Dental pain may result from gingivitis, which can lead to dental abscess.
- Pulmonary. Dyspnea, cough, and fever suggest pneumonia. Fever without pulmonary complaints may be the presenting symptom of PCP or pneumococcal and *H. influenzae* pneumonias.
- Abdominal complaints. Diarrhea may suggest *Salmonella,* which is frequently associated with bacteremia.
- Neurologic. Symptoms such as headache, neck stiffness, and seizures should be pursued. Cryptococcal infection is common and may present with fever and no CNS symptoms.
- Vascular access devices. Bacteremia is common when indwelling catheters are in place in AIDS patients. *S. aureus* and *S. epidermidis* are the most common organisms.

Recommended Diagnostic Approach

Review of the most recent CD_4 lymphocyte count is important in assessing the likelihood of fever representing opportunistic infection. If the CD_4 count is $>500/mm^3$, certain diagnoses including PCP and MAI infection are very unlikely.

In addition to the clinical evaluation, the following laboratory studies should be considered:

- Chest X-ray
- Blood cultures. If fever is acute, blood cultures for bacteria and cryptococcus should be obtained; if fevers are recurrent, obtain blood cultures for mycobacteria as well
- CBC
- Sinus X-rays or CT scan
- Hepatic enzymes
- TB skin test with controls
- Serum cryptococcal antigen

EVALUATION OF THE HIV POSITIVE PATIENT WITH HEADACHE OR SEIZURES

Differential Diagnosis

- Cryptococcal meningitis is the most common cause of meningitis in AIDS patients and usually presents with headache and fever. Nausea is common.
- Toxoplasmosis can present as headache, but presents more commonly as encephalopathy or with seizures. It is the most common cause of CNS mass lesion in AIDS patients.
- Aseptic meningitis. HIV meningitis can occur at the time of infection and can subsequently recur.
- Metabolic disturbances. Hypoglycemia (most frequently as a complication of IV or IM pentamidine) and hyponatremia can cause seizures.
- CNS lymphoma commonly presents with seizures or headache.

- Drugs. AZT is associated with headaches, particularly at higher (e.g., 1200 mg daily) doses.
- HIV encephalitis. Most patients present with seizures, memory loss, decreased attention span, and problems with activities of daily living.

Clinical Features

SYMPTOMS/HISTORY

- Motor dysfunction/weakness. Focal seizures or localized weakness suggest a CNS mass lesion (e.g., toxoplasmosis, CNS lymphoma, tuberculoma).
- Travel history. The risk of toxoplasmosis is much higher in patients who have resided in Africa or Haiti than for patients who have never left the United States.
- Medications

SIGNS/EXAMINATION

- Fever is common with crypotococcus and toxoplasmosis.
- Skin. Cryptococcal infection is systemic, and may involve the skin.
- Neurologic. A focal neurologic exam suggests a CNS mass lesion (toxoplasmosis, CNS lymphoma, tuberculoma).
- Mental status exam. Confusion, memory loss, and mental dulling suggest HIV encephalopathy (AIDS dementia complex), which can be associated with seizures.

LABORATORY STUDIES

- CSF analysis
  1. Cell counts are frequently noninflammatory in AIDS patients with cryptococcal meningitis. In a recent series only 20% had >20 leukocytes/mm^3 in the CSF.
  2. Cryptococcal antigen is positive in 90% of patients with cryptococcal meningitis and AIDS.
  3. Protein is often elevated, but is nonspecific.
- Non-CSF cultures. Sixty-eight percent of patients with cryptococcal meningitis also have a positive culture from an extrameningeal source. Common sites include lung, kidney, and blood.
- Toxoplasma titers. The absence of antibody to toxoplasma makes CNS toxoplasma infection extremely unlikely. A 4-fold rise in IgM or IgG titers allows for a presumptive diagnosis. Most patients with toxoplasmosis do not have high titers.
- Radiographic examination
  1. CT scan. The most common finding is cortical atrophy associated with HIV encephalopathy. The presence of multiple ring-enhancing lesions with surrounding edema suggests toxoplasmosis. Most toxoplasmosis lesions are located in the basal ganglia and gray matter.
  2. MRI is more sensitive than CT scans but probably less

specific. Abnormalities can be found in most HIV-infected patients.

Recommended Diagnostic Approach

- Head CT scan should be done on all patients with CNS complaints to exclude CNS mass lesions before doing a lumbar puncture.
- Lumbar puncture with CSF studies
  1. Cell count
  2. Protein
  3. Glucose
  4. India ink prep
  5. Cryptococcal antigen
  6. Culture for cryptococcus, mycobacteria, bacteria
- Toxoplasma titer (if CNS mass lesion present on CT scan).
- Serum electrolyte and glucose levels.

EVALUATION OF THE HIV-POSITIVE PATIENT WITH RESPIRATORY SYMPTOMS

Differential Diagnosis

- Infectious
  1. *Pneumocystis carinii*
  2. Pyogenic bacteria, particularly *S. pneumoniae* and *H. influenzae*
  3. Mycobacteria, both *M. tuberculosis* and MAI
  4. *Cryptococcus neoformans*
  5. *Histoplasma capsulatum*
  6. CMV
- Noninfectious
  1. Lymphocytic interstitial pneumonitis
  2. Kaposi's sarcoma

Symptoms/History

- Cough. A productive cough suggests pyogenic bacterial infection. Cough due to PCP is a dry persistent cough. Tuberculosis in AIDS patients can be associated with a productive or nonproductive cough or no cough at all.
- Pleuritic chest pain. This may be seen with bacterial pneumonia, spontaneous pneumothorax (which is associated with PCP), or pleural involvement with KS.
- Dyspnea. The insidious onset and progression of dyspnea is highly suggestive of PCP. Lymphocytic interstitial pneumonia is less common than PCP, but presents in a similar fashion.
- Travel history. Several pulmonary pathogens are common in HIV-infected patients who have resided or traveled to endemic areas.
  1. Haitians or Africans: tuberculosis
  2. Midwest (Ohio River Valley): histoplasmosis
  3. Southwestern United States: coccidioidomycosis

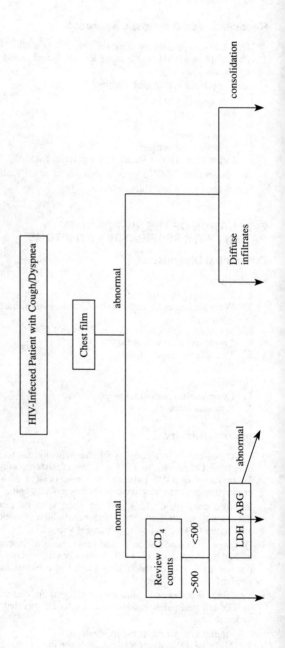

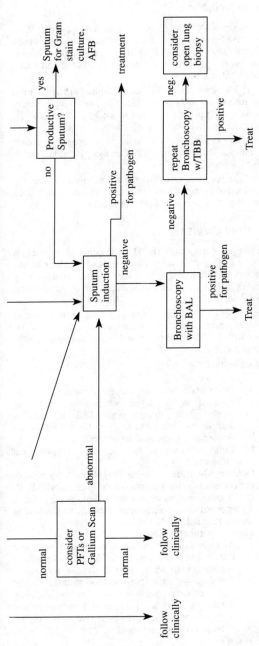

Figure 74–1. Diagnosis for HIV-infected patient.

649

Signs/Examination

In most cases of PCP the physical exam is nonspecific. Most patients have fever, tachycardia, and an unremarkable pulmonary exam. Other signs on physical exam that indicate immunosuppression suggest an increased likelihood of opportunistic pulmonary infection.

- Fever. The acute onset of fever, particularly in association with rigors, suggests acute bacterial pneumonia. Fevers that have been present for days to weeks are more consistent with opportunistic lung infections.
- Pulmonary exam. Signs of consolidation suggest bacterial pneumonia. Patients with PCP often lack abnormal auscultative findings.
- Skin. The presence of multifocal KS lesions increases the likelihood of pulmonary involvement. Nodular skin lesions may suggest disseminated cryptococcus.

Laboratory Studies

- Lactate dehydrogenase (LDH). Elevation of the serum LDH in PCP is attributed to uncontrolled B-cell proliferation and destruction of lung tissue. It is elevated in many patients with PCP and may be used as a predictor of severity of disease.
- Arterial blood gases. Blood gases are frequently abnormal in AIDS patients with pulmonary complaints. Most patients with PCP have hypoxia and an increased A-a gradient even with a normal chest X-ray.
- Radiographic tests
  1. Chest X-ray
     a. PCP usually presents with diffuse interstitial infiltrates. It is associated with pneumothorax and, rarely, cavitary disease, isolated hilar adenopathy and pleural effusions. Early in the course of the disease the X-ray may be normal.
     b. Lobar infiltrates suggest bacterial or cryptococcal pneumonia.
  2. Gallium 67-citrate scanning. A gallium scan reveals abnormalities in the vast majority of patients with PCP. It is most useful in evaluating symptomatic patients with normal chest radiographs. A normal gallium scan makes PCP extremely unlikely.
  3. Pulmonary function tests
     a. Abnormalities in pulmonary function tests are common in patients with PCP. They can be used as screening tests when chest X-rays are normal.
     b. The diffusing capacity for carbon monoxide is the most sensitive parameter. A decreased diffusing capacity is most likely due to PCP but can be due to CMV pneumonia, pulmonary KS, and lymphocytic interstitial pneumonitis.
  4. Microbiology
     a. Induced sputum
        i. Induced sputum or expectorated sputum samples frequently are positive for bacterial

pathogens when a bacterial pneumonia is present.
    ii. In experienced hands, induced sputum can be positive for pneumocystis in 50 to 75% of patients with PCP.
  b. Bronchoalveolar lavage (BAL) fluid
    i. Staining BAL fluid for *Pneumocystis carinii* is very sensitive. If both BAL and transbronchial biopsy are done, the sensitivity for PCP is 95%.
    ii. Acid-fast staining of BAL fluid gives a good yield for mycobacteria as well.
  c. Open lung biopsy is rarely needed; it should be reserved for the difficult case where PCP is not strongly suspected.

Recommended Diagnostic Approach (Figure 74–1)

- The chest X-ray is the cornerstone of diagnosis in evaluation of the HIV-infected patient with cough and dyspnea.
- If the onset is acute and a lobar infiltrate is present, bacterial pneumonia is the most likely diagnosis.
- In patients with a normal X-ray, the likelihood of PCP is low with a CD_4 count over 500/mm³, but with a CD_4 count under 200/mm³, PCP is common.
- In addition to the clinical evaluation, arterial blood gases and serum LDH should be determined.
1. Sputum examination
  a. If productive cough: Gram's and acid-fast stains and cultures. If X-ray pattern consistent with PCP, then pneumocystis stain.
  b. If nonproductive cough: induced sputum for pneumocystis and acid-fast stains.
  c. If induced sputum is negative, refer for bronchoscopy.
  d. If BAL, bronchial brushings, and transbronchial biopsy are negative and clinical suspicion for PCP is low, then consider an open lung biopsy. If clinical suspicion for PCP is high, then repeat bronchoscopy or treat empirically with antipneumocystis drugs.

Bibliography

Centers for Disease Control. Update: Acquired immunodeficiency syndrome—United States, 1981–1988. MMWR 1989;38:229–250.

Centers for Disease Control. Update: Acquired immunodeficiency syndrome—United States, 1989. MMWR 1990;39:81–86.

Chuck SL, Sande MA. Infections with *Cryptococcus neoformans* in the acquired immunodeficiency syndrome. N Engl J Med 1989;321:794–799.

Clement MT, et al. Diagnosis of pulmonary diseases. Clin Chest Med 1988;9(3):497–505.

Dalakas M, et al. AIDS and the nervous system. JAMA 1989;261:2396–2399.

Garay SM, Greene J. Prognostic indicators in the initial presentation of *Pneumocystis carinii* pneumonia. Chest 1989;95:769–772.

Glatt AE, Chirgwin K. *Pneumocystis carinii* pneumonia in human immunodeficiency virus-infected patients. Arch Intern Med 1990;150:271–279.

Holtzman DM, et al. New-onset seizures associated with human immunodeficiency virus infection: Causation and clinical features in 100 cases. Am J Med 1989;87:173–177.

Lopez AP, Gorbach SL. Diarrhea in AIDS. Inf Dis Clin North Am 1988;2(3):705–718.

Smith PD, Janoff EN. Infectious diarrhea in human immunodeficiency virus infection. Gastro Clin North Am 1988;17(3):587–598.

Steckelberg JM, Cockerill FR. Serologic testing for human immunodeficiency virus antibodies. Mayo Clin Proc 1988;63:373–380.

Ward JW, et al. Laboratory and epidemiologic evaluation of an enzyme immunoassay for antibodies to HTLV-III. JAMA 1986;256:357–361.

MALARIA AND THE FEBRILE PATIENT FROM THE TROPICS

ELAINE C. JONG, *and*
RUSSELL McMULLEN

He is so shak'd of a burning quotidian tertian that it is most lamentable to behold.

SHAKESPEARE (1564–1616) Henry V,II, i, 123

DEFINITION

Malaria is a severe febrile illness caused by infection with bloodborne protozoan parasites that are transmitted from person to person in endemic areas by biting female anopheline mosquitoes.

EPIDEMIOLOGY

- Malaria is widespread in tropical and developing areas of the world such as Mexico, Haiti, Central America, South America, Africa, the Middle East, the Indian subcontinent, Southeast Asia, and Oceania. Almost all cases in North America are diagnosed in recent immigrants or returning travelers.
- Malaria transmission by mosquitoes has been recorded in North America and Western Europe around international airports, military bases, and in areas where large numbers of people from malaria-endemic areas (who may have undiagnosed infections) live.
- Other modes of malaria transmission include:
  1. At birth from infected mother to infant through cord blood.
  2. By accidental transfusion of infected blood.
  3. From sharing of contaminated needles and syringes by IV drug users.
- Many species of malaria infect warm-blooded animals, but only 4 species commonly cause disease in humans:
  1. *Plasmodium vivax* (worldwide distribution).
  2. *Plasmodium falciparum* (worldwide distribution).
  3. *Plasmodium ovale* (Western Africa).
  4. *Plasmodium malariae* (worldwide distribution).
- Of malaria infections diagnosed in North America, in 1988,

(1023 cases), *P. falciparum* accounted for 45.5% and *P. vivax* for 42.7%.

- In all types of malaria, the incubation period before the first clinical manifestation of disease is usually 1 or more weeks. *P. vivax* and *P. ovale* may lie dormant in the hepatocytes of the liver for months to years before the patient becomes ill. *P. malariae* may also remain dormant for years.

THE LIFE CYCLE OF PLASMODIA

- The life cycle of the malaria parasite involves a stage of sexual reproduction in the female mosquito vector and an asexual reproductive cycle in the human host (Figure 75–1).

- Sexual development in the gut of the female mosquito results in the production of sporozoites, which then migrate to the salivary gland of the mosquito; from there they are injected into the capillaries of a human host during a blood meal (i.e., a bite).

- Once in the human host the sporozoites lodge within hepatocytes and undergo an exoerythrocytic stage. The parasites develop into hepatic schizonts, which can then differentiate into thousands of merozoites.

- After a variable incubation period in the liver, merozoites are released into the peripheral circulation and invade erythrocytes (RBCs). Generally, 1 merozoite invades 1 RBC, except in falciparum malaria, where more than 1 merozoite per RBC is common.

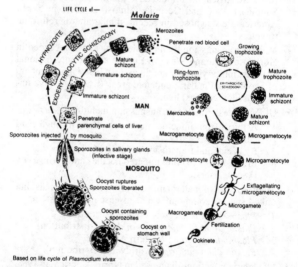

Figure 75–1. The life cycle of plasmodia based on *P. vivax*. (From Strickland GT, ed. Hunter's Tropical Medicine, 7th ed. Philadelphia, W.B. Saunders, 1991, p. 588.)

- *P. vivax* and *P. ovale* may also persist in the liver for months to years as dormant hypnozoites. Hypnozoites can eventually reactivate and differentiate into merozoites, causing late primary infections.
- After binding to and invading the RBC, the merozoite develops into a ring form, then a trophozoite, and eventually into the reproductive form, the RBC schizont, which then divides to form merozoites.
- When the RBC ruptures, merozoites are released which can invade other RBCs. This is the point where the classic malaria paroxsym ensues.
- In some RBCs the merozoites develop into gametocytes, which, while not infective to other RBCs, can perpetuate the sexual reproductive cycle in the female mosquito once they are ingested during a blood meal.
- *P. vivax* and *P. ovale* preferentially infect reticulocytes, and *P. malariae* infects mature RBCs. *P. falciparum,* however, can infect all RBCs. This, plus the higher number of merozoites that can develop in RBCs infected with *P. falciparum,* account for the rapid development of high levels of parasitemia (and higher morbidity) often seen in falciparum malaria.

CLINICAL FEATURES OF THE FEBRILE PATIENT FROM THE TROPICS

- History
  1. If the patient's risk factor for malaria is travel, the following historical information should be elicited:
     a. Geographic area(s) visited. Are the areas visited endemic for malaria, especially chloroquine- or multiple drug-resistant falciparum malaria?
     b. Pretravel immunizations received; in particular, typhoid fever, immune globulin for hepatitis A, hepatitis B, measles, yellow fever, and meningococcal meningitis.
     c. Malaria chemoprophylaxis used: medications, doses, intervals, and for how long after leaving the malarious area (important especially in considering the possibility of chloroquine-resistant *P. falciparum*). No current chemoprophylactic regimen is 100% effective.
     d. Illnesses sustained during travel, medical care received, and medications used.
     e. Exposure to insects and recollection of bites sustained (mosquitoes, flies, fleas, and ticks). Other insect-transmitted illnesses of concern include dengue fever, viral hemorrhagic fevers, filariasis, plague, leishmaniasis, African trypanosomiasis, and Chagas' disease.
     f. Close occupational, social, or sexual contact with natives.
     g. Swimming or immersion in bodies of fresh water, such as rivers, streams, or lakes, may put one at

risk of contracting schistosomiasis, leptospirosis, or amebic meningoencephalitis.

h. Unusual exposures such as raw or undercooked food, unpasteurized dairy products, water, drink, dust, animal exposure, or bites. (Disease risks include hepatitis A, enteric fever, trichinosis, brucellosis, amebiasis, melioidosis, Q fever, rabies, and erlichiosis.)

2. If the patient is not a traveler, consider malaria if there is a history of blood transfusion, being born to a mother from a malaria endemic area, IV drug use, or residence near an international airport, military base, or in an area with many immigrants from malaria endemic areas.

- Signs and symptoms
  1. The febrile illness of a malaria attack can last a week or more if left untreated. The fever pattern tends to be irregular and noncyclical during the initial attack in a nonimmune person, especially if the infecting strain is *P. falciparum;* absence of the classic tertian (48 hr) or quartan (72 hr) fever pattern cannot be used to rule out malaria. The fever spike, which may be as high as 39 to 40°C, is usually preceded by a period of shaking chills; defervescence occurs after a period of several hours and is marked by drenching sweats. If the initial attack is untreated, the fevers tend to become cyclical after the first week.

  2. Natives and recent immigrants from malaria-endemic areas are likely to have had previous infections with malaria. As a consequence, they may have partial immunity (which is species specific).
     a. In partially immune individuals, the fever tends to be cyclical, recurring every 48 hr (*P. vivax, P. falciparum, P. ovale*) or every 72 hr (*P. malariae*). The attack is milder than in a nonimmune person.
     b. Relapses disappear within 1 to 3 yr for infections with *P. falciparum* and 3 to 5 yr for infections with *P. vivax* and *P. ovale*. *P. malariae* infection may persist for many years.

  3. The patient with malaria may have fever as the sole sign of disease (Table 75–1).
     a. In severe malaria caused by *P. falciparum,* the patient may develop lethargy which can progress rapidly to obtundation and coma.
     b. Physical findings commonly seen in malaria include splenomegaly and tender hepatomegaly. Care should be exercised when palpating the spleen, as rupture of the distended capsule can occur.
     c. Lymphadenopathy or rashes are uncommon in malaria and should lead the clinician to consider other diagnoses.

  4. Severe malaria, generally due to *P. falciparum*, may present with many symptoms typical of septicemia including multiple end-organ failure. ARDS, renal failure ("blackwater fever"), and/or heart failure may all be seen in severe malaria.

TABLE 75–1. Clinical Signs and Symptoms in Acute Malaria

Fever	Abdominal pain
Headache	Myalgias
Chills	Diarrhea
Nausea	Jaundice

5. Cerebral malaria can also occur as a complication of infection with *P. falciparum;* symptoms may include somnolence or coma, psychosis, and major motor seizures. Findings on lumbar puncture are usually normal.

DIFFERENTIAL DIAGNOSIS (Table 75–2)

The length of time between potential exposure to malaria and the onset of symptoms is often helpful in organizing the differential diagnosis. Septicemia and bacterial meningitis should

TABLE 75–2. Incubation Periods for Tropical Infectious Diseases

Short (less than 10 days)
  Arboviral infections, including dengue and yellow fever
  Typhus fevers (louse-borne and flea-borne)
  Plague
  Paratyphoid fever
  Gastrointestinal bacterial pathogens
  Anthrax
  Acute melioidosis
  Leptospirosis
Intermediate (10–21 days)
  Malaria (*P. falciparum*)
  Malaria (*P. vivax, P. malariae, P. ovale*)
  Hemorrhagic fevers, including Lassa fever
  Scrub typhus, Q fever
  Spotted fever group
  Typhoid fever
  Brucellosis
  African trypanosomiasis
  Leptospirosis
Prolonged (greater than 21 days)
  Viral hepatitis
  Rabies
  Tuberculosis
  Malaria (*P. vivax, P. malariae, P. ovale*)
  Amebic abscess of the liver
  Filariasis
  Schistosomiasis
  Visceral leishmaniasis

Source: Strickland GT, Fever in travelers, in Strickland GT, ed. Hunter's Tropical Medicine. Philadelphia, W.B. Saunders, 1984, p. 945.

always be considered in the gravely ill patient from whom one cannot obtain an adequate history.

LABORATORY STUDIES

- CBC with white cell differential and platelet count. Leukopenia, thrombocytopenia, and a relative monocytosis are common in all forms of malaria.
- Thick and thin smear for malaria examination (may also reveal babesiosis, African trypanosomiasis, or *Borrelia recurrentis*, the causative organism for relapsing fever).
- Serum electrolyte and chemistry panel. Hyponatremia, hypoglycemia, and lactic acidosis are often seen in severe malaria.
- Serum bilirubin and hepatic enzyme levels. Consider checking hepatitis A and B serologies if the patient's previous immune status is negative or unknown.
- Urinalysis may detect hemoglobinuria or signs of acute tubular necrosis.
- Blood cultures (at least 2 sets).
- Chest X-ray should be performed if pulmonary symptoms are present.
- Glucose-6-phosphate dehydrogenase (G6PD) level. Patients with G6PD deficiency may develop severe hemolytic anemia if treated with primaquine, which is used to eliminate the hepatic phase organisms in infection due to *P. vivax* and *P. ovale*.
- Draw 1 to 2 extra tubes of blood so that acute phase serum can be frozen and available for future diagnostic testing.
- Serologic tests for all 4 malaria species are available on a nonemergency basis from commercial specialty laboratories. However, serologic testing is useful only to demonstrate *previous* infection with a particular strain of malaria.
- If meningeal signs or altered mental status are present, a lumbar puncture should be performed, and the CSF analyzed for glucose, protein, cell count, and microbiologic studies.
- The gold standard of malaria diagnosis is identifying the parasites on "thick" and "thin" smears of the peripheral blood stained with Giemsa stain (Table 75–3).
    1. Parasites can often be identified on standard peripheral blood smears stained with Wright's stain and examined manually.
    2. Thick and thin blood smears of heparinized or EDTA-treated blood should be examined for any febrile patient who has been to a malarious area. The thick smear is more sensitive in cases of low levels of parasitemia.
    3. The species of malaria may be determined by the morphology of the ring forms, the size and morphology of the RBCs that are parasitized, the appearance of RBCs containing malaria schizonts, and by the morphology of the malaria gametocytes.

TABLE 75-3. Preparation of Blood Smears for Malaria Detection

THIN SMEARS

Thin smears for evaluation of the blood for malarial parasites are made the same way that routine blood smears for hematologic evaluation are made. A small drop of blood is placed at one end of a clean glass microscopic slide. A second slide is held at a 45 degree angle to the first slide, contacting the drop of blood, and spreading it out in a thin smear as the second slide is pushed along the surface of the first slide to the opposite end. After air-drying, the slide is fixed and stained in a standard manner for Wright's or Giemsa stain.

THICK SMEARS

A thick smear for detection of malarial parasites in the blood when the parasitemia is very low is made by placing one drop of blood on a clean glass microscopic slide and using the corner of a second slide to spread the blood around to create a spot about the size of a dime. After air-drying, the slide *is not fixed* but stained directly with an aqueous stain (Wright's or Giemsa stain). Exposure of the thick smear to an aqueous stain without prior fixation causes the red cells to rupture and enables visualization of parasite forms in the thick layer of organic material on the slide.

Source: White NJ, Jong EC. Malaria diagnosis and treatment. In: Jong EC, ed. The Travel and Tropical Medicine Manual. Philadelphia, W.B. Saunders, 1987, p. 83.

4. The purple-staining ring stages of the malaria parasite can be seen within infected RBCs and are one-fifth to one-third the diameter of the cells. *P. vivax* and *P. ovale* preferentially infect reticulocytes, so the cells containing the trophozoites are often larger in diameter than neighboring noninfected cells, and the number of parasitized cells is low, usually less than 1%.

5. *P. malariae* preferentially infects older RBCs, which typically results in a relatively low degree of parasitemia.

6. *P. falciparum* will infect RBCs of any age, thus, the level of parasitemia will rapidly increase in the untreated patient, going from 1–2% to 10–15% or higher during the course of an attack. The banana-shaped gametocytes of *P. falciparum* seen within RBCs or free on the smear confirm the diagnosis of *P. falciparum* infection.

- Speciation of a malaria infection may not be possible during the initial laboratory investigation. If the species is unclear, and the patient has been in an area where chloroquine-resistant *P. falciparum* (CRPF) is present, the clinician should initiate treatment for CRPF.

- Malaria smears are often reported as negative in a patient who is likely to have malaria based on geographic and clinical features. If the patient is seriously ill, he or she should be hospitalized, and, in addition to other diagnostic and supportive measures, thick and thin smears should be done at 6-hr intervals. It may require up to 6 sets of smears to confirm the diagnosis.

- Fluorescent antibody techniques are beginning to allow more efficient diagnosis of malaria infections in endemic areas, but this technology is not widely available in community hospitals and laboratories in North America at this time.

RECOMMENDED DIAGNOSTIC APPROACH

- Take a careful history, considering the likelihood of malaria according to the countries and times visited. Consider epidemiologic factors that would make alternative diagnoses likely.
- Physical findings may be limited to fever. Hepatomegaly and splenomegaly may be present, but lymphadenopathy or rash should suggest alternative diagnoses. In any patient who may have malaria, and who is severely ill, consider septicemia or meningitis as alternative diagnoses.
- Laboratory studies
  1. CBC with manually examined peripheral blood smear
  2. Thick and thin blood smears
     a. These should be done at the time the patient is febrile (ideally during the ascending curve of the fever).
     b. Several sets at frequent intervals should be performed in patients who remain febrile despite negative smears, or who have negative smears in the face of possible partially treated infection.
  3. Serum electrolyte, glucose, bilirubin, and liver enzyme levels should be checked. Consider checking hepatitis serologies, blood cultures, and a chest X-ray.
  4. Obtain a urinalysis to rule out infection and detect hemoglobinuria.
  5. Lumbar puncture should be performed on patients in whom meningitis is a possible diagnosis.
  6. Malaria serologies should only be performed to confirm previous infections with malaria; they are not reliable in the diagnosis of acute malaria.
  7. Recorded general advice from the CDC regarding malaria prophylaxis, diagnosis, and treatment can be obtained by calling (404) 639-1610. The malaria specialists at the Centers for Disease Control are available for emergency telephone consultation 24 hours a day. Telephone (404) 639-3311 Monday through Friday during normal business hours EST, or (404) 639-2888 on weekends and at night. The consultants can assist with the diagnostic and therapeutic recommendations, especially if an investigational treatment protocol (e.g., exchange blood transfusion, intravenous quinidine) is warranted.

Bibliography

Centers for Disease Control. Health Information for International Travel, 1991. Washington DC, U.S. Government Printing Office, 1991. HHS Publication No. (CDC) 9I-8280. (May be ordered by calling (202) 783-3238.)

Steffen R, et al. Health problems after travel to developing countries. J Infect Dis 1987;156:84–91.

Strickland GT. Fever in travelers. In: Strickland GT, ed. Hunter's Tropical Medicine. Philadelphia, W.B. Saunders, 1984, pp. 944–952.

White NJ, Jong EC. Malaria diagnosis and treatment. In: Jong EC, ed. The Travel and Tropical Medicine Manual. Philadelphia, W.B. Saunders, 1987, pp. 79–89.

Wyler DJ. Plasmodium species (malaria). In: Mandell GL, Douglas RG, Bennett JE ed. Principles and Practice of Infectious Diseases, 3rd ed. New York, Churchill Livingstone, 1989, pp. 2056–2066.

76

LYME DISEASE

RANDALL CULPEPPER

Every man carries a parasite somewhere.

JAPANESE PROVERB

DEFINITION

Lyme disease is a systemic, multistage disease with protean manifestations, including dermatologic, rheumatic, neurologic, and cardiac abnormalities. It is caused by the spirochete *Borrelia burgdorferi* and is transmitted to people by the bite of infected ticks, principally *Ixodes dammini* and *I. pacificus* in the United States.

EPIDEMIOLOGY

- Lyme disease was first described in the United States in 1975 in association with a cluster of juvenile rheumatoid arthritis cases in Old Lyme, Connecticut.
- Between 1982 and 1989, over 15,000 cases were reported to the CDC, making Lyme disease the most common vector-borne infection in the United States.
- Lyme disease occurs worldwide. The infection has spread, particularly in the coastal areas of the northeastern United States, in Wisconsin and Minnesota in the midwest, and, to a lesser degree, in the far west from California northward to British Columbia (Figure 76–1).
- All age groups are affected, but most reported cases occur in young adults and children, who are most likely to be exposed to the tick.
- The acute infection is typically acquired in the early summer months when the nymphal (juvenile) form of the tick is feeding. Chronic disease is identified year-round. The white-footed mouse is the preferred host for both the larval and nymphal stages of *I. dammini;* however, the adult ticks feed on a variety of wild animals, including birds. On the west coast, Lyme disease is less prevalent, and only 1 to 3% of *I. pacificus* ticks are infected.
- Lyme disease also occurs in domestic animals, including dogs, horses, and cattle, but there is no documented transmission from these animals to people.

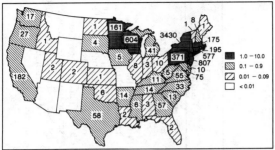

*Data for Oregon and California are for 1987 only.

Figure 76–1. Number and average annual incidence rates of reported Lyme disease cases, per 100,000 population—United States, 1987–1988. Data for Oregon and California are for 1987 only. (From Lyme Disease—United States, 1987 and 1988. MMWR 1989;38:669.)

DIFFERENTIAL DIAGNOSIS

- Syphilis. Many possible signs and symptoms of Lyme disease are similar to syphilis, another spirochetal disease.
- Lyme borreliosis may mimic other disorders, many of which are not due to infectious agents. Examples include pauciarticular arthritis, radiculopathy, fibromyalgia, and extreme chronic fatigue.
- The clinical spectrum of late neurologic complications of Lyme disease is incompletely defined. Infection with *B. burgdorferi* does *not* cause classic clinical pictures of multiple sclerosis, amyotrophic lateral sclerosis, or Alzheimer's disease.
- The nonspecific symptoms of fatigue, headache, or musculoskeletal pain should not be confused with Lyme disease if there are no objective signs of the disease.

CLINICAL FEATURES

- Background
    1. A history of residence or travel in an area with documented local transmission of Lyme disease (endemic area) should be sought.
    2. Lyme disease occurs in stages with different organ systems affected at each stage. It is best characterized as an illness which progresses from early to late disease without reference to an arbitrary staging system (Table 76–1).
        a. The early phase of infection begins within a few days to several months after a tick bite.
        b. The late phase of disease occurs several months to 2 years after acute infection.

TABLE 76–1. Manifestations of Lyme Disease by Stage[a]

SYSTEM[b]	EARLY INFECTION		LATE INFECTION Persistent (Stage 3)
	Localized (Stage 1)	Disseminated (Stage 2)	
Skin	Erythema migrans	Secondary annular lesions, malar rash, diffuse erythema or urticaria, evanescent lesions, lymphocytoma	Acrodermatitis chronica atrophicans, localized sclerodermalike lesions
Musculoskeletal system		Migratory pain in joints, tendons, bursae, muscle, bone; brief arthritis attacks; myositis[c]; osteomyelitis[c]; panniculitis[c]	Prolonged arthritis attacks, chronic arthritis, peripheral enthesopathy, periostitis or joint subluxations below lesions of acrodermatitis
Neurologic system		Meningitis, cranial neuritis, Bell's palsy, motor or sensory radiculoneuritis, subtle encephalitis, mononeuritis multiplex, myelitis[c], chorea[c], cerebellar ataxia[c]	Chronic encephalomyelitis, spastic parapareses, ataxic gait, subtle mental disorders, chronic axonal polyradiculopathy, dementia[c]
Lymphatic system	Regional lymphadenopathy	Regional or generalized	

Heart		lymphadenopathy, splenomegaly
		Atrioventricular nodal block, myopericarditis, pancarditis
Eyes		Conjunctivitis, iritis[c], choroiditis[c], retinal hemorrhage or detachment[c], panophthalmitis[c]	Keratitis
Liver		Mild or recurrent hepatitis
Respiratory system		Nonexudative sore throat, nonproductive cough, adult respiratory distress syndrome[c]
Kidney		Microscopic hematuria or proteinuria
Genitourinary system		Orchitis[c]
Constitutional symptoms	Minor	Severe malaise and fatigue	Fatigue

[a] The classifications by stages provides a guideline for the expected timing of the illness's manifestations, but this may vary from case to case.
[b] Systems are based from the most to the least commonly affected.
[c] The inclusion of this manifestation is based on one or a few cases.

Source: Steere AC. Lyme disease. New Engl J Med 1989; 321:586–596. Used with permission.

- Early infection
  1. Erythema migrans (EM)
     a. This pathognomonic skin lesion of early Lyme disease occurs in 60 to 80% of patients infected with the spirochete.
     b. The lesion first appears as a red papule at the site of the tick bite, most commonly, the axilla, groin, and thigh. An expanding area of erythema around the bite develops over days to weeks, attaining a median diameter of 15 cm. Central fading typically gives EM a ringlike or bulls-eye appearance.
     c. The lesion is often flat and usually asymptomatic, but tender, warm, or pruritic lesions are also quite common. It usually fades without treatment in 3 to 4 weeks.
     d. Facial EM is more common in children.
  2. Flu-like symptoms often occur early after tick exposure. Malaise and fatigue usually persist long after the other symptoms have faded.
  3. Musculoskeletal manifestations (see Table 76–1)
     a. Sixty percent of untreated patients develop joint symptoms ranging from migratory arthralgias and myalgia to a chronic destructive arthritis a mean of 6 months after EM.
     b. Commonly found symptoms include asymmetric, oligoarticular arthritis (especially knee joints), large joint effusions, Baker's cysts, and temporomandibular joint pain.
  4. Neurologic abnormalities (see Table 76–1)
     a. These occur in 15% of untreated patients, usually within 2 to 8 weeks after disease onset.
     b. Commonly found symptoms include unilateral or bilateral facial palsy (10%), peripheral neuritis, severe headache, and mild neck stiffness.
  5. Cardiac abnormalities (see Table 76–1)
     a. Cardiac disease occurs in 8% of untreated patients within 2 to 6 weeks following infection.
     b. Commonly found abnormalities include AV block, especially first degree and Mobitz Type I block. The cardiac conduction abnormalities usually last days to weeks and generally do not require permanent cardiac pacing.
- Late infection
  1. Late or chronic infection is characterized by persistent, episodic arthritic and neurologic symptoms. They may last months rather than weeks and occur during the second and third years of the disease.
  2. The chronic neurologic syndromes of Lyme disease may include:
     a. Subtle symptoms of CNS dysfunction, such as memory loss, somnolence, or behavioral changes
     b. Progressive encephalomyelitis
     c. Intermittent distal paresthesia
     d. Radicular pain

LABORATORY FEATURES

- Patients with Lyme disease produce IgM antibodies during the first several weeks after onset of EM and produce IgG more slowly. Antibody titers can remain elevated for months or years, especially in patients with chronic manifestations.
- Serologic tests
  1. The most widely used testing procedures (ELISA and indirect fluorescent antibody [IFA]) generally suffer from frequent false-positive and false-negative reactions. The ELISA method is preferred over IFA methods.
  2. False-positive results can occur in patients with syphilis, Rocky Mountain spotted fever, relapsing fever, autoimmune diseases, and some neurologic disorders.
- Culture or direct visualization of *B. burgdorferi* is difficult and usually a low-yield process. DNA probes and polymerase chain reaction techniques are under development, but are not yet widely available.

RECOMMENDED DIAGNOSTIC APPROACH

- A careful history should be taken to evaluate the patient for:
  1. Residence or travel to an endemic area
  2. Possible tick exposure or bite
  3. Onset of rash consistent with erythema migrans
  4. Other nonspecific constitutional symptoms consistent with early Lyme disease
- Physical examination should concentrate on the dermatologic, rheumatologic, neurologic, and cardiac systems (see Table 76–1).
- Laboratory analysis should be limited to providing confirmation of suspicious clinical cases. Indiscriminate use of currently available imperfect serologic assays may confound the diagnostic process.
- Empiric therapy. A trial of antibiotic therapy may be appropriate for the few patients who are a diagnostic dilemma and in whom all other diagnostic possibilities have been eliminated.

Bibliography

Burgdorfer W, et al. The western black-legged tick, *Ixodes pacificus:* A vector of *Borrelia burgdorferi*. Am J Trop Med Hyg 1985;34: 925–930.

Halperin JJ, et al. Lyme neuroborreliosis: Central nervous system manifestations. Neurology 1989;39:753–759.

Steere AC. Lyme disease. New Engl J Med 1989;321:586–596.

Steere AC, et al. Lyme carditis: Cardiac abnormalities of Lyme disease. Ann Intern Med, 1980;93:8–16.

Trock DH, et al. Clinical manifestations of Lyme disease in the United States. Conn Med 1989;53(6):327–330.

77

INFECTIOUS MONONUCLEOSIS

DAVID C. DUGDALE

The fact that your patient gets well does not prove that
your diagnosis was correct.

SAMUEL J. METTZER (1851–1921)

DEFINITION AND GENERAL COMMENTS

- Infectious mononucleosis (IM) is a specific infection
  caused by the Epstein-Barr virus (EBV). The clinical syndrome may be mimicked by many other infectious diseases.
- Criteria for diagnosis. The presence of the classic clinical,
  hematologic (atypical lymphocytosis), and serologic (heterophil antibody) picture is sufficient for diagnosis. Five to
  ten percent of patients with documented EBV mononucleosis
  have negative heterophil tests (''heterophil-negative IM'').
  Unequivocal diagnosis is established if specific anti-EBV
  antibodies are identified.
- Epidemiology
  1. IM is found worldwide. In economically under-
     developed areas a subclinical or mild infection occurs
     in virtually all young children. In middle and upper
     socioeconomic groups half of adolescents have anti-
     bodies to EBV.
  2. Sixty percent of clinical cases in the United States
     occur in persons 15 to 24 years old.
  3. Transmission usually occurs by salivary exchange dur-
     ing close personal contact. The disease is not very
     contagious, with an annual incidence of less than 15%
     among susceptible college students.

DIFFERENTIAL DIAGNOSIS

- Pharyngitis. IM causes less than 2% of the sore throat cases
  seen by most clinicians. If suggestive historical and physical findings are absent, the pharyngitis is probably not due
  to IM, and tests for heterophil antibodies are not indicated.

Adapted with permission of authors and publisher from Cummins RO.
Infectious mononucleosis. In: Cummins RO, Eisenberg MS, eds. Blue
Book of Medical Diagnosis. Philadelphia, W.B. Saunders, 1986.

- Prolonged malaise, low-grade fever, upper respiratory infections, and lymphadenopathy. Causes other than IM that should be considered include:
    1. Febrile pharyngotonsilitis. This can be caused by streptococcal or viral infection, diphtheria, or Vincent's angina.
    2. Hematologic malignancy.
    3. Rubella. The rash of IM spares the face, whereas the rash of rubella regularly affects the face.
    4. Cytomegalovirus (CMV) infection. Fever, splenomegaly, hepatitis, and atypical lymphocytosis occur with CMV infection. An older age group is usually involved, pharyngitis and cervical adenopathy are rare, and a history of multiple blood transfusions is often present. Specific complement-fixing antibody tests are needed to confirm this diagnosis.
    5. Toxoplasmosis. Fever, generalized lymphadenopathy, atypical lymphocytosis, splenomegaly, and malaise occur with toxoplasmosis, but pharyngitis is absent or minimal.
    6. "Heterophil-negative" IM. This term is applied to patients who have the classic signs and symptoms of IM but who have negative heterophil reactions (Table 77–1).

CLINICAL MANIFESTATIONS

- History
    1. Clinicians usually first suspect IM when patients who complain of sore throat are noted to have prominent lymphadenopathy associated with fever and malaise.
    2. In the typical case a 3- to 5-day prodrome of fatigue, myalgia, and malaise occurs. Then a 7- to 20-day period occurs in which the major symptoms are sore throat, fever, headache, and weakness. The fever lasts over a week in 90% of the febrile cases and over 2 weeks in 50%.
- Classic features (Table 77–2)

TABLE 77–1. Causes of Heterophil-Negative Infectious Mononucleosis

EBV infection (30 to 50% of cases)
CMV infection (20 to 40% of cases)
Miscellaneous (10% of cases)
 Viruses: hepatitis (A, B, C), mumps, adenovirus, HIV
 Bacteria: listeriosis, subacute bacterial endocarditis,
    brucellosis, chronic meningococcemia,
    syphilis, cat-scratch disease
 Other infections: toxoplasmosis, trichinosis
 Noninfectious: serum sickness, SLE, polyarteritis
    nodosa, and drug reactions (isoniazid,
    para-aminosalicylic acid, sulfasalazine,
    phenytoin, and rubella vaccine)

TABLE 77–2. Classic Features of Infectious Mononucleosis

Clinical signs and symptoms
  Lymphadenopathy (90%)
  Splenomegaly (50 to 60%)
  Sore throat (70%)
  Exudative pharyngitis (40%)
  Malaise (50%)
  Fever: >38.3°C (75%)
Hematologic picture
  Absolute lymphocytosis: >4000/mm^3 (>90%)
  Relative lymphocytosis: >50% (> 90%)
  Atypical ("Downy cell") lymphocytes: >10% of total WBC (>90%)
Elevated titers of heterophil antibody

- Pharyngitis. In patients with pharyngitis, the following findings occur significantly more often in heterophil-positive patients than in heterophil-negative patients (frequency in heterophil-positive patients in parentheses):
  1. Inguinal adenopathy (53%)
  2. Posterior auricular adenopathy (33%)
  3. Palatal petechiae (27%)
  4. Marked axillary adenopathy (20%)
- Other signs and symptoms. These are generally nonspecific but may cause significant morbidity when present (expected frequency in parentheses):
  1. Hepatic signs: hepatomegaly (20%); jaundice (4%). The frequencies are 42 and 27%, respectively, in patients over 40 years old.
  2. Rash (2%): urticarial and morbilliform.
  3. Neurologic symptoms (2%): aseptic meningitis, encephalitis, cranial nerve paralysis, transverse myelitis, and Guillain-Barré syndrome.
  4. Miscellaneous (each less than 1%):
     a. Pericarditis, myocarditis
     b. Pulmonary infiltrates and effusions
     c. Glomerulonephritis
     d. Pancreatitis
     e. Hilar adenopathy
     f. Hemolytic anemia, thrombocytopenia, and splenic rupture (0.5%).

LABORATORY TESTS

- Hematologic picture. Lymphocyte levels noted in Table 77–2 generally occur at some stage of the disease, but may not be continuously present.
- The serology of IM. In 1932 Paul and Bunnell demonstrated that the serum of patients with IM agglutinated the RBCs of sheep and horses (heterophil agglutination test).
  1. Other diseases that may produce sheep cell agglutinins include serum sickness, hepatitis, Hodgkin's disease,

rubella, leukemia, sarcoidosis, rheumatoid arthritis, and adenovirus infections. Normal people may have low titers (the nonspecific Forssman antibody).

2. Monospot® Test. The Monospot® test (with horse RBCs; manufactured by Ortho Diagnostic Systems, Inc., Raritan, NJ) is generally used to detect heterophil antibodies. A positive reaction is 1:80 in titer. Monospot®-negative IM is more common in children and the elderly. Monospot® test parameters in young adults (prevalence of probable EBV infection 25 to 30%) include:
   a. Sensitivity and specificity of 95%.
   b. Positive and negative predictive values of 95%.
   c. The false-positive tests probably represent low titers from previous infection.
   d. The false-negative tests are usually positive when repeated. During the first week of clinical signs, 38% of patients have a positive result, 60% are positive during the second week, and 80% during the third week.
   e. Five to ten percent of patients with IM never develop a positive test.

3. Specific anti-EBV antibodies
   a. Patients generate antibodies to viral capsid antigen (VCA; IgM and IgG), early antigen (diffuse [anti-D] and restricted [anti-R]), and EB nuclear antigen (EBNA).
   b. The presence of IgM antibodies to VCA or high-titer IgG antibodies to VCA (titer $\geq$ 1:320 or 4-fold rise) and the absence of antibodies to EBNA (titer $\leq$ 1:2) indicate current or recent IM.

RECOMMENDED DIAGNOSTIC APPROACH

- WBC and differential counts should be performed.
- If the following are found, the Monospot® test should be done:
   1. Elevated (>10%) atypical lymphocytes, plus
   2. Absolute lymphocytosis (>4000/mm^3), or
   3. Relative lymphocytosis (>50%).
- Many clinicians order a Monospot® test and CBC simultaneously if IM is suspected.
- If the Monospot® test result is $\geq$1:80, the diagnosis is confirmed. Thirty percent of patients with this peripheral blood picture have positive Monospot® test results.

Bibliography

Aronson MD, et al. Heterophil antibody in adults with sore throat: Frequency and clinical presentation. Ann Intern Med 1982;96: 505–508.

Axelrod P, Finestone AJ. Infectious mononucleosis in older adults. Am Fam Pract 1990;42:1599–1606.

Begovac J, et al. Cytomegalovirus mononucleosis in children compared with the infection in adults and with Epstein-Barr virus mono-nucleosis. J Infect 1988;17:121–125.

Bergman MM, Gleckman RA. Heterophil-negative infectious mononu-cleosis-like syndrome. Postgrad Med 1987;81(1):313–326.

Cohen JI, Correy GR. Cytomegalovirus infection in the normal host. Medicine 1985;64:100–114.

Horwitz CA, et al. Clinical and laboratory evaluation of cytomegalovi-rus induced mononucleosis in previously healthy individuals. Medi-cine 1986;65:124–134.

Horwitz CA, et al. Long-term serological follow-up of patients with Epstein-Barr virus after recovery from infectious mononucleosis. J Infect Dis 1985;151:1150–1153.

Sumaya CV. Serologic testing for Epstein-Barr virus—developments in interpretation. J Infect Dis 1985;151:984–987.

SECTION XI

RHEUMATOLOGY

78

ARTHRALGIAS AND MYALGIAS

JAN HILLSON

I don't deserve this award, but I have arthritis and I
don't deserve that either.

JACK BENNY

DEFINITION

"Arthralgias" and "myalgias" refer to the *symptoms* joint
pain and muscle pain. These symptoms arise in disorders
affecting joints, periarticular structures, muscles, bones, soft
tissues, and associated nerves and blood vessels. They also
occur in systemic inflammation and in clinical syndromes
characterized by a lack of recognizable pathology (Table
78–1). Arthritis, myositis, and other rheumatologic syndromes are discussed in chapters 79 to 86.

DIAGNOSTIC FEATURES OF
SELECTED SYNDROMES

- Fibromyalgia. The American College of Rheumatology defines fibromyalgia by these criteria:

  1. History of widespread musculoskeletal pain
  2. "Mild or greater" tenderness of at least 11 of 18 specific
     sites (Figure 78–1)
  3. No exclusion for concomitant disease

  The prevalence of this clinical entity is estimated at 2 to
  10% in general medicine clinic populations, with a 3:1 female predominance.

  1. Clinical features. The second criterion is met when
     pain is reported on palpation with a 4-kg force at the
     sites shown in Figure 78–1. Fatigue, nonrestorative
     sleep, and stiffness are each reported by 75% of pa-
     tients. Coexistent systemic disease is common.
  2. Laboratory and imaging
     a. Exclusionary lab tests are not required for diagno-
        sis. Because fibromyalgia often occurs with other
        disorders, evaluation should include stool occult
        blood, mammogram if older than 35, CBC, urinal-
        ysis, and tests for systemic inflammation (ESR or
        C-reactive protein [CRP]) and thyroid function.
     b. When arthralgias and stiffness are prominent, anti-

675

TABLE 78–1. Disorders Characterized by Arthralgias or Myalgias

DISORDER	PREVALENCE PER 1000
Functional pain syndromes	
Fibromyalgia	10–100
Myofascial Pain Syndromes	100
Diagnostic and Statistical Manual III-R:	
Somatization Disorder	rare
Somatiform Pain Disorder	100
Overuse and chronic impingement syndromes	
Tendinitis	Common
Bursitis	Common
Other (stress fractures, cartilage damage, muscle rupture, etc.)	Common
Trauma	
Rupture of bone, cartilage, ligament, tendon, muscle	Common
Peripheral nerve damage	350
Systemic connective tissue diseases (CTD)	
Rheumatoid arthritis	15
Polymyalgia rheumatica	0.5 in adults over 50 yr
Systemic lupus erythematosus	0.5
Polymyositis/Dermatomyositis	0.05
Sjögren's syndrome	10
Systemic sclerosis	0.05
Primary vasculitis syndromes	0.1
Undifferentiated/overlap CTD	25% of CTD pts
Sarcoidosis (synovitis, osteolysis, myositis)	0.2
Others (including relapsing polychonditis, adult Still's disease, eosinphilic fasciitis, familial Mediterranean fever, panniculitis)	
Spondyloarthropathies	
Ankylosing spondylitis	1–5
Psoriatic arthritis	1
Reiter's syndrome	1
Enteropathic arthropathies	20% of pts with enteropathy
Crystal deposition diseases	
Gout	15
Pseudogout (calcium pyrophosphate deposition disease)	60
Degenerative diseases	
Osteoarthritis	350
Degenerative disc disease	350
Disuse atrophy	Unknown
Neuropathy	
Reflex sympathetic dystrophy	Unknown
Entrapment neuropathy	Common

DISORDER	PREVALENCE PER 1000
Other (peripheral neuropathy, CNS disease, etc.)	Unknown
Bone disorders	
Osteoporosis	
Osteonecrosis	
Paget's disease	
Osteochondritis dessicans	
Diffuse idiopathic skeletal hyperostosis	
Hypertrophic osteoarthropathy	
Endocrine diseases	
Diabetes (neuropathy, cheiroarthropathy, scleredema, tendinitis)	
Acromegaly (osteoarthritis, CTS, myopathy)	
Hypothyroidism (synovitis, myopathy, CTS, osteonecrosis)	
Hyperthyroidism (myopathy, periostitis, osteoporosis, adhesive capsulitis)	
Hyperparathyroidism (crystal synovitis, osteoporosis, myopathy, neuropathy)	
Hypoparathyroidism (enthesitis, muscle cramps)	
Cushing's syndrome (osteoporosis, osteonecrosis, myopathy)	
Infection	
Acute viral syndromes	
Chronic postviral syndromes (hepatitis B, parvovirus, rubella)	
Chronic postbacterial syndromes (rheumatic fever, intestinal bypass, dysenteric)	
Spirochetes (Lyme disease, syphilis)	
Bacteria, mycoplasma, fungus, parasites	
Neoplasm	
Paraneoplastic syndromes	
Metastatic disease	
Primary tumors of musculoskeletal structures (includes osteochondromatosis, villonodular synovitis, multiple myeloma, osteosarcoma, synovioma)	
Other	
Cryoglobulinemia (vasculitis, secondary neuropathy, arthropathy)	
Amyloidosis (myopathy, arthropathy, peripheral nerve compression)	
Drugs (myopathy, neuropathy, induction of CTD)	
Dialysis (osteoporosis, crystal synovitis, myopathy, amyloidosis)	
Coagulopathy (venous thrombosis, ischemia, hematoma)	
Atherosclerosis (ischemia of muscle/nerve)	
Electrolyte disorder (muscle cramps)	
Biochemical disorders (includes vitamin deficiency, hyperlipidemias, hemochromatosis, ochronosis, Gaucher's disease, inherited abnormalities of collagen, hemoglobinopathies, hemophilia, complement deficiency, and coagulopathy).	

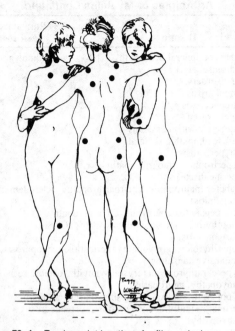

Figure 78–1. Tender point locations for fibromylagia.

Occiput: at the suboccipital muscle insertions.

Low cervical: at the anterior aspects of the intertransverse spaces at C5–C7.

Trapezius: at the midpoint of the upper border.

Supraspinatus: at origins above the scapular spine near the medial border.

Second rib: at the second costochondral junctions.

Lateral epicondyle: 2 cm distal to epicondyles.

Gluteal: in upper outer quadrants of buttocks in anterior fold of muscle.

Greater trochanter: posterior to the trochanteric prominence.

Knee: at the medial fat pad proximal to the joint line.

(From Wolf F, et al. The American College of Rheumatology 1990 criteria for the classification of fibromyalgia. Arth Rheum 1990;33:160.)

nuclear antibody (ANA), rheumatoid factor, and Lyme titer measurements may be useful. Significant myalgias warrant checking the serum creatine kinase (CK) and aldolase levels, and often electromyography. Radiographs are useful to evaluate localized pain.

3. Differential diagnosis. Polymyalgia rheumatica, polyarthritis, polymyositis, hypothyroidism, chronic infection, and neoplasm may cause similar symptoms. Fibromyalgia is not distinguishable from the "somatiform pain disorders," of which it comprises a subset.

· Polymyalgia rheumatica (PMR) is an idiopathic systemic

inflammatory disease causing limb girdle pain and stiffness in the elderly. The disorder is more common in women (2:1) and in those of Scandinavian descent.

1. Clinical features
   a. The onset may be acute or insidious. Fatigue, weight loss, anorexia, low-grade fever each occur in about 50% of patients.
   b. Exam reveals discomfort on rising from a squat and on resisted shoulder movement. True weakness or synovitis do not rule out PMR, but should broaden the differential diagnosis.
   c. Dramatic, rapid response to low-dose steroids (5 to 15 mg prednisone/day) is diagnostic. Because giant cell arteritis is reported in 0.1 to 80% of PMR patients, a history of cranial artery compromise (visual loss, diplopia, ptosis, headache, transient ischemic attacks, jaw claudication) and signs of temporal artery tenderness, bruits, or decreased pulses must be sought.
2. Lab and imaging. Lab values are normal except for a marked elevation in the ESR. Any symptom suggestive of arteritis mandates temporal artery biopsy.
3. Differential diagnosis
   a. Neoplasm should be excluded with a physical exam with survey studies (stool occult blood, pelvic exam, mammogram, chest X-ray in smokers, CBC, urinalysis, liver function tests).
   b. PMR is distinguished from seropositive rheumatoid arthritis (RA) by the absence of rheumatoid factors, but may be indistinguishable from late-onset seronegative RA. PMR is differentiated from polymyositis by normal CK, aldolase, and EMG. PMR is differentiated from fibromyalgia by the high ESR and clinical response to steroids.
   c. PMR with fever must be differentiated from chronic infection by blood and urine cultures, CBC, CXR, tuberculin skin test, and immune serologies indicated by exposure history.

- Bursitis is inflammation of closed mesenchymal-cell-lined sacs that lie between tissue planes.
  1. Clinical features. Localized pain occurs with movements or stresses the bursae normally buffer. Pain is aggravated by contraction of overlying muscles. Tenderness and swelling occur directly over bursa. Reduction of symptoms on instillation of local anesthetic is diagnostic. Trauma and overuse are the most common causes of bursitis.
  2. Lab and imaging
     a. Accessible fluid should be aspirated and examined for color, clarity, WBC count and differential, crystals, atypical cells, and organisms. These tests distinguish crystal-induced, infectious, or rheumatoid bursitis from the more common, less inflammatory bursitis associated with acute and chronic trauma.

    b. MRI and ultrasound are useful to establish disease of deep bursae.

3. Common clinical syndromes (Table 78–2)

- Tendinitis. This term encompasses both inflammation of the cellular lining of the tendon sheath and proliferation of the fibrous wall of the sheath.

1. Clinical features. Pain is greatest with tendon movement or stretch. Exam shows focal tenderness. Focal or fusiform swelling, crepitation or rub with motion, warmth, erythema, and decreased range of motion may also be present. Chronic trauma and overuse are the most common causes of tendinitis. Rheumatoid arthritis frequently involves synovial-lined tendon sheaths, as may the spondyloarthropathies. A characteristic dorsal tenosynovitis of the wrists is seen in disseminated gonococcal infections.

2. Lab and imaging studies are often unnecessary. Exceptions include radiographic evaluation of the shoulder in advanced rotator cuff tendinitis and work-up for infection systemic inflammation in marked or multifocal inflammatory tenosynovitis.

3. Common clinical syndromes

    a. Lateral epicondylitis (tennis elbow) results from violent or repetitive rotation of the extended forearm. The tender point is at the epicondyle. Pain is reproduced by resisted wrist extension and supination.

    b. Medial epicondylitis (golfer's elbow) presents with tenderness over the medial epicondyle at the insertion of flexor carpi radialis. Pain is reproduced by resisted wrist flexion and pronation.

    c. De Quervain's disease of the abductor pollicis longus and extensor pollicis brevis occurs with repetitive radial deviation of the wrist while grasping with the thumb. Pain, tenderness, and sometimes swelling are present over the radial styloid. There may be sharp pain on Finkelstein's test: have the patient make fist with thumb inside fingers, then ulnarly deviate wrist.

    d. Volar flexor tenosynovitis usually involves the middle or index flexor digitorum tendon sheath. Flexion causes pain in the palm. Trigger finger may develop due to fibrotic narrowing of the sheath over the metacarpal heads, with formation of a tendon nodule distal to constriction.

    e. Achilles tendinitis presents with painful ankle motion, tenderness, and crepitus along the distal third of the tendon. Hyperlipidemia may cause tendinous xanthomas that mimic tendinitis.

    f. Posterior tibial tendinitis causes pain and tenderness posterior to the medial malleolus that is aggravated by passive eversion and resisted inversion.

    g. Popliteal tendinitis produces pain in the posterolateral aspect of knee, aggravated by running downhill, and focal tenderness and pain on straight leg raising.

TABLE 78–2. Clinical Features of Bursitis

NAME	CAUSE	LOCATION OF PAIN	COMMENT
Olecranon	Usually traumatic	Point of elbow	May be due to rheumatoid arthritis, crystal-induced arthropathy, or infection
Subacromial	Friction between coracoacromial arch and rotator cuff	Poorly localized to shoulder	Positive impingement sign: pain on forced elevation of arm while immobilizing scapula
Iliopectineal	Iliopsoas friction with inguinal ligament	Groin pain radiating to knee; tender lateral to femoral pulse, below inguinal ligament	Pain worse with hip extension
Ischial	Gluteus maximus friction with ischial tuberosity	Ischial pain may radiate down thigh; tender ischial tuberosity	Often related to prolonged sitting
Trochanteric	Friction between greater trochanter and tensor fascia lata	At or posterior to the greater trochanter of hip	Pain greatest on active abduction
Prepatellar	Usually traumatic	Over lower patella or patellar tendon	Often related to prolonged kneeling
Anserine	Friction between medial tibial metaphysis and medial hamstring tendons	Medial knee 5 cm below joint line	Pain aggravated by stair climbing
Retrocalcaneal	Friction between calcaneus and Achilles tendon	Tender over Achilles tendon insertion.	Pain worse with ankle dorsiflexion
Calcaneal	Friction between calcaneal spur and soft tissue	Over a calcaneal spur	Usually in older persons
Plantar fasciitis	Overuse or spondyloarthropathy	Insertion of plantar fascia on calcaneus	Frequently seen in young athletes

    h. Bicipital tendinitis results from chronic abrasion of the long head of the biceps against the humeral head. Tenderness migates with bicipital groove on abduction and external rotation of arm. Yergason's sign is positive: pain on resisted pronation of the forearm with elbow at 90 degrees.

    i. Rotator cuff tendinitis/impingement syndrome. Supraspinatus tendinitis and inflammation of related structures results from chronic impingement between the humerus, acromion, and coracoacromial ligament. Pain characteristics vary, but the impingement sign is positive. Late sequelae include rupture of the rotator cuff, with weakness of abduction and external rotation. Narrowing of the acromiohumeral gap, superior migration of the humeral head, and acromial erosion may be evident on plain film. Rotator cuff tear may be confirmed by US or arthrography.

    j. Calcific tendinitis of the supraspinatus tendon may occur with or without impingement. Symptoms are similar to those of impingement, but inflammation may be marked. Calcium is evident on plain X-ray.

- Entrapment neuropathy
  1. Clinical features
     a. There is a history of pain, dysesthesia, paresthesia, weakness, aggravated by activities that increase impingement. Nocturnal symptoms are common.
     b. Work-up is directed toward (1) demonstrating a sensory deficit or weakness (maneuvers that compress the affected nerve at the site of injury may reproduce transient symptoms), (2) determining the distribution of deficit, thus the level of nerve involvement, and (3) identifying the factors contributing to nerve damage.
  2. Lab and imaging: Nerve conduction velocity (NCV) studies confirm early disease and the level of damage. Advanced disease causes electromyographic (EMG) abnormalities reflecting denervation.
  3. Common syndromes
     a. Peripheral nerve entrapment can occur anywhere a peripheral nerve passes through a fibrous opening or osseofibrous canal. Conditions that decrease the size of the canal causing entrapment include small stature, synovitis, myxedema, amyloid deposition, spur formation in osteoarthritis, acromegaly, pregnancy, and tumor. Compression may also result from extrinsic trauma or pressure. Nerves already compromised by ischemia or metabolic disease are more vulnerable to entrapment damage.
       i. Median nerve entrapment usually occurs between the tranverse carpal ligament and the carpus bone, causing carpal tunnel syndrome (CTS).

(a) Pain or tingling in the hand, usually localized to thumb, index, middle, and radial half of ring finger, often referred to the forearm, worse after sustained grasp and at night.

(b) Tinel's sign (symptoms elicted by tapping nerve at site of lesion) is positive in 50%. Phalen's (symptoms with passive wrist flexion for 1 min) is positive in 80%.

(c) Sensory NCV is abnormal early. EMG abnormalities, thenar wasting, abductor pollicus brevis weakness occur late.

(d) Occasionally entrapment occurs within the pronator teres causing pain in forearm and hand that is aggravated by pronation, as in tennis or hammering, and absent at night. The tender point is in the proximal pronator teres.

ii. Ulnar nerve entrapment

(a) This may occur at the wrist in Guyon's canal between the pisiform and the hook of the hamate, but is more common at the elbow in the medial condylar groove or in the cubital tunnel between the medial ligament of the elbow joint and the aponeurosis of the flexor carpi ulnaris. It is localized by NCV tests or Tinel's sign.

(b) Entrapment at any site may cause sensory symptoms in the fifth finger, ulnar half of the fourth finger, and palm, weakness in apposition of the fourth and fifth fingers, and first dorsal intraoseus, and hypothenar wasting.

iii. Radial nerve compression occurs at the axilla with prolonged pressure, as from crutches or stuporous sleep, and produces wrist drop and triceps weakness. Entrapment of the posterior interosseous branch just distal to the lateral epicondyle of the humerus leads to elbow pain and weakness in the extensors of digits 3–5.

iv. Meralgia paresthetica is due to entrapment or stretch of the lateral cutaneous nerve of the thigh as it exits the pelvis beneath the lateral inguinal ligament. Burning paresthesias along the lateral aspect of the thigh, worse with standing or prolonged adduction or extension of the leg. Motor function and EMG are normal.

v. Peroneal nerve compression is due to external pressure at the neck of the fibula (e.g., leg crossing).

(a) Involvement of the deep (anterior tibial) branch causes foot drop and hypesthesia between the first and second toe.

Involvement of the superficial (musculocutaneous) branch produces weak foot eversion and sensory changes over the lateral leg and dorsal foot.

(b) Tinel's sign or NCV tests, normal foot inversion, and ankle reflex differentiate this from L-5 radiculopathy and sciatic neuropathy.

vi. Posterior tarsal tunnel syndrome. Entrapment of the posterior tibial nerve behind and inferior to the medial malleolus causes burning pain and paresthesias in toes and the sole of the foot, often worse at night and reproducible by forcibly inverting and medially rotating foot. Tinel's sign and NCV tests are helpful.

vii. Morton's neuroma may reflect entrapment of an interdigital nerve, most commonly that between the third and fourth toes, causing paresthesias, burning, and aching aggravated by walking. Local tenderness, occasionally with swelling, may occur.

b. Spinal nerve root compression may occur within the spinal canal, the neuroforamen, or in the extraforminal nerve canal.

i. Impingement is usually ascribed to herniated disc, disc degeneration with settling of the rami, or facet joint disease. Clinical features are variable, as peripheral nerves include contributions from multiple roots. NCV and EMG are helpful (Table 78–3).

ii. When impingement is due to distal narrowing of the spinal canal, the patient presents with spinal stenosis syndrome: leg pain and weakness aggravated by postures that extend and thus shorten the spine, such as walking downhill.

- Reflex sympathetic dystrophy (RSD). A regional pain syndrome, hypothesized to involve abnormal activity in the sympathetic nervous system.

1. Clinical features. Four of the following 10 features, plus alleviation of the symptoms by sympathetic block, establish the diagnosis: pain (burning, sustained or lancinating, nondermatomal); abnormal temperature (hot early, cold late); abnormal color (red early, cyanotic late); abnormal sweating (dry early, moist late); edema; atrophy of hair, nails, skin; hyperpathia (overreaction to repetitive stimulation); osteopenia; weakness; psychologic disorder.

2. Lab and imaging. Early in the disease course technetium pyrophosphate bone scans show diffusely increased uptake on delayed phase images. Plain films show patchy osteopenia later in the course.

3. Clinical syndromes. RSD usually follows trauma, but may occur in neurologic and visceral disorders and following exposure to certain drugs.

TABLE 78-3. Clinical Features of Radiculopathy

ROOT	LOCATION OF PAIN	MUSCLES WEAK	REFLEX DIMINISHED
C5	Medial scapula, lateral arm	Deltoid, rhomboids, supraspinatus, infraspinatus	Biceps
C6	Lateral forearm, thumb, and index finger	Biceps, brachioradialis, pronators and supinators of arm	Supinator
C7	Posterior arm, lateral parts of hand, mid-forearm, scapula	Wrist flexors and extensors, triceps, pectoralis major and minor	Triceps
C8	Medial forearm and hand	Flexor carpi ulnaris and finger flexion and extension	
T1	Shoulder with radiation to olecranon	Hand intrinsics	
L4	Posterolateral thigh and anteromedial leg	Quadriceps	Patellar
L5	Posterior thigh, anterolateral leg, medial foot	Dorsiflexors of toes and foot	
S1	Posterior thigh and leg, posterolateral foot	Plantar flexor, foot evertor	Achilles
S2–S4	Buttocks, posterior thigh and leg, and plantar foot	Sphincters, hamstrings, toe and heel walk	Achilles

a. Shoulder-hand syndrome, with adhesive capsulitis of the shoulder and RSD-related atrophy of the hand, is seen following myocardial infarction. RSD-related shoulder pain may also occur in the hemiparetic side after a stroke.

b. Causalgia is a severe form that follows partial injury, usually by gunshot or shrapnel, to nerves proximal to the elbow or knee.

- Myofascial pain syndromes (MPS) are regional pain disorders characterized by an area of deep muscle tenderness, termed a "trigger point," palpation of which creates pain in a predictable reference zone. Alleviation of pain by acupuncture, injection of anesthetic or saline, or transcutaneous electrical nerve stimulation at the trigger point is a diagnostic feature. Diagnosis requires the exclusion of other causes of pain. Syndromes include:

1. Temporomandibular (TM) pain and dysfunction is characterized by pain in the periauricular region aggravated by jaw movement, limited or irregular jaw movement, and tenderness of jaw muscles. Diagnosis requires absence of TM joint tenderness or radiographic changes. Nocturnal bruxism is common. Trigger point is in the lateral pterygoid.

2. Occipital neuralgia has been ascribed to MPS with trigger point in the trapezius. Temporal headache may result from MPS with trigger point in the temporalis, masseter, or sternocleidomastoid.

3. Lumbago, nonradiating low back pain, has been ascribed to MPS with trigger points in the rectus abdominus, paraspinals, glutei, piriformis, or quadratus lumborum. MPS may also cause pain in limbs, chest, or shoulders.

RECOMMENDED DIAGNOSTIC APPROACH

- When confronted with a patient complaining of musculoskeletal pain, the clinician must first localize the anatomic site of the abnormality, then define the pathology, and finally identify underlying contributing factors or diseases. Structures that are present and the pathologic processes to which they are vulnerable include intraarticular and extraarticular (bursae, tendon) structures, bone, muscle, and nerve.

- Cardinal symptoms include pain, stiffness, loss of function, and sleep disturbance.

1. Pain in intraarticular disease is made worse by joint motion and relieved by rest. Pain in periarticular disease relates more closely to use of specific muscle groups than to joint motion. Bone pain increases with weight-bearing. Regional pain that is unremitting, nocturnal, burning or tingling, or associated with numbness suggests neuropathy. Generalized unremitting pain raises the question of functional disorder.

2. Stiffness on awakening or after sitting implies inflammation regardless of the structure involved; its dura-

tion is closely related to severity in synovitis and myositis.

3. Loss of function, distinguished from painful function, is often described as decreased range of motion in intraarticular disease ("can't bend my wrist") or in fibrosing soft tissue disease ("can't straighten my fingers"), but as decreased power in muscle or nerve disease ("keep dropping my glass").

4. Sleep disturbance is common in neuropathy and the functional pain syndromes; its occurrence in disease of other structures suggests severe pathology, tumor, or infection.

- Cardinal signs include swelling, tenderness, limited range of motion, weakness, and deformity.

1. Joints may have distention of the capsule, the thickened tender tissue characteristic of synovitis, or minimally tender nodules reflecting osteoarthritic spurs.

2. Muscle palpation may find generalized tenderness, trigger points, and tender points suggestive of myopathy, myofascial pain syndromes, or fibromyalgia, respectively. Muscle strength is tested for evidence of generalized weakness suggestive of myopathy or localized weakness suggestive of neuropathy or disuse.

3. Percussion along the length of the nerve (or maneuvers to stretch inaccessible nerves) may elicit symptoms (Tinel's signs) of entrapment neuropathy.

4. Joint movement may elicit crepitation in cartilage damage, "catching" suggestive of intraarticular loose bodies, limited range reflecting osteoarthritic spurs or loss of cartilage, or pain suggestive of inflammation.

- Laboratory evaluation may include:

1. Aspiration of effusions to distinguish crystal disease, infection, rheumatic disease, and acute internal derangements from more benign syndromes.

2. Further evaluation of clinical synovitis may include rheumatoid factor, ANA, cultures and serologies if infectious exposures suspected, thyroid function tests, and, when crystal synovitis is evident, serum creatinine, urate, calcium, and phosphate measurements.

3. Diffuse muscle tenderness, weakness, or wasting is evaluated with serum CK and aldolase levels, with muscle biopsy to follow. NCV and EMG are useful in evaluating suspected neuropathy.

4. Fever, weight loss, diffuse or multifocal inflammation, or other clinical suggestions of systemic illness warrant CBC, ESR, or CRP, screening tests for neoplasm appropriate to age, and cultures and serologies indicated by exposure history.

- Imaging

1. Plain X-rays will reveal fracture, dislocation, gross bone disease, joint space narrowing in cartilage disease, osteophytes, and marginal erosions in synovitis. CT is more sensitive to subtle abnormalities of bone, including osteopenia, osteomyelitis, tumor, and small fractures.

2. MRI is most useful in evaluating deep soft tissue disease and is the preferred method for imaging early osteonecrosis. Ultrasound is less expensive and often helpful in rotator cuff disease, synovial cysts, effusions of the hip joint, and intramuscular hematomas.

3. Bone scintigraphy permits very sensitive detection of early disease and is most often applied to evaluation of osteoarthritis, aseptic necrosis, early reflex sympathetic dystrophy, disc space infection, osteomyelitis, septic arthritis, and sickle cell disease.

4. Arthrography is used to visualize dissection, rupture, and loose bodies of the joint capsule. Arthroscopy has largely replaced this procedure for evaluation of mechanical disruption in the knee.

Bibliography

Campbell SM. Regional myofascial pain syndromes. Rheum Dis Clin North Am 1989;15:31.

Dawson DM, et al. Entrapment Neuropathies. Boston, Little, Brown, and Co., 1983.

Hadler NM. Medical Management of the Regional Musculoskeletal Diseases. Orlando, FL, Grune and Stratton, 1984.

Hunder GG, Michet CS. Giant cell arteritis and polymyalgia rheumatica. Clin Rheum Dis 1985;11:471.

Kozin F. The reflex sympathetic dystrophy syndrome. Bull Rheum Dis 1986;36:1.

Wolf F, et al. The American College of Rheumatology 1990 criteria for the classification of fibromyalgia. Arth Rheum 1990;33:160.

79

POLYARTHRITIS

CARIN E. DUGOWSON, *and*
THOMAS D. KOEPSELL

I never indulge in poetics
Unless I am down with rheumatics

QUINTUS ENNIUS (239–169 B.C.)

DEFINITION

- "Polyarthritis" is defined as pain and inflammation present simultaneously in 2 or more joints.
- An acutely inflamed joint exhibits swelling, warmth, and/or erythema. Other signs of inflammation include joint tenderness to palpation, joint effusion, restricted range of motion, pain with active or passive range of motion and crepitus, which is a grating felt or heard when the joint is moved.

DIFFERENTIAL DIAGNOSIS (Table 79–1)

The term "osteoarthritis" is a misnomer, since "arthritis" or the presence of inflammation is not a prominent feature of osteoarthritis (OA; see chapter 80).

EPIDEMIOLOGY (Table 79–2)

HISTORY (Table 79–3)

- All of the polyarthritides can occur with abrupt or gradual onset. Reiter's disease and gout have acute onset.
- Peripheral joint involvement is the rule in gout, rheumatoid arthritis (RA), and SLE; it is variably present in the other diseases.
  1. Ankylosing spondylitis always affects the axial skeleton.
  2. Reiter's syndrome is characterized by sacroiliitis.
  3. Psoriatic arthritis can cause a spondyloarthropathy or mimic rheumatoid arthritis.
  4. Gout has a marked predilection for the great toe, other metatarsophalangeal (MTP) joints, ankle, knee, and wrist.
  5. RA and SLE are characterized by symmetric, peripheral small joint involvement.

689

TABLE 79–1. Diseases That Can Cause Polyarthritis

Most common
Rheumatoid arthritis
SLE
AS
Psoriatic arthritis
Reiter's syndrome
Crystal-induced arthritis: gout, pseudogout
Less common
Arthritis associated with inflammatory bowel disease
Systemic sclerosis (scleroderma)
Rheumatic fever
Virus-associated arthritis (hepatitis B, rubella, HIV)
Mixed connective tissue disease (MCTD)
Polyarteritis nodosa
Sarcoidosis
Hemochromatosis
Gonococcal arthritis
OA

- Nonarticular features can also be very useful in the differential diagnostic process (see Table 79–3). Evidence of enthesopathy (inflammation at the attachment of ligaments to bone) suggests a spondyloarthropathy.

SIGNS

- By definition, arthritis is seen in all 6 illnesses. Symmetry and the specific joints involved are of great value in the diagnostic process.
- In patients with longer-standing or more severe disease, there are fairly specific joint deformities (Table 79–4).
- A careful search for extraarticular features is also rewarding.
  1. Rheumatoid nodules are seen almost only in RA and some overlap syndromes. They are found over the extensor surfaces of joints, particularly the fingers and elbows.
  2. Malar skin rash and alopecia are helpful in diagnosing SLE.
  3. Of patients with psoriatic arthritis, 84% have skin manifestations; the scalp and gluteal folds may be the only affected areas in mild skin disease.

LABORATORY STUDIES (Table 79–5)

- The erythrocyte sedimentation rate (ESR), though inexpensive and rapid, is of little diagnostic value because it is elevated in all of the inflammatory polyarthritides.
- A rheumatoid factor titer of 1 : 80 or greater by the latex fixation method is suggestive of RA. However, it is neither

Text continued on page 695

TABLE 79–2. Epidemiologic Characteristics of Selected Polyarthritides

FEATURE	RA	SLE	AS	GOUT	PSORIATIC ARTHRITIS	REITER'S SYNDROME
Prevalence	10–30/1000	0.1–1.0/1000	1–10/1000	1–3/1000	0.2–1.4/1000	1/1000
Sex	Females predominate 3:1	Females predominate 8–9:1	Males predominate 3:1	Marked male predominance	No gender predominance	Male predominance
Age	Steady increase with age	Peaks in 2nd to 4th decades	Peaks at age 15–30	Peak incidence 40–60 years old	Peaks at age 15–45	Peaks at age 15–45
Race	Little variation	Threefold higher risk for blacks	Fourfold higher risk for whites	Unknown	Unknown	Unknown
Other high risk groups	HLA-DR4	HLA-DR2, DR3, positive family history	HLA-B27– positive patients, certain Indian tribes	Obese and alcoholic	HLA-B27– positive patients	HLA-B27– positive patients

691

TABLE 79-3. Typical Symptoms of Selected Polyarthritides

FEATURE	RA	SLE	AS	GOUT	PSORIATIC ARTHRITIS	REITER'S SYNDROME
Onset	Gradual (80%)	Usually gradual	Usually gradual	Acute	Gradual or acute	Usually acute
Skeletal symmetry	Symmetric (> 80%)	Symmetric (> 80%)	Affects axial; asymmetric if peripheral joints affected	Usually asymmetric	Asymmetric (80%)	Asymmetric (95%)
Joints commonly affected	MCP, wrist, elbow, knee, shoulder, hip	PIP, MCP, knee, wrist, ankle, elbow	Spine, sacroiliac, costovertebral, hip, knee, shoulder	MTP, arch of foot, ankle, knee, wrist, hand	Hand and foot joints, axial skeleton, sacroiliacs	Knees, sacroiliac, ankle, feet
Morning stiffness	90–100%	20%	15%	Rare	Common	Common
Extraarticular symptoms	Fatigue, weight loss, sicca symptoms	Photosensitivity, CNS symptoms, renal disease, Raynaud's disease, pleuritis, sicca symptoms	Iritis	None	Skin lesions	Urethritis, iritis, enthesopathy, back pain

TABLE 79–4. Physical Signs of Selected Polyarthritides

FEATURE	RA	SLE	AS	GOUT	PSORIATIC ARTHRITIS	REITER'S SYNDROME
Deformities	Ulnar deviation at MCP, wrist, swan-neck and buttoniere deformities	Reducible soft tissue deformities of hand joints	Loss of spine motion	Joint erosion or fusion	Sausage digit, rheumatoid-like deformities	Rare
Extraarticular signs	Subcutaneous nodules on extensor surfaces, cutaneous vasculitis, carpal tunnel syndrome, pulmonary fibrosis	Malar rash, mucosal ulcers, discoid lupus, alopecia	Iritis, aortic regurgitation	Tophi	Psoriasis with nail pitting	Urethritis, circinate balanitis, oral ulcers, keratoderma blennorhagica

693

TABLE 79-5. Laboratory Features of Selected Polyarthritides

FEATURE	RA	SLE	AS	GOUT	PSORIATIC ARTHRITIS	REITER'S SYNDROME
ESR	Usually elevated	Usually elevated	Usually elevated	Elevated in acute phase	Elevated in acute phase	Elevated in acute phase
Rheumatoid factor (Latex fixation)	Usually positive (titer ≥ 1:80) after first year of disease	Positive in 20–40%	Normal for age	Normal for age	Normal for age	Normal for age
Antinuclear antibody	15–20% positive, usually low titer	>90% positive, usually titer ≥ 1:80	Normal for age	Normal for age	Normal for age	Normal for age
Anti-double-stranded DNA	Negative	Positive in 80–90%	Negative	Negative	Negative	Negative
HLA-B27 positive	6–8% (population frequency)	6–8%	90–95%	6–8%	20%	75–80%
X-ray	Periarticular osteopenia, symmetric erosion without new bone formation	Soft-tissue swelling, periarticular osteopenia	Vertebral ankylosis, sacroiliitis	Joint erosion with overhanging margin, joint destruction, ankylosis, tophi	Distal phalangeal tuft resorption, erosion with sclerosis, pencil-in-cup deformity	Sacroiliitis, plantar spur

perfectly sensitive nor specific for RA. Particularly in early rheumatoid arthritis, the rheumatoid factor may be negative.

- The antinuclear antibody (ANA) test, in titers of 1 : 80 or greater, is sensitive and specific for SLE. Primary Sjögren's syndrome and mixed connective tissue disease (MCTD) may also be associated with a positive ANA. Some ethnic groups have an increased prevalence of positive ANAs in healthy individuals.

- Antibodies to double-stranded DNA are essentially pathognomonic for SLE, though they are far less sensitive than the ANA.

- An X-ray of joint(s) most frequently clinically affected is among the most valuable tests for differential diagnosis, provided the disease process has been sufficiently chronic.
    1. Hand X-rays can show characteristic joint abnormalities in gout, RA, and the spondyloarthropathies.
    2. Sacroiliac and lumbar spine X-rays will identify the majority of patients with AS; however, sacroiliac X-rays can also be abnormal in Reiter's and psoriatic arthritis.

- A bone scan can be extremely useful in the early diagnosis of inflammatory joint disease, although it may not be able to distinguish among them. The bone scan has increased uptake in affected joints before the X-ray is abnormal.

- Arthrocentesis of an affected joint is also extremely helpful in confirming the diagnosis of inflammatory arthritis.
    1. Turbidity usually correlates with leukocyte count and can be abnormal in the inflammatory syndromes. Marked turbidity raises the question of joint infection.
    2. Viscosity is inversely related to inflammation and inflamed joints show watery joint fluids.
    3. All joint fluids should be cultured, since infection is more common in joints with an underlying abnormality and because signs of infection can be subtle.
    4. Crystal examination of the joint fluid can definitively diagnose gout (uric acid) or pseudogout (calcium pyrophosphate).

RECOMMENDED DIAGNOSTIC APPROACH

- Historical points of interest include the presence of systemic symptoms (especially morning stiffness), inflammatory bowel symptoms, eye symptoms, or mucocutaneous symptoms which may not have been previously diagnosed.

- The physical examination should include careful scrutiny of both small and large joint for swelling, pain, decrease in range of motion, and deformity. The pattern of joint involvement should be noted. The presence of extraarticular signs should also be sought including skin lesions, pleuropericarditis, rheumatoid nodules, and mucosal ulcerations.

- If an arthritic process has been present for more than 6 to 8 weeks, an X-ray of the affected joint(s) is indicated.

1. Hand X-rays can be diagnostic if gout, RA, or psoriatic arthritis are suspected.
2. AS or Reiter's syndrome is possible, sacroiliac and/or lumbar spine films are appropriate.

- Arthrocentesis is indicated if there is a significant effusion in a joint and the diagnosis is not certain.
- Careful choice of serologies will minimize the false-positives due to the nonspecificity of these tests.

1. A rheumatoid factor should be done if RA is considered.
2. A negative ANA is uncommon in SLE. A positive Smith antigen or anti-double stranded DNA confirms the diagnosis of SLE.

Bibliography

Beary FJ III, et al. Manual of Rheumatology and Outpatient Orthopedic Diseases. Boston, Little, Brown, 1981.

Getter RA. A Practical Handbook of Joint Fluid Analysis. Philadelphia, Lea & Febiger, 1984.

Kelley WN, et al., eds. Textbook of Rheumatology, 3rd ed. Philadelphia, W. B. Saunders, 1989.

Spiegel TM, ed. Practical Rheumatology. New York, Wiley, 1983.

80

OSTEOARTHRITIS

CARIN E. DUGOWSON, *and*
THOMAS D. KOEPSELL

Pain wanders through my bones like a lost fire.
THEODORE ROETHKE (1908–1963)

DEFINITION

- Osteoarthritis (OA), also called degenerative joint disease (DJD), is a clinical syndrome of joint symptoms and signs associated wth defective integrity of cartilage and changes in underlying bone at the joint margin. OA results in joint space narrowing, osteophyte formation and the clinical syndrome of joint pain, stiffness, and restricted range of motion.

- Although the pathogenesis is not known, OA appears to be partly a consequence of changes in bone and articular cartilage seen with aging.

- OA can be either primary (idiopathic) or secondary, when it is associated with a predisposing condition such as trauma or a congenitally abnormal joint.

EPIDEMIOLOGY

- OA is the most common musculoskeletal disease, with an overall prevalence of almost 10% of the U.S. population.
- Risk factors (Table 80–1)
  1. Age. OA is more common in the older age groups. This corresponds to the increased prevalence of X-ray findings of OA with increasing age. However, there is a poor correlation between X-ray findings and clinical symptoms.
  2. Underlying joint abnormality. Any event or condition that causes incongruity or damage to a joint surface will predispose to OA, including trauma, congenital joint abnormality, and inflammatory or infectious joint disease.
  3. Obesity. Increased weight is a risk factor for knee OA.
  4. Occupations. Those with significant stress on a limited number of joints may have an increase in OA over the general population.
  5. Handedness. OA is more common in the dominant extremity.

697

TABLE 80–1. Some Preexisting Conditions Thought to Predispose to Secondary DJD

Previous joint disease or injury
    Trauma
    Infectious arthritis
    Aseptic necrosis
    Menisectomy (knee)
    Intraarticular steroids
    Rheumatoid arthritis
    Gout
    Pseudogout
    Spondyloarthropathy
    Congenital hip dysplasia
    Neuropathic joint (Charcot's arthropathy)
Endocrine or metabolic disease
    Diabetes mellitus
    Paget's disease
    Hyperparathyroidism
    Acromegaly
    Ochronosis
    Hemochromatosis
    Wilson's disease
    Homocystinuria
Other
    Hemophilia
    Sickle cell disease
    Many heritable syndromes: mucopolysaccharidoses, Ehlers-Danlos syndrome, Marfan's syndrome, multiple epiphyseal dysplasia, and others

CLINICAL FEATURES

- Historical
  1. Joint pain in one or a limited number of joints.
  2. Systemic signs and symptoms should not be present or should be attributable to another condition.
  3. Morning stiffness is shorter than 30 min.
  4. Character of pain:
     a. Pain increases with or following activity.
     b. Pain is more common late in the day.
     c. Rest and sleep improve symptoms.
  5. Pattern of joint involvement
     a. Hips, knees, distal interphalangeal joints (DIPs), lumbar, and cervical spine commonly involved.
     b. Wrist, metacarpophalangeal joints, and shoulders rarely involved in the absence of a predisposing condition.
     c. Can be asymmetrical.
- Physical examination
  1. Pain is localized to the joint and especially the joint margin on palpation or movement.
  2. Range of motion is often decreased.
  3. Bony enlargement is common. When present at the DIPs they are called Heberden's nodes.

4. Crepitus (joint grating with movement) is often heard or felt with movement.
5. Heat and erythema are generally absent. There is a subgroup of patients with inflammatory OA, also called erosive OA, where both heat and erythema can be seen in affected joints. This is most common in the hands.
6. Joint effusions, if present, are generally small.

LABORATORY EVALUATION

1. No abnormalities characteristic of OA are found in blood tests. The ESR, blood counts, and routine blood chemistries are not altered by OA.
2. Joint fluid in OA patients is clear, viscous, and non-clotting.
   a. Total white cell count is:
      <500 cells/mm^3 in 52% of cases
      <1000 cells/mm^3 in 86% of cases
      <2000 cells/mm^3 in 93% of cases
      Cell differential is generally mononuclear cells.
   b. Protein content is nearly always <3 g/dl.
   c. Microscopic examination shows few cells and no bacteria. Occasionally, urate crystals, generally not phagocytosed, can be seen in joints without apparent crystal-related symptoms.
3. X-ray. Characteristic findings include loss of joint space, marginal osteophytes, sclerosis of the subchondral bone, and bone cysts. Periarticular osteopenia, as seen in inflammatory arthritis, is absent.

DIFFERENTIAL DIAGNOSIS

Two of the most important differential diagnoses:
- Crystal-induced arthropathy (gout and pseudogout)
  1. Can co-exist with OA.
  2. Usually has an abrupt onset of symptoms.
  3. Swelling, erythema, and exquisite tenderness of affected joint are common.
  4. Laboratory: elevated serum uric acid in 80% of gout patients.
  5. X-rays
     Gout: periarticular bony erosions
     Pseudogout: calcification of the cartilage in knees and wrists (chondrocalcinosis)
- Rheumatoid arthritis
  1. Causes a symmetric, systemic inflammatory arthritis.
  2. Morning stiffness and fatigue are common systemic symptoms.
  3. The small joints of the feet and hands are most commonly involved. Older patients may have shoulder, knee, and hip involvement. Joint swelling, erythema, and heat are common.

4. Laboratory. Rheumatoid factor and ESR are often abnormal.
5. X-rays. Periarticular osteopenia occurs in early disease. Later disease shows joint erosions and joint space narrowing.

RECOMMENDED DIAGNOSTIC APPROACH

- A careful history and physical examination should allow tentative diagnosis of OA.
- X-ray of the affected joint(s) should be done if the diagnosis is uncertain or initial therapy is unsuccessful.
- Arthrocentesis is indicated if there is any significant effusion or the joint is warm or red. The fluid should be evaluated for appearance (turbidity and viscosity), cell count and differential, total protein, crystals, and culture.

Bibliography

Acheson RM, et al. New Haven survey of joint diseases. XII. Distribution of symptoms of osteoarthrosis in the hand with reference to handedness. Ann Rheum 1970;29:275–286.

Hamerman D. Mechanisms of disease: The biology of osteoarthritis. N Engl J Med 1989;320:1322–1330.

Kelsey JL. The Epidemiology of Musculoskeletal Conditions. New York, Oxford University Press, 1983.

Moskowitz RW. Clinical and laboratory findings in osteoarthritis. In: McCarty DJ, ed. Arthritis and Allied Conditions, 11th ed. Philadelphia, Lea & Febiger, 1989.

National Center for Health Statistics. Osteoarthritis in Adults by Selected Demographic Characteristics. United States, 1960–1962. Vital and Health Statistics, Series 11, No. 20, 1966.

81

GOUT AND PSEUDOGOUT

ANTHONY SAWAY

Be temperate in wine, eating, girls, and sloth, or the gout will seize you and plague you both.

Poor Richard's Almanac (1734)
BEN FRANKLIN (1706–1790)

GOUT

Definitions

Gout refers to the clinical syndromes produced by monosodium urate (MSU) crystal deposition.

Epidemiology

Primary gout is most common in men 30 to 59 years old and is uncommon in women before menopause. The incidence in postmenopausal women is similar to that in men. Primary gout occasionally occurs in adolescent males with a large body mass.

Gout can coexist with calcium pyrophosphate dihydrate deposition disease (CPDD) and, uncommonly, with infectious arthritis.

Clinical Manifestations

Gout occurs in 3 stages.
- Acute gout
  1. Acute gout most often presents as a mono- or oligoarthritis. It can be polyarticular.
  2. The attack often begins at night. In a person receiving therapy for gout, improper use of medications or noncompliance can precipitate an attack.
  3. The joint involvement in gout is usually asymmetric with a propensity to "migrate."
     a. The joints most commonly affected include the first metatarsophalangeal (MTP) ("podagra"), tarsals, ankles, wrists, and elbows. Involvement of the shoulders or hips is uncommon.
     b. In postmenopausal women with primary osteoarthritis of the hands, acute gout can occur in preexisting Heberden's nodes, especially in patients using diuretics.

4. The joint inflammation is intense with prominent erythema.
   a. Tenosynovitis and cutaneous inflammation can be prominent features of acute gout and suggest infection when accompanied by fever and leukocytosis.
   b. Acute bursitis, especially of the olecranon and prepatellar bursae, can also occur.
5. Acute gout is self-limited, usually lasting less than 2 weeks; however the symptoms are severe enough that patients seek treatment.

- Intercritical gout
  1. Recurrent attacks with symptom-free intervals (that may be long) occur in most patients.
  2. In untreated gout, recurrent attacks tend to become more frequent and can cause a chronic arthropathy.
- Chronic gout
  1. In some persons, persistent hyperuricemia leads to tophaceous deposits, usually preceded by recurrent attacks of acute gout. Tophi can be subcutaneous, periarticular, intraarticular, intraosseus, or nonarticular (helix of pinna) and may cause chronic joint inflammation, destruction, and deformity.
  2. Although nephrolithiasis from urate stones is common and can precede gout, urate nephropathy is uncommon.

Laboratory Studies

- Hyperuricemia precedes gout but is not always evident during acute attacks.
- Synovial fluid
  1. Synovial fluid analysis is the most important diagnostic test in a patient who may have gout.
  2. The synovial fluid has an elevated WBC count (5000 to 100,000/mm^3).
  3. Monosodium urate (MSU) crystals, which appear negatively birefringent and needle-shaped by polarized microscopy, are detectable in most cases of gout. In 15% of initial aspirates, crystals are not seen. Repeated arthrocenteses may be indicated.
- Synovial tissue. Biopsy is rarely necessary for the diagnosis of gout. Tissue sections can demonstrate gouty granulomata but require special processing.
- Radiographic studies (Table 81–1)
  1. In the initial attack, soft tissue swelling is usually the only radiographic finding. Intraosseus gout can cause bony destruction that mimics tumor or infection.
  2. The radiographic differential diagnosis of gout includes OA, amyloidosis, hyperlipoproteinemia, pannus-producing arthropathies (e.g., RA), and multicentric reticulohistiocytosis.

TABLE 81–1. Radiographic Findings of Gout and Pannus-producing Arthropathies

RADIOGRAPHIC FEATURE	GOUT	PPA
Soft tissue swelling	Asymmetric	Symmetric
Joint space	Often preserved	Usually lost or narrowed
Periarticular osteopenia	Uncommon	Common
Erosions	Yes	Yes
Corticated	Common	Uncommon
Location relative to the joint	Nonmarginal or marginal	Marginal
Overhanging margin	Yes	No
Bony overgrowth	Yes	No

Differential Diagnosis

1. The classic presentation of gout, podagra, is often viewed as synonymous with gout. Pseudogout, psoriatic arthritis, sarcoidosis, and RA can all present with podagra *and* hyperuricemia.
2. OA or inflamed bunions can be mistaken for gout.
3. Besides gout, the most common causes of acute mono- or oligoarthritis are infectious arthritis, pseudogout, a seronegative spondyloarthropathy, sarcoidosis, or trauma.
4. Chronic arthritis in gout is usually oligo- or polyarticular. The differential diagnosis includes RA, CPDD, polymyalgia rheumatica, generalized OA, the seronegative spondyloarthropathies (especially Reiter's syndrome and psoriatic arthritis), sarcoidosis, amyloidosis, hemochromatosis, and multicentric reticulohistiocytosis.

Recommended Diagnostic Approach

- Establish the diagnosis
  1. Gout is confirmed when MSU crystals are recovered from the site of inflammation or a tophus. Crystal confirmation of the diagnosis is recommended in *all cases* initially.
  2. In the absence of crystal confirmation, the diagnosis of acute gouty arthritis can be made from clinical criteria (Table 81–2). Confirmation by crystal analysis is preferred.
  3. Patients with intercritical or chronic gout can have subcutaneous nodules or radiographic evidence of tophi from which MSU crystals can be readily recovered. In the absence of an acute presentation, aspiration of a tophus is usually preferred since the yield of

TABLE 81–2. Clinical Criteria for Diagnosis of Gout[a]

More than one attack of acute arthritis
Maximal inflammation developing within 1 day
Monarticular arthritis
Joint redness
Painful or swollen first MTP joint
Unilateral attack in a first MTP joint
Unilateral attack in a tarsal joint
Suspected tophi
Hyperuricemia
At radiography, asymmetric joint swelling
At radiography, subcortical cysts without erosions
Negative results of microbial culture of joint fluid

[a] Six or more of the listed criteria required for a clinical diagnosis of gout.

Source: Wallace SL, et al. Preliminary criteria for the classification of the acute arthritis of primary gout. Arth Rheum 1977; 20(3):895–900.

MSU crystals is high and because aspiration of tophi is often less traumatic than arthrocentesis.

- Classify the mechanism of gout (Table 81–3)
  1. A 24-hr urine collection for uric acid and creatinine should be done to distinguish uric acid overproduction from underexcretion.
  2. A healthy person on a purine-restricted diet has a 24-hr urine uric acid of about 600 mg. Strict adherence to a purine-restricted diet is difficult and the study is often conducted without dietary restriction.
  3. Impaired renal excretion of uric acid is present in 95% of patients with hyperuricemia. Underexcretors have low or normal 24-hr urine uric acid levels and overproducers have levels > 800 to 1000 mg. This distinction can guide therapy.

PSEUDOGOUT

Definitions

- Calcium pyrophosphate dihydrate deposition disease (CPDD) refers to the musculoskeletal syndromes produced by the deposition of calcium pyrophosphate dihydrate (CPPD) crystals (Table 81–4).
- Chondrocalcinosis refers to cartilage calcification evident radiographically or pathologically
  1. It can result not only from CPPD deposition, but also from dicalcium phosphate dihydrate and hydroxyapatite crystals.
  2. It is seen with aging and following trauma, is frequently asymptomatic, and is not synonymous with CPDD.
- Pseudogout is one manifestation of CPDD that clinically resembles acute gout.

TABLE 81–3. Disorders and Disturbed Physiological States Associated with Gout and/or Hyperuricemia

Hyperuricemia due to excessive uric acid production
1. Inherited enzyme defects
   a. Hypoxanthine-guanine phosphoribosyl transferase deficiency
   b. 5-Phosphoribosyl-1-pyrophosphate synthetase superactivity
   c. Glucose-6-phosphatase deficiency
2. Increased cell turnover
   a. Malignant diseases, especially myeloproliferative and lymphoproliferative disorders
   b. Nonmalignant diseases: hemolytic anemias, psoriasis, obesity
3. Increased purine nucleotide catabolism
   a. Tissue hypoxia
   b. Glycogenoses types III, V, VII
   c. Drug-induced: ethanol, fructose, cytotoxic agents
4. Increased purine ingestion
   a. Purine-rich diets
   b. Pancreatic extract
Hyperuricemia due to impaired renal uric acid excretion
1. Renal disease
   a. Chronic renal failure
   b. Lead nephropathy
   c. Polycystic kidney disease
   d. Hypertension
2. Abnormal metabolic states
   a. Starvation
   b. Dehydration
   c. Salt restriction
   d. Lactic acidemia
   e. Glycogenosis type I
   f. Diabetic ketoacidosis
   g. Eclampsia
   h. Bartter's syndrome
3. Endocrinopathies
   a. Hyperparathyroidism
   b. Hypothyroidism
   c. Nephrogenic diabetes insipidus
4. Drug-induced
   a. Diuretics
   b. Low-dose salicylates
   c. Ethanol
   d. Ethambutol
   e. Pyrazinamide
   f. Levodopa
   g. Methoxyflurane
   h. Laxative abuse (alkalosis)
5. Other
   a. Sarcoidosis
   b. Berylliosis
   c. Down syndrome

Source: Becker MA. Clinical aspects of gout. Rheum Dis Clin North Am 1988;14(2): 377–394.

TABLE 81–4. Classification of CPPD Crystal Deposition Disease

Hereditary
Sporadic (idiopathic)
Associated with metabolic disease
  Hyperparathyroidism
  Familial hypocalcuric hypercalcemia
  Hemochromatosis
  Hemosiderosis
  Hypothyroidism
  Gout
  Hypomagnesemia
  Hypophosphatasia
  Amyloidosis
Associated with joint trauma or surgery

From: Schumacher HR, ed.: Primer on the Rheumatic Disease, 9th ed. Atlanta, Georgia: The Arthritis Foundation, 1988, p. 207.

Epidemiology

- CPDD is less common than gout and uncommon before the age of 50. Its prevalence increases with age. Males are affected slightly more often than females.
- CPDD may result from a metabolic disorder. Uncommonly, CPDD may coexist with gout or infectious arthritis.

Clinical Features

Several clinical syndromes may result from CPDD.
- Many patients with radiographic or pathologic evidence of CPPD deposition remain asymptomatic.
- Pseudogout
  1. Clinically mimics gout. Like acute gout, attacks can be precipitated by surgery or acute medical illness. It can coexist with gout and infectious arthritis.
  2. May involve any synovial joint, but the knee accounts for one-half of all cases.
  3. Occurs in 25% of cases of CPDD.
  4. Patients can have hyperuricemia.
- Pseudo-rheumatoid arthritis
  1. Chronic symmetric polyarthritis affecting small and large joints that clinically resembles RA.
  2. Erosions, nodules, and deformities similar to those in RA are not seen unless CPDD and RA coexist.
  3. Accounts for 5% of cases of CPDD.
  4. Approximately 10% of patients have a positive rheumatoid factor.
- Pseudo-osteoarthritis
  1. Clinical syndrome is similar to OA. A severe destructive arthropathy resembling a neuropathic joint can occur.
  2. Commonly affected joints include the knees, wrists, metacarpophalangeals (MCPs), hips, shoulders, el-

bows, ankles, and first MTP. CPDD should be suspected when OA-like changes occur in joints not commonly affected with primary osteoarthritis (such as the wrists, MCPs, shoulders, elbows, and ankles).

3. Accounts for one-half of cases of CPDD.

- Other
  1. Achilles tendonitis
  2. Olecranon, infrapatellar, and retrocalcaneal bursitis

Laboratory Studies

- Synovial fluid analysis
  1. As in gout, this is the most important laboratory study in the diagnosis of CPDD. The fluid may be minimally inflammatory or grossly purulent.
  2. CPPD crystals are typically rhomboid shaped but can be pleomorphic (including needle shaped). CPPD crystals have weak positive birefringence under polarized light unlike the strongly negatively birefringent crystals of gout.
- Synovial tissue is rarely required for diagnosis. The CPPD crystals are preserved during routine processing of synovial tissue.
- Radiographic features of CPDD (Table 81–5).
- Additional laboratory studies are intended to diagnose conditions that are associated with CPDD.
  1. In the absence of clinical or radiographic findings suggesting an underlying metabolic disorder, routine laboratory screening in CPDD is unnecessary. It should be considered in patients under 50.
  2. Tests that should be considered include the serum cal-

TABLE 81–5. Radiographic Features of CPDD That May Distinguish It From Osteoarthritis

1. Unusual articular distribution: can involve joints not commonly affected in primary osteoarthritis, i.e. wrists, elbows, shoulders, MCP joints.
2. Unusual intraarticular distribution: isolated involvement of the:
   a. Radiocarpal or trapezioscaphoid articulations of the wrist
   b. Patellofemoral articulation of the knee
   c. Talocalcaneal articulation of the midfoot
3. Prominent subchondral cyst formation. Multiple cysts of variable size.
4. Severe progressive destructive arthropathy that may be extensive or associated with intraarticular osseous bodies.
5. Variable osteophyte formation.

Adapted from: Resnick D, Niwayama G: Crystal-induced and related diseases. In Resnick D, Niwayama G: Diagnosis of Bone and Joint Disorders, 2nd ed. Philadelphia: W.B. Saunders, 1988, pp. 1703–1705.

cium, phosphorus, magnesium, alkaline phosphatase, ferritin, iron, transferrin, TSH, and uric acid.

Differential Diagnosis

1. Due to the older patient group, the differential diagnosis of acute CPDD (pseudogout) differs somewhat from gout. Possible diagnoses include gout, calcium hydroxyapatite crystal deposition disease, infectious arthritis, RA, carcinomatous arthritis, and polymyalgia rheumatica.
2. Chronic CPDD (pyrophosphate arthropathy) most closely resembles primary osteoarthritis. It should also be considered in patients with extensive joint destruction as seen in neuropathic arthropathy but who lack neurologic abnormalities.

Recommended Diagnostic Approach

- Establish the diagnosis
  1. The diagnosis of CPDD is based upon demonstration of CPPD crystals in synovial fluid from a symptomatic joint or the characteristic radiographic findings.
  2. In the acute arthropathy of CPDD (pseudogout), the radiographic findings are often confined to soft tissue swelling.
     a. The diagnosis often depends upon demonstration of CPPD crystals. These small, weakly positive birefringent crystals can be difficult to identify and frequently occur in small numbers.
     b. Infectious arthritis must be excluded by Gram's stain and culture of the synovial fluid.
  3. In chronic CPDD, synovial fluid is often not available or CPPD crystals are not recovered. The diagnosis is then based upon the distribution of joint involvement and radiographic findings.
- Categorize the CPDD. If the patient is under 50, a careful search for an underlying metabolic disease should be done. Most patients over 50 have idiopathic CPDD.

Bibliography

Gatter RA. A Practical Handbook of Joint Fluid Analysis. Philadelphia, Lea and Febiger, 1984.
Kelley WN, et al. eds. Gout and related disorders of purine metabolism. In: Kelley WN, et al. Textbook of Rheumatology, 3rd ed. Philadelphia, W.B. Saunders, 1989. pp. 1395–1448.
McCarty DJ, ed. Crystalline deposition diseases. Rheum Dis Clin North Am, 1988;14(2)253–495.
Moskowitz RW. Diseases associated with deposition of calcium pyrophosphate or hydroxyapatite. In: Kelley WN, et al., eds. Textbook of Rheumatology, 3rd ed. Philadelphia, W.B. Saunders, 1989. pp. 1449–1467.

82

SPONDYLO-ARTHROPATHIES

BRUCE GILLILAND

The rheumatism is a common name for many aches and pains, which have yet got no peculiar appelation, through owing to very different causes.

WILLIAM HEBERDEN (1710–1801)

DEFINITION AND GENERAL COMMENTS
(see Tables in Chapter 79)

- Spondyloarthropathies are a group of disorders that have in common the following features:
  1. Spine inflammation: sacroiliitis and spondylitis.
  2. Peripheral joint arthritis: usually 5 or less joints are involved in an asymmetric pattern. There is a predilection for the lower extremity joints.
  3. Enthesopathy: inflammation at sites of insertion of tendons, ligaments, and fascia into bone (collectively called entheses).
  4. Extraarticular manifestations, the most common of which are:
     a. Acute anterior uveitis
     b. Aortic valve insufficiency
     c. Cardiac conduction abnormalities
     d. Mucocutaneous lesions
  5. Young adults, especially men, are more often affected.
  6. Haplotype B27 of the histocompatibility antigen complex (HLA-B27) is found in a high percentage of patients with spondyloarthropathy.
  7. Rheumatoid factor is not found in patients with this group of disorders (thus the term "seronegative").
- Disorders classified as spondyloarthropathies include:
  1. Ankylosing spondylitis (AS)
  2. Reiter's syndrome, including reactive arthritis associated with nongonococcal urethritis, and intestinal infection by strains of *Shigella, Yersinia, Salmonella,* and *Campylobacter*
  3. Psoriatic arthritis
  4. Arthritis associated with inflammatory bowel disease: Crohn's disease and ulcerative colitis.

ANKYLOSING SPONDYLITIS

- Definition. AS is an inflammatory arthritis predominantly of the spine. Both sacroiliac joints are affected and peripheral arthritis may be present.
- Epidemiology
  1. The male to female ratio is 3 : 1. The prevalence of AS in Caucasians is 0.1 to 0.2%. It is less common in blacks and rare in patients of Asian descent.
  2. The frequency of HLA-B27 in AS patients is 90%. The occurrence of AS in those who are HLA-B27 positive is 20%.
- Clinical features
  1. Onset. The disease begins between puberty and age 35. The peak age of onset is in the mid-20s.
  2. Sacroiliac joints and spine symptoms
     a. Symptoms begin insidiously as pain and/or stiffness in the low back.
     b. Morning stiffness which lasts 30 min or longer is often present in the lower back. It usually improves with physical activity.
     c. Deep buttock pain and pain radiating into the posterior thighs may be experienced. Pain can alternate from side to side.
     d. Back symptoms ascend from the lumbar spine to involve the thoracic and cervical spine.
     e. With time, back and neck mobility decrease. Fusion occurs involving part or most of the spine which becomes osteoporotic. The spine fuses in varying degrees of flexion.
     f. Chest expansion may become limited due to involvement of costovertebral and costosternal joints.
  3. Peripheral arthritis. Arthritis is usually monarticular involving a hip or knee.
  4. Enthesopathy
     a. The most common sites of enthesopathy are at the insertions of the Achilles tendon and plantar fascia into the calcaneus.
     b. Pleuritic chest pain may result from inflammation at intercostal muscle insertions.
  5. Extraarticular manifestations
     a. Acute anterior uveitis is usually unilateral and recurrent. It may antedate signs and symptoms of spine disease. Delay in treatment may lead to acute glaucoma.
     b. Aortic insufficiency and heart block result from inflammation of the aortic valve and atrioventricular conduction bundle, respectively. They usually appear after several years of disease.
     c. Neurologic complications
        i. The fused and osteoporotic cervical spine is susceptible to fracture, which can result in spinal cord compression.
        ii. Chronic arachnoiditis around the sacral nerves may cause a cauda equina syndrome

manifest by pain and sensory loss in the lower extremities and bladder or bowel dysfunction.
   d. Pulmonary. Fibrobullous apical disease occurs in 1% of patients.
   e. Renal. Secondary amyloidosis occurs in 4% of patients. IgA nephropathy is a rare manifestation.
- Laboratory features
  1. Blood studies. A mild hypoproliferative anemia is occasionally present. The sedimentation rate is usually elevated. The HLA-B27 antigen is found in greater than 90% of patients.
  2. Radiographic examination
     a. Sacroiliac joints. Early in the disease, blurring of margins, irregular subchondral erosions, and patchy sclerosis are present. Later, the joints become fused.
     b. Spine. Initially, there is straightening of the lumbar spine with squaring of the vertebral bodies. Syndesmophytes form along the lateral and anterior sides of the intervertebral disc and bridge adjacent vertebrae.
     c. Enthesis. Erosions, sclerosis, fluffy new bone, and spurs are observed at sites of tendon insertions.
  3. ECG. In patients with cardiac involvement, varying degrees of heart block may be present.
- Diagnostic clues
  1. The diagnosis is evident in the patient with advanced stages of disease by the characteristic immobile spine and bent-over posture. It should be considered in a young adult male who experiences low back pain and greater than 30 min of morning stiffness that typically decreases with physical activity.
  2. The diagnosis of AS is strengthened by a positive family history. A history of prior or current episodes of anterior uveitis in a patient with low back pain should also suggest the diagnosis of AS.
  3. Low back pain due to disc or facet joint disease differs from that of AS by the lack of significant duration of morning stiffness and the worsening of symptoms with physical activity.
  4. When peripheral joint arthritis is the predominant feature, confusion with RA may occur. The asymmetric pattern of arthritis, negative rheumatoid factor, and radiographic evidence of bilateral sacroiliitis differentiates AS from RA.
  5. AS is distinguished from other spondyloarthropathies by bilateral sacroiliitis and other clinical features.

REITER'S SYNDROME

- Definitions
  1. Reiter's syndrome is characterized by the triad of urethritis, conjunctivitis, and arthritis which appear in sequence over time.

2. Incomplete Reiter's syndrome is a diagnosis given to patients with a characteristic oligoarticular arthritis, usually of the lower extremity joints, who do not have urethritis or conjunctivitis.

3. Reactive arthritis applies to patients with features of Reiter's syndrome in whom a discrete triggering organism can be identified. Microorganisms that can trigger reactive arthritis include *Salmonella typhimurium*, *Salmonella enteritidis*, *Shigella flexneri*, *Yersinia pseudotuberculosis*, *Camplyobacter fetus*, *Chlamydia trachomatis*, chronic cutaneous infection (acne fulminans), HIV infection, and *Mycobacterium avium-intracellulare*.

· Epidemiology. Young adults are affected with a male-to-female ratio of 9 : 1.

· Clinical features

1. Reiter's syndrome typically follows sexual exposure or a diarrheal illness.

2. Urethritis is often the first sign and is characterized by transient mucopurulent or mucoid discharge and dysuria, but it can be asymptomatic.
   a. Prostatitis may be present in 80% of male patients.
   b. In women, vaginitis or cervicitis may be present.

3. Conjunctivitis is bilateral and usually mild. Uveitis can also develop during the illness.

4. Arthritis is oligoarticular with a predilection for the lower extremity joints, particularly knees and ankles.
   a. The onset is often acute or subacute. An episode usually lasts several months.
   b. One-third of patients have recurrent episodes over years and about 20% develop a chronic arthritis; joint damage can occur in these patients. A few patients have self-limited illnesses.
   c. Unilateral sacroiliitis occurs and causes buttock and back pain. Spinal involvement above the sacroiliac joints is unusual.
   d. Enthesopathy leads to Achilles tendonitis, plantar fasciitis, and chest wall pain. Patients may present complaining of a tender heel.
   e. Dactylitis produces a sausagelike digit, resulting from inflammation of the joints and the adjacent tendon sheath fascia.

5. Mucocutaneous lesions
   a. Keratoderma blennorrhagicum describes cutaneous lesions that occur most often on the soles of the feet, toes, and glans penis. Lesions also can appear on the palms, scalp, scrotum, and trunk. They begin as small vesicles which become opaque papules. The papules become hyperkeratotic, and may coalesce to form plaques.
   b. Circinate balanitis is characterized by painless superficial erosions of the glans penis. Lesions may begin as small vesicles that rupture to produce shallow erosions and coalesce to form a circinate pattern. In circumcised patients, lesions become crusted; in uncircumcised patients, they

remain moist and can become infected. Circinate balanitis can antedate other features of Reiter's syndrome.

c. Mucosal lesions present as painless superficial ulcerations which occur on the palate, tongue, buccal mucosa, and lips.

d. Nail involvement appears as brownish-orange discoloration of the nail caused by the accumulation of subungual hyperkeratotic material. Periungual erythema may be present.

- Laboratory evaluation
  1. Blood studies. A mild hypoproliferative anemia and/or leukocytosis may be present. The ESR is elevated. HLA-B27 is present in 60 to 75% of patients.
  2. Synovial fluid studies. Leukocyte counts range from 5000 to 50,000/mm^3 and are predominantly neutrophils.
  3. Radiographic features
     a. Peripheral joint X-rays are initially normal. Spurs and fluffy periosteal new bone form at sites of tendon insertions, particularly the calcaneus.
     b. Sacroiliac X-rays shows unilateral involvement.
     c. Spine X-rays may detect syndesmophytes that are not symmetrically distributed along the spine and are not as extensive as in AS. They arise from near the middle of the vertebral body rather than from its margin as seen in AS.

- Diagnostic clues
  1. The diagnosis of Reiter's syndrome should be considered in a sexually active young man who presents with an acute or subacute onset of arthritis which is asymmetric and involves predominantly the lower extremities. Dactylitis (sausage toe) and/or heel tenderness may be present.
  2. The arthritis is usually preceded within a month by nongonococcal urethritis. Reiter's syndrome or reactive arthritis may follow a diarrheal illness.
  3. When only arthritis is present, other spondyloarthropathies or rheumatoid arthritis should be considered. Septic arthritis should be excluded by arthrocentesis when arthritis is acute and involves only 1 or 2 joints in the absence of other features of Reiter's syndrome.

PSORIATIC ARTHRITIS

- Definition. Psoriatic arthritis is a seronegative inflammatory arthritis which occurs in association with psoriasis. Peripheral joints and the spine are affected. Arthritis develops in about 5% of patients with psoriasis.
- Epidemiology. The male-to-female ratio is 1:1. HLA-B27 is present in 50% of patients with spinal involvement. Peripheral arthritis is associated with HLA haplotypes Bw38 and Bw39 and not with B27.

- Clinical features
  1. Arthritis affects predominantly young adults but can occur in children and older patients.
  2. Skin disease usually precedes arthritis. The severity of arthritis does not correlate with extent or activity of skin disease. Nail pitting is more common in patients with arthritis.
  3. Arthritis and skin disease can be triggered by HIV infection.
  4. Five clinical patterns of arthritis are recognized:
     a. Distal interphalangeal joint involvement of fingers and/or toes.
     b. Asymmetric oligoarthritis of peripheral joints.
     c. Symmetric polyarthritis with negative rheumatoid factor.
     d. Arthritis mutilans, which is a deforming arthritis that causes severe destruction of peripheral joints.
     e. Sacroiliitis with or without spondylitis.
  5. Asymmetric oligoarthritis is the most common pattern. Arthritis mutilans is often associated with spinal involvement. For most patients with arthritis, the course tends to be indolent and slowly progressive.

- Laboratory features
  1. Blood studies. The CBC is usually normal and the rheumatoid factor is negative. The sedimentation rate may be elevated.
  2. Radiographic features
     a. Whittling of the proximal phalangeal tuft shaft at the distal and proximal interphalangeal joints and hypertrophic cupping of the distal phalanx gives the appearance of a "pencil in cup" deformity. This feature may also be seen in other spondyloarthropathies, but is less frequent.
     b. New bone formation adjacent to periarticular bone erosions occurs more often with psoriatic arthritis than with other types of spondyloarthropathy.
     c. The axial skeletal findings are similar to Reiter's syndrome.

- Diagnostic clues
  1. The diagnosis of psoriatic arthritis should be considered with any one of the above described patterns of arthritis occurring in a patient with psoriasis. The lesions of psoriasis may be very subtle and hidden in the scalp, intergluteal fold, or umbilicus.
  2. Occasionally, an oligoarticular arthritis with a sausage digit(s) occurs in the absence of psoriatic lesions or features of Reiter's syndrome, but psoriasis may subsequently appear.
  3. Acute dactylitis or monarticular arthritis can mimic septic arthritis or gout.
  4. Psoriatic arthritis is distinguished from rheumatoid arthritis by the absence of rheumatoid factor.

ARTHRITIS ASSOCIATED WITH INFLAMMATORY BOWEL DISEASE

- Definition. A peripheral and/or spine arthritis may occur in patients with IBD (ulcerative colitis, Crohn's disease). Arthritis may precede symptoms of bowel disease especially in patients with Crohn's disease.

- Clinical features
  1. Peripheral arthritis
     a. Approximately 20% of patients have joint symptoms. Arthralgias are the most common manifestation, but patients may develop an acute arthritis affecting one or a few joints.
     b. The most commonly involved joints are the knees, ankles, or wrists. Arthritis lasts for a few weeks and does not usually result in residual joint damage.
     c. Acute arthritis may be accompanied by fever, oral ulcers, erythema nodosum, or pyoderma gangrenosum.
     d. Acute arthritis usually indicates active bowel disease and may herald the appearance of bowel symptoms. Effective treatment of the bowel disease (including by colectomy in patients with ulcerative colitis) leads to disappearance of the arthritis.
  2. Spine arthritis
     a. Sacroiliitis with or without higher spinal involvement occurs in approximately 10% of patients with IBD. The pattern of spondylitis is indistinguishable from AS.
     b. The spinal disease progresses independently of bowel inflammation. Treatment of the bowel disease or a colectomy does not affect the course of the spondylitis.

- Laboratory features
  1. Blood tests reflect the underlying IBD. HLA-B27 is present in only half of patients with spondylitis. Peripheral arthritis is not associated with HLA-B27.
  2. The radiographic findings of spondylitis associated with IBD are indistinguishable from those of AS. X-rays of peripheral joints are usually normal.
  3. The joint fluid of patients with acute peripheral arthritis is characteristic of acute inflammation.

- Diagnostic clues. It may initially be difficult to distinguish reactive arthritis following a diarrheal illness from the peripheral arthritis of IBD. The latter is often accompanied by aphthous stomatitis, erythema nodosum, uveitis, or pyoderma gangrenosum. When these symptoms are not present, the subsequent clinical course of IBD clearly distinguishes these disorders.

RECOMMENDED DIAGNOSTIC APPROACH

In a patient presenting with features suggesting one of the spondyloarthropathies, the following work-up is recommended.

- History
  1. Ask the patient about low back pain, buttock pain, and whether pain radiates down the back of the leg to the knee.
  2. Question the patient about prior episodes of peripheral arthritis.
  3. Ask about previous episodes of acute conjunctivitis or uveitis, bowel symptoms, urethral discharge, painful urination, vaginal discharge, and skin or oral lesions.
- Physical examination
  1. Note the pattern of arthritis and the presence of dactylitis (sausage digit).
  2. Examine the sacroiliac joints by palpation and maneuvers that move the sacroiliac joint (causing pain when the joint is inflamed).
     a. Compress the iliac wings together.
     b. Patrick's maneuver, in which, with the patient supine, one foot is placed on the opposite knee causing flexion, abduction, and external rotation of the leg. One hand is placed on the opposite superior iliac crest to stabilize the pelvis while the other hand applies downward pressure on the externally rotated knee. This maneuver torques the sacroiliac joints.
  3. Inspect the back for loss of lumber lordosis and atrophy of paravertebral muscles which give the lower back an "ironed-out" or flattened appearance. Baseline clinical measurement should be made.
     a. Schober's test measures flexion of the lumbosacral spine: a 10-cm vertical line is measured upward, along the vertebrae, from the level of the posterior iliac spines. The patient is asked to bend forward, and the amount of distraction of the line is measured; more than 5 cm is considered normal.
     b. Chest expansion with respiration should be measured. It should be 2.5 cm or greater when measured in the 4th intercostal space.
  4. Examine the skin and nails for evidence of psoriasis. The soles and palms may have lesions of keratoderma blennorrhagicum.
  5. On examination of the genitourinary tract, look for balanitis, urethral discharge, prostatitis, vaginitis, and cervicitis.
  6. Examine the eye for conjunctivitis and iritis (past or present).
  7. The mouth should be examined for oral ulcers on the tongue, palate, and buccal mucosa.
- Laboratory evaluation should include the following:
  1. CBC and ESR.
  2. Rheumatoid factor.

3. An HLA-B27 test should be ordered only when the history and physical examination are suggestive of one of the HLA-B27–associated spondyloarthropathies. HLA-B27 is present in 6% of Caucasian individuals, and it is of little diagnostic value in a patient with vague back symptoms or arthralgias.

4. Synovial fluid examination should be performed in a patient with an acute monarticular arthritis where the possibility of septic or crystal-induced arthritis cannot be excluded.

5. Radiographic studies should include X-rays of affected peripheral joints when the diagnosis is in doubt or for evaluation of joint damage and X-rays of the sacroiliac joints and spine when spondylitis is suggested clinically.

Bibliography

Arnett FC. Seronegative spondyloarthropathies. Bull Rheum Dis 1987;37:1.

Calin A, ed. Spondyloarthropathy. New York, Grune and Stratton, 1984.

Kaye BR. Rheumatologic manifestations of infection with human immunodeficiency virus. Ann Intern Med 1989;111:158–167.

Keat A. Reiter's syndrome and reactive arthritis in perspective. N Engl J Med 1983;309:1606–1615.

Khan MA. Medical and surgical treatment of seronegative spondyloarthropathy. Curr Opin Rheumatol 1990;2:592.

Khan MA, Khan MK. Diagnostic value of HLA-B27 testing in ankylosing spondylitis and Reiter's syndrome. Ann Intern Med 1982;94:70–76.

83

SYSTEMIC LUPUS ERYTHEMATOSUS

BRUCE C. GILLILAND

What you should put first in all the practice of our art is how to make the patient well; and if he can be made well in many ways, one should choose the least troublesome.

HIPPOCRATES

DEFINITION AND GENERAL COMMENTS

- Systemic lupus erythematosus (SLE) is an immunologically mediated multisystem disorder most often affecting the skin, joints, serosal membranes, kidneys, and CNS. There are hematologic and immunologic abnormalities and antinuclear antibodies (ANAs) in virtually all patients.
- SLE affects predominantly women of child-bearing age (female-to-male ratio is 9 : 1). It occurs in the very young and old of both sexes and is more frequent in black Americans.
- Environmental factors may aggravate or induce SLE. Ultraviolet light may precipitate skin lesions or exacerbate cutaneous disease.

CLINICAL FEATURES (Table 83–1)

- Constitutional symptoms. Fever, anorexia, weight loss, or fatigue are frequent, especially with active disease.
- Musculoskeletal manifestations
  1. Arthralgias or myalgias occur in 95% of patients.
  2. A nonerosive symmetric polyarthritis affecting the small joints of the hands, feet, wrists, and knees is present in 60% of patients.
  3. Arthritis may be migratory and transient, resolving within 24 hr. In a few patients arthritis causes damage to the joint capsule resulting in flexion contractures and reducible joint subluxation.
  4. Muscle pain and weakness may be due to myositis.
- Cutaneous manifestations
  1. A fixed erythematous malar ("butterfly") rash over the cheeks and bridge of the nose occurs in half of patients. The rash may also involve the chin or ears.
  2. Discoid lesions occur in 15% of patients and appear on the head and neck, extremities, and, less often, the

TABLE 83–1. Clinical Features of SLE

FEATURE	FREQUENCY (%)
Constitutional	
Fever	80
Anorexia and weight loss	60
Fatigue	90
Musculoskeletal	
Arthralgia or myalgia	95
Symmetric polyarthritis	60
Cutaneous	
Malar rash	50
Photosensitive rash	40
Alopecia	40
Oral ulcer	40
Raynaud's phenomenon	30
Discoid lesion	15
Renal disease	50
Pulmonary	
Pleuritis	50
Pneumonitis	10
Cardiac	
Pericarditis	30
Myocarditis	10
Neuropsychiatric disease	50–75
Hematologic	
Lymphadenopathy	50
Splenomegaly	10–20

trunk. These lesions cause scarring and are disfiguring:
3. Other types of skin lesions in SLE patients are urticaria/angioedema, erythema multiforme, petechiae, maculopapules, and vesiculobullae.
4. Rashes are photosensitive in 40% of patients.
5. Alopecia occurs in 40% of patients. It may be patchy or diffuse and permanent or reversible.
6. Oral ulcers, which may be painful, occur in 40%.
7. Vasculitic skin lesions manifest as nailfold or volar pad infarcts, palpable purpura, ulcers, or livedo reticularis. Raynaud's phenomenon occurs in 30% of patients.
8. Panniculitis (lupus profundus) occurs in 10%.
9. Subacute cutaneous lupus erythematosus (SCLE)
   a. This is a subset of SLE characterized by a photosensitive rash that is erythematous, annular, or papulosquamous (psoriasiform).
   b. Healing of skin lesions results in hypopigmentation but not scarring.
   c. Patients usually do not have significant renal disease. Antibodies to Ro (SS-A) are present and the patients usually have the HLA-DR3 haplotype.
- Renal manifestations
  1. Clinical renal disease occurs in half of all SLE patients. It is classified into 4 types:
     a. Mesangial: 25%.
     b. Segmental focal glomerulonephritis (GN): 15%.

      c. Diffuse proliferative GN: 45%.

      d. Membranous GN: 15%.

  2. Segmental focal GN progresses to diffuse GN in 20 to 30% of cases. Diffuse proliferative GN carries the worst prognosis.

  3. Renal vein thrombosis and hypertension are complications of renal disease. Renal disease is the leading cause of death due to SLE.

- Pulmonary manifestations

  1. Pleurisy is common, occurring in 50% of patients. Pleural effusions are usually small and a pleural friction rub may be present.

  2. Lupus pneumonitis is seen in 10% of cases and manifests as fever, cough, and dyspnea. Pulmonary infiltrates and hypoxemia are usually present.

  3. Chronic interstitial pneumonitis may occur but is not common.

  4. Pulmonary hypertension may result from pulmonary arteritis.

  5. SLE predisposes to thrombophlebitis, which may cause pulmonary embolism.

- Cardiac manifestations

  1. Pericarditis occurs in one-third of patients. Chest pain or a pericardial friction rub may be present. Myocarditis occurs in 10% of cases.

  2. Libman-Sacks endocarditis (verrucous vegetations) is present in many patients but usually does not produce symptoms.

  3. Valvular lesions occur in 20% of patients and may produce aortic or mitral regurgitation.

  4. Coronary arteritis may cause myocardial infarction. The presence of anticardiolipin antibodies is associated with MI.

  5. Glucocorticoid therapy is associated with coronary artery atherosclerosis and MI.

- GI manifestations

  1. Vasculitis of the mesentery or bowel wall produces abdominal pain, diarrhea, and bleeding. It may progress to bowel infarction or perforation.

  2. Acute pancreatitis may be a manifestation of SLE or due to glucocorticoid therapy.

- Neurologic manifestations

  1. Neuropsychiatric symptoms occur in 50 to 75% of patients.

  2. CNS symptoms include headaches which may simulate migraine, behavioral abnormalities including psychosis, cognitive dysfunction, seizures, strokes, chorea, ataxia, aseptic meningitis, transverse myelitis.

  3. Peripheral or cranial neuropathies may also occur.

  4. Antineuronal antibodies, especially if present in the CSF, correlate with the presence of CNS lupus.

- Hematologic manifestations (see Table 83–2). Lymphadenopathy is present in half of patients and is more common in active SLE. Splenomegaly is present in 10 to 20%.

TABLE 83-2. Laboratory Features of SLE

FEATURE	FREQUENCY (%)
Hematologic	
Hypoproliferative anemia	50
Hemolytic anemia	10
Leukopenia	50–60
Thrombocytopenia	25–30
Antiphospholipid antibody	50
Immunologic	
Antinuclear antibody	95–100
Anti-double strand DNA antibody	70
Anti-Sm antibody	20–30
Anti-Ro (SS-A) antibody	30
Anti-La (SS-B) antibody	10
Anti-RNP antibody	40
Anti-histone antibody	70–95

- Ocular manifestations
  1. Patients may experience dry eyes as a manifestation of Sjögren's syndrome.
  2. Other features include episcleritis, optic neuritis, and retinal vasculitis.
- Antiphospholipid antibody syndrome
  1. Antiphospholipid antibodies occur in 40 to 50% of cases. Antiphospholipid antibodies include:
     a. The lupus anticoagulant
     b. Anticardiolipin antibodies
     c. The antibody responsible for the biologic false-positive test for syphilis that is seen in patients with SLE.
  2. Antiphospholipid antibodies are associated with arterial and venous thrombosis, recurrent fetal loss, thrombocytopenia, and hemolytic anemia.
  3. Patients may experience strokes and transient ischemic episodes. Recurrent deep vein thrombosis may lead to pulmonary emboli.
- Drug-induced SLE
  1. Many drugs may induce a positive ANA test, but only some of these patients develop symptoms of SLE. The most frequently implicated medications are procainamide, hydralazine, phenytoin, D-penicillamine, and alpha-methyldopa.
  2. The most common symptoms are arthralgias, arthritis, pleuritis, and pericarditis. Renal and CNS manifestations are rare.

DIFFERENTIAL DIAGNOSIS

- Patients with SLE may present with one or several clinical features. The clinical expression and course of disease is highly variable.

1. The most common presenting features are fatigue, arthralgias, arthritis, butterfly (malar) rash, and pleurisy.
2. Almost all patients have a positive ANA. When anti-double strand DNA or anti-Sm antibodies are present in a patient with consistent clinical features, the diagnosis is established.
3. The American College of Rheumatology revised criteria for the classification of SLE are listed in Table 83–3. These criteria are for the primary purpose of identifying SLE patients for clinical studies. To be classified as SLE, a patient must have 4 or more of the 11 criteria at some point in their illness.

- Many of the clinical features of SLE are also seen in other connective tissue disorders:
    1. Rheumatoid arthritis (RA)
        a. Both RA and SLE may have a symmetric peripheral polyarthritis.
        b. SLE can be differentiated by the following:
            i. Joint fluid is usually noninflammatory.
            ii. Lack of periarticular bone erosions and fixed joint deformities.
            iii. Presence of nephritis, rash, or CNS disease.
    2. Systemic sclerosis
        a. Both disorders may cause Raynaud's phenomenon and musculoskeletal symptoms.
        b. SLE is differentiated by the lack of sclerodactyly and other skin changes of systemic sclerosis.
    3. Dermatomyositis (DM)
        a. Rashes (including photosensitivity), arthritis, and muscle weakness may be present in both disorders.
        b. SLE is usually associated with normal muscle enzymes. The rash of SLE usually does not occur over the extensor surfaces of joints (as does the rash in DM).
    4. Mixed connective tissue disease (MCTD)
        a. Serious renal disease is uncommon in patients with MCTD.
        b. Patients with MCTD have high titers of anti-ribonucleoprotein (anti-RNP) antibodies.
    5. Sjögren's syndrome
        a. Patients with SLE may have dry eyes and/or mouth; in this case they are considered to have secondary Sjögren's syndrome.
        b. Patients with primary Sjögren's syndrome usually do not have significant GN. Anti-double strand DNA and anti-Sm antibodies are not present.
    6. Drug-induced SLE. The drug history of all patients with SLE should be reviewed. The finding of ANAs restricted to anti-histones suggests drug-induced lupus.
    7. Multiple sclerosis (MS). Patients with MS usually do not have positive ANAs. SLE may be distinguished when other clinical features of SLE appear.

TABLE 83–3. The 1982 Revised Criteria for Classification[a] of SLE

CRITERION	DEFINITION
1. Malar rash	Fixed erythema, flat or raised, over the malar eminences, tending to spare the nasolabial folds.
2. Discoid rash	Erythematous raised patches with adherent keratotic scaling and follicular plugging; atrophic scarring may occur in older lesions.
3. Photosensitivity	Skin rash as a result of unusual reaction to sunlight, by patient history or physician observation.
4. Oral ulcers	Oral or nasopharyngeal ulceration, usually painless, observed by a physician.
5. Arthritis	Nonerosive arthritis involving 2 or more peripheral joints, characterized by tenderness, swelling, or effusion.
6. Serositis	a. Pleuritis: convincing history of pleuritic pain or rub heard by a physician or evidence of pleural effusion. OR b. Pericarditis: documented by electrocardiography or rub or evidence of pericardial effusion.
7. Renal disorder	a. Persistent proteinuria greater than 0.5 g/day or greater than 3+ if quantitation not performed. OR b. Cellular casts: may be red cell, hemoglobin, granular, tubular, or mixed.
8. Neurologic disorder	a. Seizures: in the absence of offending drugs or known metabolic derangements e.g., uremia, ketoacidosis, or electrolyte imbalance. OR b. Psychosis: in the absence of offending drugs or known metabolic derangements e.g.,

Table continued on following page

TABLE 83–3. The 1982 Revised Criteria for Classification[a] of SLE *Continued*

CRITERION	DEFINITION
	uremia, ketoacidosis, or electrolyte imbalance.
9. Hematologic disorder	a. Hemolytic anemia: with reticulocytosis.
	OR
	b. Leukopenia: $<4000/mm^3$ total on 2 or more occasions.
	OR
	c. Lymphopenia: $<1500/mm^3$ total on 2 or more occasions.
	OR
	d. Thrombocytopenia: $<100,000/mm^3$ in the absence of offending drugs.
10. Immunologic disorder	a. Positive LE cell preparation.
	OR
	b. Anti-DNA: antibody to native DNA in abnormal titer.
	OR
	c. Anti-Sm: presence of antibody to Sm nuclear antigen.
	OR
	d. False positive serologic test for syphilis known to be positive for at least 6 months and confirmed by *Treponema pallidum* immobilization or fluorescent treponemal antibody absorption test.
11. Anti-nuclear antibody	An abnormal titer of antinuclear antibody by immunofluorescence or an equivalent assay at any point in time and in the absence of drugs known to be associated with "drug-induced lupus" syndrome.

[a] The proposed classification is based on 11 criteria. For the purpose of identifying patients in clinical studies, a person shall be said to have SLE if any 4 or more of the 11 criteria are present, serially or simultaneously, during any interval of observation.

Source: Reprinted with permission from Tan EM, et al. The 1982 revised criteria for the classification of systemic lupus erythematosus. Arthritis Rheum 1982;2511:1271.

LABORATORY STUDIES (see Table 83–2)

- Urine tests. Urinalysis in patients with nephritis may show proteinuria that is mild or in the nephrotic range. An active urine sediment contains red cells or casts (red cell, white cell, or hyaline).
- Blood tests
  1. Hematologic studies
     a. Hypoproliferative anemia (anemia of chronic disease) is present in half of SLE patients.
     b. In patients with a Coombs' positive hemolytic anemia (10% of all SLE patient), IgG, and/or C3 is found on the red cell membrane. Frank hemolysis occurs in only a few patients.
     c. Leukopenia occurs in 50 to 60% of patients, but only 15% have a leukocyte count less than $4000/mm^3$.
     d. Thrombocytopenia (platelet count $<100,000/mm^3$) is present in 25 to 30% of patients but severe thrombocytopenia with purpura and bleeding occurs in less than 5% of patients.
  2. Renal function. Elevated levels of serum creatinine and BUN indicate renal dysfunction.
  3. Coagulation studies
     a. Antiphospholipid antibodies are present in half of patients with SLE. They are associated with thrombosis.
        i. The lupus anticoagulant is detected by a prolonged partial thromboplastin time and is present in 15% of patients.
        ii. Anticardiolipin antibodies are found in 40% of patients.
        iii. A biologic false-positive serologic test for syphilis occurs in 25% of patients.
     b. Antibodies to coagulation factors VIII, IX, XI, XII, or XIII may occur in patients with SLE and may be associated with bleeding.
  4. Antinuclear antibodies
     a. Almost all patients with SLE have a positive ANA test with a standard immunofluorescence screening assay.
        i. This test, while sensitive, is not specific for SLE and is positive in a small number (less than 5%) of normal people and patients with other diseases.
        ii. The frequency of a positive ANA in apparently healthy persons increases with age in older patients.
        iii. The likelihood of SLE or another connective tissue disease increases when the ANA titer is ≥ 4 times the threshold value for defining a positive test.
     b. Anti-double strand (native) DNA is found in 70% of patients and is seldom seen in other connective tissue diseases. Anti-DNA antibodies are often associated with renal disease.
     c. Anti-Sm ("Sm" stands for Smith) occurs in only

20 to 30% of SLE patients, but is highly specific for SLE.

d. Anti-Ro (SS-A) occurs in 30% of SLE patients and is associated with SCLE and neonatal lupus. Anti-Ro is also seen in patients with primary Sjögren's syndrome.

e. Anti-La (SS-B) is present in 10% of SLE patients and is seen in conjunction with anti-Ro.

f. Anti-RNP occurs in 40% of SLE patients. High titers are associated with MCTD.

g. Anti-histone antibodies are present in 70% of SLE patients and 95% of patients with drug-induced SLE.

5. Complement studies

a. Blood levels of total hemolytic complement (CH_{50}), C3, and C4 are reduced in active SLE, especially when renal disease is present. Low levels usually reflect consumption of complement by immune complexes.

b. A CH_{50} level that is zero or undetectable with normal C3 and C4 levels suggests an hereditary deficiency of a complement component. C2 deficiency is the most common hereditary complement deficiency.

6. Immunologic tests

a. Immune complex assay. Immune complexes are most often measured by the C1q binding assay. Elevated levels of immune complexes correlate with clinical activity in some patients.

b. Rheumatoid factor is found in 25% of SLE patients.

c. Polyclonal hypergammaglobulinemia is frequent.

- CNS studies

1. The CSF in patients with CNS lupus has elevated protein and levels of IgG and a mild pleocytosis. Anti-neuronal antibodies in the CSF may correlate with active CNS disease.

2. CT or MRI may show abnormalities in patients with CNS lupus.

3. EEG may reveal focal CNS abnormalities.

- Synovial fluid analysis. Joint fluid in patients with SLE is clear or slightly cloudy with low cell counts.

RECOMMENDED DIAGNOSTIC APPROACH

- When a patient presents with features suggesting SLE, an ANA screening test should be obtained.
- If the ANA is positive, specific antinuclear antibody tests should be obtained:

1. Anti-double strand DNA
2. Anti-Sm
3. Anti-Ro (SS-A)
4. Anti-RNP
5. Anti-histone when drug-induced SLE is suspected

- Serum complement studies are useful to evaluate for complement consumption by immune complexes or the possibility of an hereditary complement deficiency.
- A CBC with ESR, urinalysis, and serum creatinine and BUN levels should be obtained. Other laboratory studies should be obtained based on the clinical picture.

Bibliography

Asherson RA, et al. The "primary" antiphospholipid syndrome: Major clinical and serological features. Medicine 1989;68:366–374.

Klippel JH (ed.). Systemic lupus erythematosus. Rheum Dis Clin North Am 1988;14:1–252.

Swaak T, et al. Clinical significance of antibodies to double-stranded DNA (dsDNA) for systemic lupus erythematosus (SLE). Clin Rheumatol 1987 (June, Suppl.):56–73.

Tan EM. Antinuclear antibodies: Diagnostic markers for autoimmune disease and probes for cell biology. Adv Immunol 1989;44:93.

Tan EM, et al. The 1982 revised criteria for the classification of systemic lupus erythematosus. Arthritis Rheum 1982;2511:1271.

Wallace DJ, DuBois EL, eds. Dubois' Lupus Erythematosus, 3rd ed. Philadelphia, Lea and Febiger, 1987.

84

POLYMYOSITIS AND DERMATOMYOSITIS

ANTHONY SAWAY

The skin calls for faculty of close observations.

LOUIS DUHRING (1845–1913)

DEFINITION

- Polymyositis (PM) is an inflammatory disorder of unknown cause affecting primarily the muscles of the shoulder and pelvic regions.
- In dermatomyositis (DM), a characteristic rash is also seen.
- PM/DM can also occur in childhood and in association with connective tissue disorders. The association of PM/DM with malignancy is controversial.

EPIDEMIOLOGY

The annual incidence of PM is 3–6 cases per million. Women are affected more often than men. There is a bimodal age distribution. In childhood, DM is more common; in adults, PM is seen more often.

DIFFERENTIAL DIAGNOSIS
(See Table 84-1)

CLINICAL FEATURES

- Common presenting symptoms of PM/DM include the following:
  1. Dysfunction from proximal muscle weakness
     a. Shoulder girdle: difficulty reaching overhead, combing hair, shaving, brushing teeth, picking up objects
     b. Pelvic girdle: difficulty getting out of a chair, off of toilet, out of tub, going up steps, getting in and out of car
     c. Neck weakness: flexor involvement greater than extensor involvement
  2. Myalgia is usually not severe and is usually less prominent than weakness.

TABLE 84–1. Differential Diagnosis of Polymyositis/Dermatomyositis

Drug-induced myopathy
  Glucocorticosteroids
  Penicillamine
  Chloroquine derivatives
  Colchicine
  Cimetidine
  Clofibrate
  Emetine
  Lovastatin
  Alcohol
Myositis associated with other connective tissue diseases
  (including overlap syndromes)
  Scleroderma
  SLE
  MCTD
  Sjögren's syndrome
  RA
Inclusion body myositis
Eosinophilic fasciitis
Infectious myositis
  Viral
    Influenza
    HIV
    Coxsackie
    Echovirus and adenovirus (in patients with congenital
      agammaglobulinemia)
    Epstein-Barr virus
    Rubella
  Bacterial
    Staphylococcus
    Streptococcus
    Clostridium
    Salmonella typhi
    Mycobacterium leprae
  Spirochetal: *Borrelia burgdorferi*
  Protozoal: *Toxoplasma gondii*
  Parasitic: *Trichinella spiralis*
Endocrine
  Hypothyroidism
  Hyperthyroidism
  Cushing's syndrome
  Hyperparathyroidism
  Hypoparathyroidism
  Diabetic amyotrophy
Metabolic
  Hypokalemic periodic paralysis
  Carnitine deficiency
  Myophosphorylase deficiency (McArdle's disease)
  Phosphofructokinase deficiency
  Carnitine palmityl transferase deficiency
  Mitochondrial myopathies
  Adult acid maltase deficiency

Table continued on following page

TABLE 84–1. Differential Diagnosis of Polymyositis/Dermatomyositis *Continued*

Neurologic
  Noninflammatory myopathies: muscular dystrophies
  Diseases of the neuromuscular junction
    Myasthenia gravis
    Eaton-Lambert syndrome
  Proximal neuropathies
    Porphyria
    Diabetes mellitus
  Motor neuron disease: amyotrophic lateral sclerosis

3. Dysphagia
4. Arthralgias or arthritis (more common in overlap syndromes)
5. Raynaud's phenomenon (more common in overlap syndromes)
6. Rash
   a. Gottron's papules: Specific for DM, these are erythematous to violaceous patches, often scaly, that overlie the dorsum of the metacarpophalangeal and proximal interphalangeal joints of the hand, elbows, knees, or medial malleoli.
   b. Heliotrope rash: A violaceous rash on the upper eyelids, which are often edematous and which is strongly suggestive of DM in the appropriate clinical setting.

- The association of PM/DM and malignancy is controversial. An exhaustive search for malignancy is not warranted beyond a comprehensive history and physical examination (including examination of stools for occult blood, pelvic examination with cervical cytology, complete blood count and chemistry screen, chest X-ray, and, possibly, mammography).

LABORATORY FEATURES

- Measures of muscle injury
  1. Serum levels of enzymes released from muscle are elevated.
  2. Creatine phosphokinase (CPK)
     a. This is usually elevated in cases of PM/DM but the level does not correlate with the degree of muscle weakness or inflammation seen on biopsy.
     b. The total CPK level is useful in monitoring response to therapy. Because regenerating muscle fibers contain significant levels of the isoenzyme CPK-MB, as much as 20% of the total CPK may be of the MB type even when there is no cardiac involvement.
  3. Aldolase
     a. This enzyme level can be elevated when the CPK is normal.

    b. Increased serum levels occur with muscle inflammation but also in disorders affecting the heart, liver, and bone marrow.

4. Other studies
    a. The lactate dehydrogenase (LDH) and serum glutamic-oxaloacetic transaminase (SGOT or AST) can also be elevated in PM/DM. They are less useful due to their low specificity.
    b. Myoglobinemia and myoglobinuria are usually present but their measurement does not add information to measurements of the serum enzymes.

- Immunologic abnormalities (autoantibodies)
1. Antinuclear antibody (ANA, by immunofluorescence) is detected in one-fourth of patients with either PM or DM. It is more frequent in patients with an associated connective tissue disease.
2. PM is often associated with a distinctive group of antibodies directed against transfer-RNA synthetases.
    a. Anti-Jo-1 is an antibody that reacts with histidyl-transfer-RNA. It is present in 30% of patients with PM and 70% of patients with PM and interstitial lung disease.
    b. Other autoantibodies have been detected in patients with PM/DM, however their clinical usefulness has not been determined.

- Electrophysiologic studies
1. Electromyography (EMG) is useful in confirming the presence of a myopathy. Nerve conduction studies can exclude denervation as a cause of the patient's symptoms.
2. A positive EMG occurs in 90% of patients with PM/DM. Paraspinous muscles may be abnormal when limb muscles are normal.
3. Characteristic electrophysiologic findings of PM include:
    a. Small amplitude, short duration, polyphasic motor unit potentials.
    b. Spontaneous fibrillations, positive spike waves at rest, with increased insertional irritability.
    c. Bizarre high frequency repetitive discharges.
    d. Absence of neuropathy.
4. EMG can assist in the selection of a muscle biopsy site.

- Muscle biopsy
1. The positive histopathologic findings in acute PM/DM consist of either focal or diffuse inflammatory infiltrates containing lymphocytes and macrophages surrounding muscle fibers and blood vessels. The muscle cells may have features of degeneration and regeneration.
2. Sampling error (i.e., false-negative results) can occur if the inflammatory process is focal.
3. Common biopsy sites include the deltoid, biceps, and quadriceps muscles.
    a. The muscle to be biopsied should be weak but not atrophic.

b. The biopsied muscle must have had no recent intramuscular injections or needle insertions. A common strategy is to perform EMG on one side and to biopsy the contralateral side.

4. A muscle biopsy is indicated in all cases initially. Additional biopsies may be helpful in cases refractory to treatment.

RECOMMENDED DIAGNOSTIC APPROACH

• PM/DM is a clinicopathologic diagnosis supported by laboratory and electrophysiologic findings. In suspected cases, the serum CPK and aldolase levels should be measured. If both are normal, PM is unlikely.

• If elevated levels are present, an EMG should be done to confirm the presence of a myopathic process and to assist in selecting the muscle group for biopsy.

1. The EMG is performed unilaterally and the muscle biopsy is performed contralaterally.

2. Paraspinous muscles should be studied if the limb EMG does not confirm a myopathy.

• A directed muscle biopsy should be taken from patients with myopathic findings. In patients who have negative EMG findings, a random muscle biopsy may be taken from the biceps, deltoid, or quadriceps muscles.

• A definitive diagnosis depends on a positive biopsy.

Bibliography

Bohan A, et al. A computer-assisted analysis of 153 patients with polymyositis and dermatomyositis. Medicine 1977;56:255–286.

Bradley WG, et al. Inflammatory diseases of muscle. In Kelley WN, et al., eds. Textbook of Rheumatology, 3rd ed. Philadelphia, W.B. Saunders Company, 1989.

Bunch TW. Polymyositis: A case history approach to the differential diagnosis and treatment. Mayo Clin Proc 1990;65:1480–1497.

Dalakas MC. Medical progress: polymyositis, dermatomyositis, and inclusion-body myositis. N Engl J Med 1991;325:1487–1498.

85

SYSTEMIC SCLEROSIS (SCLERODERMA)

BRUCE C. GILLILAND

Physicians think they do a lot for a patient when they give his disease a name.

IMMANUEL KANT (1724–1804)

DEFINITION

- Systemic sclerosis (scleroderma) is characterized by fibrosis of skin, blood vessels, and internal organs, including the GI tract, lungs, heart, and kidneys.
    1. It occurs in several forms, which have different prognoses. Some features of this disorder may occur in conjunction with other connective tissue diseases.
    2. This disorder occurs in all races and is more common in women.
    3. The disease is associated with immunologic abnormalities. Vascular damage may contribute to organ dysfunction.
    4. Diffuse cutaneous scleroderma
        a. In these patients, skin involvement can be rapidly progressive and extensive.
        b. Internal organ disease is more likely to occur, especially in the kidneys. The prognosis is determined by the degree of visceral involvement.
    5. Limited cutaneous scleroderma
        a. These patients have cutaneous involvement restricted to the distal extremities and face.
        b. This form is also referred to as the CREST syndrome: calcinosis, Raynaud's phenomenon, esophageal dysmotility, sclerodactyly, and telangiectasias.
        c. Pulmonary hypertension or biliary cirrhosis may occur.
- Mixed connective tissue disease (MCTD)
    1. Patients with MCTD have some features of scleroderma, SLE, RA, and polymyositis.
    2. High titers of autoantibodies to ribonucleoprotein (RNP) may be present.
- Overlap syndrome. Patients have diagnostic criteria for systemic sclerosis as well as for another connective tissue disease such as Sjögren's syndrome, polymyositis, or SLE.
- Drug-induced or chemically induced scleroderma (or scleroderma-like illness)

1. Polyvinyl chloride: Raynaud's phenomenon, acroosteolysis, and sclerodermatous skin changes.
2. Pentazocine: scleroderma-like skin changes.
3. Bleomycin: fibrotic skin nodules and pulmonary fibrosis.
4. L-Tryptrophan: eosinophilia-myalgia syndrome, which is characterized by myalgias and diffuse fasciitis affecting predominantly the lower extremities. Scleroderma-like skin may result as well as peripheral neuropathy, diarrhea, and respiratory symptoms.

- Localized scleroderma (morphea) indicates cutaneous involvement without internal organ disease. The lesions may be small and circumscribed.

CLINICAL FEATURES

- Raynaud's phenomenon. Episodic (usually cold-induced) blanching of the fingers or toes occurs in at least 90% of patients with systemic sclerosis and may antedate other features by months or years.
- Skin
  1. The fingers, distal extremities, and face are swollen in the early stages of systemic sclerosis. Later, the skin becomes firm, thickened, and hide-bound. In the late phase of disease, the skin becomes atrophic.
  2. Small ulcers may develop on the fingertips. Resorption of the distal digits may also occur.
  3. Skin changes in the distal extremities usually progress proximally. The face is usually involved as is, in some patients, the trunk.
- Gastrointestinal
  1. Patients may complain of dysphagia and heartburn. Esophageal reflux is common, and esophageal strictures may develop. The esophagus may subsequently become distended and atonic.
  2. Atony of the small bowel may lead to bacterial overgrowth causing a malabsorption syndrome with weight loss, bloating, steatorrhea, and anemia.
  3. Large bowel involvement produces constipation and episodes of obstruction.
- Musculoskeletal
  1. Most patients complain of stiffness and swelling of their fingers and knees. Leathery crepitation may be appreciated over moving joints and/or tendons.
  2. Patients may have symmetrical polyarthritis resembling RA. Destructive arthritis is uncommon. An inflammatory myositis may lead to proximal muscle weakness.
- Cardiac
  1. Cardiomyopathy due to fibrosis leads to heart failure, heart block, and arrhythmias.
  2. Acute or chronic pericarditis may occur.
  3. Left ventricular failure can result from severe hyper-

tension. Pulmonary hypertension and fibrosis may cause right ventricular failure.

- Pulmonary
  1. Bilateral pulmonary fibrosis usually begins in the lower lobes and causes exertional dyspnea. Pulmonary hypertension with right-sided heart failure is a late finding.
  2. Patients with the CREST syndrome may develop pulmonary hypertension in the absence of pulmonary fibrosis. Exertional dyspnea is the earliest symptom.

- Renal
  1. Renal failure is the most common cause of death in patients with scleroderma and is more likely to occur in patients with rapidly progressive diffuse cutaneous scleroderma.
  2. Renal crisis is characterized by malignant hypertension, proteinuria, microscopic hematuria, and rapidly progressive renal failure.
  3. Microangiopathic hemolytic anemia and chronic pericardial effusion may be harbingers of impending renal crisis.

DIAGNOSIS

- The diagnosis of systemic sclerosis is based on clinical features that appear and evolve over time (months to years). Diagnosis is further strengthened by the presence of specific ANAs.
- Raynaud's phenomenon is usually the initial symptom followed by sclerodermatous skin changes in the distal extremities, which progress proximally and spread to the trunk. Facial skin tightening occurs simultaneously.
- Systemic features subsequently develop, including arthralgias and arthritis, esophageal dysmotility, pulmonary fibrosis, hypertension, heart failure, renal failure, dry eyes and/or mouth (Sjögren's syndrome).

DIFFERENTIAL DIAGNOSIS

- Raynaud's phenomenon may be an early feature of other connective tissue diseases including SLE, Sjögren's syndrome, and RA.
  1. The majority of patients with only Raynaud's phenomenon do not develop a connective tissue disease.
  2. When Raynaud's phenomenon is accompanied by changes in the vasculature of the nailfolds (decrease in the number of capillary loops along with capillary dilation) observed by wide angle microscopy or with an ophthalmoscope, systemic sclerosis is more likely.
  3. The presence of ANAs in a patient with only Raynaud's phenomenon increases the likelihood that the patient may develop a connective tissue disease.

- Arthralgias and arthritis are also observed in other connective tissue disorders, especially SLE and RA.
- Muscle weakness due to scleroderma is differentiated from polymyositis by the absence of elevated muscle enzymes. However, systemic sclerosis and polymyositis can coexist or be features of MCTD.
- Primary amyloidosis and scleromyxedema are rare disorders in which skin involvement may mimic systemic sclerosis.

LABORATORY STUDIES

- Blood and urine tests
  1. Hematologic studies
     a. Hypoproliferative anemia is common.
     b. A microangiopathic hemolytic anemia can occur in patients with renal involvement, especially renal crisis.
  2. Renal studies
     a. Urinalysis may show proteinuria. Red cells are seen in malignant hypertension.
     b. Elevated creatinine and BUN indicate renal failure.
  3. ANA studies. A positive ANA test is an indication for more specific tests.
     a. Anti-topoisomerase 1 (anti-Scl 70) is found in 20% of patients with systemic sclerosis and relatively rarely in other connective tissue diseases.
     b. Anticentromere antibodies are strongly associated with limited systemic sclerosis (CREST syndrome).
     c. Antinucleolar antibodies are found in 20 to 30% of patients but are not sensitive.
     d. Anti-RNP also occurs in systemic sclerosis and, when in high titer, points to the diagnosis of MCTD.
  4. Other immunologic studies
     a. Hypergammaglobulinemia occurs in one-third of patients.
     b. Rheumatoid factor is found in 25% of patients.
     c. Serum complement levels are normal.
- Radiographic studies
  1. Chest X-ray. Bilateral lower lobe pulmonary fibrosis is the earliest radiographic sign of pulmonary disease in patients with systemic sclerosis.
  2. Barium studies
     a. Esophageal dysmotility is seen early, followed later by esophageal dilation. Strictures from esophagitis can also develop.
     b. Gastric and/or small bowel atony can be present.
     c. Barium enema may detect large mouth diverticula of the colon.
- ECG. Heart block and arrhythmias occur in systemic sclerosis and may be asymptomatic.

- Pulmonary function studies
  1. Arterial blood gases. Ventilation-perfusion abnormalities that are found in patients with pulmonary fibrosis or pulmonary hypertension may cause hypoxemia.
  2. Spirometry may disclose a restrictive defect.
  3. The diffusing capacity is diminished even in early pulmonary involvement with systemic sclerosis.

RECOMMENDED DIAGNOSTIC APPROACH

- In a person with only Raynaud's phenomenon, no further work-up is recommended.
- When features such as persistent hand swelling, sclerodactyly, arthralgias, arthritis, dysphagia, or telangiectasia are present, further studies should be performed.
  1. An ANA test should be performed. If positive, the specificity of the ANA should be determined to aid in classification of the patient's disease.
  2. Other studies as noted in the laboratory section above should be done as clinically indicated to quantify organ system dysfunction in patients with systemic sclerosis.

Bibliography

Black CM, et al. Scleroderma. Rheum Dis Clin North Am 1989;15: 193–212.

Gilliland BC. Systemic sclerosis (scleroderma). In: Wilson JD, et al., eds. Harrison's Principles of Internal Medicine, 12th ed. New York, McGraw-Hill, 1991, pp. 1443–1448.

LeRoy EC, et al. Scleroderma (systemic sclerosis): Classification, subsets, and pathogenesis. J Rheumatol 1988;15:202–5.

Maricq HR, et al. Diagnostic potential of *in vivo* capillary microscopy in scleroderma and related disorders. Arthritis Rheum 1980;23: 183–189.

Sullivan WD, et al. A prospective evaluation emphasizing pulmonary involvement in patients with mixed connective tissue disease. Medicine 1984;63:92.

Tuffanelli DL. Systemic scleroderma. Med Clin North Am 1989;73:1167–1180.

86

VASCULITIS

GREGORY C. GARDNER

The blood burns in my veins!

WALT WHITMAN (1819–1892)

DEFINITION

Vasculitis is a process characterized by inflammation and necrosis of blood vessels, which occurs in a wide spectrum of clinical syndromes and diseases. Vasculitis is the result of immune complex deposition within or around blood vessels.

CLASSIFICATION

A common classification of the vasculitic syndromes is on the basis of size of the vessel affected (Table 86–1).

VASCULITIC SYNDROMES

- Large vessel vasculitis
  1. Takayasu's arteritis
     a. This disease most often affects women aged 15 to 45 years.
     b. It has 2 phases with the acute phase characterized by nonspecific systemic symptoms and the chronic phase marked by vascular occlusion.
     c. Vessels commonly involved include the aorta and aortic arch vessels, renal arteries, and pulmonary arteries. Mortality is most often due to occlusion of coronary or CNS vessels.
     d. Diagnosis
        i. Consider Takayasu's arteritis in a young woman with a nonspecific systemic illness, anisophygmia (unequal pulses or blood pressures), and an elevated ESR. The initial systemic phase may not be remembered.
        ii. Angiography of the entire aorta is the most important diagnostic test and typically shows areas of smooth-walled tapering of affected vessels.
        iii. Duplex ultrasound may be useful for an initial evaluation and to follow patients under therapy.
        iv. For obvious reasons, tissue diagnosis is difficult in this disease and often is not obtained.

TABLE 86–1. Topological Classification of Vasculitis

Predominantly large and medium-sized vessels
   Takayasu's arteritis
   Temporal arteritis
Predominantly medium and small-sized vessels
   PAN group
      Classic and microscopic polyarteritis
      Allergic angiitis and granulomatosis (Churg-Strauss)
      Overlap syndrome of necrotizing vasculitis
   Wegener's granulomatosis
   Lymphomatoid granulomatosis
   Isolated CNS vasculitis
   Vasculitis associated with other rheumatic diseases
Predominantly small-sized vessels
   Hypersensitivity vasculitis group
      Serum sickness–like reactions and drug
        hypersensitivity
      Henoch-Schönlein purpura
      Essential mixed cryoglobulinemia
      Hypocomplementemic vasculitis
      Vasculitis associated with malignancy
      Vasculitis associated with infectious diseases
Miscellaneous
   Thromboangiitis obliterans (Buerger's disease)
   HIV-associated vasculitis

2. Temporal arteritis
   a. This condition generally affects people over 55. It is rare in blacks.
   b. Symptoms may include weight loss, fever, anorexia, and fatigue, as well as unilateral headache, scalp tenderness, visual changes, and jaw claudication. Fifty percent may have associated polymyalgia rheumatica.
   c. Vascular inflammation may lead to permanent blindness. If suspected, treatment should be initiated before diagnostic biopsy (3 to 5 days of prednisone therapy will not affect the biopsy result).
   d. The ESR is often quite high (see Table 86–2), and patients may be anemic.
   e. Ten to fifteen percent of patients may have arteritis of other large vessels especially those of the aortic arch.
   f. Diagnosis
      i. Temporal artery biopsy of the symptomatic side is the procedure of choice.
      ii. The length of the biopsy specimen is important (3 to 4 cm), and multiple cuts are needed as skip lesions are a feature of this disease. A positive biopsy may show only inflammation but classically contains giant cells.
      iii. Not infrequently, both sides may have to be biopsied to make the diagnosis.

TABLE 86-2. Laboratory Evaluation of Vasculitis

PARAMETER	UTILITY
WBC count	Elevated in many syndromes Leukopenia in SLE
Eosinophilia	Seen in Churg-Strauss vasculitis
ESR	Level reflects activity in PAN, WG, TA, and Takayasu's arteritis
Urine sediment	Red cell casts indicate glomerulonephritis Abnormal in many syndromes
ANA	Present in SLE, SS, MCTD
RF	Present in rheumatoid vasculitis, SS, mixed cryoglobulinemia, and 50% of patients with WG
Serum protein electrophoresis (SPEP)	Identify monoclonal gammopathy Hypergammaglobulinemia (polyclonal) in many syndromes
Immunoglobulins	IgA elevated in Henoch-Schönlein purpura
Cryoglobulins	Present in rheumatoid vasculitis, mixed cryoglobulinemia, myeloma, hepatitis B vasculitis and other infectious diseases
Antineutrophil cytoplasmic antibody	WG, microscopic polyarteritis
Complement levels	Decreased in SLE, mixed cryoglobulinemia, hypocomplementemic vasculitis
Blood cultures	Positive in SBE and septicemia, which may mimic vasculitis

WG = Wegener's granulomatosis; TA = temporal arteritis; SS = Sjögren's syndrome; SBE = subacute bacterial endocarditis.

      iv. Angiography is useful if aortic arch involvement is suspected.
- Medium and small vessel vasculitis
    1. Polyarteritis nodosa (PAN) group: Classic PAN
       a. A necrotizing vasculitis of muscular medium and small arteries occurs, generally in people between 40 and 60 years old. Men outnumber women 2 : 1.
       b. Arteries in the following organ systems are frequently involved: CNS, peripheral nerves (mononeuritis multiplex), bowel, muscle, and kidneys.

c. The microscopic variant of PAN affects mainly arterioles and target organs tend to be skin, lung, and kidney. Patients with microscopic polyarteritis can develop a rapidly progressive glomerulonephritis and pulmonary hemorrhage. This group of patients also have a positive antineutrophil cytoplasm antibody (ANCA) test.

d. Classic PAN has been associated with hepatitis B antigenemia, CMV infection, hairy cell leukemia, HIV infection, Crohn's disease, and amphetamine abuse.

e. The overlap syndrome of necrotizing vasculitis may contain characteristics of PAN, Churg-Strauss vasculitis, and small vessel vasculitis.

f. Diagnosis
   i. The initial evaluation should include biopsy of a symptomatic nerve or muscle (Table 86–3). If either is negative or neither site is symptomatic, then angiography is done, which typically demonstrates visceral or renal aneurysms or vessel narrowing. Testicular biopsy may also be useful.
   ii. The most useful diagnostic tests for microscopic polyarteritis is biopsy of the affected organ system, especially kidney, which shows necrotizing vasculitis, and a positive ANCA. Angiography is generally not useful in the diagnosis of microscopic polyarteritis.

2. Allergic angiitis and granulomatosis (Churg-Strauss vasculitis)
   a. The vessels affected are similar to PAN except for less renal disease and more pulmonary involvement. Patients classically have preceding history of asthma.
   b. Distinctive features include formation of intra- and extravascular granulomas, eosinophilia, and eosinophilic tissue infiltrates.
   c. Diagnosis
      i. This is suggested by the correct clinical setting and peripheral eosinophilia (up to 50% of the white cells).
      ii. Biopsy of the affected tissue (lung, skin, nerve) is confirmatory.

3. Wegener's granulomatosis
   a. Classically, this disease involves the triad of upper respiratory tract (especially sinuses), lung, and

TABLE 86–3. Diagnostic Evaluation of Suspected PAN

1. Biopsy symptomatic nerve or muscle.
2. If negative or if neither site symptomatic, proceed with angiography.
3. If angiography negative, consider:
   testicular biopsy in males.
   muscle biopsy in females.

kidney with granulomatous vascular inflammation.

b. Disease limited to the upper respiratory tract also occurs. Eyes, skin, and joints may also be involved.

c. Rapidly progressive renal failure may occur and is the major cause of morbidity.

d. Diagnosis

   i. The evaluation should include sinus X-rays, a chest X-ray (looking for infiltrates or nodules that may be cavitary), ESR, serum creatinine, and urinalysis.

   ii. Recently, serum ANCA has emerged as a sensitive and specific test for this disease. The most specific pattern is a diffuse cytoplasmic immunofluorescence. This test can also be done serially to follow the course of the disease and to differentiate infection from disease flare.

   iii. A tissue diagnosis is still important if aggressive therapy is contemplated. The highest yield biopsy material comes from an open lung procedure, but nasal mucosa is easier to obtain and may be diagnostic. Renal biopsy is rarely distinctive enough to make a firm diagnosis.

4. Lymphomatoid granulomatosis

   a. This is a rare disease characterized by granulomatous angiocentric and angiodestructive vasculitis due to infiltrating cells that are atypical lymphocytes and plasma cells.

   b. The upper and lower airways are predominantly involved, but the skin and kidneys may also be affected.

   c. Fifty percent of patients eventually develop a malignant lymphoma.

   d. Diagnosis

      i. Nodular densities may be present on chest X-ray.

      ii. The diagnosis rests on biopsy of involved tissue.

5. Isolated CNS vasculitis

   a. This is a rare disorder in which vascular inflammation is restricted to the small and medium-sized vessels of the CNS.

   b. It occurs in males slightly more often than females, and possible predisposing factors include herpes zoster ophthalmicus, amphetamine abuse, HIV infection, and lymphoma.

   c. Patients may present with nonspecific CNS dysfunction, such as confusion or memory disorder, or focal neurologic deficits, such as cranial neuropathy or aphasia.

   d. Diagnosis

      i. Consider this possibility in a young person with a stroke or other CNS symptoms.

    ii. MRI may be useful to identify areas of edema or infarct.

    iii. Cerebral angiography typically shows tapering, aneurysms, or beading of the affected arteries. If only small vessels are affected, the angiogram may be normal and biopsy of the leptomeninges may be necessary. With definite angiographic changes biopsy is probably not required.

6. Vasculitis associated with other rheumatic diseases

    a. Many of the rheumatic diseases can have associated vasculitis (usually medium and small vessels) including RA, SLE, relapsing polychondritis, Sjögren's syndrome, Behçet's disease, and Cogan's disease.

    b. Behçet's disease, RA, and the HLA-B27–associated spondyloarthropathies can cause an aortitis.

    c. Behçet's disease affects veins as well as arteries.

    d. Vasculitis complicating rheumatoid arthritis usually occurs in patients with longstanding seropositive disease and often when the joint disease is quiet. It is more common in men.

    e. Cogan's disease is a rare form of vasculitis. A typical patient has an acute onset of interstitial keratitis and vestibular dysfunction often associated with a large vessel vasculitis.

- Small vessel vasculitis (hypersensitivity vasculitis group)

1. This group encompasses a wide variety of disorders that cause a leukocytoclastic vasculitis which affects postcapillary venules.

2. It is characterized by vascular infiltration with polymorphonuclear leukocytes with leukocytoclasis (nuclear debris), fibrinoid necrosis, and extravasation of red cells.

3. Generally, only the skin is involved, but there are exceptions.

4. It is often traced to an infectious organism or drug and occurs 1 to 10 days after exposure to the antigen.

5. Lesions generally present in crops as palpable purpura, especially on the lower extremities. Biopsy of the affected skin is an important procedure in all of the syndromes discussed below.

6. Serum sickness–like reactions and drug hypersensitivity.

    a. Drugs (Table 86–4) account for a large portion of all cases of hypersensitivity vasculitis. Penicillin and sulfa antibiotics are major culprits.

    b. Symptoms can include urticaria, fever, arthralgias, and lymphadenopathy.

    c. Diagnosis is based on the above symptom complex and skin biopsy.

7. Henoch-Schönlein purpura

    a. This occurs most frequently in children but can be seen in adults.

TABLE 86–4. Drugs Associated with a Vasculitis Syndrome

Penicillin	Phenylbutazone
Sulfonamides	Thiazides
Propylthiouracil	Amphetamines
Allopurinol	Phenytoin

    b. Patients can have GI symptoms (diarrhea, GI bleeding), arthritis/arthralgias, and renal disease (glomerulonephritis) in addition to purpura.

    c. The symptoms often follow a viral illness and may recur but the illness is generally self-limited.

    d. The diagnosis is based on symptom complex, demonstration of IgA immunofluorescence on skin or kidney biopsy, or elevated serum IgA levels.

8. Essential mixed cryoglobulinemia

    a. This disease is most often seen in middle-aged females.

    b. Features include purpura, Raynaud's phenomenon, arthralgias, hypergammaglobulinemia, and glomerulonephritis.

    c. The hypergammaglobulinemia usually includes a polyclonal IgM rheumatoid factor directed against IgG.

    d. Diagnosis is by symptom complex and laboratory demonstration of cryoglobulins in the serum. Blood must clot at body temperature to avoid losing the cryoglobulins.

    e. Cryoglobulins are seen in a variety of conditions including infectious, connective tissue, lymphoproliferative, and chronic liver diseases. The term "essential" indicates there is no identifiable stimulus to cryoglobulins production.

9. Hypocomplementemic vasculitis

    a. This uncommon form of vasculitis is associated with recurrent episodes of urticarial skin eruptions, fever, symmetric polyarticular arthralgias or arthritis, and abdominal pain. The kidneys are occasionally involved.

    b. Typically, all complement component levels are low.

10. Vasculitis associated with malignancy

    a. Myeloproliferative disorders are most often associated with this form of vasculitis.

    b. Cutaneous vasculitis may occur in acute and chronic myelogenous leukemia and myelofibrosis. It may antedate the appearance of the malignancy and is frequently associated with polyarthritis.

    c. Treatment of the underlying malignancy does not always improve the cutaneous vasculitis.

11. Vasculitis associated with infectious diseases

    a. A variety of agents including hepatitis B, CMV, streptococci, rickettsia, and organisms that cause subacute bacterial endocarditis can cause a cutaneous vasculitis.

   b. The resultant vascular lesions are indistinguishable from other forms of cutaneous necrotizing vasculitis. The etiology is most likely on the basis of immune complex disease.

   c. Diagnosis is by identification of the offending organism.

- Miscellaneous vasculitic syndromes
  1. Thromboangiitis obliterans
     a. This is a segmental inflammatory obliterative vascular disease that affects young adults, generally men, who are heavy cigarette smokers.
     b. The affected vessels are the small and medium-sized arteries and veins of the extremities.
     c. The symptoms of thromboangiitis result from vascular occlusion and include Raynaud's phenomenon, thrombophlebitis, claudication, and ulceration or gangrene of the fingertips and toes.
     d. Diagnosis is by Doppler studies of the extremities, which demonstrate the large vessel disease. Angiography is needed to study the small and medium vessels.
  2. Vasculitis associated with HIV disease. HIV infection has been associated with several types of vasculitis. The most common type is a PAN-like disease but isolated CNS vasculitis, leukocytoclastic vasculitis, lymphomatoid granulomatosis, and eosinophilic vasculitis have all been reported.

DISEASES MIMICKING SYSTEMIC VASCULITIS

- Atrial myxoma
  1. Patients with this disorder may have fever, weight loss, purpuric rash, Raynaud's phenomenon, claudication, and stroke-like features involving the CNS.
  2. The ESR or serum globulins may be elevated.
  3. The diagnosis is made by echocardiogram.
- Cholesterol emboli
  1. Patients with cholesterol emboli may present with livedo reticularis, cutaneous infarcts, leukocytosis, eosinophilia, thrombocytopenia, abnormal urinary sediment, and hypocomplementemia.
  2. Aortic aneurysms are usually the source of such emboli.
  3. The diagnosis can be made by biopsy of the involved tissue which demonstrates vascular occlusion by cholesterol emboli.
- Septicemia
  1. Disseminated gonococcal infection, meningococcemia, staphylcoccal septicemia, and pseudomonas septicemia may produce an illness which simulates vasculitis.

2. For this reason blood cultures are important in the initial evaluation of the patient with a febrile systemic illness thought to be a vasculitis.

- Ergotism. Patients using high doses of ergots over a prolonged period of time may develop peripheral vascular insufficiency. The diagnosis is made by angiography and the medication history.

RECOMMENDED DIAGNOSTIC APPROACH

- Vasculitis should be considered in any patient presenting with a systemic illness especially if it includes evidence of active glomerulonephritis, palpable purpura or necrotic skin lesions, mononeuritis multiplex, asymmetry of pulses, or fever without an established cause.
- A variety of laboratory abnormalities can be seen in patients with vasculitis, but a tissue diagnosis is required in most cases.

Bibliograpy

Albert DA, et al. The diagnosis of polyarteritis nodosa: I. A literature-based decision analysis approach. Arthritis Rheum 1988;31:1117–1127.

Conn DL, Hunder GG. Vasculitic syndromes. In: Kelley WN, et al., eds. Textbook of Rheumatology, 3rd ed. Philadelphia, W. B. Saunders, 1989.

Cupps TR, et al. Isolated angiitis of the central nervous system. Am J Med 1983;74:97–105.

Fauci AS, et al. The spectrum of vasculitis. Ann Int Med 1978;89:660–676.

Haynes BF, et al. Diagnostic and therapeutic approach to the patient with vasculitis. Med Clin North Am 1986;70:355–369.

Kaufman LD, Kaplan AP. Microscopic polyarteritis. Hosp Pract (June) 1989:85–104.

Kaye BR. Rheumatologic manifestations of infection with human immunodeficiency virus (HIV). Ann Int Med 1989;111:158–167.

Longley S, et al. Paraneoplastic vasculitis. Am J Med 1986;80:1027–1030.

Swerlick RA, Lawley TJ. Cutaneous vasculitis: Its relationship to systemic disease. Med Clin North Am 1989;73:1221–1235.

SECTION XII

NEUROLOGY

87

COMA

ARTHUR KELLERMAN, *and* CURTIS SAUER

Ignore death up to the last moment; then, when it can't be ignored any longer, have yourself squirted full of morphine and shuffle off in a coma.

ALDOUS HUXLEY (1894–1963)

DEFINITION

- Coma is a state of sleeplike unresponsiveness from which a patient cannot be awakened. The comatose individual lacks all awareness of self or environment. Coma must be distinguished from several similar conditions, especially the persistent vegetative state and the locked-in syndrome. In the former condition, wakefulness and response to environmental stimuli are preserved but there is no evidence of cognitive functioning. In the latter, generalized motor impairment precludes response to stimuli. Psychogenic coma is superficially similar to coma but has no known organic basis.

- Coma is a symptom, not a disease. It is a manifestation of some severe underlying pathologic process. Other clinical terms such as "lethargy," "obtundation," and "stupor" represent a continuum of disorders involving the level of consciousness, the most severe of which is coma. Delirium and related alterations in the content of consciousness are discussed separately (see Chapter 89).

DIFFERENTIAL DIAGNOSIS

- Causes of coma (Table 87–1). Grouping the causes of coma into three major categories is useful in the initial evaluation and treatment of coma and helps to guide subsequent diagnostic tests and therapy. These general causes include:

  1. Supratentorial mass lesions. These lesions lead to coma by several mechanisms, including increased intracranial pressure, lateral displacement of the midline of the hemispheres, and compression or displacement of the diencephalon and brainstem reticular activating system (RAS).

  2. Subtentorial lesions. These lesions in the posterior fossa or brain stem either ablate or directly compress the RAS.

  3. Diffuse, toxic, and metabolic processes. These

TABLE 87–1. Causes of Coma[a]

	PERCENT OF CASES
Diffuse, toxic, and metabolic causes	50–65
Toxic (drugs, poisons)	25–50
Anoxic ischemia	3–5
Infectious (meningitis, encephalitis)	3–5
Hypoglycemia	3–5
Hepatic coma	3–5
Subarachnoid hemorrhage	2–4
Hyperosmolarity	<3
Hyponatremia	<3
Other endocrine disorders (Addison's hypopituitarism, myxedema)	<3
Hypercalcemia	<1
Uremia	<3
Postictal (seizures)	<3
Disorder of temperature regulation	<3
Nutritional deficiencies	<1
Hypercarbia	<1
Structural causes	35–50
Supratentorial	25–30
Hemorrhage	
Intracerebral	8–10
Subdural	3–5
Epidural	<1
Pituitary apoplexy	<1
Trauma (contusion or occult)	<3
Infarction (massive)	<3
Infectious (abscess)	<3
Tumor	
Primary	<1
Metastatic	<3
Subtentorial	
Infarction	
Pontine or brainstem	10–15
Cerebellar	8–10
Epi- or subdural	<1
Hemorrhage	
Pontine or brainstem	2–4
Cerebellar	<3
Tumor	<1
Abscess	<1
Demyelination	<1
Basilar migraine	<1

[a] Following identification of obvious trauma, drug ingestion, and postarrest anoxia.

processes widely damage or impair neuronal function in the cortex and brain stem.

- Drugs and poisons. Drugs and poisons are the single most common cause of coma of unknown origin even after known cases of self-poisoning have been excluded (Table

87–1). Ethanol and barbiturates remain the most common causes of drug-induced coma in the United States.

- Head injury. Following exclusion of "obvious head injuries" (such as from high-speed vehicular accidents and penetrating wounds), closed head trauma and its sequelae (epidural and subdural hematomas) remain a common cause of coma of unknown origin (4 to 6%).

CLINICAL FEATURES

- History. Information should be obtained from all available sources, including family, friends, bystanders, and ambulance personnel.
    1. Onset
        a. Sudden onset suggests drug overdose, trauma, or intracranial bleed. In older persons, brainstem or cerebellar hemorrhage or infarction must also be excluded.
        b. A more gradual onset suggests an evolving toxic or metabolic encephalopathy, brain tumor, or chronic subdural hematoma.
    2. Associated symptoms
        a. Headache or recent history of head trauma (no matter how trivial) suggests a supratentorial mass lesion. Asymmetric motor or sensory complaints are supportive.
        b. An occipital headache, especially if it is associated with vertigo, ataxia, diplopia, or vomiting, suggests a subtentorial lesion.
        c. Confusion, disorientation, and somnolence preceding coma suggest a toxic or metabolic cause. Motor findings are usually symmetric, although old focal pathology can be unmasked by an evolving process.
    3. Associated medical problems. A history of a previous seizure disorder or liver, renal, or endocrine disease may be important. Patients may be wearing a medical alert tag or carrying a card in their wallet or purse.
    4. Surroundings. Circumstances at the time of discovery may provide valuable clues, such as pill bottles, drug paraphernalia, evidence of a struggle, or a cold room suggest potential diagnoses.
    5. Medications. All drugs prescribed to the patient as well as those to which he or she may have had access should be reviewed.
- Directed general physical examination
    1. Observation
        a. The patient should be observed undisturbed for several moments. Body position, spontaneous movements, and respiratory rate and pattern should be noted.
        b. Comatose patients with acute hemiplegia may lie with the affected leg externally rotated.
        c. Myoclonic jerks and tremor may suggest a toxic or metabolic cause.

    d. Jacksonian or generalized seizures should be noted and aggressively treated.

2. Skull palpation. The physician should carefully inspect and palpate the skull for lacerations, hematomas, edema, or skull depressions.

3. Hemorrhage and ecchymoses. The physician should search for subconjunctival hemorrhages, sharply demarcated periorbital ecchymoses (''raccoon eyes''), mastoid ecchymoses (Battle's sign), and blood in the external auditory canal or hemotympanum. If eardrum perforation is suspected, caloric stimulation should be deferred.

4. CSF rhinorrhea or otorrhea. CSF rhinorrhea or otorrhea appears as a clear watery discharge. A positive test for glucose in the fluid is nonspecific and unhelpful. CSF mixed with blood may separate when placed on filter paper. This ''rim sign'' is strongly suggestive of a basilar skull fracture. If it is present, caloric stimulation should be deferred.

5. Mouth and facial bones. The mouth and facial bones should be examined and palpated. Loose teeth should be removed to prevent aspiration. Tongue lacerations, especially laterally, are suggestive of recent seizure activity. The patient's breath should be noted for the odor of ketones, alcohol, paraldehyde, and uremic or hepatic fetor.

6. Evidence of fracture or soft tissue injury. The remainder of the body should be examined for evidence of fractures or soft tissue injury. Breath sounds should be symmetric and confirm good ventilatory exchange. A pneumothorax should be excluded.

7. Core temperature. Core temperature should be checked with a rectal temperature probe. Disordered thermoregulation can cause coma and requires urgent treatment.

8. Skin. Skin should be inspected for needle tracks, abscesses, stigmata of chronic liver disease, petechiae, purpura, and evidence of prolonged pressure injury.

9. Nuchal rigidity. Once cervical trauma has been excluded, the neck should be flexed to detect nuchal rigidity.

10. Optic fundi
    a. The optic fundi must be examined to detect papilledema (which develops after several hours of increased intracranial pressure), optic neuritis (suggesting methanol intoxication), retinal artery spasm, and subhyaloid hemorrhage (often associated with subarachnoid bleeds).
    b. Mydriatic agents should be avoided, since their use obscures subsequent determination and monitoring of pupillary reflexes.
    c. Changes in pupillary responses are more sensitive than papilledema for detection of increasing intracranial pressure.

- Directed neurologic examination. Evaluation of the following five neurologic functions provides invaluable information on the level of neurologic impairment (Table 87–2).

TABLE 87–2. Anatomic Localization of Neurologic Signs

EXAMINATION FINDINGS	NEUROANATOMIC SUBSTRATE
Cognition	Cortex
Conscious behaviors	Cortex and reticular activating system
Pupils	Midbrain
Extraocular movements (oculocephalic response)	Brainstem (midbrain to medulla)
Motor responses	Pons or medulla (if flaccid)
Respiration	Medulla (if ataxic)

This information, combined with the short-term clinical course, should provide an initial presumptive diagnosis and guide further laboratory evaluation.

1. Level of consciousness. Although the comatose patient is unresponsive, subsequent improvement in level of consciousness as well as patterns of speech serve as good measures of clinical improvement.
2. Pupillary response
   a. Normal pupillary function implies that the midbrain and third cranial nerves are intact.
   b. Symmetric or diffuse diencephalic processes produce small reactive pupils.
   c. Preservation of the pupillary light reflex in the presence of other signs of brainstem impairment strongly supports a toxic or metabolic cause of the coma. Abnormal pupillary reflexes are uncommon (less than 5% of cases) in hepatic and other metabolic encephalopathies.
   d. Mild anisocoria with intact bilateral reactivity is most likely congenital. Asymmetric reactivity suggests an acute structural process.
   e. Enlarging supratentorial mass lesions can produce uncal herniation. Subsequent compression of the peripheral pupilloconstrictor fibers of the third cranial nerve produces a dilated unresponsive pupil on the same side as the lesion.
   f. Midbrain damage can produce midposition and unreactive pupils. Severe hypothermia and barbiturate intoxication can also produce midposition unreactive pupils, simulating brain death.
   g. Pontine bleeds or infarction can produce small to pinpoint pupils. The pupillary light reflex is generally preserved when the eyes are examined with a magnifying glass. Small to pinpoint pupils can also be seen with opiate or anticholinesterase intoxication.
   h. Dilated unreactive pupils are often seen after an agonal release of norepinephrine following anoxia or ischemia. Atropine, scopolamine, and glutethimide intoxication can also produce dilated pupils that are unreactive to light.

3. Oculocephalic and oculovestibular reflexes
   a. The doll's eye reflex becomes easy to elicit when consciousness is lost and the brain stem centers for conjugate gaze are released from the control of the frontal gaze centers. (Evaluations should be delayed until cervical spine injury is excluded).
   b. A normal symmetric response indicates that the tegmentum of the midbrain, pons, and medulla is largely structurally intact. Loss of the oculocephalic response suggests brain stem dysfunction and a greater risk of subsequent respiratory arrest.
   c. Asymmetric responses are more commonly seen with structural than with metabolic lesions.
   d. Cold calorics (irrigation of the external auditory canal with 50 cm³ of ice water while elevating the head at 30 degrees) is a more potent stimulus for eye deviation than the oculocephalic reflex. Observed abnormalities have the same pathophysiologic significance.
   e. Cortical mass lesions may produce ipsilateral conjugate deviation of the eyes, which can be overcome with the doll's eye maneuver or caloric stimulation.
   f. Brainstem lesions produce contralateral conjugate deviation of the eyes. Since the pontine centers for lateral gaze are affected, oculocephalic maneuvers and calorics do not reverse the deviation.
   g. If deviation is associated with hemiplegia, the eyes tend to look away from cortical hemiplegia but toward pontine brainstem hemiplegia.
   h. Deep metabolic coma and midbrain lesions produce midline immobile eyes. Eyes directed straight ahead have no localizing value.
   i. Jerk nystagmus with the fast phase directed away from the side of cold caloric irrigation, in a seemingly comatose patient, is diagnostic of psychogenic unresponsiveness.
4. Motor response
   a. Abnormal responses should be described and noted. Use of diagnostic labels such as "decorticate" and "decerebrate" are potentially confusing and neuroanatomically inaccurate.
   b. Abduction to a noxious stimulus is not observed in withdrawal reflexes and represents purposeful movement.
   c. Abnormal but symmetric motor responses may be seen in midline structural or toxic and metabolic coma and have no localizing value.
   d. Asymmetric motor responses at any level suggest a structural cause of coma.
   e. Previously occult focal motor deficits may be unmasked by toxic or metabolic impairment.
   f. Abnormal posturing may be subtle and intermittent or produced only by noxious stimulation.
   g. An upper extremity flexor and lower extremity

extensor response implies cortical or high diencephalic dysfunction.

h. Flaccidity appears with progressive involvement of the pons or medulla and is also seen with acute spinal cord injury.

i. Asymmetric resting muscle tone or deep tendon reflexes, or Babinski's signs, suggest a structural lesion. Bilateral upgoing toes are commonly seen in toxic and metabolic coma.

j. Tremor, asterixis, and myoclonus are characteristic of toxic and metabolic coma.

5. Respiratory pattern

a. Several patterns or respiratory abnormality may occur in the comatose patient and have localizing significance.

b. Periodic (Cheyne-Stokes) respiration is a nonspecific finding associated with cortical and high diencephalic dysfunction. Sedatives, metabolic encephalopathies, CHF, and cerebrovascular disease can also produce this respiratory pattern.

c. Grossly irregular (ataxic) respirations suggest medullary involvement, while inspiratory pauses (apneustic breathing) maybe seen with pontine lesions. Both patterns may precede sudden respiratory arrest.

d. Central neurogenic hyperventilation has little localizing significance. When present, however, it is usually a predictor of poor outcome.

• Clinical course

1. Rostral-caudal progression of neurologic dysfunction is characteristic of supratentorial mass lesions and toxic and metabolic encephalopathy. Midline mass lesions or bilateral lesions may produce few or no focal signs. Laterally placed lesions may demonstrate focal signs early in the clinical course that are masked by progressive pressure and damage to lower brain centers. Thus, structural lesions can mimic toxic/metabolic coma.

2. Absence of an orderly rostral-caudal progresssion, especially with impaired oculovestibular and pupillary responses, suggests a subtentorial structural lesion.

3. Toxic encephalopathies can mimic subtentorial lesions. For example, opiate overdose can cause small pupils and apnea resembling medullary damage, while anticholinesterase poisoning can cause coma, small pupils, extraocular palsy, and a flaccid quadriparesis similar in pattern to pontine hemorrhage.

4. When confronted with obvious clinical deterioration, measures to treat potentially increased intracranial pressure (including hyperventilation and administration of mannitol) may be indicated prior to definitive diagnostic tests.

The typical clinical features for general diagnostic categories are summarized in Table 87–3.

TABLE 87–3. Typical Signs in Coma[a]

	History (Prior to Coma)	Pupils	Oculocephalic Response and Calorics	Motor	Rostal to Caudal Progression	Best Test
Supratentorial mass lesions	Trauma, headache, focal signs	Unilateral enlargement with cranial nerve III dysfunction[b]	Deviate away from hemiplegia; calorics overcome conjugate gaze, or are absent	Focal signs present (early) or flaccid	Present	CT scan
Subtentorial mass lesions	Occipital headache,[b] nausea, vomiting, vertigo, diplopia, ataxia (truncal)	Commonly impaired, often asymmetric	Deviate toward hemiplegic; calorics[b] fail to overcome disconjugate gaze, or are absent	Signs usually symmetric or flaccid	Absent	CT scan
Diffuse toxic or metabolic	Confusion, apathy, delirium, somnolence	Preserved despite other brain stem signs[b]	Generally symmetric or absent	Seizures, myoclonus, possible signs usually symmetric or flaccid	Often present	Blood chemistries, LP (if infection is suspected)
Psychogenic unresponsiveness	Previous psychiatric history	Intact, normal	Absent, nystagmus with normal calorics[b]	Flaccid or avoidance	None	EEG (if unsure)

[a] Exceptions occur and differentiation may be especially difficult late in clinical course.
[b] Most helpful in differential diagnosis.
Source: Modified from Plum F, Posner J. The Diagnosis of Stupor and Coma, 3rd ed. Philadelphia, F. A. Davis Company, 1982, pp. 353–362.

LABORATORY STUDIES

- Immediate laboratory tests. Laboratory tests that should be obtained in the initial evaluation of coma include:
  1. Serum electrolytes, glucose, BUN, creatinine, calcium, and measured serum osmolarity. Observation of an "osmolar gap" (measured osmolarity greater than calculated osmolarity) suggests an additional significant solute such as ethanol or methanol.
  2. Arterial blood gas
     a. Spontaneous hypocarbia ($PaCO_2 < 30$ mm Hg) is associated with a worse prognosis.
     b. A terra cotta color of the blood sample may suggest methemoglobinemia or sulfhemoglobinemia.
     c. The cherry red color described for carboxyhemoglobinemia (carbon monoxide poisoning) is infrequently seen and not clinically useful.
     d. A difference between measured and calculated hemoglobin oxygen saturation suggests carbon monoxide poisoning.
  3. ECG. The ECG can diagnose cardiac arrhythmias and show evidence of myocardial ischemia. Metabolic and electrolyte disturbances may be suspected from the ECG before results of blood chemistry analyses are available.
- Subsequent laboratory tests. Subsequent tests should be guided by the results of the initial clinical and laboratory evaluation. These tests should be obtained as rapidly as possible but only if specifically indicated.
  1. Specific blood tests
     a. Blood alcohol determination. Additional clinical chemistry analysis includes a blood alcohol determination (in certain clinical settings, this is a part of the immediate laboratory evaluation). Alcohol remains the most common drug cause of coma, either alone or in combination with other agents.
     b. Drug screen. Qualitative tests can be run on blood, urine, and gastric contents. These tests are not very sensitive (0.60 to 0.70) and do not detect a number of important drugs, and wide variability exists among laboratories.
     c. Specific drug levels. Serum levels of anticonvulsant medication and barbiturates may roughly correlate with a patient's clinical condition. Salicylate and acetaminophen levels may be helpful in subsequent management. Drug levels are expensive and should not be ordered without appropriate clinical suspicion or a positive drug screen.
     d. Liver enzymes, prothrombin time, and bilirubin determinations. Elevations of these tests may suggest hepatic encephalopathy. Blood arterial ammonia levels correlate roughly with clinical symptoms.
     e. Carboxyhemoglobin level. This test is mandatory for diagnosis of carbon monoxide poisoning because clinical signs are insensitive and nonspecific.

f. Serum creatine phosphokinase isoenzyme (CPK BB). Elevation of this enzyme for 6 hr or longer following cardiac arrest is associated with severe anoxic brain injury.

g. Additional metabolic studies may include thyroid function tests and levels of adrenocorticotropic hormone and cortisol levels.

h. Other toxicologic tests. These include serum iron, heavy metals, and methemoglobin.

2. CT Scan

a. The CT scan is the radiographic procedure of choice for detecting intracranial mass lesions.

b. Resolution depends on the generation of the scanner and the density of any lesion. High-density intracranial bleeds as small as a few millimeters may be detected. CT has a sensitivity of 0.95 and a specificity of 0.90 for detecting mass lesions in the cerebral hemispheres, diencephalon, and cerebellum.

c. Lesions in the midbrain, pons, and medulla are more easily missed owing to interference from adjacent bone, although CT may still detect up to 85% of these lesions. MRI is rapidly becoming the procedure of choice for evaluation of these areas.

d. CT will detect approximately 90% of subarachnoid hemorrhages, especially if performed within 24 hr of onset. If clinical suspicion exists and CT is negative, lumbar puncture (LP) should be performed.

e. Administration of contrast material prior to the initial CT scan may obscure diagnosis by CT of subarachnoid hemorrhage.

f. Subacute and chronic subdural hematomas may evolve through an isodense phase and be suspected only by their mass effects. Reexamination following administration of contrast material can confirm the diagnosis.

g. CT is not useful for detecting toxic or metabolic coma, meningitis, or many cases of encephalitis. Brain contusion, small subtentorial lesions, brain stem infarction, pituitary apoplexy, and disseminated tumor may also be missed by CT.

3. LP

a. The LP is essential in the evaluation of suspected meningitis and encephalitis and may be needed to confirm the diagnosis of subarachnoid hemorrhage.

b. Lumbar puncture can be hazardous with increased intracranial pressure and may precipitate herniation.

c. When an intracranial mass lesion is suspected, an emergency CT scan should be obtained prior to an LP.

d. In cases of suspected acute bacterial meningitis or brain abscess, administration of antibiotics should not be delayed beyond 30 min. If delay is unavoidable, antibiotics should be given prior to CT scanning and lumbar puncture.

e. Papilledema is a relatively late sign of increased intracranial pressure and may be absent in acute processes. Venous pulsations in the optic discs virtually assure normal pressure but are absent in many normal patients.

f. True blood in the CSF can be distinguished from a traumatic tap by the presence of xanthochromia, no decrease in RBC count between the first and last tubes, or a final sample RBC count >1000/mm^3.

g. Gram's stain counterimmunoelectrophoresis (CIE) for bacterial antigens, India ink preparation, cultures for bacteria, fungi, and tuberculosis, cell count and differential, glucose, and total protein measurements should be considered in the evaluation of CSF.

h. CSF protein, sugar, and cell counts may be normal with brain tumors or abscess, although the opening pressure is commonly elevated.

i. Specific additional studies of CSF may include glutamine (elevated in hepatic encephalopathy), creatine phosphokinase (present in anoxic encephalopathy), viral studies, and fungal antigens.

4. EEG

a. The EEG has a relatively minor role in the emergent evaluation of the comatose patient and is far less helpful than CT in discriminating structural from metabolic lesions.

b. Metabolic disease most commonly produces symmetric slowing.

c. The EEG is probably most helpful in distinguishing repetitive or subclinical seizure activity and in confirming brain death. Seizures rarely cause coma without overt convulsions.

d. Coma can be reliably differentiated from psychogenic unresponsiveness by the EEG. However, most cases can be distinguished on clinical grounds.

e. Severe toxic or metabolic encephalopathy and hypothermia can produce an isoelectric EEG and must be excluded prior to a diagnosis of brain death.

5. Skull films

a. CT scanning has largely replaced skull films in the evaluation of suspected intracranial mass lesions after head trauma.

b. Skull films can still provide valuable inferential evidence regarding the severity of head injury and are a more sensitive test for detecting skull fracture.

c. High-yield criteria have been developed for ordering skull films, of which coma, focal neurologic signs, and a decreasing mental status are the most predictive.

d. Regardless of whether skull films or a CT scan are obtained, the importance of cervical radiographs to exclude spinal injury cannot be overemphasized.

6. Cerebral angiography
   a. Angiography is rarely indicated for the early evaluation of the comatose patient.
   b. Angiograms are sensitive (>0.95) but less specific (0.85) than CT for detecting mass lesions and much more hazardous to perform.
   c. The primary utility of angiography in coma is to locate aneurysms and confirm vascular spasm, although the value of surgery in patients comatose from subarachnoid hemorrhage is uncertain.

RECOMMENDED DIAGNOSTIC APPROACH

- Life-threatening aspects of the patient (airway, arrhythmias, hypotension) must be cared for while the diagnostic process is initiated.
- Historical features should be sought from friends and witnesses, especially if an aggravation of a preexisting medical problem or drug intoxication is suspected.
- The directed physical neurologic exam should be systematic, with the differential diagnosis in mind. Level of consciousness, pupillary response, oculocephalic/oculovestibular reflex, motor response, and respiratory pattern should be rapidly assessed.
- The "immediate laboratory tests" should be initiated as attention is directed to management of life-threatening problems. Subsequent laboratory testing should be guided by clinical judgment rather than a "shotgun" approach.

Bibliography

Adams H, et al. CT and clinical correlations in recent aneurysmal subarachnoid hemorrhage: A preliminary report of the cooperative aneurysm study. Neurology 1983;33:981–988.

Baker H, et al. National Cancer Institute Study: Evaluation of computed tomography in the diagnosis of intracranial neoplasms. Radiology 1980;136:91–96.

Fishman R. Brain edema. N Engl J Med 1975;293:706–711.

Kellermann A, et al. Utilization and yield of drug screening in the emergency department. Am J Emerg Med 1988;6:14–20.

Levy D, et al. Predicting outcome from hypoxic-ischemic coma. JAMA 1985;253:1420–1426.

Longstreth W, et al. Neurologic recovery after out of hospital cardiac arrest. Ann Intern Med 1983;98 (Part I):588–592.

Masters S, et al. Skull x-ray examinations after head trauma: Recommendations by a multi-disciplinary panel and validation study. N Engl J Med 1987;316:84–91.

North J, Jerrett S. Abnormal breathing patterns associated with acute brain damage. Arch Neurol 1974;31:338–344.

Plum F. Mechanisms of "central" hyperventilation. Ann Neurol 1982;11:636–637.

Plum F, Posner J. The Diagnosis of Stupor and Coma, revised 3rd ed. Philadelphia, F. A. Davis Company, 1982.

Ropper A. Lateral displacement of the brain and level of consciousness in patients with an acute hemispheral lesion. N Engl J Med 1986;314:953–958.

Sabin T. Coma and the acute confusional state in the emergency room. Med Clin North Am 1981;65:15–32.

88

SYNCOPE

TERRY J. MENGERT

Prithee do not turn me about. My stomach is not constant.

SHAKESPEARE (1564–1616) The Tempest II, II

DEFINITION

Syncope is a sudden temporary loss of consciousness. Inherent elements of the definition are:

1. The patient regains consciousness spontaneously.
2. The patient is unable to maintain postural tone during the episode.
3. The loss of consciousness was not due to either head trauma or a seizure.

In the vast majority of cases the underlying mechanism is cerebral hypoperfusion.

- Epidemiology. Syncope is a common symptom, and accounts for 3% of emergency room visits and 1% of hospital admissions. One-third of people will complain of at least one episode of syncope in their lifetime. The incidence of syncope increases with age.
- Difficulties in the diagnosis of syncope
  1. It is a common complaint, experienced by a large number of patients.
  2. Syncope has a tremendous number of possible causes.
  3. A large array of expensive diagnostic tests may be utilized in an attempt at diagnosis.
  4. Even with an aggressive and expensive work-up, the etiology may still not be apparent in as many as 48% of patients.
  5. Though a diagnosis is not possible in every case, an aggressive work-up is mandatory in those patients in whom a cardiovascular or suspected life-threatening etiology is likely.

DIFFERENTIAL DIAGNOSIS

Syncope must be distinguished from other causes of transient loss of consciousness (Table 88–1).

- Seizure versus syncope
  1. With *both* seizures and syncope the patient may lose bladder control and may have myoclonic jerking. Con-

TABLE 88–1. Causes of Transient Loss of Consciousness

Syncope
Seizures
  Generalized Seizures
    Absence
    Myoclonic
    Clonic, tonic, and tonic-clonic
    Atonic
  Partial complex seizures
  Status epilepticus
Drug-induced
  Alcoholic blackouts
  Sedatives
  Other
Metabolic-hypoglycemia
Head trauma
Other central nervous system
  Cerebral vascular insufficiency
  Subarachnoid hemorrhage
  Narcolepsy and other sleep disorders
  Brain tumors/metastasis
Hysterical-psychogenic

vulsive movements in the setting of cerebral hypoperfusion (in the absence of an underlying seizure disorder) have been well described. Unusual muscular movements during the episode of unconsciousness do not necessarily mean that the patient has suffered a seizure.

2. The most reliable clue that a patient has had a true seizure rather than a syncopal episode is a delayed return of an alert mental status (postictal state) or the occurrence of a Todd's paralysis. The syncopal patient may not feel well or normal after the event, but he or she should be alert with clear mentation.

3. Additional clues that a seizure has occurred include brief aura (deja vu, olfactory, gustatory, visual, etc.) just prior to the event, preceding stimulus of monotonous music or blinking lights, occurrence during sleep, cyanosis or stertorous breathing during the episode, and tongue biting.

4. Partial seizures, absence seizures, and atonic or akinetic seizures occur with little or no motor activity. Therefore, the absence of convulsive movements with the loss of consciousness does not rule out a seizure.

- Syncope
  1. Syncope is the most common cause of transient loss of consciousness.
  2. There are many potential causes of syncope (Table 88–2).
  3. In those cases where the cause of syncope is determined, syncope due to vasovagal mechanisms is the most common.

TABLE 88–2. Causes of Syncope

Vagal mechanism
  ''Simple faint''
  Carotid sinus hypersensitivity
  Glossopharyngeal syncope
  Micturition syncope
  Swallow syncope
  Post-pain (trigeminal neuralgia)
Cardiovascular
  Dysrrhythmia
    Sick-sinus syndrome
    Bradycardia
    Atrioventricular block (Mobitz type II or complete
      heart block)
    Pacemaker malfunction
    Supraventricular tachycardia
    Ventricular tachycardia
    Drug-induced dysrhythmias
    Congenital prolonged QT interval
  Valvular heart disease
    Aortic stenosis
    Mitral stenosis
    Pulmonic stenosis
    Tricuspid stenosis
    Mitral valve prolapse
    Prosthetic valve thrombosis or malfunction
  Cardiomyopathy
    Obstructive cardiomyopathy
    Restrictive cardiomyopathy
  Ischemic heart disease
    Angina pectoris
    Myocardial infarction
  Nonvalvular obstructive disease
    Atrial myxoma
    Pulmonary hypertension
    Pulmonary embolus
  Other
    Aortic dissection
    Pericardial disease
    Anemia
Orthostatic hypotension
  Drug-induced
  Hypovolemia
  Autonomic insufficiency
  Adrenal insufficiency
  Idiopathic
Metabolic
  Hypoxemia
  Hypocapnia
  Poisoning (e.g., carbon monoxide)
  Other drug toxicity
Cerebrovascular and neurologic
  Posterior circulation transient ischemic attack
  Migraine
  Imminent stroke

Table continued on following page

TABLE 88–2. Causes of Syncope *Continued*

Subclavian steal syndrome
Neurocirculatory asthenia
Multiple sclerosis
Hypertensive encephalopathy
Miscellaneous
  Hyperventilation
  Hysteria
  Allergic reaction
Cause unknown

4. Syncope of cardiovascular origin ultimately has a significant mortality.

CLINICAL EVALUATION

- History
  1. Obtain a thorough description of the episode from patient, family, and witnesses (if possible). Important aspects include:
     a. Preceding events (change in position, fearful or painful stimulus, hyperventilation, coughing, micturition, swallowing, use of medication, chest pain, palpitations, nausea, dizziness, abdominal pain, exertion).
     b. Body habitus and movements during the unconscious episode.
     c. Duration of unconsciousness.
     d. Return to consciousness (immediate or prolonged).
  2. Have similar episodes occurred before, and under what circumstances?
  3. What other symptoms accompanied the loss of consciousness?
  4. What other health problems does the patient have (e.g., coronary artery disease, valvular heart disease, cerebrovascular disease, known risk factors for pulmonary embolism, and diabetes mellitus)?
  5. Take a thorough medication history, including over-the-counter medications. Antihypertensive medications, nitrates, and other drugs known to cause orthostatic hypotension are potential causes. Be especially alert to any recently started medications or ones whose dosage has been changed recently.
- Physical exam
  1. Observe the patient closely. Are they awake, oriented, and appropriate or do they appear postictal? True syncope is associated with rapid, spontaneous return to baseline mental status.
  2. Obtain vital signs. Checking for postural changes should be routine in the evaluation of any syncopal patient. As many as 30% of elderly patients, however, have postural vital sign changes "normally." Even

when a patient is shown to be postural, this does not necessarily establish the cause of syncope.

3. Perform a thorough examination, with special emphasis on the cardiopulmonary exam.
4. Perform a detailed neurological examination: mental status, cranial nerves, musculoskeletal (including deep tendon reflexes), cerebellar function, and sensation.

- Laboratory evaluation
  Pursuit of further laboratory evaluation should *not* be considered routine in the evaluation of the patient suffering from syncope (with the exception of the electrocardiogram and rhythm strip). Specific tests should be ordered only as guided by the results of the history and physical examination above.

  1. ECG and rhythm strip. This is the only test that should be considered routine in the evaluation of the syncopal patient. It is mandatory in any patient with known cardiac disease or if the patient is 40 or older.
  2. CBC. Consider in the postural patient, patient with history of blood or volume loss, or patient clinically suspected of being anemic.
  3. Glucose. Mandatory in the diabetic or the alcoholic patient with syncope.
  4. Electrolytes. Mandatory in the patient who is postural, has a history of volume loss, or takes a diuretic. Strongly consider obtaining these in the elderly patient as well or the patient in whom alcohol abuse is suspected.
  5. Calcium, magnesium, phosphorus should not be routinely ordered unless the history and physical exam reveal a concomitant medical condition likely to result in an abnormality in one of these (e.g., starvation, alcoholism, parenteral nutrition), or if after a thorough history and physical exam a seizure disorder is still a likely possibility.
  6. Chest X-ray is unlikely to be helpful unless history and physical exam reveal a likely cardiopulmonary abnormality (e.g., pulmonary hypertension).
  7. ABG may be useful if history and physical exam are suspicious for significant cardiopulmonary abnormality (e.g., pulmonary embolus).

FURTHER DIAGNOSTIC TESTING

None of the many, and often expensive, tests below are either routine or mandatory in the majority of patients presenting with syncope. The clinician should proceed further only as justified by the clinical information obtained as outlined above.

- ECG monitoring in search of a dysrhythmic cause of syncope probably should be done over at least a 48-hr period. It is especially useful in the patient with suspected or known cardiac disease. Special devices are available for prolonged monitoring. There are also patient activated recording devices, which the patient turns on when symptomatic.

- Echocardiography is usually ordered to further evaluate a cardiac abnormality (e.g., aortic stenosis) identified or suspected on the basis of history (e.g., exertional or postexertional syncope) or physical exam. Other cardiac causes of syncope that may be silent on exam, but present on echocardiogram, include asymmetric septal hypertrophy, pericardial effusions, and atrial myxomas or thrombi.

- Signal averaged ECG. This relatively new technique is used to detect patient susceptibility to malignant ventricular dysrhythmias. It evaluates the surface ECG for high-frequency, low-amplitude signals in the terminal portion of the QRS complex, which have been correlated with the risk of sustained ventricular dysrhythmias. It should be considered in consultation with a cardiologist, in the patient with suspected cardiac syncope, prior to pursuing electrophysiologic testing.

- Stress testing. Though generally of low yield, exercise stress testing can provide evidence of stress-induced cardiac block or dysrhythmias responsible for syncope. In the occasional patient with syncope induced by severe ischemic heart disease, it may also be useful. Consider it in the patient with syncope that has occurred due to exertion.

- Head-up tilt table test has proven useful in the induction of a vasovagal cause of loss of consciousness in patients with syncope that has been otherwise nondiagnosed. A special motorized tilt table with a footplate support is used to travel from 0 degrees to 60 degrees in 15 sec. ECG monitoring is performed continuously, and blood pressure is measured every 5 min with an automatic sphygmomanometer. This head-up tilt is maintained for a maximum of 45 min (or until syncope and bradycardia are reproduced in a shorter time).

- Electrophysiologic testing is expensive and invasive. Its use is recommended in the patient with recurrent syncope, a negative noninvasive work-up, and a suspected cardiac dysrhythmic origin to the syncope. It is not yet clear whether treatment of suspected dysrhythmias identified by electrophysiologic testing changes mortality in syncope patients.

- Cardiac catheterization is pursued in the setting of a highly abnormal stress test or when echocardiography reveals significant aortic stenosis.

- Ventilation/Perfusion lung scan is appropriate when pulmonary embolism is felt to be a likely cause of syncope on the basis of history and physical exam and a suggestive ABG.

- Carotid sinus massage can be performed at the bedside in patients in whom carotid sinus hypersensitivity is felt to be a cause of syncope (e.g., syncope that occurs, usually in the older individual, with neck hyperextension or head turning). The patient must have both blood pressure and pulse continuously monitored, IV access established with atropine at the bedside, and no carotid bruits or history of cerebrovascular disease. There are two types of carotid hypersensitivity: 1) cardioinhibitory with ventricular asystole of greater than 3 sec with carotid massage, and 2) vasodepressor with a 50 mmHg or more drop in systolic blood pressure with carotid massage. Documenting carotid sinus hypersensitivity does not necessarily prove it is the cause of syncope. Important questions are: Did it reproduce the patient's symptoms? Was the clinical setting in which the syncope occurred compatible with a carotid sinus hypersensitivity mechanism?

- EEG is performed in search of a seizure disorder as a cause of transient loss of consciousness. It should be ordered only if the clinical setting and description of the event (e.g., prolonged return of consciousness) strongly suggest a seizure disorder.

- Head CT scan is a very low yield procedure in the work-up of syncope. Do it in the patient who describes focal neurologic symptoms in association with syncope, or if the neurologic examination reveals focal abnormalities.

- Skull films and lumbar puncture are generally unhelpful in the work-up of the syncope patient.

RECOMMENDED DIAGNOSTIC APPROACH

- Be precise. Make certain at the outset that the patient had syncope. Was there actual loss of consciousness, postural tone, and spontaneous recovery as outlined in the definition above?

- History and physical examination. Perform very carefully with the differential diagnosis of both transient loss of consciousness and syncope in mind. Special emphasis must be placed on the cardiopulmonary and neurologic examination. Always obtain postural vital signs.

- ECG and rhythm strip is the only diagnostic test that is routine.

When a diagnosis of syncope is possible, the information obtained with the above simple steps will provide that diagnosis in the majority of patients. Specific tests often are indicated by the clinical circumstances:

1. Syncope with exertion—stress test and echocardiogram
2. Cardiac murmur—echocardiogram
3. Focal neurologic examination—EEG and Head CT
4. Syncope with turning of the head or working overhead (with head hyper-extended)—carotid sinus massage
5. Syncope with dyspnea—ABG, CXR, ventilation/perfusion scan
6. Syncope with postural vital signs—CBC, serum electrolytes

- Further testing. If the cause of syncope remains undetermined, then further evaluation should be based on the following stratification:
  1. Low-risk patients: Patients 30 years or younger with no history of syncope and no evidence of cardiac syncope, or patients 70 or younger with clinically suspected vasovagal syncope—no further testing necessary, but clinical followup recommended.

2. Intermediate-risk patients: Patients not suspected of having suffered from cardiac syncope, but who do have a history of cardiac disease, or patients over 30 and up to 70 with syncope of unknown cause; or patients older than 70—further work-up must be individualized, but should probably include ambulatory ECG monitoring for at least 48 hr.

3. High-risk patients: Patients with frequent episodes of syncope that occur with little or no warning, or syncope while recumbent, or syncope with cardiac symptoms, or an abnormal electrocardiogram. Further aggressive diagnostic testing is mandatory in this group of patients and consultation with a cardiologist is appropriate. Further testing, at the least, should include cardiac monitoring for at least 48 hr (in-hospital cardiac monitoring should be considered). Additional tests on an individual basis may include stress test, echocardiogram, signal averaged ECG, and electrophysiologic testing.

Bibliography

Branch WT, Jr. Approach to syncope. J Gen Int Med 1986;1:49–58.

Day SC, et al. Evaluation and outcome of emergency room patients with transient loss of consciousness. Am J Med 1982;248:1185–1189.

Dohrmann ML, Cheitlin MD. Cardiogenic syncope: Seizure versus syncope. Neurol Clin 1986;4(3):549–562.

Fitzpatrick A, Sutton R. Tilting towards a diagnosis in recurrent unexplained syncope. Lancet 1989(Mar. 25):658–660.

Kapoor WN. Evaluation and outcome of patients with syncope. Medicine 1990;69:160–175.

Kapoor WN. Diagnostic evaluation of syncope. Am J Med 1991;90:91–106.

Kapoor WN, et al. Prolonged electrocardiographic monitoring in patients with syncope. Am J Med 1987;82:20–28.

Kapoor WN, et al. A prospective evaluation and follow-up of patients with syncope. N Engl J Med 1983;309(4):197–204.

Manolis AS, et al. Syncope: Current diagnostic evaluation and management. Ann Int Med 1990;112:850–863.

Mozes B, et al. Cost-effectiveness of in-hospital evaluation of patients with syncope. Israel J Med Sci 1988;24:302–306.

Strasberg B, et al. The noninvasive evaluation of syncope of suspected cardiovascular origin. Am Heart J 1989;117(1):160–163.

89

DELIRIUM

ARTHUR KELLERMAN, and
CURTIS SAUER

Brain. An apparatus with which we think that we think.

AMBROSE BIERCE (1842–1914)

DEFINITION

- General description. Delirium is an organic mental disorder characterized by a generally transient but global impairment in cerebral function. Impaired consciousness of some degree is essential to the diagnosis.
- Criteria for diagnosis. Delirium should be considered a symptom, not a disease (Diagnostic and Statistical Manual of Mental Disorders, IIIR).
  1. Reduced ability to maintain attention to external stimuli and to appropriately shift attention to new external stimuli.
  2. Disorganized thinking, as indicated by rambling, irrelevant, or incoherent speech.
  3. At least two of the following:
     a. Reduced level of consciousness: difficulty keeping awake during the examination.
     b. Perceptual disturbances: misinterpretations, illusions, or hallucinations.
     c. Disturbance of sleep-wake cycle with insomnia or daytime sleepiness.
     d. Increased or decreased psychomotor activity.
     e. Disorientation to time, place, or person.
     f. Memory impairment: inability to learn new material or to remember past events.
  4. Clinical features develop over a short period of time (usually hours to days) and tend to fluctuate over the course of a day.
  5. Either (a) or (b):
     a. Evidence from the history, physical examination, or laboratory tests of a specific organic factor (or factors) judged to be etiologically related to the disturbance.
     b. In the absence of such evidence, an etiologic organic factor can be presumed if the disturbance cannot be accounted for by any nonorganic mental disorder (e.g., manic episode accounting for agitation and sleep disturbance).
- Clinical subtypes. The confusional state may be hyperalert

or hypoactive and somnolent. Individuals may move from one state to the other.

- Delirium with an organic brain syndrome. Delirium may be superimposed on a chronic organic brain syndrome. Such individuals are usually identified by a relatively abrupt change in awareness and cognition from a previously stable level of functional impairment.
- Pathogenesis
  1. Level vs. content of consciousness. While the level of consciousness is a function of both the cerebral cortex and the reticular activating system, the content of consciousness is largely a cortical function.
  2. Causes of delirium vs. causes of coma (Table 89–1). As with coma, most cases of delirium are related to metabolic imbalances or intoxication.
  3. Focal lesions. Focal lesions in the frontal, temporal, and occipital lobes as well as infarction in the distribution of the right middle cerebral artery may produce acute confusional states as their only manifestation.
  4. Complex partial seizures. When prolonged (i.e., "status"), they may cause only behavioral and cognitive change and require an EEG for diagnosis.
- Epidemiology
  1. Prevalence. Delirium of some degree occurs in 5 to 15% of all patients hospitalized on general medical and surgical floors. Estimates are higher for patients on psychiatric floors (5 to 40%) and in intensive care units (20 to 50%).
  2. Relative risk. Elderly patients are twice as likely to develop delirium following a given physiologic stress.
  3. Mortality. The 1-year mortality for patients admitted with delirium has been estimated at 30 to 50%.

DIFFERENTIAL DIAGNOSIS

- Delirium vs. functional psychiatric disorders (Table 89–2)
  1. Psychiatric symptoms (agitation, apathy, psychosis, combative or inappropriate behavior) commonly predominate in delirium and can lead to inappropriate triage or premature psychiatric referral.
  2. Roughly 3% of patients "medically cleared" for psychiatric admission are found to have delirium. Delirium may coexist with a previously diagnosed psychiatric disorder, making evaluation even more difficult.
  3. Disorientation, clouding of consciousness, age over 40 without a previous psychiatric history, and abnormal vital signs all raise the suspicion of delirium.
- Delirium vs. dementia in the elderly
  1. Delirium commonly has an onset of hours to days rather than months to years, as in dementia. Alterations in consciousness, fluctuation in clinical course, and lucid intervals are characteristic of delirium.
  2. Delirium may coexist with dementia and should be

considered in the event of rapid deterioration or abnormal vital signs in a previously stable patient.

- Other conditions mistaken for delirium. Wernicke's aphasia, Korsakoff's syndrome, denial states following certain cerebrovascular accidents, mental retardation, and Ganser syndrome ("pseudoinsanity") may be mistaken for delirium.

CLINICAL FEATURES

- Abnormal vital signs. Abnormal vital signs should not be dismissed as secondary to agitation. An associated medical condition such as infection, drug withdrawal, intoxication, or metastatic disturbance should be sought.
- Disordered wakefulness or sensorium. This finding is required for the diagnosis of delirium. The level of consciousness may be either increased or decreased, but concentration is impaired and attention cannot be sustained. Insomnia is common.
- Impaired cognition. Impaired cognition may be manifest as disorientation, illusions, hallucinations (most commonly visual), delusions, and defects in short-term memory.
- Emotional lability. Emotional lability is characteristic of delirium. Hallucinations are commonly perceived as foreign ("ego-dystonic") and frightening to the patient, in contrast to those associated with schizophrenia.
- Psychomotor disturbance. Psychomotor disturbance ranges from quiet apathy to gross agitation. Picking at clothes and IV tubing, wandering from bed or ward, and combative behavior may occur. Gross tremors, seizures, ataxia, myoclonic jerks, asterixis, and choreoathetoid movements are common manifestations of delirium.
- Varying degrees of impairment. Fluctuation from moment to moment is common. Symptoms are generally more severe at night, when organizing sensory input is decreased.

RECOMMENDED DIAGNOSTIC APPROACH

- Initial stabilization
  1. Initial assessment and stabilization should precede a definitive diagnostic evaluation in a manner analogous to the methods outlined in Chapter 87 for coma. The patient's airway, breathing, and circulatory status should be immediately assessed and supported if necessary.
  2. If hypoglycemia is suspected, glucose and thiamine should be provided while initial laboratory tests are pending.
  3. When necessary, the patient should be gently restrained to avoid injury to himself or others. Sedation with drugs should be avoided until the underlying diagnosis is established.

TABLE 89-1. Causes of Delirium

	DIAGNOSIS	PERCENT
Toxic	Alcohol	25–50
	Drugs (illicit, prescribed, over-the-counter)	
	Inhalants (gasoline, glue, ether, liquid paper)	
	Poisons (solvents, carbon monoxide, organophosphates, heavy metals)	
Infections	Systemic (sepsis, pneumonia, pyelonephritis, typhoid, Legionnaires' disease)	10–20
	Intracranial (meningitis, encephalitis, abscess)	
Withdrawal syndromes	Alcohol, sedative hypnotics, amphetamines	10–15
Epilepsy	Status epilepticus, postictal states	10–15
Fluid and electrolytes	Hypo- or hypernatremia	10–15
	Hypo- or hypercalcemia	
	Acidosis or alkalosis	
	Hypo- or hypermagnesemia	
Metabolic	Hepatic encephalopathy	5–10
	Uremia and dialysis syndromes	
	Respiratory failure (hypercarbia, hypoxia)	
	Circulatory failure (hypertensive encephalopathy, shock, congestive heart failure)	
	Porphyria	
	Wilson's disease	

Category		
Endocrine	Hypo- or hyperglycemia	2–5
	Hypo- or hyperthyroidism	
	Addison's disease or Cushing's syndrome	
	Hypo- or hyperparathyroidism	
	Hypopituitarism	
Trauma	Head (concussion, contusion, epi- or subdural and intracerebral hematomas)	2–5
	Systemic (burns, surgery, intensive care unit status, multiple injuries, fat embolism)	
Cerebrovascular disease	Transient ischemic attacks	2–5
	Cerebrovascular accident	
	Subarachnoid hemorrhage	
	Complex migraine	
Nutritional	Deficiency (thiamine, niacin, vitamin B_{12}, pyridoxine, folate)	(<3)
	Hypervitaminosis A or D	
Neoplastic	Primary intracranial neoplasms	(<3)
	Cerebral and meningeal metastases	
	Carcinoid and paraneoplastic syndromes	
Autoimmune	SLE, polyarteritis, rheumatic fever	(<3)
Miscellaneous	Hypo- or hyperthermia	(2–5)
	Sleep or sensory deprivation	
	Hospitalization (intensive care unit and postoperative delirium)	
	Toxemia of pregnancy	

TABLE 89–2. Differential Diagnosis of the "Confusional" State

Delirium
Dementing disorders[a]
Psychiatric disorders
   Acute schizophrenia
   Acute manic and paranoid states
   Depression
   Acute grief reaction
   Hysterical psychosis
   Ganser syndrome
   Conversion disorder
Korsakoff's syndrome
Fluent aphasia
Denial syndromes (past cerebrovascular accident)
Mental retardation

[a] See Chapter 90.

- History. A history should be obtained from all available sources. Despite confusion, the patient may provide valuable clues. These should be corroborated whenever possible. All available pill containers should be identified, since virtually any drug can produce delirium. Coincident head trauma and intoxication demand a high level of suspicion for an intracranial process.

- Physical examination. Special emphasis should be placed on the vital signs. Fever, tachycardia, or hypertension should prompt a particularly careful evaluation for an underlying medical condition. Cardiopulmonary problems and occult infections are common causes of delirium in the elderly.

- Mental status examination. The Mini Mental State evaluation outlined in Chapter 90 may be helpful. Fluctuation is common, and frequent reevaluation is mandatory until the diagnosis is established.

- Laboratory evaluation. The laboratory evaluation should be tiered, with an initial limited battery of tests designed to screen for major physiologic derangements. Further evaluation should be guided by the results of these preliminary tests as well as by clinical findings.

  1. Initial screening tests should be obtained early during the initial assessment of the patient
     a. CBC with white cell differential
     b. Serum electrolyte, urea nitrogen, creatinine, glucose, and calcium determinations
     c. ECG
     d. Chest X-ray
     e. Urinalysis
     f. Stool for occult blood
     g. Arterial blood gas or hemoglobin oxygen saturation by pulse oximetry
  2. Subsequent confirmatory tests should only be done when dictated by clinical suspicion
     a. Emergency toxicology

i. "STAT" qualitative toxicologic screens of blood, gastric contents, and urine take time to perform, have limited sensitivity, and fail to screen all potentially important drugs. Drug screens should supplement but not overrule clinical suspicion.

ii. Blood or breath alcohol level determinations are fast, inexpensive, and reasonably accurate. Quantitative drug levels may be extremely important in certain clinical situations such as suspected overdoses of aspirin, acetaminophen, theophylline, lithium, diphenylhydantoin, or digoxin but should only be ordered selectively.

b. Lumbar puncture should be performed and antibiotics administered at the slightest suspicion of meningitis. Both are mandatory when delirium is accompanied by fever or other signs of infection.

c. An immediate CT scan is indicated if there is a history of head trauma, focal abnormalities on neurologic exam, or if an intracranial mass is suspected.

d. Further laboratory tests, including liver enzymes, serum ammonia, endocrine studies, ANA assay, serum protein electrophoresis, bromide level, CSF glutamine, and urine for porphyria or heavy metals, should only be obtained when there are specific indications and appropriate clinical suspicion.

e. The EEG has little place in emergent evaluation but may confirm the presence of complex partial status epilepticus.

f. Radionuclide brain scanning and MRI have no place in the emergent evaluation of delirium but may be useful if herpes encephalitis is suspected and the CT scan is not diagnostic.

Bibliography

American Psychiatric Association. Diagnostic and Statistical Manual of Mental Disorders (DSM-III-R). Washington, DC, American Psychiatric Association. 1987.

Dubin WR, et al. Organic brain syndrome. The psychiatric imposter. JAMA 1983;249:6062.

Francis J, et al. A prospective study of delirium in hospitalized elderly. JAMA 1990;263:1097–1101.

Lipowski ZJ. Delirium in the elderly. N Engl J Med 1989;320:578–582.

Mori E, Yamadori A. Acute confusional state and agitated delirium. Occurrence after infarction in the right middle cerebral artery territory. Arch Neurol 1987;44:1139–1143.

Rabin P, Folstein M. Delirium and dementia: Diagnostic criteria and fatality rates. Br J Psychiatr 1982;140:149–153.

90

DEMENTIA

BEVERLY M. PARKER, and
BARRY J. CUSACK

Our brains are seventy year old clocks. The angel of life
winds them up once for all, then closes the case, and
gives the key into the hand of the angel of the resurrec-
tion.

OLIVER WENDELL HOLMES (1857)

DEFINITION

Dementia is a syndrome characterized by intellectual impairment. It can affect persons of any age, but is most common in
those over 65. In that group, the prevalence is 5 to 10%. In
those over 85 the prevalence is 30 to 40%, but does not rise
thereafter.

DIAGNOSTIC CRITERIA

The clinical definition of dementia is (DSM-IIIR; all criteria
must be present):

- A state of acquired global cognitive impairment severe
  enough to interfere with social or occupational performance.
- There is impairment of short- (e.g., 3 objects at 3 min) and
  long-term memory (e.g., past information such as what
  happened yesterday, birthplace, previous occupations).
- There is at least one of the following: impaired abstract
  thinking, impaired judgment, dysphasia, motor dyspraxia,
  agnosia, constructional difficulties (e.g., drawing a clock),
  or personality change.
- The changes are not occurring exclusively during the
  course of delirium.
- There is clinical or laboratory evidence of an organic cause.
- If there is no such clinical or laboratory evidence, an organic cause may be presumed if the condition is not due to a
  nonorganic disorder such as major depression.

DIFFERENTIAL DIAGNOSIS (Table 90–1):

Alzheimer's dementia (DAT), multi-infarct dementia (MID),
or a combination of the 2 account for 80 to 85% of all cases of
dementia in persons over 65. DAT is a less common, but still

TABLE 90–1. Causes of Dementia

Primary CNS disorders
  DAT
  Pick's disease
  Parkinson's disease
  Huntington's disease
Vascular
  MID
  Vasculitides: e.g., granulomatous vasculitis, SLE,
    temporal arteritis
  Cerebral hypoxia or anoxia
Systemic/Metabolic
  Endocrine disorders: e.g., hypothyroidism,
    hypercalcemia, Cushing's syndrome
  Chronic hepatic encephalopathy
  Uremia
  Uremic encephalopathy (dialysis dementia)
  Vitamin deficiencies: e.g., B_{12}, folate
  Drugs and toxins: e.g., alcohol, sedatives/hypnotics,
    anticholinergic medications
Intracranial mass lesions
  Tumor: primary or metastatic
  Chronic subdural or epidural hematoma
Infection
  Viral: e.g., human immunodeficiency virus (HIV)
    encephalopathy, Creutzfeld-Jakob disease
  Fungal: e.g., cryptococcal meningitis, coccidioidomycosis
  Bacterial: e.g., tuberculosis, neurosyphilis
Miscellaneous
  Normal pressure hydrocephalus
  Sarcoidosis
  Mixed dementia (DAT and MID)
  Trauma (serious head injury)

important cause of dementia in those under 65 years. DAT is currently a diagnosis of exclusion.

MAJOR DEMENTIA SYNDROMES

- Alzheimer's disease (Dementia of the Alzheimer's Type—DAT)
  1. This accounts for up to 60% of cases in those over 65. It occurs sporadically, but is inherited as an autosomal dominant disease in a small minority of cases. Pick's disease is a clinically similar but rare form of dementia mainly involving the frontal lobes.
  2. The disease is insidious in onset and progresses slowly with development of total functional disability. Death occurs within 10 to 15 years, usually from intercurrent infection or metabolic dysfunction.
  3. Dysphasia is a common symptom which can occur early and may portend a relatively rapid cognitive decline.

4. Patients develop agnosias and task apraxias.
5. Motor dysfunction occurs and extrapyramidal signs are present in 30 to 60% of patients. They are preceded by cognitive decline.
6. Depression is common, especially in early disease, and can worsen cognition. Patients with DAT are susceptible to delirium.
7. Laboratory studies
   a. The head CT scan may show atrophy of the anterior and medial temporal lobes which does not correlate with the clinical severity.
   b. The head MR scan shows atrophy and a smooth periventricular halo on T2-weighted images.
   c. Positron emission tomographic (PET) scanning shows a global decrease in cerebral glucose and oxygen metabolism, especially in the temporal and parietal lobes.

- Vascular dementia
  1. This term encompasses several marginally distinct syndromes, including
     a. Subacute arteriosclerotic encephalopathy (Binswanger's disease)
     b. Lacunar dementia
     c. MID
  2. MID is most common after the age of 60. It is strongly associated with hypertension, diabetes mellitus, cardiac disease, tobacco use, hyperlipidemia, and hypotensive episodes.
  3. MID is most commonly caused by small lacunar infarcts due to lipohyalinosis. Extracranial occlusive disease and cardiac emboli are less common causes.
  4. The course usually has an abrupt onset, a stepwise progression, and associated focal neurologic signs and symptoms.
  5. The Hachinski Ischemia Score and the Modified Ischemia Score are useful in diagnosing MID (Table 90–2).
  6. Laboratory studies
     a. The head CT scan characteristically shows 1 or more hypodensities, typically in periventricular white matter or subcortical areas.
     b. The head MR scan shows periventricular white matter lesions. It may show an intense halo of periventricular density on T2-weighted images with patchy distribution and irregular margins.

- Parkinsonism
  1. Parkinson's disease may result in dementia, depression, and psychosis. The dementia is often mild but may occur in up to 40% of cases. It is most common in elderly patients and occurs relatively late in the disease.
  2. Progressive supranuclear palsy is the most common of the rare multisystem parkinsonoid disorders, and is characterized by an extension posture, ophthalmoplegia, rigidity, and subcortical dementia.

- Huntington's disease

TABLE 90–2. Multi-infarct Dementia Scales

HACHINSKI ISCHEMIC SCALE[a]		MODIFIED ISCHEMIA SCORE[b]	
Abrupt onset	2	Abrupt onset	2
Stepwise deterioration	1	History of stroke	1
Fluctuation	2	Focal symptoms	2
Nocturnal confusion	1	Focal signs	2
Relative preservation of		CT hypodensities	
personality	1	single	2
Depression	1	multiple	3
Somatic complaints	1		
Emotional lability	1		
Hypertension	1		
History of stroke	2		
Focal symptoms	2		
Focal signs	2		
Other signs of atherosclerotic	1		
vascular disease			

[a] 0–4 = Low probability of MID; 5–6 = indeterminant; ≥7 = high probability of MID.
[b] 0–2 = Low probability of MID; 3–4 = indeterminant; ≥5 = high probability of MID.

1. This is a genetic syndrome of progressive dementia and chorea with autosomal dominant inheritance.
2. Its onset is in the 4th or 5th decade, with rapid progression of choreiform movements and dementia.
3. Laboratory studies
   a. Atrophy of the caudate is seen on CT scanning.
   b. PET scanning demonstrates a marked decline in caudate metabolism.

POTENTIALLY TREATABLE FORMS OF DEMENTIA

Up to 20% of demented patients under 65 have a potentially treatable cause of dementia, but only 5% of those over 65 have any likelihood of response.

- Pseudodementia (Table 90–3).
  1. This is most commonly due to depression and occasionally to psychosis.
  2. Depression is superimposed on dementia far more often than acting as a cause of pseudodementia.
  3. Depression scales such as the Zung or Beck Depression Inventory may be helpful evaluation tools.
- Normal pressure hydrocephalus
  1. This is a rare disorder of CSF reabsorption which causes communicating hydrocephalus. A history of subarachnoid hemorrhage, meningitis, or head injury should heighten suspicion.
  2. Principal clinical features include dementia, gait dis-

TABLE 90–3. Differences Between Pseudodementia and Dementia

PARAMETER	PSEUDODEMENTIA	DEMENTIA
Onset	<6 months	>6 months
Memory loss	Tend to emphasize	Often deny
Cognitive decline	Complain of decline	Deny decline
Depression symptoms	Present	Absent
Test performance	Do poorly because of poor motivation or fail marginally	Try to answer but fail
Antidepressant response	Good	Poor: may cause confusion

turbance, and urinary incontinence. The gait typically is slow, shuffling, wide-based, and ataxic.

3. The CT scan shows a bulbous-appearing enlargement of the ventricular system out of proportion to the size of the sulci.

4. The MR scan shows similar ventricular enlargement, increased periventricular thinning, and a CSF void sign (decreased image of the cerebral aqueduct due to increased flow of CSF).

- Vitamin deficiencies

1. The association of B_{12} and folate deficiencies with dementia has been reported, although in the latter case, reports are anecdotal. Dementia from B_{12} deficiency may precede hematologic and peripheral neurologic disorders.

2. An RBC folate is a much better index of body stores than serum folate, which correlates with recent dietary folate intake.

- Alcoholism

1. In addition to acute Wernicke's encephalopathy and the chronic Korsakoff's syndrome, dementia is associated with alcoholism. Cerebral atrophy is common.

2. Alcoholism may be overlooked, particularly in older white female patients or those with higher levels of education.

- Endocrine/Metabolic

1. Cognitive deficits, often with a delirium-type picture, are associated with electrolyte disorders.

2. Both hypothyroidism and hyperthyroidism have been associated with cognitive deficits. Screening with a highly sensitive serum TSH assay can detect either abnormality and may be preferred to serum T4 levels.

- Infections

1. Neurosyphilis, encephalitis, chronic meningitis due to tuberculosis or fungal infection, and viral infections

(e.g., Creutzfeldt-Jakob disease) are the infectious diseases most likely to cause dementia without other clinical clues. HIV infection is an increasingly important cause of dementia. Few viral diseases are treatable.

2. A lumbar puncture should be performed when active CNS infection is suspected. Since it is expensive and invasive with a low yield, it should not be routinely performed.

- Structural lesions
  1. Resectable CNS tumors (meningioma, glioma) which arise in the "silent" areas of the brain—midline structures, frontal lobes, or right temporal lobe—are rare causes of unexplained dementia.
  2. Chronic subdural hematoma must be ruled out in older or alcoholic patients with a subacute onset of dementia. A history of falls and localizing neurological signs often are absent.

- Toxic
  1. In addition to alcohol, toxins such as heavy metals and medications may cause dementia.
  2. *It is always valuable to attempt reducing or stopping possible offending medications.*
  3. Aluminum toxicity contributes to "dialysis dementia."

- Inflammatory
  1. The vasculitides cause a dementia syndrome, often in association with other neurologic findings.
  2. A sedimentation rate and serologic studies are appropriate initial studies.
  3. Tissue biopsies or cerebral angiography may be indicated in unresolved cases if the clinical suspicion is high.

RECOMMENDED DIAGNOSTIC APPROACH

- Establish that the diagnosis is dementia, according to DSM-IIIR criteria. Other causes of altered mental status such as psychosis, delirium, and depression should be excluded. Conditions that may aggravate dementia (e.g., urinary tract infection) should be excluded.

- Initial procedures in the diagnosis of dementia
  1. History (from different sources if necessary) including medication and substance abuse history.
  2. Physical examination. Particularly note signs of vascular, pulmonary, and hepatic disease, focal neurologic signs, and gait abnormalities.
  3. Check clinical findings against DSM-IIIR criteria.
  4. Do Folstein Mini-Mental Status Score (Table 90–4) or one other validated dementia score.
  5. Formal neuropsychologic testing should be considered if there is doubt about the presence of significant cognitive impairment.
     a. Such testing will provide a measure of the degree of dementia present, and serial studies may be

TABLE 90–4. Folstein Mini-Mental Status Examination

	MAX. SCORE
Orientation	
1. What is the (year) (season) (date) (day) (month)?	5
2. Where are we (state) (county) (city) (hospital) (floor)?	5
Registration	
Immediately repeat 3 objects	3
Attention/Calculation	5
Count serial 7s backwards from 100 (5 times) or spell WORLD backwards	
Recall	
Remember above 3 objects at 2 minutes	3
Language	
Name a pen and a watch	2
Repeat "No ifs ands or buts"	1
3-stage command: Take this piece of paper in your right hand, fold it in half, and put it on the floor	3
Written command "Close your eyes"	1
Write a sentence	1
Visual/Spatial	
Copy intersecting pentagon design	1
Maximum total[a]	30

[a] 25–30 = Normal; 21–24 mild impairment; 16–20 moderate impairment; ≤15 severe impairment.

Source: Used with permission from Folstein MF, et al. Mini-Mental State. A practical method for grading the cognitive state of patients for the clinician. J Psychiatry Res 1975;12:189–198.

              useful in the early stages of doubtful cases to document any decline in cognition.

    b. Specific "dementia batteries" are also available that can help separate Alzheimer's disease from other causes of dementia.

  6. Laboratory studies

    a. CBC, ESR ("rule-out" anemia, vasculitis, infection).

    b. Chemistry screen ("rule-out" renal, metabolic, hepatic disease).

    c. Urinalysis ("rule-out" urinary tract infection).

    d. Thyroid function studies.

    e. Chest X-ray ("rule-out" neoplasm).

    f. ECG.

    g. Serum B_{12} and red cell folate levels.

    h. Serologic test for syphilis.

    i. Head CT scan (with and without contrast). The yield is low except in cases with a short history (less than 6 months), headache, or focal signs (including speech difficulty). An MR scan may be the study of choice in some centers.

- Secondary procedures
  1. EEG is useful only in cases of suspected encephalitis, delirium, or toxic encephalopathy.
  2. Lumbar puncture should be reserved for cases with suspected CNS infection. Clinical features that predict a high yield include subacute onset, fever, and signs of meningeal irritation.
- Tertiary procedures
  1. Heavy metal screen: e.g., lead.
  2. Serologic studies: e.g., antinuclear antibody.
  3. HIV antibody test: should be performed in persons considered to be at increased risk of HIV infection.
  4. Tissue biopsy: e.g., liver biopsy, temporal artery biopsy. Brain biopsy is rarely required, but may help diagnose disorders such as CNS lymphoma, granulomatous angiitis, or chronic infection.

Bibliography

American Psychiatric Association. Diagnostic and Statistical Manual of Mental Disorders, 3rd ed. (revised). Washington, DC, 1987, p. 107.

Clarfield AM. The reversible dementias: Do they reverse? Ann Int Med 1988;109:476–486.

Johnson KA, et al. Comparison of magnetic resonance and roentgen ray computed tomography in dementia. Arch Neurol 1987;44:1075–1080.

Katzman R. Alzheimer's disease. N Engl J Med 1986;314:964–973.

Larson EB, et al. Diagnostic tests in the evaluation of dementia. Arch Intern Med 1986;146:1917–1922.

Martin DC. B_{12} and folate deficiency dementia. Clin Ger Med 1988;4(4):841–852.

McKhann G, et al. Clinical diagnosis of Alzheimer's disease: Report of the NINCDS-ADRDA Work Group. Neurology 1984;34:939–944.

National Institutes of Health Consensus Development Conference Statement. Differential diagnosis of dementing diseases. 1987; 6(11):1–9.

Turner DA, McGeachie RE. Normal pressure hydrocephalus—evaluation and treatment. Clin Ger Med 1988;4(4):815–829.

Van Horn G. Dementia. Am J Med 1987;83:101–110.

91

HEADACHE

HASI M. VENKATACHALAM

Lord, how my head aches! What a head have I! It beats as it would fall in twenty pieces.

SHAKESPEARE (1564–1616) Romeo and Juliet, II, v, 49

GENERAL COMMENTS

Headache is a symptom, not a disease. Each year, 45 million Americans seek help for headache complaints, and approximately half of the U.S. population has had at least one severe headache.

DIFFERENTIAL DIAGNOSIS

- "Headache" commonly refers to head pain at or above brow level (Table 91–1).
- One-third of ambulatory patients with headache have tension-type headaches. Migraine accounts for 20 to 25% of cases. The remainder consist mostly of the "combination" variety of the older classification (tension-muscle contraction and migraine). Fewer than 0.5% are related to brain tumors.
- The key issue in diagnosis is the differentiation of headaches with benign prognoses and those with serious consequences (e.g., tumor, vascular accidents).

CLINICAL FEATURES

A careful history is essential to diagnosis and when coupled with a focused neurologic examination, leads to diagnosis in over 90% of patients. (Figure 91–1 and Table 91–2).

- Migraine
  1. Migraine with aura (includes previously used categories of classic migraine, ophthalmic, hemiplegic, or complicated migraine)
     a. Classic migraine
        i. Twenty percent of migraines fall in this category.
        ii. Onset is usually by the third decade of life and is rare after age 40. The incidence is higher in males before puberty and in females after puberty. There is a positive family history in at least 60% of cases.

TABLE 91–1. International Headache Society Classification of Headache

Primary headache
1. Migraine
2. Tension-type headache
3. Cluster headache and chronic paroxysmal hemicrania

Other headache
4. Miscellaneous headaches not associated with structural lesion
5. Headache associated with trauma
6. Headache associated with vascular disorders
7. Headache associated with nonvascular intracranial disorder
8. Headache associated with substance abuse or substance withdrawal
9. Headache associated with noncephalic infection
10. Headache associated with metabolic disorder
11. Headache or facial pain associated with disorders of the cranium, neck, eyes, ears, nose, sinuses, teeth, mouth, or other cranial structures
12. Cranial neuralgias, nerve trunk pain, and deafferentation pain
13. Headaches not classifiable

Source: Headache Classification Committee of the International Headache Society: Classification and diagnostic criteria for headache disorders, cranial neuralgias, and facial pain. Cephalalgia 1988;8(suppl 7):9–96.

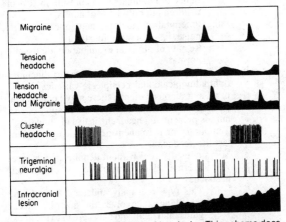

Figure 91–1. Temporal patterns of headache. This scheme does not bring out the difference in duration between the pain of trigeminal neuralgia (repeated jabs lasting a fraction of a second) and that of cluster headache (each lasting 20 to 120 minutes). Reproduced with permission from Lance JW. Mechanism and Management of Headache. Fourth edition. London: Butterworths, 1982.

TABLE 91–2. Temporal Classification of Headache

Acute, recurrent: e.g., migraine
Acute, sudden: e.g., acute sinusitis, subarachnoid hemorrhage
Chronic, nonprogressive: e.g., tension-type headache
Chronic, progressive: e.g., intracranial mass lesion

   iii. Patients experience an aura which consists of visual (in one-third), auditory, or other sensory symptoms. The aura develops gradually over 5 to 20 min and usually lasts less than 60 min. Generally, it precedes the headache.

   iv. Examples of visual auras include photophobia, fortification spectra, teichopsia (zigzag lines of light) with scintillating scotomata (10%), and photopsia (unformed flashes of light, 25%).

   v. The headache is unilateral in two-thirds. Initially the pain is dull and progresses to severe or intense throbbing. The duration ranges from 4 hr to 3 days, but most migraine headaches last several hours. Attacks prohibit usual daily activities and the patient prefers to "sleep off" the headache.

   vi. The headache phase may be completely absent in a few cases (acephalgic migraine).

   vii. Nausea or vomiting occurs in 68% of patients. Abdominal pain is present in 20% of children but only 1.5% of adults.

   viii. Precipitating factors may include diet, noise, light, or stressful stimuli.

   ix. Results of physical examination are usually normal.

  b. Complicated migraine. This category includes ophthalmoplegic and hemiplegic varieties. In 4% of all migrainous patients, there may be unilateral paresthesias with hemiparesis or dysphasia. An aura is present and headache is usually unilateral. Temporary or permanent neurologic deficits outlast the headache.

  c. Migrainous disorder without definite criteria (previous terms: facial migraine or lower-half headache)

   i. This type is usually unilateral and may be throbbing. It involves the nostrils, cheek, gums, and teeth and may spread to the neck, ear, or eye.

   ii. It differs from cluster headache in that remissions (which usually occur between bouts of cluster headache) are absent and episodes last from 4 hr to several days (while cluster headaches last 2 hr or less).

2. Migraine without aura (previously used term: common migraine). This is more common than migraine with aura. Except for the lack of aura, it is clinically similar to the migraine with aura.

3. Status migrainosus. This is a migraine attack with the headache phase lasting more than 72 hours. Headache is continuous throughout the attack or interrupted by less than 4 hours of headache-free intervals. Status migrainosus is usually associated with ergotamine tartrate or analgesic overuse.

- Tension-type headache (previously used terms: tension headache, muscle contraction headache)

  1. Pain is constant or pressing and initially episodic, but some become chronic or daily.
  2. Headache is bilateral in 90% with a "hatband" distribution of pressing, dull, undulating pain during the day, usually waxing with the day's progression.
  3. Nausea is absent, but photophobia or phonophobia may be present.
  4. Results of physical examination are usually normal.

- Coexisting migraine and tension-type headache (previously used terms: mixed headache, tension-vascular headache, combination headache)

  1. Migraine and tension-type headache often occur in the same patient.
  2. A headache pattern chronicle kept by the patient is helpful in evaluating the relative importance of the 2 conditions and thus establishing priority for treatment.
  3. Results of physical examination are usually normal.

- Cluster headache and chronic paroxysmal hemicrania (previously used terms: Horton's histamine headache, migrainous neuralgia)

  1. In this syndrome, each headache has a sudden onset, with severe, boring, throbbing, or pulsating pain that is centered over one eye and the adjacent head and/or face. Untreated, an attack may last 15 to 180 min. There may be associated ipsilateral rhinorrhea or blocked nostril.
  2. The term "cluster" is used because the headaches occur daily, usually once per day, over a period of 1 to 8 weeks and then cease abruptly. The patient may remain symptom-free for years with subsequent recurrence of a cluster. Alcohol may precipitate headaches in a susceptible individual during a "cluster."
  3. Age at onset is typically from 20 to 40 years. The ratio of male to female patients is about 6:1.
  4. During an attack the patient is usually restless and pacing (in contrast to a migrainous patient, who prefers to lie quietly, curled up, in a dark and silent room).

- Miscellaneous headache not associated with structural lesions include the following:

  1. Idiopathic stabbing headache lasting a fraction of a second, seen in migrainous patients. The distribution of pain is over the first division of the trigeminal nerve, on the side of migraine in about 40%.

2. External compression headache, e.g., "swim-goggle headache."
3. Cold stimulus headache: e.g., following exposure to subzero weather or diving into cold water.
4. Benign cough headache: precipitated by cough in the absence of any cranial disorder. Onset is sudden and duration is less than 1 min. Physical examination is normal. May be diagnosed only after a thorough history and after structural lesions such as posterior fossa tumor have been excluded by neuroimaging.
5. Benign exertional headache: usually bilateral and more common in migrainous patients.
6. Headache associated with sexual activity: usually bilateral with increasing severity becoming intense at orgasm, in the absence of any intracranial pathology such as aneurysm.

- Headache associated with head trauma. These may be acute or chronic. Objective physical findings may be absent. These cases must have follow-up evaluation to exclude intracranial pathology.
- Headaches due to serious underlying disease. These patients are more likely to have neurologic findings on physical examination. The more common causes include subarachnoid hemorrhage, chronic subdural hematoma, intracranial mass lesions, temporal arteritis, and infections such as meningitis.

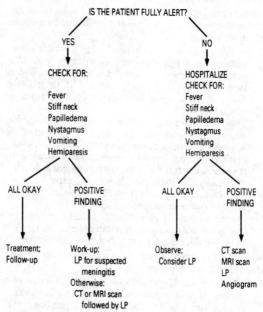

Figure 91–2a. Evaluations of patients with Acute headache.

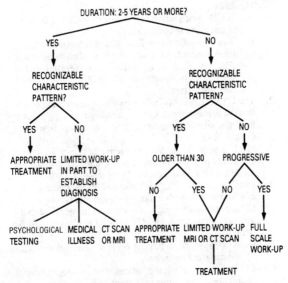

Figure 91–2b. Evaluation of patients with Chronic recurring headache.

RECOMMENDED DIAGNOSTIC APPROACH (Figure 91–2)

- History. The history is paramount, and includes:
  1. Age and sex of the patient.
  2. Number and types of headaches present.
  3. Circumstances and age of onset.
  4. Family history.
  5. Characteristics of pain: location, frequency, duration, radiation, quality of pain, and time of onset. A headache diary may help clarify these.
  6. Prodromal symptoms and precipitating factors.
  7. Medical history: past illnesses, concurrent disease, trauma, surgery, alcohol use, sleep pattern, and allergies.
  8. Response to medication.
  9. Psychosocial factors.

- Physical examination. Focal neurologic signs, as well as papilledema, altered mental status, and personality changes, especially in older or debilitated patients, or in patients with high alcohol intake or a history of head trauma, should alert the physician to the possibility of intracranial lesions.

- Laboratory evaluation. This usually adds little to the history and physical examination. When underlying organic disease is suspected or abnormal neurologic findings are present, further testing is warranted. Negative laboratory results do not rule out specific medical causes of headache. Appropriate clinical reassessments are *essential*.

1. Hematology
   a. A CBC with white cell differential should be done if infection is suspected.
   b. The ESR should be determined if temporal arteritis is suspected (in new onset headaches after age 50). The ESR is almost always elevated and is greater than 40 mm/hr in 70% of patients with temporal arteritis.
2. The CT scan is useful when results of neurologic examination are abnormal but has a low yield of significant findings when the neurologic examination is normal (Table 91–3).
3. MRI. The yield of MRI is higher in the presence of abnormal physical findings. It is the preferred imaging modality in selected cases (Table 91—4).
4. Lumbar puncture (LP) is indicated for headaches (usually acute) in which bacterial meningitis is suspected. LP is potentially dangerous when an intracranial mass lesion is suspected, and CT or MRI studies should be done first.
5. Skull X-rays are indicated only in selected cases of posttraumatic headache.
6. EEG is useful only if the patient has neurologic deficits or seizures, or in some infections (e.g., herpes simplex encephalitis).
7. Cerebral angiogram can be used to confirm the presence of specific vascular lesions, including small aneurysms, angiomas, or masses.
8. Biopsy. Temporal arteritis should be suspected in new onset headaches starting after age 50. Temporal artery tenderness may be absent, and prompt temporal artery biopsy is necessary to establish the diagnosis.

TABLE 91–3. Frequency of Abnormal Findings in Headache Patients

| | DIAGNOSTIC YIELD | | |
PROCEDURE	Overall Abnormal Findings (%)	Abnormal with Abnormal Findings on Neurologic Examination (%)	Abnormal with Normal Findings on Neurologic Examination (%)
Neurologic examination (n = 161)	10		
EEG (n = 161)	12	44	9
CT scan (n = 40)	2	11	0
Cerebral angiogram (n = 7)	29	40	0
Skull X-rays (n = 93)	1	0	0

Source: Adapted from Larson EB, et al. Diagnostic evaluation of headache: Impact of computerized tomography and cost-effectiveness. JAMA 1980;243:359–362.

TABLE 91–4. First Choice of Imaging Procedure for Headache Evaluation

CT PREFERRED	MRI PREFERRED
Acute onset severe headache	Chronic headache
Acute head trauma	Chronic head trauma
Stroke	Headache with visual disturbance
	Headache with symptoms and signs of increased intracranial pressure
	Headache associated with dementia

Bibliography

Allen NB, Studenski SA. Polymyalgia rheumatica and temporal arteritis. Med Clin North Am 1986;70:369–385.

Clough C. Non-migrainous headaches. Br Med J 1989;299:70–72.

Cooper BC, Lucente FE. Management of Facial, Head, and Neck Pain. Philadelphia, W.B. Saunders, 1989.

Diehr P, et al. Acute headaches: Presenting symptoms and diagnostic rules to identify patients with tension and migraine headaches. J Chron Dis 1981;34:147–158.

Fontanarosa PB. Recognition of subarachnoid hemorrhage. Ann Emerg Med 1989;18:1199–1205.

Larson EB, et al. Diagnostic evaluation of headache: Impact of computerized tomography and cost-effectiveness. JAMA 1980;243:359–362.

Raskin NH. Headache, 2nd ed. New York, Churchill Livingstone, 1988.

92

CEREBROVASCULAR DISEASE

PHILLIP D. SWANSON

O, then how quickly should this arm of mine, now prisoner to the palsy, chastise thee.

SHAKESPEARE (1564–1616)

DEFINITION

- Cerebrovascular disease includes conditions that primarily or secondarily affect the blood vessels of the brain. The major outcome of cerebrovascular disease is generically termed "stroke."
- Patients with cerebrovascular disease seek medical attention for transient symptoms of cerebral dysfunction or for the rapid onset of neurologic symptoms such as unilateral weakness, loss of consciousness, or loss of language abilities, suggesting a rapidly progressing problem involving the brain.

EPIDEMIOLOGY

- The average annual incidence rate for stroke rises with age, from 106 per 100,000 for those between 45 and 54 years to 1825 per 100,000 for those over 85.
- Of strokes with a known cause, thrombotic infarction accounts for about 60%. Other categories (subarachnoid hemorrhage, intracerebral hemorrhage, definite embolic infarction) each account for 10 to 15% of cases. About 15% of cases are reported to be "of unspecified type."
- Factors that determine the degree of risk for cerebrovascular disease include age and genetic factors and identifiable risk factors including hypertension, diabetes mellitus, heart diseases, use of high estrogen contraceptives, and smoking.

DIFFERENTIAL DIAGNOSIS

- Transient ischemic attacks (TIA)
  1. Most definitions of TIA use a 24-hr cut-off point for the duration of symptoms and signs. Beyond that, the diagnosis changes to reversible ischemic neurologic deficit

(RIND), stroke-in-evolution, or completed stroke. The usual duration of a TIA is between 8 and 14 min.

2. To be classified as a TIA, the episode must be understandable as an ischemic event in the territory of a cerebral vessel. In the absence of additional symptoms, dizziness, faintness, or loss of consciousness are usually excluded from this diagnosis.

3. Several conditions can mimic TIA (Table 92–1). Migraine is usually associated with headache. The term "migraine accompaniment" refers to episodes of cerebral dysfunction due to cerebral ischemia during a migraine attack. Migraine episodes usually last longer (15 to 25 min) than typical TIAs, and the symptoms often evolve to include other parts of the body.

4. TIAs are usually classified as "carotid" or "vertebrobasilar" according to the likely arterial system producing the symptoms.

- Evolving or completed stroke (Table 92–2). The symptoms and signs of stroke evolve within minutes to hours. They indicate localized dysfunction within the cerebral hemispheres or brain stem that can be understood as resulting from occlusion or rupture of blood vessels.

    Brain tumors, degenerative diseases, and multiple sclerosis are conditions whose time courses usually differ from those of stroke syndromes.

CLINICAL FEATURES

- Transient ischemic attacks
    1. Historical information from the patient (Table 92–3) is far more important than are physical findings, since most TIAs are not witnessed.
    2. The symptoms should be classified as carotid or vertebrobasilar in origin.
    3. It is particularly important to differentiate amaurosis fugax, which indicates ischemia in a carotid artery territory, from transient hemianopia, which is often

TABLE 92–1. Features of Conditions Producing TIA-Like Symptoms

CONDITION	FEATURES
Presyncope	Lightheadedness, upright position
Hyperventilation	Breathlessness, finger or lip tingling
Partial seizures	Aura, stereotyped episodes, altered awareness, sensory or motor progression ("march")
Episodic or positional vertigo	Spinning sensation, nystagmus during attack, vertigo with positional change
Migraine	Longer duration, scintillations, headache by history

TABLE 92–2. Classification of Stroke

Intracranial hemorrhage
  Subarachnoid hemorrhage due to ruptured berry
    aneurysm
  Intracerebral hemorrhage
    Primary, associated with hypertension
    Rupture of an arteriovenous malformation
    Lobar, associated with congophilic (amyloid)
      angiopathy
    Lobar, associated with intravenous drug abuse
    Contusions from head trauma
    Hemorrhagic infarction from cerebral embolism or
      cerebral vein thrombosis
    Hemorrhage into a brain tumor
Ischemic stroke
  Thrombotic stroke
    Associated with atherosclerosis
    Associated with hematologic disease
      Polycythemia vera
      Essential thrombocytosis
      Consumptive coagulopathies
      Dysproteinemias (cryoglobulinemia)
      Hemoglobinopathies (sickle cell disease)
      Lupus anticoagulant
    Associated with inflammatory disease
      Specific infections (meningovascular syphilis,
        tuberculous or fungal meningitis)
    Collagen vascular diseases
      SLE, periarteritis nodosa
    Granulomatous angiitis
    Associated with amphetamine or cocaine use
  Infarct associated with migraine
  Miscellaneous
    Fibromuscular dysplasia
    Dissecting aneurysm of ascending aorta, or of large
      arteries (carotid or vertebral)
    Moya-moya arteriopathy
    Trauma (vertebral occlusion associated with neck
      manipulation)
  Embolic stroke
    Bacterial endocarditis
    Rheumatic heart disease
    Atrial fibrillation
    Left ventricular mural thrombus with acute MI,
      ventricular aneurysm, or dilated cardiomyopathy
    Atrial myxoma
    Marantic (nonbacterial, thrombotic) endocarditis
      associated with malignancy
    Libman-Sacks endocarditis associated with SLE
    Paradoxical embolism associated with patent foramen
      ovale or septal defect
    Air or fat emboli
    Mitral valve prolapse
    Artery to artery emboli

TABLE 92–2. Classification of Stroke *Continued*

Embolism associated with arteriography or cardiac
surgery
Venous thrombosis (often causes hemorrhagic stroke)
  Septic
  Nonseptic
    Postpartum
    Associated with dehydration

---

due to ischemia in the territory of a posterior cerebral
artery (usually vertebrobasilar system).

- Evolving or completed stroke
  1. Evolving or completed infarcts (Table 92–4).
  2. Lacunar infarcts are usually due to occlusions of small
     perforating arterioles in individuals with chronic hy-
     pertension or diabetes mellitus. Clinical presentations
     include:
     a. Pure motor hemiparesis.
     b. Pure hemisensory syndrome.
     c. Dysarthria–clumsy hand syndrome.
     d. Ataxic hemiparesis syndrome.
  3. Ruptured berry aneurysm may have the following:
     a. Presentation with headache and neck stiffness,
        since bleeding is usually first into the subarachnoid
        space.
     b. Subhyaloid retinal hemorrhages.
     c. With aneurysms on the internal carotid artery at
        the junction with the posterior communicating ar-
        tery, an ipsilateral third cranial nerve palsy (ptosis, dilated pupil that is poorly reactive, exter-
        nally rotated eye with inability to look medially,
        up, or down) is common. Since cranial nerve four
        is intact, the superior oblique muscle intorts the
        eye with downward gaze.
     d. Loss of consciousness.

TABLE 92–3. Features of TIA in Carotid or Vertebrobasilar Territories

	CAROTID		VERTEBROBASILAR
	L	R	
Transient amnesia	0	0	+
Dysphasia	+	0	0
Dysarthria	+	+	+
Diplopia	0	0	+
Visual loss	+	+	+
Unilateral weakness	+	+	+
Bilateral weakness	0	0	+
Dizziness	0	0	+
Loss of consciousness	0	0	+

TABLE 92–4. Clinical Features of Stroke

ANATOMIC LOCATION	COMMON CLINICAL FEATURES
Left cerebral hemisphere	Dysphasia, hemiparesis, hemianopia
Right cerebral hemisphere	Unilateral neglect, hemiparesis, hemianopia
Cerebellum	Ataxia, vertigo, stupor, nystagmus
Pons	Stupor or coma, bilateral weakness, bilateral gaze paresis
Lateral medulla	Ataxia, vertigo, hoarseness, dysphagia, sensory loss to pain and temperature that is ipsilateral on face and contralateral on body

    e. Signs of secondary ischemia due to spasm of middle cerebral, anterior cerebral, or, occasionally, basilar artery.

4. Venous sinus or cortical vein thrombosis
    a. Seizures, often partial, are frequent in patients with cortical vein thrombosis. Focal findings may occur.
    b. Increased intracranial pressure may accompany thrombosis of the superior sagittal or lateral venous sinuses.
    c. Cavernous sinus thrombosis is often associated with proptosis, retinal hemorrhages, and ophthalmoplegias.

LABORATORY STUDIES

- TIA. Laboratory studies should be more comprehensive in young individuals in whom atherosclerotic disease is unlikely. Tests to consider include:
1. CBC with platelet count.
2. ANA, ESR, lupus anticoagulant, complement levels, and other autoantibodies to search for evidence of collagen vascular diseases.
3. Echocardiography to evaluate the possibility of valvular disease, mitral valve prolapse, nonbacterial thrombotic endocarditis, or patent foramen ovale.
4. Ultrasonic duplex scanning, to assess the degree of stenosis of extracranial arteries, especially if carotid endarterectomy might be contemplated.
5. Cerebral angiography is indicated only if further anatomic detail is necessary prior to endarterectomy.
6. CT or MRI of the brain to exclude arteriovenous malformation, unsuspected brain tumor, or evidence of previous small infarctions.
7. Electroencephalography to rule out the possibility of

partial seizures manifest by episodes of sensory loss or aphasia.

- Evolving or completed stroke
  1. CT without contrast is the most important initial study because it detects hemorrhage.
  2. If a subarachnoid hemorrhage is demonstrable, and if aneurysm clipping would be favored, cerebral angiography is done to locate and demonstrate size, shape, and presence or absence of an aneurysmal neck. Transcranial Doppler studies are useful for demonstrating spasm of large arteries.
  3. Lumbar puncture is rarely necessary with acute stroke patients, unless the stroke may be associated with an infectious process such as meningovascular syphilis.
  4. Assessment of cardiac function is important in patients with ischemic stroke to look for clues to a source of emboli.
     a. ECG should be routine.
     b. Echocardiography is recommended in young individuals or in others where cardiac disease is strongly suspected.

RECOMMENDED DIAGNOSTIC APPROACH

- Transient ischemic attacks
  1. The history of the episodes gives the most important information leading to the correct diagnosis. The extent of assessment depends on whether the patient is a candidate for carotid endarterectomy.
  2. Basic approach to evaluate TIA:
     a. History to establish the diagnosis of TIA and to determine the arterial distribution of the symptoms.
     b. Physical examination to assess for hypertension, persistent neurologic signs, evidence of retinal emboli, the presence or absence of carotid or supraclavicular bruits, unequal arm blood pressures, cardiac murmurs, or arrhythmias.
     c. Ultrasonic duplex examination of the extracranial vessels.
     d. ECG.
     e. Head CT to exclude unsuspected mass lesion.
     f. Consider EEG if partial seizure is possible.
     g. Consider cerebral angiography if the patient is a candidate for carotid endarterectomy.

- Evolving or completed stroke
  1. History and physical examination to assess the symptoms at onset and the likely location of the event.
  2. Immediate head CT without contrast to assess for the presence of hemorrhage.
  3. CBC with platelet count, ESR, serum glucose and lipoprotein levels, and a serologic test for syphilis should be performed initially.
  4. If a collagen vascular disease is suspected, ANA,

rheumatoid factor, and lupus anticoagulant should be checked.

5. Toxicology screen if drug abuse is suspected.
6. ECG.
7. Chest X-ray.
8. Blood cultures if endocarditis is suspected.
9. Echocardiography if a cardiac source of emboli is suspected.
10. Ultrasonic duplex examination of the extracranial arteries.
11. Cerebral angiography should be done if:
    a. The stroke is minor and noninvasive studies suggest an extracranial stenosis amenable to surgery.
    b. There is a suspicion of arterial dissection, fibromuscular dysplasia, or cerebral angiitis.
    c. Subarachnoid hemorrhage has been demonstrated.
12. If cerebral angiitis is strongly suspected, and angiography is not diagnostic, meningeal biopsy should be considered.

Bibliography

Adams RD, Victor M. Principles of Neurology, 4th ed. New York, McGraw-Hill, 1989.

Dyken ML, et al. Cooperative study of hospital frequency and character of transient ischemic attacks. I. Background, organization, and clinical survey. JAMA 1977;237:882–886.

Fisher CM. Late-life migraine accompaniments as a cause of unexplained transient ischemic attacks. Can J Neurol Sci 1980;7:9–17.

Futty DE, et al. Cooperative study of hospital frequency and character of transient ischemic attacks. V. Symptom analysis. JAMA 1977;238:2386–2390.

Hart RG, Miller VT. Cerebral infarction in young adults: A practical approach. Stroke 1983;14:110–114.

Posner JD, et al. Stroke in the elderly: I. Epidemiology. J Am Geriatr Soc 1984;32:95–102.

Report of the WHO Task Force on Stroke and Other Cerebrovascular Diseases. Stroke 1989. Recommendations on stroke prevention, diagnosis, and therapy. Stroke 1989;20:1407–1431.

93

MULTIPLE SCLEROSIS

JAMES D. BOWEN

Variability is the law of life, and as no two faces are the same, so no two bodies are alike, and no two individuals react alike and behave alike under the abnormal conditions which we know as disease.

SIR WILLIAM OSLER (1849–1919)

DEFINITION

- Multiple sclerosis (MS) is a disease affecting the CNS. Characteristic sclerotic plaques occur throughout the white matter of the brain and spinal cord.
- Microscopically, plaques consist of sharply demarcated areas of demyelination. Neurons, axons, and vascular structures are relatively spared, whereas oligodendrocytes are damaged and glial cells proliferate.

PATHOGENESIS

- Autoimmune theory. The autoimmune theory is supported by HLA linkage, inheritance patterns, immunocytes found in plaques and changes in peripheral blood immunocytes. Experimental allergic encephalomyelitis is an animal model of autoimmunity with remarkable similarity to MS.
- Viral theory. The viral theory is supported by animal models of infectious diseases of myelin, an increasing incidence of disease at higher latitudes, clustering of cases within families, and geographic clustering. Human T-cell lymphotrophic virus, type I (HTLV-1) associated myelopathy results from a retrovirus infection and has remarkable similarities to MS.
- Combined theory. An environmental exposure (toxin or virus) in early life might trigger an autoimmune disorder.

EPIDEMIOLOGY

- Demographics. Incidence peaks in the late third and early fourth decades, but age ranges from childhood to senescence. Those of northern European descent have a higher rate of disease than Blacks or Asians.
- Geography. The increasing incidence of MS with higher latitude is independent of race. The risk associated with residing at a particular latitude is fixed by late childhood.

799

- Genetics. Up to 20% of MS patients have another relative with the disease. For relatives of MS patients, the lifetime risk of developing MS is 1 to 2% for parents, children, siblings, and dizygotic twins. Monozygotic twins have a 35 to 50% risk.

CLINICAL FEATURES

- Course of disease. The clinical course of MS is frequently punctuated by acute deterioration. Exacerbations occur in an unpredictable pattern. They are at least 24 hr in length. Although all symptoms occurring within 1 to 3 months are often considered within a single relapse, a typical relapse develops over several hours or a few days, then slowly improves over several weeks.
  1. Benign. About 20% of patients have a course with infrequent exacerbation and little disability.
  2. Exacerbating-remitting. About 25% follow a course of more frequent exacerbation, intermediate periods of stability, and mild to moderate disability.
  3. Chronic-exacerbating. About 40% have a course with frequent exacerbations superimposed upon progressive disability.
  4. Chronic-progressive. About 15% have a steadily progressive course without exacerbation.
- Symptoms. Symptoms are often worsened by elevated body temperatures. Fatigue may worsen underlying symptoms.
  1. White matter symptoms. Since MS involves primarily the white matter, symptoms most commonly affect information transfer from one area of the CNS to another.
     a. Visual symptoms. Optic neuritis with acute loss of visual acuity is the most common symptom of the optic pathway. At least one-half of MS patients develop optic neuritis. Internuclear ophthalmoplegia, which may be unilateral, is also common.
     b. Motor symptoms include weakness, spasticity, clonus, and flexor spasms of the legs.
     c. Sensory symptoms include numbness and paresthesias.
     d. Cerebellar symptoms include ataxia, nystagmus, incoordination, and dysarthria.
     e. Autonomic pathway involvement is associated with urinary urgency and incontinence; fecal urgency, incontinence or constipation; and impotence.
  2. Nonlocalized symptoms include:
     a. Fatigue is frequently the primary source of disability.
     b. Cognitive changes may be widespread but are often overshadowed by long-tract symptoms. Affective changes include euphoria and depression.
  3. Episodic symptoms are occasionally encountered.
     a. Epilepsy has been noted in 1 to 8% of cases.

b. Tonic seizures are episodic spasms which resemble extensor posturing. They are often preceded by sensory symptoms. The spasms are often painful, and consciousness is maintained.

c. Sensory phenomena may occur episodically with pain, itching or paresthesias. Lhermitte's sign is an episodic sensation of "electric tingling" radiating down the spine or limbs. It is precipitated by neck flexion.

d. Episodic ataxia or vertigo are occasionally seen.

4. Painful symptoms. Pain occurs in 11 to 35% of patients. Trigeminal neuralgia is found in 1 to 2% of cases. Painful paresthesia or musculoskeletal pain due to mechanical dysfunction may be disabling.

LABORATORY STUDIES

- MRI changes are found in 85 to 90% of clinically definite cases. High-signal-intensity lesions are found in the white matter on T2-weighted scans. Specificity is poor. CT scanning has much less sensitivity.

- Evoked potentials are useful in characterizing subclinical lesions. Visual evoked responses are abnormal in 75 to 97% of definite MS cases. Somatosensory evoked potentials are abnormal in 72 to 96% of cases. Brain stem auditory evoked responses are abnormal in 57 to 65% of cases. These tests also have low specificity.

- CSF may contain oligoclonal bands (OCBs) and myelin basic protein (MBP). OCBs are found in 90 to 98% of definite cases. OCBs denote activation of the immune system within the CNS and are positive in a number of neurologic diseases. MBP is commonly found in CSF. It indicates myelin damage and is found in a wide array of CNS disorders. An elevated IgG level or IgG index indicate activation of the immune system within the CNS.

CRITERIA FOR DIAGNOSIS

There is currently no test specific for MS. Cases are classified as definite or probable.

- Definite MS
  1. Clinically definite MS requires the demonstration of 2 or more lesions and 2 or more separate relapses. The number of lesions may be determined clinically or with laboratory assistance.
  2. Laboratory-supported definite MS must have CSF oligoclonal bands or CSF IgG abnormalities (elevated IgG or IgG Index)

$$\text{IgG Index} = \frac{\text{CSF IgG/Serum IgG}}{\text{CSF albumin/Serum albumin}}$$

Additional criteria include either: (a) 2 attacks involving separate parts of the nervous system, but clinical or laboratory documentation of only 1 is required (the other being undocumented historical information); or (b) a single attack occurring with clinical or laboratory documentation of 2 lesions.

- Probable MS
  1. Clinically probable MS includes cases with either: (a) 2 attacks, but only a single lesion; or (b) cases having 1 attack, but 2 lesions (defined by laboratory or clinical means). CSF is normal.
  2. Laboratory-supported probable MS includes cases with 2 attacks involving different parts of the nervous system, but without demonstrable lesions through clinical or laboratory means. CSF studies must show oligoclonal bands or IgG abnormalities.

DIFFERENTIAL DIAGNOSIS

- Multiple small strokes are commonly confused with MS. Optic nerve and spinal cord lesions are unusual in stroke syndromes. In the elderly, multiple periventricular lesions on MRI often have uncertain clinical significance.
- Vasculitic conditions may affect small vessels of the CNS including SLE, polyarteritis nodosa, Behçet's disease, sarcoidosis, and the meningovascular form of syphilis.
- Neurodegenerative diseases such as olivopontocerebellar degeneration and the hereditary ataxias typically have steadily progressive courses. MRI shows atrophic changes, but not the high-signal intensity lesions seen in MS. Paraneoplastic disorders include ataxia, limbic encephalitis, and retinal degeneration.
- Viral, postinfectious, and postvaccination demyelinations are diseases with multiple lesions, but only a single unimodal course. HTLV-1 is expected in patients from endemic locations.
- Inherited disorders such as adrenoleukodystrophy, metachromatic leukodystrophy, and other leukodystrophies must be considered.

RECOMMENDED DIAGNOSTIC APPROACH

- Patients with appropriate symptoms and signs should be evaluated by MRI.
  1. If multiple high signal lesions are seen in the white matter, then several disorders must be considered including MS, stroke, vasculitis, and age-related changes of uncertain significance.
  2. If MRI findings are typical of MS and clinical setting is supportive, then the evaluation can often cease at this point. Equivocal cases require additional testing such as evoked potential studies or CSF analysis.
- Evoked potential studies may identify additional subclinical lesions. Use of these tests to confirm already-identified lesions is not helpful to the diagnostic process. Sequential

use of visual, somatosensory, or auditory evoked potential tests is more cost-effective than batteries of all three. The visual evoked potential test is usually used first.

- If MRI and evoked potential tests do not diagnose definite MS, then CSF should be examined for OCBs or IgG. A matched serum sample often enhances the accuracy of CSF OCB and IgG determinations.

- Tests to exclude other disorders may be helpful including: FTA-Abs, sedimentation rate, screens for clinically suspected vasculitic disorders, and HTLV-1 serology.

Bibliography

Koetsier JC, ed. Handbook of Clinical Neurology, vol. 47, Demyelinating Diseases. New York, Elsevier Science Publishers, 1985.

Matthews WB, et al. McAlpine's Multiple Sclerosis. New York, Churchill Livingstone, 1985.

McDonald WI, Silberberg D. Multiple Sclerosis. London, Butterworth, 1986.

Rationale for immunomodulating therapies of multiple sclerosis. Symposium. Los Angeles, August 1–2, 1986. Proceedings. Neurology 1988 (July);38(7 Suppl 2):1–89.

Sibley WA. Therapeutic Claims in Multiple Sclerosis. New York, Demos, 1988.

94

NEUROPATHY AND MYOPATHY

JAMES D. BOWEN

As to diseases, make a habit of two things—to help, or at least to do no harm.

HIPPOCRATES

Diseases of the peripheral nervous system and muscles are relatively rare disorders. The diseases discussed in this chapter are systemic disorders which affect sensation or strength in a symmetric manner. Myopathic disease affects only motor function, whereas neuropathies usually have at least some sensory loss. Neuropathy usually begins distally, while myopathy initially involves proximal muscles. Reflexes are often relatively spared in myopathy, but lost in neuropathy.

POLYNEUROPATHIES

Definitions and General Comments

Peripheral nerves contain several types of fibers. Motor fibers are large and myelinated. Several types of sensory fibers exist. Large myelinated fibers convey position sense and light touch. Medium-sized, lightly myelinated fibers subserve vibration and light touch. Small unmyelinated fibers are small and lightly myelinated; postganglionic fibers are small and unmyelinated.

Clinical Features

Polyneuropathies typically affect long nerves first. Thus, symptoms begin in the feet and spread proximally. When symptoms reach just above the knees, the hands become involved, followed shortly by the anterior trunk (intercostal nerves) and crown of the head.

- Motor nerves. Involvement of motor nerves causes weakness, atrophy, cramps, and loss of reflexes.
- Sensory nerves
  1. Involvement of large myelinated sensory nerves cause light touch and proprioceptive loss. Numbness, sensations of "walking on thick carpet," or imbalance in the dark are common complaints.
  2. Medium-sized, lightly myelinated fiber loss causes

numbness with loss of light touch and vibratory sensations.

3. Small unmyelinated fiber involvement is associated with decreased pain and temperature sensation, and unpleasant paresthesias.

- Autonomic nerves. Autonomic involvement usually is recognized as impotence or postural hypotension. Bladder dysfunction, altered sweating, and GI dysmotility are occasionally encountered.
- Other symptoms. Trophic skin changes and hair loss in involved areas should be noted. High arches and hammer toes are important clues of longstanding disease. Some disorders cause palpable enlargement of nerves.

Laboratory Studies

- Electrodiagnostic tests. These are an extension of the physical examination. Nerve conduction velocities (NCVs) can assist in classifying polyneuropathies as axonal vs. demyelinating. Axon loss causes a mild slowing of the NCV with a disproportionate loss of amplitude. Demyelination causes mild loss of amplitude with disproportionate slowing of the NCV. If motor axons are lost, EMG will detect fibrillations, positive sharp waves, and decreased numbers of motor unit potentials.
- Nerve biopsy. Nerve biopsies have limited utility in the clinical evaluation of polyneuropathy. They are helpful in hereditary cases, and some organic solvent toxicities. Biopsy is occasionally helpful in Guillain-Barré syndrome, leprosy, amyloidosis, polyarteritis nodosa, and sarcoidosis.

Differential Diagnosis

Hyperventilation may cause distal paresthesias. Somatization disorders usually have an inappropriate distribution of sensory loss and sharp borders of anesthetic areas. Entrapment neuropathies are differentiated clinically and electrodiagnostically. Central nervous system causes of distal sensory loss include syphilis, multiple sclerosis or compressive myelopathy. Signs of upper motor neuron involvement are present, and electrodiagnostic signs of peripheral involvement are absent.

- Predominantly motor neuropathies include Guillain-Barré syndrome, porphyria, diabetes, hereditary disorders, toxins, lead, mercury, and paraproteinemias.
- Predominantly sensory neuropathies include diabetes, alcohol, hereditary disorders, amyloidosis, leprosy, toxins, B_{12} deficiency, and paraneoplastic disorders.
- The differential diagnosis of polyneuropathy is (except for uremia and hepatic failure) included in the mnemonic DANG THERAPISTS.

1. Diabetes can cause virtually any combination of motor, sensory, or autonomic involvement.
2. Alcohol can cause virtually any combination of mo-

tor, sensory, or autonomic involvement. Burning feet is a common presentation.

3. Nutritional deficiencies are often found with dietary inadequacies. Thiamine, pyridoxine, and B_{12} deficiencies have been implicated in polyneuropathy.

4. Guillain-Barré syndrome is an inflammatory demyelinating disorder with predominant loss of motor function. The hallmark of the disease is an elevated CSF protein without elevation of CSF leukocytes. Chronic forms are recognized.

5. Toxins are important reversible causes of polyneuropathy. Both industrial toxins (e.g., lead, mercury, or arsenic) and drugs must be considered.

6. Hereditary disorders may affect motor or occasionally sensory nerves. High arches and hammer toes may be the only manifestation in some family members.

7. Endocrine. Hypothyroidism, acromegaly, and occasionally hyperthyroidism join diabetes in this category.

8. Refsum disease is an autosomal recessive disorder manifested by polyneuropathy associated with retinitis pigmentosa, ichthyosis, and hearing loss.

9. Amyloidosis frequently involves autonomic and pain fibers.

10. Porphyria is also associated with abdominal pain and psychiatric illness. Neuropathy often begins as pain followed by acute weakness. Proximal involvement occurs before distal.

11. Infection. Leprosy afflicts cooler areas of the body. Cutaneous modalities are lost before deeper modalities. Diphtheria causes an acute motor neuropathy, which often involves proximal regions initially. Polyneuropathy may be associated with HIV infection.

12. Systemic disorders include sarcoidosis, RA, SLE, and polyarteritis nodosa.

13. Tumors may cause paraneoplastic syndromes, paraproteinemia, and antibodies to myelin-associated globulin (anti-MAG antibody) or ganglioside (anti-GM antibody).

14. Severely ill patients (sepsis, ARDS, trauma) may develop polyneuropathy, which resolves with improvement in the underlying disorder.

Recommended Diagnostic Approach

• If the history and physical examination do not reveal the cause of a polyneuropathy, then further tests are indicated. Electrodiagnostic tests can confirm the clinical impression of polyneuropathy, but only occasionally allow precise classification.

• Laboratory tests should include serum glucose, renal and hepatic function tests, CBC, urinalysis, thyroid function tests, serum B_{12} level, ESR, and serum protein electrophoresis or immunofixation tests.

• If these tests are unrevealing, then additional evaluation must be tailored to the particular case. A significant number of cases will remain without a specific diagnosis.

MYOPATHY

Definition and General Comments

When confronted with a myopathic pattern of weakness (e.g., predominantly proximal muscles), each part of the peripheral nervous system and muscle must be considered. Possible sites of abnormalities include:

1. Anterior horn cell.
2. Peripheral nerve.
3. Neuromuscular junction.
4. Muscle cell membrane.
5. Muscle metabolism.

Clinical Features

Weakness is the predominant symptom. Motor loss may be constant or fluctuating, acute or chronic. Symptoms may develop only on extreme exertion. Muscles may be atrophic or may have pseudo-hypertrophy. Myoglobinuria and muscle cramps are useful clues.

Laboratory Studies

- Electrodiagnostic tests
  1. Motor nerves are investigated by NCVs. The myoneural junction is evaluated by repetitive stimulation during NCV testing.
  2. Muscles are studied by EMG. Denervated muscle has fibrillations, positive sharp waves, and a decreased number of motor units. Myopathic disease is recognized by low amplitude, short duration motor unit potentials with less prominent membrane instability.
- Muscle biopsy is most useful if a clinical hypothesis is derived beforehand, and the biopsy is used to test the hypothesis.
- CK is a measure of enzyme leakage into the blood from damaged muscles. The aldolase level may occasionally be useful.

Differential Diagnosis

- Anterior horn cell disease
  1. Amyotrophic lateral sclerosis is recognized by the combination of upper motor neuron lesions associated with widespread lower motor neuron changes. Primary lateral sclerosis is a related disorder with isolated anterior horn cell loss.
  2. Spinal muscular atrophies are progressive diseases with loss of anterior horn cells. There are infantile, juvenile, and adult forms.

3. Poliomyelitis is now an uncommon cause of anterior horn cell disease.

- Peripheral nerve disease. Discussed earlier in this chapter.
- Neuromuscular junction
  1. Myasthenia gravis is characterized by fluctuating weakness and fatigability. Bulbar muscles are usually involved. There is generalized weakness in some cases. Decremental responses on repetitive nerve stimulation are found, and antiacetylcholine receptor antibodies are usually identified. Improvement following administration of edrophonium (Tensilon test) can be dramatic.
  2. Lambert-Eaton myasthenic syndrome resembles myasthenia gravis, but has an incremental response to repetitive nerve stimulation. Many cases are associated with small-cell carcinoma of the lung.
  3. Botulism produces rapidly progressing weakness. Diagnosis is confirmed by demonstration of the toxin in serum, stool, or the ingested food.
- Myotonic disorders and periodic paralysis. These diseases are due to alterations of ion channels in the muscle cell membrane.
  1. Myotonic dystrophy is an autosomal dominant disorder with myotonia (delayed relaxation after muscle contraction), slowly progressive weakness, frontal balding, cataracts, arched palate, mental deficiency, cardiac conduction abnormalities, and hypogonadism. Myotonic discharges are found on EMG.
  2. Periodic Paralysis (PP). At least three types of PP are recognized.
     a. Hypokalemic PP is associated with attacks of weakness lasting several hours. Attacks are precipitated by cold, carbohydrate ingestion, and exercise. Serum potassium is decreased during attacks. Some patients are thyrotoxic.
     b. Hyperkalemic PP is associated with brief attacks of weakness with elevated serum potassium. Attacks are precipitated by rest, fasting, cold, and potassium loading.
     c. Normokalemic PP is associated with prolonged attacks precipitated by rest, cold, and potassium loading.
- Metabolic myopathies are due to inherited defects of muscle metabolism. Carbohydrates and fat are the primary energy sources for muscle. Weakness and myoglobinuria may be most pronounced during excessive exercise. Cramps are common.
  1. Defects of carbohydrate metabolism can be divided into two groups:
     a. Acid maltase, debrancher, and brancher enzyme deficiencies cause progressive weakness without myoglobinuria.
     b. Phosphorylase, phosphofructokinase, phosphoglycerate kinase, phosphoglycerate mutase, and lactate dehydrogenase deficiencies cause episodic

myoglobinuria. Cramps and episodic weakness are also seen, but progressive weakness is not common.

2. Defects of lipid metabolism
   a. Carnitine deficiency presents with progressive weakness exacerbated by exercise. Hepatic encephalopathy is noted in systemic forms of the disease.
   b. Carnitine palmitoyl transferase deficiency causes episodic weakness and myoglobinuria after excessive exercise.

3. Mitochondrial myopathies are characterized by "ragged red fibers" on muscle biopsy. Many diseases in this category have fluctuating encephalopathy. Those in which weakness is the predominant symptom are associated with lactic acidosis, exercise intolerance, and weakness of extraocular, bulbar, limb, and trunk muscles.

4. Congenital myopathies include conditions of slowly progressing weakness with specific changes on muscle biopsy. Central core disease, multicore disease, centronuclear myopathy, and nemaline myopathy are examples.

5. Inherited myopathies (the muscular dystrophies) (see Table 94–1).

- Idiopathic inflammatory myopathies include polymyositis and dermatomyositis (see Chapter 84). Limb, trunk, and neck flexor muscles are usually affected. Bulbar musculature may be involved.
- Endocrine. Hyperthyroidism, hypothyroidism, hyperadrenocorticism, hypoadrenocorticism, acromegaly, and hyperparathyroidism are associated with myopathy.
- Toxins and drugs may cause myopathy.
- Infections with viral, bacterial, or parasitic organisms can cause myopathy.

Recommended Diagnostic Approach

- The history and physical examination often allow the diagnosis of neuromuscular disorders to be narrowed to a few possibilities.
- Blood tests for creatine kinase and aldolase should be obtained before electrodiagnostic tests or biopsy. Other tests that may be useful include thyroid function tests, serum cortisol, ESR, ANA, and anti-Jo-1 antibody. Antiacetylcholine receptor and antistriated muscle antibody levels are useful in suspected myasthenia gravis. The serum potassium should be measured during attacks of periodic paralysis.
- Electrodiagnostic tests are often diagnostic in anterior horn cell disease, peripheral neuropathy, neuromuscular junction disorders, and myotonic disorders. These tests confirm the presence of myopathic disorders, but are not often diagnostic of a specific myopathy.
- Muscle biopsy is often required to diagnose a specific cause

TABLE 94–1. Inherited Myopathies (The Muscular Dystrophies)

	Onset	Distribution	Increased Creatine Kinase	Progression	Comments
X-Linked					
Duchenne	Childhood	Pelvic girdle	3+	Rapid	Pseudohypertrophy, mildly decreased IQ, cardiomyopathy
Beckers	5–20 yr	Pelvic girdle	3+	Slow	Pseudohypertrophy, allelic w/ Duchenne
Emery-Dreifuss	Childhood	Pelvic girdle	2+	Slow	Contractures, cardiac involvement, no hypertrophy
Scapuloperoneal	Childhood	Proximal limbs, peroneal	2+	Slow	Cervical, elbow, calf contractures, cardiac arrhythmias
Autosomal recessive					
Limb girdle	2nd–4th decade	Scapulohumeral, proximal legs	2+	Slow	Likely heterogeneous
Childhood	1st decade	Pelvic girdle	3+	Slow	Resembles Duchenne, may have pseudohypertrophy
Congenital	Neonatal	Facial, others variable	3+	Variable	Heterogeneous
Autosomal dominant					
Facioscapulohumeral	2nd–3rd decade	Facial, scapular	1+	Slow	Many have mild involvement, may have normal lifespan
Scapuloperoneal	2nd–5th decade	Peroneal, upper arms	1+	Slow	Foot drop
Distal myopathy	Variable	Distal limbs	Variable	Slow	CK-level variable
Oculopharyngeal	Adult	Eyelid, extraocular, dysphagia	1+	Slow	May be sporadic

of myopathy. The clinical picture must be used to narrow the list of possibilities before biopsy. An involved muscle not traumatized by prior EMG should be selected (usually deltoid or quadriceps). Coordination of the primary care physician, surgeon, and pathologist is essential.

- Tests for specific disease include edrophonium injections for myasthenia gravis, provocative tests for periodic paralysis, or ischemic forearm exercise tests for some disorders of carbohydrate metabolism.

Bibliography

Dyck PJ, et al. Peripheral Neuropathy, 2nd ed. Philadelphia, W.B. Saunders, 1984.

Matthews WB, ed. Handbook of Clinical Neurology. Vol. 51. Amsterdam, Elsevier Science Publishers, 1987.

Morgan-Hughes JA. Disease of Striated Muscle. In: Diseases of the Nervous System. Asbury AK, et al. eds. W.B. Saunders, 1986, pp. 227–256.

Walton JN, ed. Disorders of Voluntary Muscle. Edinburgh, Churchill Livingstone, 1981.

95

ALCOHOLISM

PETER COGGAN

Long quaffing maketh a short lyfe.
JOHN LYLY (1554–1606)

DEFINITION AND CRITERIA FOR DIAGNOSIS

Alcoholism is a progressive illness characterized by loss of control over alcohol consumption and a variety of behavioral and biomedical consequences. There is no consensus on the precise definition.

- Criteria of the American Psychiatric Association. The Diagnostic and Statistical Manual (DSM-III-R) of the American Psychiatric Association distinguishes between substance abuse and substance dependence.
  1. Alcohol abuse is characterized by:
     a. A pattern of pathologic alcohol use including excessive daily drinking, binges, failed attempts to cut down, and some medical consequences.
     b. Impairment in social or occupational functioning due to alcohol use including violent episodes, poor job performance, job loss, and family dysfunction.
     c. Duration of disturbance of at least 1 month.
  2. Alcohol dependence is characterized by:
     a. A pattern of pathologic use or impairment of social or occupational functioning as above.
     b. Evidence of tolerance or withdrawal symptoms.
- Criteria of the National Council on Alcoholism. The diagnosis of alcoholism may be made if any of the following criteria apply:
  1. Blood alcohol concentration greater than 300 mg/dl (65 mmol/L) at any time.
  2. Blood alcohol concentration greater than 150 mg/dl (33 mmol/L) in an apparently unintoxicated patient.
  3. Blood alcohol concentration greater than 100 mg/dl (22 mmol/L) at a routine examination.
- Working definition. A simple working definition for busy medical practitioners defines the alcoholic as "one who experiences repeated negative consequences of drinking," where the consequences may be biomedical, psychosocial, or socioeconomic.

EPIDEMIOLOGY

- Approximately 10% of the adult population are alcohol abusers. Estimates in the elderly vary between 2 and 10%. Abuse among young people is very high, and 87% of high school students have experimented with alcohol.
- Irish-Americans, Native Americans, Hispanics, and black youth are at increased risk of alcoholism. Jewish and Italian-Americans are relatively protected.
- The risk of developing alcoholism is increased 2.5-fold if one parent is alcoholic.
- Occupations such as the catering and brewing industries carry an increased risk of alcoholism. Members of the health professions often are addicted to other drugs in addition to alcohol.

DIFFERENTIAL DIAGNOSIS

The key is careful history-taking to distinguish among:

1. Alcoholism as the primary complaint.
2. Alcohol abuse due to a primary depressive disorder, bipolar depression, sociopathic drinking, or other drug abuse.
3. Alcoholism as the underlying cause of a multitude of medical problems (Table 95–1).

CLINICAL MANIFESTATIONS

- Presentation
  1. Early alcoholism rarely presents as an overt problem. It is much more likely to appear as:
     a. A hidden diagnosis in an apparently well patient.
     b. The result of information received from a relative or another indirect source.
     c. Depression and other behavioral changes.
     d. The diagnosis underlying the presenting medical complaint.
     e. Abnormal laboratory data.
  2. Behavioral changes usually occur before medical problems supervene. The development of well-recognized medical complications takes 10 years or longer.
- Making the diagnosis
  1. Diagnostic uncertainty is frequently a factor when the patient continues to deny the problem, and there are few absolute indicators, particularly early in the development of the disease.
  2. Confrontation is always appropriate if the evidence suggests a drinking problem. Not to do so perpetuates denial and manipulative behavior, and does the patient, the family, and the physician a disservice.
- History
  1. Questionnaires
     a. Screening instruments can be valuable, particularly in the earlier stages of the disease. They

TABLE 95–1. Clinical Manifestations of Alcoholism

	EARLY (FIRST 5 YEARS)	LATE
General appearance	Excitability Irritability Nervousness Alcoholic facies	Unkempt appearance Rosacea Jaundice[a] Parotid swelling
Cardiovascular	Palpitations Hypertension, especially labile or difficult to control	Cardiomyopathy
Respiratory		Recurrent infections
Gastrointestinal	Coated tongue Alcoholic fetor Dyspepsia Morning nausea and vomiting Acute pancreatitis (sometimes)[a] Hepatomegaly[a] GI bleeding (sometimes)	Recurrent abdominal pain Acute and chronic pancreatitis[a] Splenomegaly Ascites GI bleeding
Genitourinary	Polyuria Impotence	Amenorrhea
Central nervous system	Hand tremor[a]	Peripheral neuropathy Seizures Ataxia
Mental status	Depression Poor memory for recent events	Blackouts
Musculoskeletal		Dupuytrens contracture[a] Myopathy Gout
Skin		Spider nevi Seborrhea
Miscellaneous	Frequent or unusual trauma[a] Multiple surgical or nonsurgical scars[a] Frequent office or emergency room visits or hospitalizations Family violence or dysfunction	

[a] Great diagnostic value.

are more predictive than abnormal laboratory values. Responses should be checked by the physician in person since denial is characteristic of the disease and nonverbal responses are so important.

b. Examples are the Michigan Alcohol Screening Test (MAST) and its shorter version (SMAST) (Table 95–2).

c. The "CAGE" screen is based on 4 questions:

i. Have you ever tried to Cut down?

ii. Have you ever Annoyed anyone with your drinking?

iii. Do you ever feel Guilty about your drinking?

iv. Do you have a morning Eye-opener?

TABLE 95–2. The Brief Michigan Alcoholism Screening Test

Questions	Circle Correct Answers		Points
1. Do you feel you are a normal drinker?	yes	no	N2
2. Do friends or relatives think you are a normal drinker?	yes	no	N2
3. Have you ever attended a meeting of Alcoholics Anonymous?	yes	no	Y5
4. Have you ever lost friends or girlfriends/boyfriends because of drinking?	yes	no	Y2
5. Have you ever gotten into trouble at work because of drinking?	yes	no	Y2
6. Have you ever neglected your obligations, your family, or your work for two or more days in a row because you were drinking?	yes	no	Y2
7. Have you ever had delirium tremens (DTs), severe shaking, heard voices or seen things that weren't there after heavy drinking?	yes	no	Y2
8. Have you ever gone to anyone for help about your drinking?	yes	no	Y2
9. Have you ever been in the hospital because of your drinking?	yes	no	Y5
10. Have your ever been arrested for drunk driving or driving after drinking?	yes	no	Y2

Interpretation: "Y2" means 2 points for a "yes" answer. Total score of 6 or more = probable diagnosis of alcoholism.

Source: Pokorny AP, et al. The brief MAST: A shortened version of the Michigan Alcoholism Screening Test. Am J Psychiatry 1972;129:342–345.

2. The history itself (Table 95–3). Denial, manipulation, and minimization are characteristic of the alcoholic, and any response should be carefully evaluated for verbal and nonverbal clues to problem drinking.
3. The contract. A contract negotiated with the patient to cut down on alcohol use can be helpful in breaking through denial. The exact quantity and type of alcohol to be consumed each day should be specified and the patient seen in several weeks to assess compliance. This strategy can sometimes be helpful in showing the patient that they have lost control.

• Physical examination (see Table 95–1). There is enormous variability between patients. Women are more susceptible to liver damage leading to cirrhosis than are men.

LABORATORY STUDIES (Table 95–4)

• No combination of tests is definitive, and each must be interpreted in conjunction with historical or physical examination data.
• An elevated aspartate aminotransferase (AST/SGOT) or an increase in mean corpuscular volume (MCV) provide

TABLE 95–3. Factors That Should Be Examined in Suspected Cases of Alcohol Abuse

Drinking to relieve stress	Guilt feelings about drinking
Symptoms of depression	Morning drinking
Frequency of drinking	Family, job, social, legal,
Gulping drinks	financial consequences
Increasing tolerance	Previous withdrawal symptoms
Attempts to cut down	Family history of alcoholism
Criticism from others	Occupation
	Smoking or other drug abuse

clues to alcohol abuse. The serum gammaglutamyl transferase (GGT) may be more sensitive to alcohol consumption.

RECOMMENDED DIAGNOSTIC APPROACH

- History. A history of alcohol consumption should always be recorded at any routine examination or when a problem could be alcohol-related. A positive family history places the patient at risk. Multiple behavioral or medical consequences or a history of symptoms of withdrawal are highly suggestive.

- Physical examination. Early in the development of alcoholism there may be no physical findings. The development of signs and symptoms is quite variable.

- Laboratory data. Some tests may be helpful in conjunction with information gained from the history and physical examination, but none except the blood alcohol concentration is diagnostic (Table 95–4).

TABLE 95–4. A Suggested Alcoholism Panel[a]

TEST	NORMAL VALUE	COMMENT
MCV	76–96 fl	Alcoholics commonly demonstrate a macrocytic picture
AST	8–30 U/L	Slower elevation and not as specific as GGT
GGT	Males < 11–51 U/L Females < 7–33 U/L	Most sensitive. Not available on some lab panels.
Albumin	40–50 g/L	Slight increase, but still within normal range, in alcohol abusers.
BUN	3.0–6.4 mmol/L (8–18 mg/L)	Increased in alcoholic patients

[a] Tests with $p < 0.001$ in distinguishing alcoholic outpatients from social drinkers and family medicine clinic patients.

Source: Adapted from Skinner HA, et al. Clinical versus laboratory detection of alcohol abuse: The alcohol clinic index. Br Med J 1986;292:1703–1708.

Bibliography

Fourth Special Report to Congress on Alcohol and Health. U.S. Department of Health and Human Services. Rockville, MD, NIAAA, 1981.

Holt S, et al. Early identification of alcohol abuse: 2. Clinical and laboratory indications. Can Med Assoc J 1981(May);124:1279–1294.

Skinner HA, et al. Early identification of alcohol abuse: I. Critical issues and psychosocial indicators for a composite index. Can Med Assoc J 1981(May);124:1141–1152.

Skinner HA, et al. Clinical versus laboratory detection of alcohol abuse: The alcohol clinical index. Br Med J 1986;292:1703–08.

Weinberg JR. Interview techniques for diagnosing alcoholism. Am Fam Physician 1974;3:107–115.

SECTION XIII

HEPATOLOGY

96

JAUNDICE

RICHARD A. WILLSON

Jaundice is the disease that your friends diagnose.
SIR WILLIAM OSLER (1849–1919)

DEFINITION AND GENERAL COMMENTS

Jaundice is caused by the accumulation of bilirubin in body tissues. It usually results from the failure of the liver to remove bilirubin from the circulation.

1. Biochemical classification of jaundice
   a. The bilirubin in serum can be fractionated into unconjugated and conjugated forms.
   b. Unconjugated hyperbilirubinemia results from overproduction, defective hepatic uptake, or impaired binding and conjugation within the liver.
   c. Conjugated hyperbilirubinemia results from diminished hepatic secretion or leakage of bilirubin into the plasma from hepatocellular injury or impairment of bile flow (cholestasis).
2. Clinical classification of jaundice
   a. In prehepatic jaundice, the serum bilirubin is largely unconjugated. The liver function tests, except for serum bilirubin, are normal.
   b. In hepatic jaundice, there are varying degrees of liver function abnormalities. The serum bilirubin is usually a combination of both unconjugated and conjugated bilirubin.
   c. The older term "obstructive jaundice" has been replaced by cholestatic jaundice. It results from lack of bilirubin excretion from the liver and can have both intrahepatic and extrahepatic causes. The serum bilirubin is often predominantly conjugated. Other liver function tests may be abnormal, and the serum alkaline phosphatase is often very high.

PATHOPHYSIOLOGY (Table 96–1)

1. Bilirubin is the breakdown product of heme, coming mainly from hemoglobin. Other endogenous compounds containing the porphyrin nucleus account for 20% of the approximately 250 to 300 mg of bilirubin formed each day. Cells of the reticuloendothelial system (mainly in the spleen) form bilirubin.
2. Unconjugated bilirubin is tightly bound to albumin which

TABLE 96–1. Important Steps in Bilirubin Metabolism

1. Conversion of heme to unconjugated bilirubin
2. Transport of unconjugated bilirubin in plasma, noncovalently bound to albumin
3. Active hepatocellular uptake of unconjugated bilirubin
4. Intrahepatic transport of unconjugated bilirubin by cytosolic carrier proteins
5. Hepatic conjugation of bilirubin to bilirubin diglucuronide by the enzyme glucuronyl transferase
6. Presumed active secretion of bilirubin diglucuronide into bile.
7. Enterohepatic circulation of bilirubin degradation products (e.g., urobilinogen)

prevents its filtration by the kidney. Thus, in jaundice due to unconjugated bilirubin (i.e., hemolysis), there is no bilirubin in the urine.

3. The diglucuronide form of bilirubin (conjugated) is more water soluble. It is transported out of the biliary tract through the small intestine to the colon where bacterial degradative enzymes reduce bilirubin to urobilinogen.

4. In liver disease, the urinary urobilinogen increases. Bilirubin is found in the urine when the conjugated bilirubin level is elevated.

5. A third form of bilirubin, called delta bilirubin, is covalently bound to albumin. It occurs late in the clinical course of cholestasis. Measurement of this third fraction is not widely practiced.

DIFFERENTIAL DIAGNOSIS

1. Unconjugated hyperbilirubinemia (Table 96–2)
   a. Hemolysis causes increased production of bilirubin. Serum bilirubin levels greater than 5 mg/dl are not commonly seen with hemolysis alone, and higher levels usually indicate some underlying hepatic disease.
   b. Gilbert's syndrome is the most common (prevalence up to 7%) hereditary disorder of bilirubin metabolism which causes unconjugated hyperbilirubinemia. It is caused by a deficiency in the conjugating enzyme glucuronyl transferase. The syndrome's inheritance is autosomal dominant. It appears during the second decade of life, and patients usually have serum bilirubin levels between 2 and 3 mg/dl. Liver histology and serum biochemical tests of liver function are normal.
   c. The Crigler-Najjar syndromes (Types I and II) are less common and are characterized by glucuronyl transferase deficiency. Serum bilirubin levels range from 5 to 25 mg/dl.

2. Conjugated hyperbilirubinemia (Tables 96–2 and 96–3). The hereditary disorders associated with conjugated hyperbilirubinemia are uncommon. Most patients with these

TABLE 96–2. Differential Diagnosis of Jaundice

Unconjugated Hyperbilirubinemia	Conjugated Hyperbilirubinemia
Increased bilirubin production	Hereditary disorders of bilirubin metabolism
Hemolytic anemia	Dubin-Johnson syndrome
Ineffective erythropoiesis	Rotor syndrome
Blood transfusions	Hepatocellular disease
Hematomata	Hepatitis
Hereditary disorders of bilirubin metabolism	Cirrhosis
Gilbert syndrome	Toxins (medications, alcohol)
Crigler-Najjar syndromes	Biliary tract disease
Medications	Pancreatic disease

syndromes are mildly jaundiced, and other biochemical tests of liver function are normal.

3. The etiology of jaundice varies considerably with age.
   a. In neonates, physiologic jaundice accounts for 75% of cases.
   b. In adolescents, the largest proportions are shared by Gilbert's disease (50%) and viral hepatitis (25%).
   c. In young adults, 50% of jaundice is caused by viral hepatitis.
   d. In the elderly, 50% of jaundiced patients have a malignancy involving the hepatobiliary system.

CLINICAL EVALUATION OF JAUNDICE

Jaundice is detected clinically when serum levels of bilirubin are between 2 and 3 mg/dl.

1. History
   a. In the history, one should obtain information about

TABLE 96–3. Differential Diagnosis of Cholestasis (Obstructive Jaundice)

Extrahepatic Cholestasis	Intrahepatic Cholestasis
Biliary tract disease	Medications (common)
Gallstones	Viral hepatitis (common)
Tumor	Alcoholic hepatitis (common)
Stricture	Primary biliary cirrhosis
Pancreatic disease	Primary sclerosing cholangitis
Tumor	Postoperative
Chronic pancreatitis	Parenteral nutrition
Pseudocyst	Sepsis
	Hereditary disorders

occupation, familial liver disease and hemolysis, contacts with jaundiced persons, travel, parenteral risks, food exposure, appetite, weight loss, fever, drug exposure, changes in color of stool and urine, and presence or absence of abdominal pain.

b. A flulike illness prior to the onset of jaundice suggests viral hepatitis.

c. Excessive alcohol ingestion or exposure to other drugs suggest toxic liver injury.

d. Abdominal pain with jaundice suggests extrahepatic biliary tract disease and perhaps a surgical problem.

2. Physical examination

a. The physical findings that suggest underlying hepatic disease include ascites, prominent venous pattern on the anterior abdomen, cutaneous spider angiomata, and hepatosplenomegaly.

b. Palpation of an abdominal mass or the gall bladder suggests extrahepatic biliary obstruction.

c. The presence of hepatomegaly does not help distinguish intrahepatic and extrahepatic cholestasis.

3. Laboratory studies

a. Serum biochemical tests of liver function. The serum alkaline phosphatase level is usually strikingly elevated by cholestasis. The serum transaminases are prominently elevated by acute hepatitis. The serum albumin may be decreased by chronic liver diseases.

b. The measurement of the conjugated and unconjugated bilirubin fractions is helpful only when serum bilirubin levels are between 5 and 10 mg/dl.

   i. In jaundice due to hepatic disease, both bilirubin fractions are elevated and fractionation does not help to distinguish the causes for the jaundice. Serum bilirubin levels above 30 mg/dl usually indicate severe hepatocellular disease.

   ii. With cholestasis, the serum bilirubin level is usually between 10 and 30 mg/dl and is predominantly conjugated.

c. Serologic tests are available for the viral hepatitides.

d. Imaging techniques

   i. Cholestatic jaundice is often more clinically perplexing, in part related to distinguishing intrahepatic and extrahepatic causes. The clinical and biochemical findings within the two groups is similar.

   ii. Cholescintigraphy provides poor anatomic definition. The more invasive imaging techniques, percutaneous transhepatic cholangiography (PTC) and endoscopic retrograde cholangiopancreatography (ERCP), are often required to make the diagnosis (Table 96–4).

e. Liver biopsy often fails to distinguish between intrahepatic and extrahepatic cholestasis. However, it may be of value when both intrahepatic and extrahepatic disease contribute to the jaundice. It is valuable in determining the type, extent, and potential prognosis of underlying liver disease.

TABLE 96–4. Diagnostic Studies in Evaluation of Jaundice

Test	Sens (%)	Spec (%)	PPV (%)	NPV (%)	Accuracy (%)
History and physical exam	95	76	74	96	84
US	73	88	89	73	78
CT	72	85	87	77	81
Cholescintigraphy	58	71	70	68	68

Sens = sensitivity; Spec = specificity; PPV = positive predictive value; NPV = negative predictive value.

Source: Adapted from Danovitch S. Evaluation of the jaundiced patient. In Chobanian SJ, Van Ness MM, eds. Manual of Clinical Problems in Gastroenterology. Boston, Little Brown, 1988, p. 140.

RECOMMENDED DIAGNOSTIC APPROACH

- The diagnosis of jaundice begins with a clinical evaluation and determination of transaminase, alkaline phosphatase, bilirubin, and albumin levels.
  1. In some cases, clinical observation with serial liver function tests may be all that is required.
  2. If indicated, hepatic imaging with ultrasound (US) or CT should be used to detect space-occupying lesions. Liver biopsy may be necessary to diagnose and stage the extent of the disease process.
- Following the clinical evaluation, the physician should decide whether extrahepatic cholestasis is very unlikely, possible, or very likely.
  1. Extrahepatic cholestasis very unlikely: consider additional tests (hepatitis serologies, anti-smooth muscle, or antimitochondrial antibodies) or a liver biopsy.
  2. Extrahepatic cholestasis possible:
     a. US is currently the noninvasive imaging modality of first choice, largely due to its lower cost.
     b. CT is indicated if US is technically inadequate or if there is additional extrahepatobiliary information which can be gained by this modality.
     c. If either modality does not suggest extrahepatic biliary cholestasis, then the work-up may stop, with clinical observation to follow.
  3. Extrahepatic cholestasis very likely: perform ERCP or PTC to obtain direct ductal visualization. The choice depends on:
     a. The availability of skilled personnel.
     b. Suspected location of the lesion in the biliary tree.
     c. Presence of ascites or coagulopathy.
     d. Surgically altered gastroduodenal anatomy. The two procedures may be complementary in complex settings.

Bibliography

Chopra S, Griffin PH. Laboratory tests and diagnostic procedures in evaluation of liver disease. Am J Med 1985;79:221–230.

Frank BB. Clinical evaluation of jaundice. A guideline of the patient care committee of the American Gastroenterological Association. JAMA 1989;262:3031–3034.

Lester R. Not two, but three bilirubins. N Engl J Med 1983;309:183–185.

Matzen P, et al. Ultrasound, computed tomography, and cholescintigraphy in suspected obstructive jaundice. Gastroenterology 1983;84:1492–1497.

O'Connor KW, et al. A blinded prospective study comparing four current noninvasive approaches in differential diagnoses of medical versus surgical jaundice. Gastroenterology 1983;84:1498–1504.

Scharschmidt BF, et al. Approach to the patient with cholestatic jaundice. N Engl J Med 1983;308:1515–1519.

Tiribelli G, Ostrow JD. New concepts in bilirubin chemistry, transport, and metabolism: Report of the international bilirubin workshop, April 6–8, 1989, Trieste, Italy. Hepatology 1990;11:303–313.

Van Ness MM, Diehl AM. Is liver biopsy useful in the evaluation of patients with chronically elevated liver enzymes? Ann Int Med 1989;111:473–478.

Weiss JS, et al. The clinical importance of protein-bound fraction of serum bilirubin in patients with hyperbilirubinemia. N Engl J Med 1983;309:147–150.

97

HEPATOMEGALY

JOHN HALSEY, *and* MICHAEL KIMMEY

. LIVER, n. A large red organ thoughtfully provided by
nature to be bilious with. . . . It was at one time considered the seat of life; hence its name—liver, the thing
we live with.

AMBROSE BIERCE (1842–1914)

GENERAL COMMENTS

- Usefulness of physical examination
  1. Hepatomegaly is usually first detected by physical ex-
     amination. Anatomic variations of liver shape are fre-
     quent, and examination alone is not a sensitive or spe-
     cific test of liver size.
  2. Imaging techniques, especially US, are more accurate
     but are currently not used to screen large populations
     for increased liver size.
- Physical assessment of liver size
  1. This is best accomplished by percussion in the right
     midclavicular line. The normal span of dullness is 8 to
     14 cm. Estimates of liver size increase if lighter percus-
     sion techniques are used. The liver edge is detectable
     more than 2 cm below the right costal margin with
     inspiration in 15% of normal persons.
  2. Liver size increases with height and weight, and males
     have larger livers than females.
  3. Falsely increased estimates of liver size are caused by:
     a. A depressed right hemidiaphragm (e.g., chronic
        obstructive pulmonary disease).
     b. Subdiaphragmatic lesions (abscess or hematoma).
     c. Riedel's lobe (anatomic variant with inferior
        projection of the right hepatic lobe).

DIFFERENTIAL DIAGNOSIS (Table 97–1)

- Vascular congestion
  1. Congestive heart failure
     a. The liver is enlarged in over 95% of patients with
        acute or chronic right-sided heart failure. The liver
        edge is palpable over 5 cm below the costal margin
        in half of patients.
     b. Liver pulsation may indicate tricuspid insuffi-
        ciency.

TABLE 97–1. Causes of Hepatomegaly

Vascular congestion
  Right-sided congestive heart failure (common)
  Budd-Chiari syndrome (rare)
  Veno-occlusive disease (rare)
  Tricuspid insufficiency (common)
  Constrictive pericarditis (uncommon)
Inflammatory conditions
  Hepatitis
    Viral (A, B, C, CMV, infectious mononucleosis)
      (common)
    Bacterial (rare)
    Parasitic (uncommon)
  Abscess
    Bacterial (uncommon)
    Amoebic (uncommon)
  Diseases of uncertain cause
    Autoimmune chronic hepatitis (uncommon)
    Primary biliary cirrhosis (uncommon)
    Primary sclerosing cholangitis (uncommon)
Alcoholic liver disease
  Fatty liver (common)
  Alcoholic hepatis (common)
  Cirrhosis (common)
Infiltrative liver disease
  Fatty liver (common)
  Amyloidosis (rare)
  Hematologic
    Leukemia (uncommon)
    Lymphoma (uncommon)
    Myeloid metaplasia (uncommon)
  Granulomatous
    Sarcoidosis (uncommon)
    Bacterial (tuberculosis, leprosy, brucellosis, Q fever,
      syphilis) (uncommon)
    Parasites (schistosomiasis, toxocariasis) (uncommon)
    Viral (mononucleosis, CMV, psittacosis) (uncommon)
    Drugs or foreign substances (beryllium) (rare)
Iron storage disorder
  Hemochromatosis (uncommon)
  Hemosiderosis (alcohol, transfusional) (uncommon)
  Congenital errors of metabolism
    Carbohydrate metabolism (hereditary fructose
      intolerance, galactosemia, glycogen storage disease)
      (rare)
    Protein metabolism (tyrosinemia) (rare)
    Lipid metabolism (Wolman disease, cholesterol ester
      storage disease) (rare)
    Bile acid metabolism (rare)
    Lipoid storage disease (Niemann-Pick, Gaucher's)
      (rare)
    Miscellaneous (α_1-antitrypsin deficiency, cystic
      fibrosis) (rare)
Biliary obstruction
  Carcinoma (pancreatic, ampullary, cholangiocarcinoma)
    (common)

TABLE 97–1. Causes of Hepatomegaly
Continued

Choledocholithiasis (common)
Hepatic tumors
   Metastatic carcinoma (common)
   Hepatocellular carcinoma (uncommon)
   Benign liver tumors (adenoma, focal nodular hyperplasia,
     hemangioma) (uncommon)
Cystic liver diseases
   Parasitic (echinococcal) (uncommon)
   Nonparasitic (uncommon)
     Solitary (uncommon)
     Polycystic (uncommon)
   Traumatic (uncommon)
   Neoplastic (uncommon)

    2. Budd-Chiari syndrome. Hepatomegaly is detected in 70% of patients with hepatic venous occlusion. Ascites (90%) and abdominal pain (60%) are also usually seen in this rare syndrome.

    3. Veno-occlusive disease (VOD). Approximately 70% of symptomatic patients with VOD due to chemotherapy and radiation therapy have hepatomegaly.

- Inflammatory conditions. Hepatitis. All types of viral hepatitis may be associated with tender hepatomegaly. A liver size more than 3 to 5 cm larger than normal is uncommon in acute viral hepatitis.

- Alcoholic liver disease

    1. Fatty liver. This is the most common type of liver pathology seen with alcohol ingestion. Most patients are asymptomatic. Liver tenderness from capsular distention is common.

    2. Alcoholic hepatitis. Liver biopsy is necessary to make this diagnosis with certainty. Ascites (70%), jaundice (70%), fever (50%), splenomegaly (40%), and encephalopathy (30%) may occur.

    3. Cirrhosis. Hepatomegaly is present in 75 to 95% of cases but does not help distinguish between the various causes of cirrhosis. The liver may also be shrunken or have disproportionate enlargement of one lobe.

- Infiltrative liver disease

    1. Fatty liver

       a. Although the most common cause of this condition is alcohol, it is also seen with inflammatory bowel disease (30% of cases), obesity, previous jejunoileal bypass, protein-calorie malnutrition, parenteral nutrition, and Reye's syndrome.

       b. Liver enlargement in diabetic patients is caused by glycogen and fat deposition.

       c. Acute fatty liver of pregnancy is a rapidly progressive disorder occurring in the third trimester or immediately postpartum with an 80% mortality.

2. Amyloidosis. Hepatomegaly is present in 50% of patients with systemic amyloidosis.
3. Hematologic disorders. Hepatomegaly is present in patients with leukemia (50%), agnogenic myeloid metaplasia (50%), non-Hodgkin's lymphoma (25%), and Hodgkin's disease (10%).
4. Granulomatous disorders. The most common cause of granulomatous liver enlargement is sarcoidosis. Hepatomegaly is seen at some time in the course of 20% of patients with sarcoidosis.
5. Iron storage disorders. Hepatomegaly is present in 75 to 95% of patients with hemochromatosis but less frequently in hemosiderosis related to alcoholic cirrhosis, and transfusional iron overload.
6. Congenital metabolic defects
   a. Most of these disorders appear in infancy or early childhood.
   b. Gaucher's disease is caused by a lysosomal enzyme deficiency and may present as late as the third decade of life with unexplained hepatosplenomegaly, especially in Ashkenazi Jews.
   c. In 5% of patients with the Pi ZZ phenotype of α_1-antitrypsin deficiency, the disease appears in infancy with hepatomegaly and jaundice. In another 5% it occurs in adulthood with cirrhosis and sometimes hepatomegaly. Coexistent emphysema is frequent in adult patients.

- Biliary obstruction. Bile duct obstruction from common duct stones or carcinoma may cause moderate liver enlargement in addition to jaundice.
- Hepatic tumors
  1. In the United States, metastatic liver tumors are 20 times more common than primary hepatocellular carcinoma. Metastases may cause palpable nodules or diffuse hepatomegaly.
  2. Ninety percent of patients with primary hepatocellular carcinoma have hepatomegaly. Fifty percent have ascites, and 30% have an arterial bruit over the liver.
- Cystic liver diseases. Solitary cysts, whether parasitic or nonparasitic, may be palpable as a discrete nodule. Thirty percent of patients with adult polycystic kidney disease also have multiple liver cysts, which expand with time and eventually produce nodular hepatomegaly.

CLINICAL MANIFESTATIONS

- History
  1. General. Review of systems should seek symptoms of congestive heart failure, malignancy, and infection.
  2. Symptoms referable to liver dysfunction. Such symptoms include jaundice, ascites, GI bleeding, encephalopathy, and pruritus.
  3. Other. A history of alcohol consumption, drug or toxin exposure, foreign travel, and a family history of liver disease may provide important clues.

- Physical examination
  1. General
     a. The physician should look for signs of CHF, malignancy, systemic infection, and alcohol consumption (tremor, neuropathy, cerebellar dysfunction, or Dupuytren's contractures).
     b. Extrahepatic manifestations of liver disease (ascites, icterus, splenomegaly, palmar erythema, spider angiomas, gynecomastia, or testicular atrophy) may occur.
  2. The liver should be examined for:
     a. Size. Use percussion in the midclavicular line.
     b. Tenderness is more likely with a recent onset of hepatomegaly.
     c. Nodularity suggests tumor, macronodular cirrhosis, or polycystic disease.
     d. Pulsation is present with tricuspid insufficiency or is transmitted from the abdominal aorta.
     e. Bruit occurs in hepatocellular carcinoma or acute alcoholic hepatitis.
     f. Venous hum may be caused by portal hypertension.
     g. Friction rub may be related to perihepatitis, metastatic tumor, or recent liver biopsy.

LABORATORY STUDIES

- Screening for hematologic, renal, and cardiac disease is often useful (CBC, serum creatinine level, and chest X-ray).
- Biochemical liver tests
  1. The bilirubin, alanine aminotransferase (ALT or SGPT), aspartate aminotransferase (AST or SGOT), alkaline phosphatase, prothrombin time, and albumin yield some abnormality in most patients with significant hepatic disorders which may direct further evaluation.
  2. Serologic tests
     a. Patients with abnormal liver enzymes and hepatomegaly should undergo serologic testing for viral hepatitis.
     b. If primary biliary cirrhosis or chronic active hepatitis is suspected on clinical grounds, testing for antimitochondrial and anti-smooth muscle antibodies is indicated.
- Imaging techniques
  1. Ultrasound. This is usually the initial imaging procedure in the evaluation of hepatomegaly. A qualitative estimate of liver size, the extent and quality (cystic versus solid) of mass lesions, and the presence of biliary obstruction or cholelithiasis may be determined.
  2. CT
     a. CT often provides the best evaluation of diffuse liver disease. Fatty infiltration and iron or glyco-

gen deposition may be distinguished by their different CT densities.

b. Ultrasound is better than CT in defining cystic masses, but CT detects more solid liver masses.

3. Liver-spleen scan. In this study, 99m-Technetium-labeled colloid is taken up by the reticuloendothelial (RE) cells. Any process that causes replacement of RE cells such as tumors, cysts, or abscesses cause "cold" areas on the scan.

4. MRI is useful to evaluate vascular and neoplastic hepatic lesions.

- Liver biopsy

1. Blind percutaneous liver biopsy should be performed in patients with unexplained diffuse hepatomegaly. Most diffuse liver diseases are safely diagnosed with this technique if the prothrombin time is prolonged less than 3 sec and the platelet count is greater than $60,000/mm^3$.

2. US or CT-directed biopsy of unexplained mass lesions usually provides a histologic diagnosis.

RECOMMENDED DIAGNOSTIC APPROACH

- CBC, creatinine, prothrombin time, ALT or AST, alkaline phosphatase, bilirubin, and albumin should be obtained.

- If the results of these tests are normal and the examiner is confident that hepatomegaly is present, US should be done to confirm liver enlargement and to look for mass lesions.

- If serum ALT or AST levels are significantly elevated relative to alkaline phosphatase, a hepatitis screen should be done and other causes of hepatitis sought. Imaging tests are usually unnecessary.

- If alkaline phosphatase or 5'-nucleotidase levels are elevated out of proportion to the transaminases, US or CT should be done to rule out biliary obstruction and the presence of mass lesions.

- Patients with unexplained diffuse parenchymal liver enlargement or unexplained mass lesions should undergo liver biopsy if clotting studies permit this.

Bibliography

Clouse ME. Current diagnostic imaging modalities of the liver. Surg Clin North Am 1989;69(2):193–234.

Sapira JD, Williamson KL. How big is the normal liver? Arch Intern Med 1979;139:971–973.

Schiff L, Schiff ER, eds. Diseases of the Liver. Philadelphia, J.B. Lippincott Company, 1987.

Sherlock S. Diseases of the Liver and Biliary System, 8th ed. London, Blackwell Scientific Publications, 1989.

98

VIRAL HEPATITIS

RUSSELL McMULLEN

All seem infected that th' infected spy
As all looks yellow to the jaundic'd eye.

ALEXANDER POPE (1688–1744)

DEFINITIONS AND GENERAL COMMENTS

- Viral hepatitis refers to infection of the liver by any of a number of viral agents that may cause acute and/or chronic hepatocellular inflammation, damage, and dysfunction.
- Causes of viral hepatitis
  1. Infectious hepatitis is now known to be due to hepatitis A virus (HAV); a main cause of serum hepatitis is the hepatitis B virus (HBV).
  2. Non-A, non-B hepatitis (NANBH) refers to a group of viruses. One of these, the hepatitis C virus (HCV), causes disease that is epidemiologically similar to hepatitis B and is commonly transmitted through blood exposure or transfusion.
  3. There is at least one other presently uncharacterized non-A non-B agent that is antigenically similar to HCV and is responsible for parenterally transmitted hepatitis.
  4. The hepatitis D virus (HDV or "delta agent") is a defective virus that must utilize the hepatitis B surface antigen in order to replicate. HDV causes illness in concert with hepatitis B, often increasing the severity of the acute or chronic hepatitis B infection.
  5. Enterically transmitted NANBH (hepatitis E) has not been found in the United States in epidemic form; occasional cases have been diagnosed in travelers or immigrants who have recently entered the country. The transmission and epidemiology of the hepatitis E virus (HEV) are otherwise similar to HAV.
- Criteria for diagnosis. Hyperbilirubinemia and elevated serum transaminase levels may suggest a diagnosis of viral hepatitis. "Liver function" abnormalities are not by themselves definitive evidence of viral hepatitis; other infections, toxic or drug-induced liver damage, and hepatobiliary tract disease must be considered and excluded.

EPIDEMIOLOGY

- Hepatitis A
  1. The usual mechanism of spread of HAV is fecal-oral. Waterborne infection (including infection from contaminated shellfish) can also occur.
  2. The disease is present worldwide but is most prevalent in areas with crowding and poor sanitation. Greater than half of urban adult Americans of low socioeconomic status have anti-HAV; rates for younger, nonurban, and middle class populations are lower.
  3. The incubation period is 2 to 6 weeks, with a mean of 26 days. Peak infectivity occurs in the 2 weeks prior to the onset of jaundice and during the early clinical illness. Many infections are subclinical and hence undiagnosed.
  4. There is no carrier state for hepatitis A, but 5 to 10% of infections will persist, waxing and waning over several months to a year before ultimate resolution.
- Hepatitis B
  1. Hepatitis B is composed of a surface antigen (HBsAg), which can circulate independently, and the core which contains a core antigen (HBcAg), DNA and a DNA polymerase molecule, and the "e" antigen (HBeAg).
  2. Transmission of HBV is often through parenteral exposure to blood, but many other body fluids contain the virus: saliva and semen have been demonstrated to transmit infection.
  3. The incubation period is 2 to 6 months. The size of the inoculum may determine the incubation period.
  4. Groups at risk for infection with HBV include:
     a. Patients receiving blood products: Transmission now occurs only when blood is administered that contains HBV at a level below the sensitivity threshhold of the HBsAg assay. Less than 10% of transfusion-associated hepatitis is due to HBV.
     b. Parenteral drug users.
     c. Hemodialysis patients.
     d. Organ transplant recipients.
     e. Health care workers, especially those with frequent contact with blood products, saliva, or other potentially contaminated body fluids, or who frequently treat patients who are likely to have acute or chronic HBV infection.
     f. Household or close physical contacts of infected individuals.
     g. Sexual contacts of infected individuals. Unprotected anal receptive intercourse may put an individual at particular risk of infection with HBV.
     h. Infants of infected mothers may acquire the virus by maternal-fetal transmission, either during gestation or, more likely, during parturition.
     i. Institutionalized individuals, such as the retarded or those in prison, who may be repeatedly exposed to sources of infection.
  5. Five to ten percent of the adult population of the

United States carries antibody to HBcAg (anti-HBc), indicating previous HBV infection. Hepatitis B is much more common in Africa, parts of South America, and most of Asia; some Southeast Asian populations have a prevalence of markers of past infection of 80 to 90%.

6. The rate of chronic HBV carriage for adults in the United States is 0.2%, reflecting an incidence of less than 10% after initial infection. Portions of the U.S. population who come from areas where HBV is highly endemic, such as Southeast Asian refugees, have a high carrier rate (10 to 15%). The risk of becoming a carrier is greater the younger one is at the time of infection, and most infections in areas with high endemic rates of HBV occur at birth or during early childhood.

- Hepatitis C
  1. The epidemiology of hepatitis C is similar to hepatitis B, at least with regard to blood transfusion and other parenteral exposures. In the United States, HCV causes at least 60%, and perhaps 90% of hepatitis associated with blood transfusions. Anti-HCV antibody is present in 1% of volunteer blood donors.
  2. Besides transfusion recipients, groups at risk for infection with HBV are also at risk for HCV infection.

- Hepatitis D
  1. HDV, referred to as the "delta agent" when first described in 1977, is a defective virus that requires that the HBsAg be present and wrapped around it in order to replicate. Hepatitis D may occur as a "coinfection" during acute HBV infection, but may also occur as a "superinfection" in carriers of HBV who become infected with the hybrid virus.
  2. Transmission of HDV occurs through similar mechanisms of transmission as HBV.
  3. Persistent HDV infection leads to chronic active hepatitis in 60 to 90% of cases. Fulminant hepatitis and death are more common when HDV is combined with HBV infection than when HBV occurs alone; superinfection of a chronic HBV carrier results in fulminant hepatitis in 10% of cases, a higher rate than is seen with coinfection.
  4. Hepatitis D is endemic in Italy, North Africa, and South America. Epidemics have occurred in the United States.

- Hepatitis E
  1. An additional type of NANBH referred to as waterborne or enterically transmitted NANBH has been recognized since a large outbreak of hepatitis that occurred during flooding in New Delhi in 1955–56 was later found not to have been caused by HAV.
  2. Viral particles have been demonstrated in the stool of patients with this infection; it is now usually referred to as hepatitis E.
     a. HEV has a fecal-oral transmission pattern, much

like HAV, and hepatitis E occurs in rural and urban epidemics, especially when floods occur and disrupt already poor sanitation conditions.

b. Notable outbreaks have occurred in India, Pakistan, Central Asia, and in African refugee camps. While isolated imported cases have been recognized in the United States, epidemic disease has not been seen; an outbreak did occur in rural Mexico in 1987.

3. Serologic assays for this infection exist but are not yet commercially available. In research settings, the virus can be detected in stool using immune electron microscopy.

CLINICAL FEATURES: SIGNS, SYMPTOMS, AND COURSE OF DISEASE

- Prodrome
  1. The onset of illness is fairly abrupt in hepatitis A but is frequently more indolent with HBV and HCV infections.
  2. Incubation periods following infection are different:
     a. HAV, 2 to 6 weeks (mean: 3.7 weeks)
     b. HBV, 2 to 6 months (mean: 11.8 weeks)
     c. HCV, 6 to 12 weeks (mean: 7.8 weeks)
     d. HDV, 3 to 6 weeks following superinfection
     e. HEV, 2 to 9 weeks (mean: 6 weeks)
  3. Infectivity
     a. Patients with HAV are most infectious for 2 weeks before the onset of icterus and less so for 1 week afterward.
     b. HBV-infected individuals are infectious when HBsAg can be detected in the serum, often as much as 6 weeks before symptoms develop.
     c. The onset of infectivity for HCV appears to be soon after infection.
  4. Symptoms. Early symptoms of hepatitis include fever (37.5 to 38.5°C), fatigue, and malaise (Table 98–1).
  5. Signs
     a. Physical findings include hepatomegaly (70% of cases) and right upper quadrant tenderness (90%), with splenomegaly (20%) in severe cases.
     b. Urticarial rash and mild arthritis may occur in hepatitis B (10% of cases) and is presumed to be caused by HBsAg-HBsAb immune complex formation. Similar findings are rarely seen with hepatitis A (1% of cases) and have occasionally been reported with hepatitis C.
- Icteric phase
  1. In young children, less than 15% of HAV infections are icteric, compared to perhaps 40 to 60% in adults. The rate of icteric hepatitis B in adult cases may be as low as 20%, and that of hepatitis C even lower.
  2. From the time of initial transaminase elevation, patients may show a progression from dark urine (bilirubinuria), to acholic stool, then jaundice.

TABLE 98–1. Symptoms in Acute Viral Hepatitis[a]

SYMPTOM	% OF CASES
Fatigue	70–90
Jaundice/Scleral icterus	20–70[b]
Dark urine	30–90[b]
Acholic stools	35–60[b]
Anorexia	40–65
Abdominal pain	40–65
Nausea/Vomiting	25–40[c]
Diarrhea	20–30[c]
Fever (low-level)	25–40
Myalgia/Arthralgia	15–30

[a] All types included: icteric hepatitis is less common in adults with hepatitis B or C compared to hepatitis A.
[b] Lower in young children with hepatitis A.
[c] Higher in young children with hepatitis A.

   3. In hepatitis A, systemic symptoms typically begin to resolve when the patient becomes jaundiced.
 • Fulminant hepatitis
   1. Fulminant hepatitis is an overwhelming infection that destroys large numbers of hepatocytes. Manifestations include profound jaundice with high initial transaminase levels, prolonged prothrombin time, persistent jaundice following enzyme normalization, and hepatic encephalopathy.
   2. Fulminant hepatitis is a rare complication of hepatitis but is more common in hepatitis B (1 to 3% of cases) or hepatitis D superinfection (10%) than in hepatitis A (<0.5%) or hepatitis C (rare).
 • Convalescent phase
   1. There is a gradual return to well-being in those hepatitis cases in which the patient recovers and does not become a chronic carrier.
   2. Bilirubin rapidly normalizes after HAV infection; transaminases return to baseline in 80 to 90% of cases within 4 months after onset of symptoms.
   3. Hepatitis B can have a slower resolution. The serum bilirubin level tends to vary directly with the level of HBsAg, which persists for 6 to 20 weeks in symptomatic infections which go on to resolution.
   4. Hepatitis C can resolve quickly or may show a smoldering pattern of transaminase elevation. Initial low levels of transaminase or a smoldering persistent elevation are associated with development of a chronic carrier state.
 • Chronic hepatitis
   1. Development of a carrier state may occur after acute infection with HBV or HCV; it does not occur after hepatitis A. A chronic HBV carrier can also remain positive for HDV.
   2. Five to 10 percent of adult patients with acute hepatitis

B become chronic HBV carriers. The risk of becoming a carrier is 85% if infected at birth, and 25% if infected in early childhood.

3. Chronic HBV carriers may develop diseases associated with immune-complex deposition, cirrhosis, and are 200 to 300 times more likely to develop hepatocellular carcinoma than the general population.

4. The rate of chronicity following HCV infection is as high as 50%. Between 3 and 7% of adults in the United States may be carriers and at risk of cirrhosis or possibly hepatocellular carcinoma.

5. Chronic HBV or HCV infection can cause chronic persistent hepatitis or chronic active hepatitis (CAH). Twenty percent of cases of CAH are caused by chronic HBV infection and probably more than 50% by HCV.

DIFFERENTIAL DIAGNOSIS

- Other viruses
  1. EBV. Infectious mononucleosis, typically seen in young adults, can involve the liver. Mild transaminase abnormalities are common, and hepatomegaly (10% of cases) and jaundice (4%) can occur. Significant hepatic sequelae are rare.
  2. CMV. In an immunocompetent adult, CMV infection can be similar to EBV infection and cause hepatomegaly and mild jaundice. In immunosuppressed patients, symptoms can be much more severe.
  3. Yellow fever. Jaundice is a common manifestation of the severe form of yellow fever. The incubation period is short (3 to 6 days). It should be suspected in unvaccinated recent travelers from endemic areas of Africa and South America.
  4. Herpes simplex. Disseminated infection can involve the liver and cause hepatic necrosis.
  5. Coxsackie virus. Hepatitis may be seen in severe systemic infection.
- Nonviral infections
  1. Typhoid fever. Jaundice as a result of diffuse hepatic involvement has been reported. It should be differentiated from the cholecystitis often seen in typhoid fever.
  2. Syphilis. Liver function abnormalities, typically alkaline phosphatase elevation, occur in 10% of patients with secondary syphilis.
  3. Leptospirosis. This biphasic illness is caused by a number of serotypes of *Leptospira interrogans,* especially *L. icterohemorrhagiae.* During the second, or "immune," phase, Weil's syndrome can occur; a picture of aseptic meningitis predominates, but marked hyperbilirubinemia and modest transaminase elevation may be seen.
  4. Q fever. This disease is caused by the rickettsia *Coxiella burnetti.* It is spread to humans by exposure to aerosols at the time of parturition of infected animals, most often goats, cows, and sheep. Exposure to hides

of these animals can also spread the disease. Hepatomegaly and jaundice may be prominent findings; the hepatic lesions are granulomatous.

5. Toxoplasmosis. Hepatic involvement is usually not severe unless the patient is immunosuppressed.

6. Schistosomiasis. Tender hepatomegaly, with occasional mild to moderate transaminase abnormalities, can be seen in the acute phase of Schistosomiasis.

7. Malaria. Hepatomegaly and marked jaundice may be seen in malaria, usually with severe disease due to *Plasmodium falciparum*.

8. Liver abscess. Bacterial and amebic liver abscesses usually cause focal hepatomegaly and tenderness. Serum bilirubin level may be elevated, but transaminases tend to be normal. A history of cholangitis or travel to endemic areas may suggest the diagnosis.

- Toxic hepatitis

  1. Acute alcoholic hepatitis. This usually occurs after a marked increase in ethanol intake by someone who is a regular consumer. Fever, hepatomegaly, and a leukocytosis are typical.

  2. Medications. Mechanisms by which medications produce liver damage include:

     a. Hepatocellular injury. This is microscopically similar to viral hepatitis. Important causes include:

        i. Halothane.
        ii. Isoniazid. The likelihood of injury increases with age.
        iii. NSAIDs.
        iv. Niacin. Both long-term, high-dose and short-term, low-dose time-release niacin preparations have been implicated.
        v. Phenytoin.
        vi. Sulfonamides.
        vii. Ketoconazole.
        viii. Methyldopa.

     b. Cholestatic jaundice. Medications causing this condition include:

        i. Erythromycin estolate.
        ii. Chlorpromazine.
        iii. Antithyroid agents (propylthiouracil and methimazole).
        iv. Estrogenic and androgenic steroids.
        v. Oral hypoglycemics.

     c. Fatty infiltration of hepatocytes

        i. Valproic acid.
        ii. Amiodarone.
        iii. Tetracycline. Severe hepatic injury is likely only if tetracycline is given intravenously at doses of ≥ 2 g/day.

     d. Hepatotoxic agents

        i. Acetaminophen. Hepatocellular injury, often severe, occurs as a result of suicide attempts or chronic overdose.
        ii. Vitamins A and D are hepatotoxic if given at very high doses.

      iii. Industrial chemicals, e.g., carbon tetra-
         chloride.

      iv. *Amanita phalloides* (mushroom) toxin.

- Biliary tract disease
- "Benign postoperative jaundice" or "reactive hepatopathy." This condition is seen in markedly ill patients with nonhepatic disease. It is characterized by elevation of bilirubin and akaline phosphatase levels with normal or near normal transaminase levels.
- Hypotension. Following an episode of hypotension, extreme but transient elevation of transaminase levels may occur.
- Gilbert's syndrome. Mild jaundice may be apparent but hepatic enzymes should be normal.
- Jaundice associated with pregnancy. Two conditions can occur in the third trimester:
  1. Cholestatic jaundice of pregnancy. This is a relatively benign condition. Bilirubin and transaminase elevations are mild.
  2. Acute fatty liver. This condition has a high mortality. Bilirubin and transaminase levels are usually very abnormal, as is the prothrombin time.

LABORATORY TESTS

- General tests
  1. Transaminases
     a. Aspartate aminotransferase (AST; serum glutamic oxaloacetic transaminase [SGOT]) and ALT (alanine aminotransferase; serum glutamic pyruvic transaminase [SGPT]) are markers for hepatocellular injury. Used as screening tests, they can detect otherwise subclinical hepatitis.
     b. Values in acute hepatitis may range from the low hundreds to several thousand IU.
     c. Generally, ALT is more elevated than AST; a useful exception occurs in alcoholic hepatitis, in which levels are rarely higher than 300 IU with AST > ALT.
  2. Bilirubin. Bilirubin elevation can be indicative of the degree of hepatic injury and usually parallels the increase in serum transaminases. It is not specific for viral hepatitis.
  3. Prothrombin time. The concentrations of liver-synthesized clotting factors determine the prothrombin time. It has some utility as a parameter of the severity and progression of liver dysfunction (provided parenteral vitamin K is given to rule out malabsorption as a cause of decreased coagulation factor synthesis).
  4. Alkaline phosphatase. This enzyme is of little value in diagnosis of hepatitis; it is elevated in almost all hepatobiliary and many systemic disorders. It is also found in bone: elevated 5'-nucleotidase or γ-glutamyl transpeptidase levels can confirm that the source is hepatic.

- Specific tests and diseases
  1. Hepatitis A (Figure 98–1). In acute infection with HAV, an antibody (anti-HAV) which is an IgM immunoglobulin is produced, beginning about the time that jaundice appears (or approximately two weeks after fecal shedding begins). This antibody remains detectable in serum for several months. Following acute infection, IgG anti-HAV develops and probably lasts for life.
  2. Hepatitis B. HBV serologic markers include (Figures 98–2 to 98–4):
     a. Hepatitis B surface antigen. Hepatitis B surface antigen (HBsAg) can be found in the serum several weeks before onset of symptoms, perhaps as early as 1 week after inoculation. HBsAg disappears with resolution of the infection. Persistence in serum beyond 6 months from onset of symptoms indicates the patient is a chronic carrier (the assay may be negative in a very low-level carrier state).
     b. Hepatitis B surface antibody
        i. Antibody to HBsAg (anti-HBs) is indicative of recovery from HBV infection and generally confers immunity to reinfection.
        ii. It is usually not seen until 1 to 4 months, or longer, after HBsAg is cleared from the serum.
        iii. In subclinical infections, anti-HBs appear early and HBsAg may never be detectable.
        iv. Anti-HBs is the antibody induced by the hep-

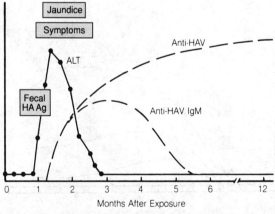

Figure 98–1. The clinical, serologic, and biochemical course of typical type A hepatitis. HA Ag = hepatitis A antigen; ALT = alanine aminotransferase; Anti-HAV = antibody to hepatitis A virus. (Reprinted with permission of publisher, from Hoofnagle JH: Perspectives on Viral Hepatitis, Vol. 2, 1st ed. Rahway, New Jersey, Abbott Laboratories, 1981, p. 4.) NOTE: This was Figure 47-1, p. 360, Cummins & Eisenberg, Blue Book of Medical Diagnosis, W.B. Saunders, Philadelphia, 1986.

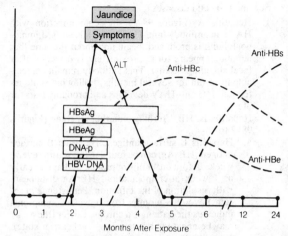

Figure 98–2. The clinical, serologic, and biochemical course of typical acute type B hepatitis. ALT = alanine aminotransferase; HBsAg = hepatitis B surface antigen; HBeAg = hepatitis B e antigen; DNA-p = serum hepatitis B virus DNA polymerase activity; HBV-DNA = serum hepatitis B virus DNA; Anti-HBs = antibody to HBsAg; Anti-HBe = antibody to HBeAg; Anti-HBc = antibody to hepatitis B core antigen. (Reprinted with permission of publisher, from Hoofnagle JH: Perspectives on Viral Hepatitis, Vol. 2, 1st ed. Rahway, New Jersey, Abbott Laboratories, 1981, p. 6.) NOTE: This figure was Figure 47-2, p. 361, Cummins & Eisenberg, Blue Book of Medical Diagnosis, W.B. Saunders, Philadelphia, 1986.

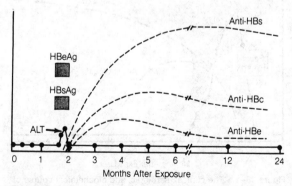

Figure 98–3. The clinical, serologic, and biochemical course of a subclinical asymptomatic hepatitis B virus infection. (Reprinted, with permission of publisher, from Hoofnagle JH: Perspectives on Viral Hepatitis, Vol. 2, 1st ed. Rahway, New Jersey, Abbott Laboratories, 1981, p. 7.) NOTE: This figure was Figure 47-3, p. 362, Cummins & Eisenberg, Blue Book of Medical Diagnosis, W.B. Saunders, Philadelphia, 1986.

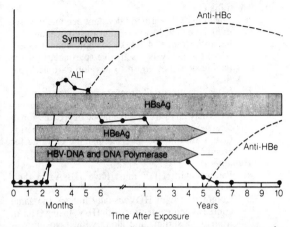

Figure 98–4. The clinical, serologic, and biochemical course of a chronic type B hepatitis infection. (Reprinted, with permission of publisher, from Hoofnagle JH: Perspectives on Viral Hepatitis, Vol. 2, 1st ed. Rahway, New Jersey, Abbott Laboratories, 1981, p. 8.) NOTE: This figure was Figure 47-4, p. 362, Cummins & Eisenberg, Blue Book of Medical Diagnosis, W.B. Saunders, Philadelphia, 1986.

atitis B vaccine; sufficiently high levels are protective against infection.

c. Hepatitis B core antibody
   i. Antibody to the core of HBV (anti-HBc) appears 3 to 4 weeks after HBsAg is found in serum, generally just before clinical illness develops.
   ii. During acute infection, a portion of anti-HBc is IgM; this finding can allow one to differentiate acute from remote infection.
   iii. After HBsAg disappears, and before anti-HBs appears, anti-HBc may be the only marker of HBV infection present (the "core window"). At this point, the anti-HBc should be of the IgM immunoglobulin class (see above).
   iv. Anti-HBc decreases after resolution of symptoms, but chronic carriers of HBV frequently have high levels.

d. Hepatitis B e antigen. The hepatitis B e antigen (HBeAg) is a portion of the core of HBV that can circulate freely. HBeAg is found in acute infection and is indicative of a high degree of infectiousness. Twenty-five to fifty percent of chronic HBsAg carriers continue to be positive for HBeAg for years.

e. Hepatitis B e antibody. If antibody to HBeAg (anti-HBe) develops, it indicates that resolution of infection will probably occur. Anti-HBe generally disappears within 1 to 2 years following acute infection.

3. Hepatitis C
   a. The anti-HCV antibody does not become positive until a mean of 15 weeks after the clinical onset of hepatitis (range: 4 weeks to more than 1 year). Also, the assay is insensitive, particularly if the patient does not go on to develop chronic hepatitis.
   b. Several patterns of transaminase elevation may occur (Figure 98–5). The biphasic and plateau patterns may have greater likelihood of progression to a carrier state, which has been defined for hepatitis C as transaminase levels remaining elevated for greater than 1 year.
4. Hepatitis D
   a. Patients with HDV must have HBsAg in their serum.
   b. Coinfection with HDV usually follows the same course as acute infection with HBV, losing HBsAg from their serum, and along with it, losing evidence for active HDV replication (Figure 98–6).
   c. Superinfection with HDV occurs in a patient who is a chronic carrier of HBsAg; patients tend to also develop chronic HDV infection. Anti-HDV levels tend to be persistently high in chronic HDV carriers (Figure 98–7).
5. Infectious mononucleosis (Epstein-Barr virus) (see Chapter 77)
6. Cytomegalovirus. Specific acute and convalescent antibody titers can confirm the diagnosis. When an individual is acutely infected, it is often possible to culture the virus from urine or occasionally from blood.

RECOMMENDED DIAGNOSTIC APPROACH

- History. Specific questioning should be directed as outlined in Table 98–2.
- Laboratory studies
  1. Initial studies
     a. Obtain AST, ALT, bilirubin, and alkaline phosphatase levels, and a CBC.
        i. If the clinical picture suggests biliary tract disease, amylase levels should be determined and appropriate imaging studies considered.
        ii. The prothrombin time should be measured if AST, ALT, or bilirubin are abnormal.

Figure 98–5. (On opposite page.) Three patterns of change in the concentration of serum glutamic pyruvic transaminase (SGPT) in patients with posttransfusion non-A non-B hepatitis. (Adapted, with permission, from Tateda A, et al.: Non-B hepatitis in Japanese recipients of blood transfusions: Clinical and serologic studies after the introduction of laboratory screening of donor blood for hepatitis B surface antigen. J Infect Dis 1979; 139:511–518.)

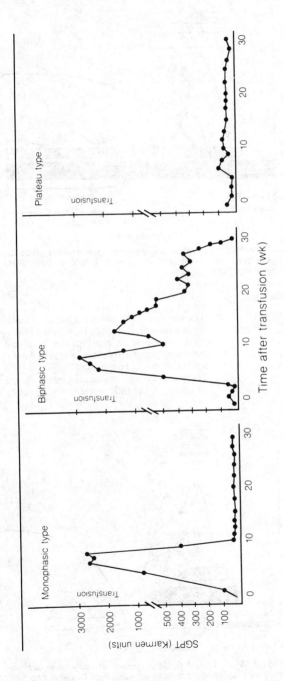

845

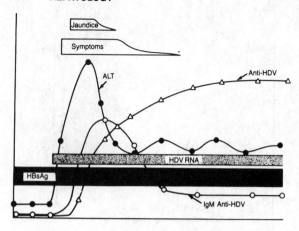

Figure 98–6. Typical serologic course of acute delta coinfection. (Reprinted from Hoofnagle JH. Type D (delta) hepatitis. JAMA 1989; 261:1321–1325.)

  iii. The CBC and differential may suggest infectious mononucleosis, in which case a Monospot test should be ordered; the Monospot may be negative early in the course of illness, and may need to be repeated.

  iv. If the history suggests an uncommon source of infectious hepatitis, acute serum should be

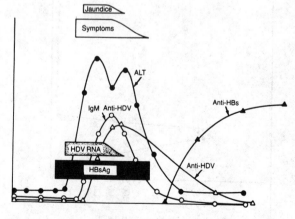

Figure 98–7. Typical serologic course of acute delta superinfection. (Reprinted from Hoofnagle JH. Type D (delta) hepatitis. JAMA 1989; 261:1321–1325.)

TABLE 98–2. Diagnosis of Hepatitis: Factors to Consider When Taking a History

Recent travel history
Ethnic background and birth place (especially Asian, Oceanic, or North African; or close exposure to these individuals)
Sexual orientation and patterns of contact
Known exposure to an infectious agent causing hepatitis (including health care workers with high risk exposure)
Past or current medical conditions
Previous hepatitis, including type (if known); other liver disease
History of or symptoms suggestive of biliary tract disease
Transfusions or administration of blood products
Hemodialysis
History of organ transplantation
History of recent surgery (benign postoperative jaundice?)
History of frequent previous jaundice (Gilbert's syndrome?)
Current pregnancy (third trimester—consider cholestatic jaundice of pregnancy or acute fatty liver of pregnancy)
Drug history
Illicit drug usage (especially parenteral)
Prescription medications (include oral contraceptives)
Over-the-counter medications (include vitamins)
Toxin exposure
Alcohol usage
Occupational exposure
Mushroom ingestion

        obtained and held for possible serologic studies.
    v. If other medical illness is suggested (e.g., Wilson's disease, sarcoidosis, complications following jejunoileal bypass, acute congestion due to heart failure), appropriate evaluation should be initiated.
  2. Hepatitis serologic screening (see Tables 98–3 and 98–4)

TABLE 98–3. Simplified Diagnosis of Acute Hepatitis

ANTI-HAV (IgM)	HBsAg	ANTI-HBc (IgM)	DIAGNOSIS
+	–	–	Acute hepatitis A
–	+	+	Acute hepatitis B
–	–	+	Acute hepatitis B ("core window")
–	+	–	Chronic hepatitis B (consider hepatitis D)
+	+	–	Acute hepatitis A chronic hepatitis B
–	–	–	Other cause

TABLE 98–4. Interpretation of Hepatitis B Serologic Tests

SEROLOGIC TEST			SUGGESTED DIAGNOSES AND FOLLOW-UP
HBsAg	Anti-HBs	Anti-HBc	
+	–	–	Early hepatitis B infection: probably preclinical or early clinical illness. HBeAg/anti-HBe testing possibly indicated. If –/– ("e window") or –/+: resolution likely. If +/–: still highly infectious. HDV testing may be considered if epidemiologically indicated. Needs follow-up testing until anti-HBs is positive (i.e., acute infection has resolved).
+	–	+	Diagnostic of any of the following: 1. Acute HBV infection: has not developed anti-HBs yet. Positive IgM subclass of anti-HBc will confirm acute infection. Consider "e" antigen testing as outlined above. Needs follow-up testing for anti-HBs until positive. 2. Chronic HBV carrier (negative IgM anti-HBc). Consider HAV or HCV as cause of the acute hepatitis. 3. HDV may be present as coinfection or superinfection; consider testing for anti-HDV and IgM of anti-HBc if epidemiologically indicated.
+	+	+	Acute hepatitis B.
+	+		Atypical pattern: usually HBsAg is gone by the time anti-HBs appears. Should resolve because anti-HBs is present, although occasionally this pattern can be seen with a second infection due to HBV of a different surface antigen serologic subtype.

HBsAg	Anti-HBc	Anti-HBs	Interpretation
−	+	+	**Remote hepatitis B infection.** Recovery is indicated by positive anti-HBs. Consider HAV, HCV, other virus, or other cause of acute hepatitis.
−	+	−	**One of the following:** 1. Remote HBV infection: anti-HBs now at undetectable level. A negative IgM anti-HBc assay can confirm that the infection is remote. In addition, HBeAg should be negative. Consider HAV, HCV, or other cause of acute hepatitis. 2. Acute or early resolving HBV infection: the "core window" after HBsAg disappears but before anti-HBs appears. A positive test for IgM anti-HBc suggests this diagnosis. While the patient may still be infectious at a low level (if HBeAg is still positive), resolution should occur because HBsAg has disappeared; follow-up is needed to be sure anti-HBs becomes positive. 3. Low-level carrier state: HBsAg is too low to measure. IgM anti-HBc should be negative. If acute hepatitis is present, consider HAV, HCV, other virus, or other cause.
−	−	+	**Either of the following:** 1. Remote HBV infection: anti-HBc now too low to detect. 2. Past immunization with hepatitis B vaccine: HBsAg is the only immunogenic antigen in the vaccine. If acute infection is present, consider HAV, HCV, other virus, or other cause of hepatitis.
−	−	−	**No evidence of HBV infection.** Consider HAV, HCV, other virus, or other cause of hepatitis.

849

a. If the history strongly suggests hepatitis A testing for anti-HAV alone may be performed. A positive IgM fraction confirms acute infection, while a negative result or positive IgG fraction rules it out.

b. It is usually advisable to obtain a full battery of hepatitis serologic studies. Besides HAV testing, this should initially include HBsAg, anti-HBs, and anti-HBc. If anti-HBc is positive, IgM fractionation can determine if the infection is acute.

c. Hepatitis C infection is likely if serologic testing fails to confirm acute hepatitis A or B. Presence of anti-HCV at the time of acute illness suggests remote rather than acute infection; the acute symptoms could be due to exacerbation of chronic hepatitis associated with HCV.

d. Serologic testing for antibody to hepatitis D (anti-HDV) is indicated only in patients in whom HDV should be epidemiologically suspected.

   i. IgM anti-HDV, which is usually present for a short time after infection, can differentiate acute from chronic hepatitis D.

   ii. Coinfection can be distinguished from superinfection of chronic HBV using the results of anti-HBc testing: coinfection occurs only in the presence of IgM anti-HBc.

e. If hepatitis E is realistically possible, as in a traveler who has returned from an endemic area and who has hepatitis not due to HAV, HBV, or some other cause, sera can be sent to reference labs (e.g., the CDC Hepatitis Branch) for possible confirmation.

3. Follow-up studies

a. If hepatitis screening does not suggest a diagnosis for an apparent acute infection, and if screening tests for mononucleosis are negative, paired sera should be obtained for EBV and CMV.

b. Liver biopsy should be reserved for cases in which significant diagnostic doubt exists, or for patients in whom more radical therapy is being considered, that is, interferon or transplant. Deteriorating condition or continued evidence of liver enzyme elevation may prompt early biopsy.

Bibliography

Alter HC, et al. Detection of antibody to hepatitis C virus in prospectively followed transfusion recipients with acute and chronic non-A, non-B hepatitis. N Engl J Med 1989;321:1494–1500.

Dienstag JL. Non-A, non-B hepatitis. I. Recognition, epidemiology, and clinical features; II. Experimental transmission, putative virus agents and markers, and prevention. Gastroenterology 1983; 85:439–462, 743–768.

Franks AL, et al. Hepatitis B virus infection among children born in the United States to Southeast Asian refugees. N Engl J Med 1989;321:1301–1305.

Gust ID, Purcell RH. Report of a workshop: Waterborne non-A, non-B hepatitis. J Infect Dis 1987;159:630–635.

Hoofnagle JH. Type D (delta) hepatitis. JAMA 1989;261:1321–1325.

Novick DM, et al. Hepatitis D virus and human immunodeficiency virus antibodies in parenteral drug abusers who are hepatitis B surface antigen positive. J Infect Dis 1988;158:795–803.

Stevens CE, et al. Epidemiology of hepatitis C virus: A preliminary study of volunteer blood donors. JAMA 1990;263:49–53.

Zimmerman HJ. Hepatotoxicity: The adverse effects of drugs and other chemicals on the liver. New York, Appleton-Century-Crofts, 1978.

99

CHRONIC HEPATITIS

DOUGLAS S. PAAUW

I can't die until the government finds a safe place to bury my liver.

PHIL HARRIS

DEFINITION

- Chronic hepatitis is defined as any condition that causes hepatic inflammation (manifest by abnormal serum transaminase levels) for at least 6 months. The range of symptom severity is very broad.
- Chronic active hepatitis and chronic persistent hepatitis are pathologic diagnoses.
    1. Chronic active hepatitis (CAH) is present when inflammatory cells are present beyond the confines of the portal area and associated patchy necrosis of hepatocytes occurs.
    2. Chronic persistent hepatitis is defined as the presence of inflammatory cells confined to the portal areas.

DIFFERENTIAL DIAGNOSIS

The most common cause is chronic viral hepatitis.
- Viral hepatitis. Hepatitis B and hepatitis C (non-A, non-B) can both cause chronic hepatitis. Risk factors for acquisition of hepatitis B and C include male homosexual contacts, IV drug use, history of blood transfusions, and country of origin (vertical transmission for hepatitis B is common in Southeast Asia and Africa).
- Alcoholic hepatitis
    1. Chronic transaminase elevations can occur with alcohol use, although not all patients who develop alcoholic liver disease have appreciable elevations of transaminases.
    2. A 2- to 10-fold elevation of transaminase levels are the rule with alcoholic hepatitis, usually with AST (SGOT) higher than ALT (SGPT).
- Drug-induced hepatitis. The most common drugs to cause CAH are alpha-methyldopa and nitrofurantoin. Other drugs reported include isoniazid, sulfonamides, dantrolene, propylthiouracil, acetaminophen, papaverine, oxyphenasitin, clometacin, and NSAIDs.
- Autoimmune chronic liver disease (lupoid hepatitis)

1. Autoimmune hepatitis is far more common in women than men (4:1) and commonly occurs perimenopausally. In as many as 30% of patients, another autoimmune disorder is present.
2. Serologic manifestations include autoantibodies to hepatocyte surface antigens. The disease is not due to SLE.

- Hemochromatosis
    1. Hemochromatosis is a disease of iron overload. It causes a chronic hepatitis which frequently progresses to cirrhosis.
    2. Primary or idiopathic hemochromatosis is an autosomal recessive disorder associated with increased iron absorption by the gut and iron deposition in different body organs. Iron overload in hemochromatosis may be more severe in chronic alcohol users due to a further increase in iron absorption due to alcohol. There is a high incidence of hepatomas in patients with cirrhosis due to hemochromatosis.
    3. Deposition of iron in the pancreas leads to diabetes, and deposition in the skin can cause a gray to bronze coloration. Gonadal failure due to pituitary iron deposition may cause impotence, and arthritis occurs due to calcium pyrophosphate deposition disease.

- Wilson's disease
    1. Wilson's disease (hepatolenticular degeneration) is an autosomal recessive metabolic disorder characterized by excessive accumulation of copper in the liver, cornea, brain, and kidney.
    2. Hepatic synthesis of ceruloplasmin is impaired and biliary excretion of copper is markedly reduced. Liver disease may occur before neuropsychiatric symptoms.

- α_1-Antitrypsin deficiency. This disease with autosomal recessive transmission is associated with liver disease, renal cysts, and emphysema. Heterozygotes frequently only manifest liver disease.

CLINICAL FEATURES

History

Many of the symptoms of chronic hepatitis are generalized (fatigue, anorexia, malaise). Patients with chronic persistent hepatitis are either asymptomatic or have only minor symptoms of fatigue or malaise. The history should determine the following:

- Medication use
- Transfusion history/Parenteral blood exposure. Multiple blood transfusions (usually for chronic hemolytic anemia) may cause secondary hemochromatosis.
- Sexual exposure. Homosexual contacts increase the risk of hepatitis B and C.
- Family history
- Presence of autoimmune disorders. Up to a third of pa-

tients with autoimmune hepatitis have other disorders with a presumed immunologic basis (thyroiditis, Sjögren's syndrome, SLE, RA, Coombs'-positive hemolytic anemia, and glomerulonephritis).

Signs/Examination

- Skin
  1. Spider angiomas and palmar erythema suggest advanced liver disease.
  2. The presence of multiple ecchymoses may indicate advanced liver disease with coexistent coagulopathy.
  3. A bronze or gray skin color can occur with hemochromatosis.
  4. Blue lunulae of the nails is an insensitive but specific finding of Wilson's disease.
- Eyes
  1. Scleral icterus is seen when serum bilirubin values are greater than 3 mg/dl.
  2. Kayser-Fleischer rings are seen in Wilson's disease. They are due to copper deposition in Descemet's membrane of the cornea. Early in the course of Wilson's disease, the rings can only be seen by slit lamp exam.
- Abdomen. Multiple firm nodules suggests metastatic tumor. Hemochromatosis is frequently associated with hepatomegaly (75 to 95% of patients) and is also associated with development of hepatoma. Patients with advanced disease (cirrhosis) may have a small liver or splenomegaly.
- Neurologic exam
  1. Hepatic encephalopathy may cause asterixis ("liver flap").
  2. Tremor, dysarthria, rigidity, and gait disturbances occur with Wilson's disease. In advanced cases of Wilson's disease, dementia may be a prominent feature.
- Joint exam. Premature osteoarthritis is seen in 25% of patients with Wilson's disease. Joint disease due to calcium pyrophosphate deposition disease (usually in the second and third metacarpophalangeal joints) is associated with hemochromatosis.

LABORATORY STUDIES

- Biochemical tests
  1. Serum transaminases
     a. Aspartate aminotransferase (AST)—also known as serum glutamic oxaloacetic transferase (SGOT)—and alanine aminotransferase (ALT)—also known as serum glutamic pyruvic transaminase (SGPT)—are the two transaminases routinely measured for evaluation of hepatocellular injury.
     b. ALT is more specific for liver, as AST is also found in muscle, kidney, and brain.

   c. Seventy percent of patients with alcoholic liver disease have an AST/ALT ratio of greater than 2.

   d. The degree of elevation of transminases does not correlate well with the extent or activity of chronic liver disease.

2. Serum albumin and prothrombin time. These parameters reflect hepatic synthetic function. A low albumin level and increased prothrombin time indicate significant hepatic damage.

3. Ceruloplasmin. Ninety-five percent of all patients with Wilson's disease have a serum ceruloplasmin level less than 20 mg/dl.

4. Iron studies

   a. In hemochromatosis the serum iron level is elevated while the total iron binding capacity is decreased or normal. The percent saturation is >60%.

   b. Serum ferritin levels are also elevated, with each 100 mg/dl of ferritin being equivalent to roughly 1 g of stored iron. Patients with hemochromatosis usually develop symptoms when their total body iron is 20 g or greater (200 mg/dl of ferritin).

- Serology and immunology

  1. Hepatitis B surface antigen. The presence of hepatitis B surface antigen suggests chronic hepatitis B infection.

  2. Hepatitis C antibody. This test measures antibody to hepatitis C which is the predominant cause of transfusion associated non-A, non-B hepatitis.

  3. Serum protein electrophoresis. Serum gamma globulin levels are elevated in 97% of patients with autoimmune hepatitis. Other types of chronic hepatitis are also associated with hypergammaglobulinemia, but the degree is less.

  4. Autoantibodies

   a. Antibodies to smooth muscle are present in 70% of patients with autoimmune hepatitis.

   b. High titer (>1 : 80) IgG antinuclear antibodies are present in 80%.

   c. Antimitochondrial antibodies are seen in 30% of patients with autoimmune hepatitis.

- Liver biopsy is the definitive tool for diagnosis of chronic hepatitis. Quantification of hepatic iron or copper are essential for the diagnosis of hemochromatosis or Wilson's disease.

RECOMMENDED DIAGNOSTIC APPROACH

- Specific risk factors or findings on the physical exam should guide the initial diagnostic approach. Hepatitis B and C serologies should be obtained before other lower yield and more expensive tests are done.

- If hepatitis serologies are negative, then pursue rarer diseases (hemochromatosis, Wilson's disease, autoimmune hepatitis) by measuring serum iron, transferrin, and ferritin levels, serum protein electrophoresis, and antinuclear antibody. If the patient is under the age of 40, check the serum ceruloplasmin level.

- If the serum ceruloplasmin level is <20 mg/dl, then a slit lamp exam should be done to detect Kayser-Fleischer rings. If the ceruloplasmin level is normal but the diagnosis is suggested on clinical grounds (neuropsychiatric abnormalities, Coombs'-negative hemolytic anemia), then perform a 24-hr urine copper measurement and slit lamp exam.
- Liver biopsy should be performed when tests do not reveal a clear diagnosis. If Wilson's disease or hemochromatosis are suggested by laboratory tests, confirmation with liver biopsy is recommended.

Bibliography

Alter HJ, et al. Detection of antibody to hepatitis C virus in prospectively followed transfusion recipients with acute and chronic non-A, non-B hepatitis. N Engl J Med 1989;321:1494–1500.

Bolt RJ. Hepatolenticular degeneration (Wilson's disease). Med Rounds 1989;2:16–21.

Bruckstein AH. Chronic hepatitis: The challenge of diagnosis and treatment. Post Grad Med 1989;85(7):67–74.

Czaja DM, et al. Clinical features and prognostic implications of severe corticosteroid-treated cryptogenic chronic active hepatitis. Mayo Clin Proc 1990;65:23–30.

Fairbanks VF, Baldus WP. Hemochromatosis: The neglected diagnosis. Mayo Clin Proc 1986;61:296–298.

Payne JA. Chronic hepatitis: Pathogenesis and treatment. Dis Mon 1988;34(3):109–159.

Stevens CE, et al. Epidemiology of hepatitis C virus. JAMA 1990;263:49–53.

Stremmel W. et al. Wilson disease: Clinical presentation, treatment, and survival. Ann Intern Med 1991;115:720–726.

100

GALLBLADDER DISEASES

ANDREW K. DIEHL

Let there be gall enough in thy ink.

SHAKESPEARE (1564–1616)
Twelfth Night III, ii, 54

DEFINITIONS

- Most gallbladder diseases are related to gallstones. "Silent" gallstones may be discovered during the work-up of GI symptoms due to other conditions. Twenty to forty percent of persons with asymptomatic cholelithiasis eventually develop biliary symptoms.
- Biliary "colic" is an attack of upper abdominal pain caused by the impaction of a gallstone in the gallbladder infundibulum or in the cystic or common ducts.
- Acute cholecystitis is characterized by prolonged biliary pain, vomiting, and fever and is associated with severe inflammation of the gallbladder wall. Ninety-five percent of attacks of cholecystitis are related to cholelithiasis.
- Eighty percent of patients with gallbladder cancer have co-existing gallstones.

EPIDEMIOLOGY

- Prevalence
  1. Ten to fifteen percent of white women in their 40s and more than 20% over age 50 have gallstones.
  2. For adult men, the corresponding numbers are 5 to 10% and over 10%.
- Risk factors for cholesterol gallstones
  1. These include female gender, increasing age, obesity, increasing parity, family history, and diabetes mellitus. Exogenous estrogen (inconsistently associated), and low serum levels of high-density lipoprotein cholesterol, and hypertriglyceridemia have been associated with cholelithiasis.
  2. Ethanol use may reduce the risk of cholesterol gallstone formation.
- Risk factors for pigment gallstones include chronic hemolysis, alcoholic cirrhosis, biliary infection, and age.

- Ethnic differences
  1. At highest risk are native Americans (Eskimos and American Indians). Pima Indian women have a gallstone prevalence of 70% by age 30.
  2. Mexican-American women have a prevalence twice that of non-Hispanic whites. In contrast, blacks have a reduced rate of gallstone disease.
- Gallbladder cancer. Persons with calcified gallbladder walls or with gallstones that are 3 cm or greater in diameter have an elevated risk for cancer.

DIFFERENTIAL DIAGNOSIS

- Gallbladder disease
  1. Cholelithiasis usually presents with right upper abdominal or epigastric pain. Gallstones may be demonstrated by ultrasonography or by oral cholecystography (OCG).
  2. Acute cholecystitis can be distinguished from other causes of abdominal pain with ultrasonography or cholescintigraphy (nuclear imaging with Technetium-99m–iminodiacetic acid derivatives). Failure of the gallbladder to visualize on cholescintigraphy is indicative of cystic duct obstruction.
  3. Cancer of the gallbladder has a nonspecific clinical presentation. Radiologic tests cannot reliably detect gallbladder cancer, and the diagnosis is usually made at surgery.
- The differential diagnosis of upper abdominal pain includes pancreatitis, hepatitis, rib fractures, pleurisy, and peptic ulcer disease. Unusual causes of right upper quadrant pain include hepatic abscess, Fitz-Hugh-Curtis syndrome, renal stones, and acute appendicitis.

CLINICAL FEATURES

- "Silent" gallstones are by definition asymptomatic. They may be found incidentally at laparotomy or during the work-up of GI symptoms related to other conditions.
- Nonspecific symptoms. Symptoms such as indigestion, heartburn, bloating, and fatty food intolerance are found no more frequently in persons with gallstones than in persons with normal gallbladders.
- Biliary colic
  1. Biliary "colic" is usually a severe constant pain. In 30%, the pain is maximal at onset, while in 32%, maximum intensity is reached within an hour and in the remainder after several hours.
  2. Approximately half of attacks last 15 min to 2 hr, with the other half lasting longer.
  3. Pain involves the epigastrium (65% of cases) and the right hypochondrium (50%). It radiates to the right scapula in 15 to 30% of cases. Lower abdominal pain is uncommon.

- Acute cholecystitis
    1. When cystic duct obstruction is prolonged, biliary colic can progress to acute cholecystitis.
    2. In addition to the symptoms listed above, patients with acute cholecystitis may have vomiting (80%) or jaundice (25%).
    3. Physical examination reveals fever and right upper quadrant tenderness. Murphy's sign (tenderness halting inspiration during palpation over the gallbladder) is present in 27%. A distended gallbladder is palpable in one-third of cases.
- Obstruction caused by stones
    1. In 15% of patients, stones pass from the gallbladder to the common duct where they can cause obstruction of bile flow resulting in marked elevations of serum bilirubin and alkaline phosphatase levels.
    2. If stones pass through the common duct, the serum amylase may become elevated with or without associated pancreatitis. Half of patients with choledocholithiasis develop ascending cholangitis or pancreatitis.
- Gallbladder cancer. The clinical presentation of gallbladder cancer is nonspecific. Common features are abdominal pain (76%), jaundice (38%), nausea and vomiting (32%), and weight loss (39%). Sixteen percent have presentations that mimic acute cholecystitis.

LABORATORY STUDIES

- Blood tests
    1. In asymptomatic cholelithiasis, serum chemistries, including tests of liver function, are normal.
    2. Acute cholecystitis
        a. Serum transaminases may be normal or may rise to 2 to 4 times normal. The alkaline phosphatase may double or triple and the bilirubin may reach 4 mg/dl. High levels of bilirubin or alkaline phosphatase suggest obstruction of the common bile duct.
        b. The leukocyte count is usually mildly elevated in acute cholecystitis (up to 15,000/mm^3) with a shift to the left.
    3. Patients with biliary colic without acute cholecystitis have normal WBC counts.
- Plain abdominal (KUB) radiographs. About three-quarters of gallstones are composed of cholesterol and are radiolucent. Since not all pigment stones can be identified on plain radiographs, the sensitivity of the KUB is only about 15%.
- US
    1. Real-time US has supplanted OCG as the initial diagnostic test for gallstones. US does not depend on liver or gallbladder function. Stones 3 mm in diameter can be visualized.
    2. With real-time US, sensitivity is 90 to 95% and specificity is 94 to 98%.

- OCG
  1. This test is useful in patients who are not jaundiced. Its sensitivity for gallstones is 92 to 95% and its specificity is 95 to 100%.
  2. The OCG has limitations
     a. Approximately one-fourth of studies show nonvisualization of the gallbladder after a single dose of contrast material and require a second administration.
     b. Nonvisualization may be caused by prolonged fasting, malabsorption, vomiting, diarrhea, liver disease, or failure to take contrast material. If these can be excluded, then a nonvisualized gallbladder after 2 doses indicates a 90% probability of cholelithiasis.
  3. The OCG may occasionally detect stones missed by US. The OCG is indicated where information regarding gallbladder function and gallstone composition, size, and number is required.
- CT offers no advantages over OCG or US for the diagnosis of gallstones.
- Cholangiography
  1. Although US can be used to diagnose dilated biliary ducts, both it and CT have poor sensitivities for the diagnosis of common duct stones.
  2. Transhepatic or endoscopic retrograde cholangiography provides direct opacification of the biliary tree and facilitates the diagnosis of choledocholithiasis.
- Tests for acute cholecystitis
  1. Neither OCG nor US is reliable in distinguishing acute cholecystitis from other causes of severe upper abdominal pain.
     a. In acute cholecystitis, the OCG does not visualize.
     b. US may reveal gallstones and gallbladder wall abnormalities, but obstruction of the cystic duct cannot be confirmed.
     c. Focal tenderness over the gallbladder elicited by the radiologist's examining transducer ("sonographic Murphy's sign") suggests acute cholecystitis with a positive predictive value of 90%.
  2. Cholescintigraphy employing iminodiacetic acid derivatives such as DISIDA have a sensitivity of 95 to 97% and a specificity of 90 to 97% for acute cholecystitis. It is more expensive than US.

RECOMMENDED DIAGNOSTIC APPROACH

- Nonspecific complaints. Symptoms such as indigestion, belching, bloating, and fatty food intolerance are not associated with gallbladder disease and should not prompt diagnostic testing.
- Biliary colic. Patients with biliary colic should be followed up with real-time US. If gallstones are not demonstrated on

US but clinical suspicion remains high, an OCG is indicated.

- Acute cholecystitis
  1. If acute cholecystitis is suspected in a patient not known to have gallstones, US or Technetium-99m–cholescintigraphy should be performed. US may be preferred because of its capacity to evaluate other abdominal organs, its lesser expense, and because it can usually be performed more rapidly.
  2. If cholelithiasis has been demonstrated previously in a patient with the clinical picture of acute cholecystitis, cholescintigraphy may be unnecessary unless pancreatitis is also a strong consideration.
  3. A WBC count and differential count, serum amylase, bilirubin, and alkaline phosphatase are indicated.
- Choledocholithiasis. If choledocholithiasis is suspected despite a normal US, the patient should undergo transhepatic cholangiography or endoscopic retrograde cholangiography.

Bibliography

Carroll BA. Preferred imaging techniques for the diagnosis of cholecystitis and cholelithiasis. Ann Surg 1989;210:1–12.

Diehl AK, et al. Clinical evaluation for gallstone disease: Usefulness of symptoms and signs in diagnosis. Am J Med 1990;89:29–33.

Gelfand DW, et al. Oral cholecystography vs. gallbladder sonography: A prospective, blinded reappraisal. Am J Roentgen 1988;151:69–72.

Gunn A, Keddie N. Some clinical observations on patients with gallstones. Lancet 1972;2:239–241.

Marton KI, Doubilet P. How to image the gallbladder in suspected cholecystitis. Ann Int Med 1988;109:722–729.

Piehler JM, Crichlow RW. Primary carcinoma of the gallbladder. Surg Gynecol Obstet 1978;147:929–942.

SECTION XIV

OCCUPATIONAL MEDICINE

101

CLINICAL APPROACH TO OCCUPATIONAL MEDICINE

CARRIE A. REDLICH

"When you come to a patient's house, you should ask him what sort of pains he has, what caused them, how many days he has been ill, whether the bowels are working and what sort of food he eats." So says Hippocrates in his work *Affections*. I may venture to add one more question: what occupation does he follow?

BERNARDINO RAMAZZINI (1633–1714)

DEFINITION

- Occupational illnesses (Table 101–1) are those caused or aggravated by work exposures (Table 101–2).
- Although there are few data on the prevalence and incidence of occupational diseases, occupational and environmental exposures are important determinants of health.

GENERAL PRINCIPLES OF OCCUPATIONAL MEDICINE

- Most occupational illnesses are difficult to distinguish from those of nonoccupational etiologies. For example, asbestos-induced and non-asbestos-induced lung cancer are clinically and pathologically indistinguishable.
- Interactions between occupational and nonoccupational factors are common. For example, both cigarette smoking and asbestos exposure increase a patient's risk for lung cancer.
- Occupational diseases occur after the occupational exposure. However, the temporal pattern between exposure and disease can be variable.
- The dose of an exposure (both amount and length of exposure) is usually important in determining its toxicity. Individual differences in susceptibility to exposures help determine disease severity. Idiosyncratic or allergic responses are less dependent on dose.
- A given substance in the workplace may produce more than one clinical or pathologic entity. For example, cobalt exposure can result in both obstructive airways disease and interstitial fibrosis.

TABLE 101–1. Major Occupational Disorders

DISORDER	SELECTED CAUSATIVE AGENTS
Skin diseases	
Contact dermatitis	Metals, solvents
Cancer	UV radiation, arsenic
Lung diseases (see Table 101–3)	
Musculoskeletal disorders	
Cumulative-trauma disorders	Repetitive trauma
Low back pain	Lifting, twisting
Hand-arm vibration syndrome	Hand-held vibrating tools
Neurologic disorders	
Central nervous system	
Acute encephalopathy	Heavy metals, solvents, pesticides
Chronic encephalopathy	Heavy metals, solvents
Peripheral nervous system	
Toxic polyneuropathy	Heavy metals, solvents, pesticides
Neuromuscular junction blockade	Insecticides
Liver disorders	
Acute hepatic necrosis	Solvents
Angiosarcoma	Vinyl chloride
Urinary tract disease	
Acute tubular necrosis	Heavy metals, solvents
Chronic renal dysfunction	Heavy metals
Bladder cancer	Dyes
Hematologic disorders	
Anemia	Lead, arsenic, benzene
Leukemia	Benzene
Occupational hearing loss	Noise
Reproductive disorders	
Infertility-Spermatotoxicity	Heat, lead
Adverse reproductive outcomes	Lead

- It is often difficult to determine what potentially toxic substances the patient has been exposed to at the workplace, in part because exposures may be multiple and change frequently.
- Government standards for permissible levels of exposure to a given substance are important regulations but do not indicate absolute safety levels below which disease cannot occur.
- The importance of diagnosing an occupational etiology
  1. Further exposure to the etiologic agent in the workplace may cause more severe, recurrent, or irreversible disease.
  2. Making the diagnosis of an occupational etiology may allow identification of other patients similarly affected.

TABLE 101–2. Major Types of Hazardous Workplace Exposures

SELECTED EXPOSURES	TYPICAL EXPOSURE SETTING(S)
Metals	
Aluminum	Welding
Beryllium	Metal alloy processing
Cadmium	Electroplating
Cobalt	Tungsten carbide production
Lead	Battery production
Mineral dusts	
Asbestos	Construction, brake linings
Coal	Mining
Crystalline silica	Mining, foundries
Chemicals	
Organic solvents	
Petroleum derivatives	Fuels
Glycol ethers	Paints
Perchloroethylene	Dry cleaning
Trichloroethylene	Degreasers
Plastics/Synthetics	
Epoxy and acrylic resins	Paints, coatings
Vinyl chloride	Manufacture of vinyls
Isocyanates	Synthesis of polyurethane
Acids and alkalies	Chemical intermediates
Aromatic amines	Aniline dyes
Gases	
Ammonia	Fertilizer production
Chlorine	Plastics production
Carbon monoxide	Fires
Pesticides	
Organophosphates	Agriculture
Organochlorine insecticides	Agriculture
Physical agents	
Noise	Any noisy workplace
Heat	Foundry, smelting
Ionizing radiation	Nuclear industry, health care workers
Nonionizing radiation	
UV radiation	Outdoor work, arc welding
Repetitive trauma	Assembly line workers, dancers, poultry workers
Biologic agents	
Infectious agents	
Hepatitis B virus	Health care workers
HIV	Health care workers
Vegetable material	
Grain dust	Grain handlers
Cotton dust	Cotton mill workers
Animal material	
Dander, excreta	Animal handlers

3. Prevention of further cases may be possible with modification of exposures.
4. New associations between exposures and disease may be identified.
5. The patient with a work-related illness is entitled to worker's compensation.

RECOMMENDED DIAGNOSTIC APPROACH TO THE PATIENT WITH AN OCCUPATIONAL DISORDER

- Occupational history
  1. The most important diagnostic tool is the occupational history
     a. General health history/present illness
        i. Does the patient think that his problem or symptoms are related to his work?
        ii. Are the patient's symptoms temporally related to certain exposures at work?
        iii. Do they improve on vacations or weekends?
        iv. Do other workers have similar problems or symptoms?
     b. Work and exposure history: the following information should be obtained about the patient's current or most recent job and prior jobs:
        i. Job title.
        ii. Type of industry.
        iii. Description of the workplace: job performed, ventilation, protective equipment (respirator, special clothing, gloves, safety glasses).
        iv. Days missed from work and the reason.
        v. Exposure to potential hazards at work.
        vi. Other exposures: hobbies, home, neighborhood industries, cigarettes.
  2. Other important sources of occupational health and exposure data include:
     a. Material Safety Data Sheets (MSDS). Employers are required to keep these data sheets on all potentially hazardous materials used and make them available to employees and their physicians.
     b. Industrial hygiene evaluation of the workplace.
     c. Employee and union records, if available.
- Criteria for determining the work-relatedness of disease are:
  1. The clinical presentation and laboratory evaluation are consistent with the diagnosis.
  2. A causal relationship between the exposure and the diagnosed condition has been previously established or strongly suggested in the medical or toxicologic literature.
  3. There is sufficient exposure to cause the disease. Such exposure can be assessed by:
     a. Industrial hygiene measurements of workplace exposures by the company or the Occupational Safety and Health Administration (OSHA).

   b. Biologic markers of exposure for those substances which can be measured (i.e., lead).
   c. Epidemiologic data documenting disease in previous workers with similar exposures, or comorbidity in fellow workers.
   d. Description of the work process.
4. The temporal relationship between exposure and disease is consistent with known information.
5. There is no other more likely diagnosis.

MAJOR OCCUPATIONAL DISORDERS

Occupational Skin Disorders (see Table 101–1)

- Definition. Occupational skin diseases include conditions that result from skin exposure to various agents in the workplace including chemicals, metals, UV radiation, heat, and trauma.
- Epidemiology. Occupational skin diseases are the most commonly reported work-related diseases in the United States. Contact dermatitis is the most common. Others include pigmentation disorders, skin cancer, actinic changes, and acne.
- Contact dermatitis
  1. Definition. Contact dermatitis can occur following exposure to substances by either an irritant (solvents, oils, acids) or allergic (chromium, nickel, epoxy resins) mechanism. Contact irritant dermatitis is much more common than contact allergic dermatitis.
  2. Clinical features
     a. Skin erythema, scaling, vesicles, and pruritus are common in exposed areas.
     b. The clinical presentations of allergic and irritant contact dermatitis can be indistinguishable, but allergic contact dermatitis may occur at lower levels of exposure and may be more generalized.
     c. A positive skin patch test can be helpful in differentiating allergic from irritant contact dermatitis and in identifying a specific agent.
  3. Differential diagnosis includes atopic dermatitis, eczematous lesions, and psoriasis. Contact dermatitis generally improves with avoidance of further exposure.

Occupational Lung Disorders (Table 101–3)

- Definition. Occupational lung diseases are the second most common occupational disorders.
- Asbestos-related diseases
  1. Definition. Asbestos is a general term for a group of naturally occurring mineral fibrous silicates which have been widely used in construction and other industries.
  2. Pathogenesis. The pathogenesis of the different

TABLE 101–3. Classification of Occupational Lung Disorders

DISORDER	SELECTED CAUSATIVE AGENTS
Airway disorders	
Occupational asthma	(see Table 101–4)
Industrial bronchitis	Mineral dusts, fumes
Acute airway injury (toxic pneumonitis)	High exposure to irritant gases
Pneumoconioses	
Asbestosis	Asbestos
Silicosis	Crystalline silica
Coal workers' pneumoconiosis	Coal mine dust
Hard metal disease	Cobalt
Hypersensitivity disorders	
Hypersensitivity pneumonitis	Molds, fungi
Metal fume fever	Zinc, copper oxides
Chronic beryllium disease	Beryllium
Pleural diseases	
Pleural effusions	Asbestos
Pleural thickening	Asbestos
Malignancy	
Bronchogenic carcinoma of lung	Asbestos, arsenic
Malignant mesothelioma	Asbestos
Upper respiratory tract cancer	Arsenic, nickel

asbestos-induced pulmonary disorders is not fully understood, but the shape and durability of the asbestos fibers are probably important factors.

3. Epidemiology

    a. A large number of workers were heavily exposed to asbestos from the 1940s to the 1970s, especially in insulation work, the construction trades, and shipbuilding.

    b. The risk of developing asbestos-related disease increases with the intensity and duration of exposure. There is a mean latency period of about 15 to 30 yr between exposure to asbestos and the development of the various sequelae.

4. Asbestos-induced pleural disorders

    a. Definition. Benign asbestos-induced pleural abnormalities are the most common sequelae of asbestos exposure and include pleural thickening (diffuse or isolated plaques) and, less commonly, exudative pleural effusions.

    b. Clinical features

       i. Asbestos-induced pleural thickening is usually bilateral and can calcify. It has a mean latency of 15 yr after asbestos exposure.

       ii. Asbestos pleural thickening generally has little effect on pulmonary function and is usually an asymptomatic finding on a chest X-ray. Mild restrictive changes can occur.

      iii. Benign asbestos-related effusions are exudative, unilateral or bilateral effusions which usually occur within 10 to 20 yr after asbestos exposure.

    c. Diagnosis. Asbestos-induced pleural thickening can be diagnosed on the basis of an appropriate exposure history and the characteristic pleural plaques, diffuse pleural thickening, or diaphragmatic plaques on chest X-rays. High resolution CT scans may be more sensitive.

5. Asbestosis

    a. Definition. Asbestosis refers to parenchymal lung fibrosis caused by asbestos exposure.

    b. Epidemiology. Asbestosis is less frequent than asbestos-induced pleural disease. The mean latency is about 20 yr. The risk of asbestosis increases with increased dose of exposure. The disease can progress after exposure has stopped.

    c. Clinical and laboratory features

      i. Progressive dyspnea and cough are the most common symptoms of asbestosis. Bibasilar rales and clubbing may be present on physical exam, but are nonspecific.

      ii. Chest X-ray shows bilaterally increased interstitial markings, more prominent at the bases. Pleural thickening is frequently present. High resolution CT scans may be more sensitive in detecting interstitial fibrosis.

      iii. Pulmonary function tests (PFTs) typically show a restrictive disorder with reduced lung volumes and a reduced diffusing capacity. Mild airflow obstruction may occur unrelated to smoking.

    d. Diagnostic criteria. The diagnosis of asbestosis can usually be made based on the following criteria:

      i. Radiographic evidence of diffuse interstitial lung disease or a restrictive defect on PFTs.

      ii. An occupational history of significant asbestos exposure at least 10 yr previously. The finding of pleural plaques helps confirm the asbestos exposure history but is not necessary for the diagnosis.

      iii. The absence of any coexisting disease known to be associated with diffuse pulmonary fibrosis.

6. Malignant mesothelioma

    a. Definition. Malignant mesothelioma is a primary tumor arising from the pleural or peritoneal mesothelium. The tumor does not arise from benign plaques.

    b. Epidemiology. More than 90% of malignant mesotheliomas occur in those with past asbestos exposure. The mean latency period is about 30 yr following initial exposure.

    c. Clinical features. Most patients present with chest

pain. Dyspnea, cough, and weight loss are also common. There is frequently a pleural effusion at the time of presentation.

   d. Diagnosis
      i. Chest X-ray frequently shows evidence of a unilateral pleural effusion or mass, most often with associated distortion of the intrathoracic anatomy towards the side of the effusion.
      ii. Open pleural biopsy is usually required to make a tissue diagnosis. Cytologic examination of the pleural fluid frequently is not definitive.

7. Lung cancer
   a. Definition. Asbestos exposure is associated with an increased risk of bronchogenic carcinoma that is indistinguishable from lung cancer associated with other risk factors such as smoking and includes all histologic types.
   b. Epidemiology. Asbestos exposure increases the risk of lung cancer up to 5-fold in nonsmokers and about 50-fold in smokers. There is a mean latency of 25 yr following initial asbestos exposure.
   c. Clinical features/diagnosis. The clinical presentation and diagnosis of asbestos-associated bronchogenic carcinoma are the same as for any bronchogenic cancer.

• Silicosis
   1. Definition. Silicosis is a parenchymal lung disorder due to exposure to crystalline silica. It can appear in a chronic "simple" form or a rarer form called progressive massive fibrosis (PMF).
   2. Epidemiology. Silicosis is the oldest recognized pneumoconiosis and occurs throughout the United States. Free crystalline silica exposure occurs in many industries including mining, foundry work, sandblasting, and ceramic and abrasive work.
   3. Clinical manifestations
      a. Simple silicosis is frequently asymptomatic and recognized on the basis of an abnormal routine chest X-ray. Progressive cough, dyspnea, and mild restriction on PFTs may occur. Patients are at increased risk of infections, especially tuberculosis.
      b. Complicated silicosis is a rare, progressive, and frequently fatal disorder with progressive pulmonary fibrosis, loss of lung function, and dyspnea.
   4. Laboratory evaluation
      a. Chest X-ray shows bilateral diffuse small rounded opacities especially in the upper lung zones.
      b. The hilar lymph nodes may develop peripheral ("eggshell") calcifications.
      c. In complicated silicosis, conglomerate upper zone and perihilar masses form. Cavitary lesions can also occur.
   5. Diagnosis. The diagnosis of silicosis is usually made on the basis of the chracteristic chest X-ray findings and an appropriate exposure history.

- Occupational asthma (Table 101–4)
  1. Definition. Occupational asthma is defined as reversible airway obstruction which occurs following exposure(s) at the workplace. These exposures include nonspecific irritants such as dusts and specific allergens such as isocyanates.
  2. Epidemiology. Two to fifteen percent of new cases of asthma in adults may be due to work exposures.
  3. Clinical manifestations
     a. Patients usually present with typical asthmatic symptoms such as cough, dyspnea, chest tightness, and wheezing.
     b. The symptoms are temporally related to exposure to the substance(s) in the workplace with improvement of symptoms on weekends and vacations. However, the exact temporal relationship depends on the type of exposure.
     c. Symptoms generally worsen with continued reexposure, and improve with removal from the workplace. Symptoms may persist after removal from the causative agent and chronic asthma triggered by nonspecific agents can occur.
  4. Diagnosis. Occupational asthma is diagnosed by confirming the presence of airflow limitation or airway hyperresponsiveness and establishing a relationship between the asthma and work exposures.
     a. The relationship between the asthma and work exposures can be established in several ways. A

TABLE 101–4. Selected Causes of Occupational Asthma

AGENT	TYPICAL EXPOSURE SETTING
Metals	Metal industries, welding
Chromium	
Nickel	
Cobalt	
Platinum	
Chemicals	
Anhydrides	Epoxy resins, plastics
Isocyanates	Plastics, polyurethane
Plant material	
Wood dust	Carpentry
Grain dust	Grain handlers
Cotton	Cotton mill workers
Wheat flour	Bakers
Animal material	
Laboratory animals	Laboratory workers
Birds, chickens	Poultry processing
Shellfish	Fish processing
Biologic enzymes	Detergent industry
Drugs	Pharmaceutical industry
Penicillins	
Cephalosporins	

history documenting the temporal pattern of symptoms is usually key.

b. A decrement of more than 15% in the FEV_1 or peak flow following work exposure is usually diagnostic, but is frequently not seen.

c. Patients may have normal spirometry at the time of evaluation, in which case a methacholine challenge test should be done to evaluate for nonspecific bronchial hyperresponsiveness.

d. Bronchial provocation testing using the specific suspected substance(s) can more definitively identify the specific causative agent, but is not routinely done.

e. Although helpful, it is not necessary to identify the specific causative substance in the workplace to make the diagnosis of occupational asthma.

f. Skin testing and serum immunologic tests may be helpful, primarily in individuals exposed to large molecule protein antigens such as grains or animal danders. A negative finding does not rule out occupational asthma.

- Industrial bronchitis. Exposure to dusts, fumes, irritant gases, and organic solvents can cause respiratory tract irritation, primarily of the upper respiratory tract. Symptoms include sore throat, cough, eye irritation, and rhinitis and generally improve with removal from exposure. The diagnosis is made on the basis of the occupational history and the exclusion of other etiologies.

Solvent-Related Disorders

- Definition. Organic solvents comprise a large group of chemicals which are used extensively throughout industry. They are associated with disorders of the skin, central and peripheral nervous system, liver, kidney, and lungs.

- Epidemiology

  1. Organic solvents are probably the most common potentially toxic substances encountered in American workplaces.

  2. Solvents are used in painting, degreasing, printing, and cleaning operations and are used as chemical reactants in numerous manufacturing processes including plastics, resins, textiles, pharmaceuticals, and rubbers.

- Neurotoxicity

  1. Excess exposure to most organic solvents can cause an acute toxic encephalopathy. Symptoms include headache, lightheadedness, irritability, disequilibrium, incoordination, weakness, and confusion. CNS depression and death can result from severe intoxication.

  2. Symptoms generally resolve with removal from exposure, although recurrent episodes of heavy intoxication may result in persistent neuropsychologic dysfunction including fatigue, memory loss, and motor or sensory deficits.

  3. Solvent exposure can also cause a peripheral neuropa-

thy, which is usually a symmetric mixed sensory and motor process. The toxic neuropathy frequently improves with removal from exposure but may persist.

4. The diagnosis is made on the basis of a history documenting significant solvent exposure and the exclusion of other likely etiologies.

- Myelotoxicity. Benzene exposure has been associated with aplastic anemia and leukemia. Ethylene glycol ethers may also be myelotoxic.

- Nephrotoxicity. Acute heavy solvent exposure can cause acute tubular necrosis. Chronic organic solvent exposure may be associated with an increased risk of glomerulonephritis and renal failure.

- Liver toxicity

1. Many organic solvents are hepatotoxic and may cause acute hepatic necrosis and steatosis. The serum ALT level is usually elevated more than the serum AST level.

2. Diagnosis

   a. The diagnosis of occupational liver injury is usually based on the finding of elevated liver transaminases in a worker exposed to a hepatotoxic solvent and exclusion of other etiologies.

   b. The ratio of ALT to AST can be helpful in differentiating solvent from alcohol-induced liver disease.

   c. Improvement in symptoms and transaminase levels away from the workplace suggests an occupational etiology.

   d. If liver function tests remain abnormal a liver biopsy should be considered. Findings of necrosis and steatosis suggest solvent related hepatotoxicity.

Bibliography

Cullen MR, et al. Medical progress: Occupational medicine. New Engl J Med 1990;322:594–601;675–683.

Klassen CD, et al. Casarett and Doull's Toxicology: The Basic Science of Poisons, 3rd ed. New York, Macmillan, 1986.

LaDou J, ed. Occupational Medicine. Norwalk, CT, Appleton and Lange, 1990.

Levy BS, Wegman DH, eds. Occupational Health: Recognizing and Preventing Work-Related Diseases. Boston, Little Brown, 1988.

Parkes WR. Occupational Lung Disorders. London, Butterworth and Co., 1982.

Rosenstock L, Cullen MR. Clinical Occupational Medicine. Philadelphia, W.B. Saunders, 1986.

Workshop on environmental and occupational asthma. Chest 1990;98:145S–252S.

APPENDIX 1. Reference Ranges for Adults for Selected Laboratory Tests

TEST	SPECIMEN	REFERENCE RANGE (CONVENTIONAL UNITS)	REFERENCE RANGE (INTERNATIONAL UNITS)
Acetoacetate	S or P	<3 mg/dL	<0.3 mmol/L
Acid phosphatase	S		M: 2.5–11.7 U/L F: 0.3–9.2 U/L
Alanine aminotransferase (ALT, SGPT)	S		5–30 U/L
Albumin	S	3.5–5.0 g/dL	35–50 g/L
Alkaline phosphatase	S		F: 56–155 U/L M: 62–176 U/L
Ammonia nitrogen	S or P	15–45 mcg of nitrogen/dL	11–32 mcmol/L
Amylase	S		25–125 U/L
Aspartate aminotransferase (AST, SGOT)	S		10–30 U/L
Bicarbonate	S	24–30	24–30
Bilirubin	S	18–23 mEq/L	18–23 mmol/L
Calcium, total	S	0.2–1.0 mg/dL	3.4–17.1 mcmol/L
Calcium, ionized	S, P, or whole blood	8.4–10.2 mg/dL	2.10–2.55 mmol/L
Chloride	S or P	4.48–4.92 mg/dL	1.12–1.23 mmol/L
		98–106 mEq/L	98–106 mmol/L

Cholesterol (75th percentile from Lipid Research Clinics)	S or P	mg/dL	mmol/L
		20 to 29 years old	
		M: 194	M: 5.02
		F: 184	F: 4.77
		30 to 39 years old	
		M: 218	M: 5.65
		F: 202	F: 5.23
		40 to 49 years old	
		M: 231	M: 5.98
		F: 223	F: 5.78
		Greater than 50 years old	
		M: 230	M: 5.96
		F: 252	F: 6.53
Cortisol	S or P (8 A.M.)	5–23 mcg/dL	138–635 nmol/L
Creatine kinase	S		M: 38–174 U/L
			F: 96–140 U/L
Creatinine	S or P	M: 0.6–1.2 mg/dL	M: 53–106 mcmol/L
		F: 0.5–1.1 mg/dL	F: 44–97 mcmol/L
Ferritin	S	M: 15–200 ng/mL	M: 15–200 mcg/L
		F: 12–150 ng/mL	F: 12–150 mcg/L
Folate	S	1.8–9 ng/mL	4.1–20.4 nmol/L
Glucose	S	70–105 mg/dL	3.9–5.8 mmol/L
	Whole blood	65–95 mg/dL	3.6–5.3 mmol/L

Table continued on following page

APPENDIX 1. Continued

Test	Specimen	Reference Range (conventional units)	Reference Range (international units)
Gamma glutamyltransferase (GGT)	S		M: 9–50 U/L F: 8–40 U/L
HDL-cholesterol (5th percentile from Lipid Research Clinics)	S or P	M: 29 mg/dL F: 35 mg/dL	M: 0.75 mmol/L F: 0.91 mmol/L
Iron	S	M: 50–160 mcg/dL F: 40–150 mcg/dL	M: 8.95–28.64 mcmol/L F: 7.16–26.85 mcmol/L
Iron-binding capacity (total, TIBC)	S	250–400 mcg/dL	44.75–71.60 mcmol/L
LDL-cholesterol (75th percentile from Lipid Research Clinics)	S or P	mg/dL 20 to 29 years old M: 128 F: 127 30 to 39 years old M: 149 F: 143 40 to 49 years old M: 160 F: 155	mmol/L M: 3.32 F: 3.29 M: 3.86 F: 3.70 M: 4.14 F: 4.01

	Specimen		
		Greater than 50 years old M: 166 F: 170	M: 4.30 F: 4.40
L-Lactate	Whole blood	Venous: 4.5–19.8 mg/dL Arterial: 4.5–14.4 mg/dL	Venous: 0.5–2.2 mmol/L Arterial: 0.5–1.6 mmol/L
Lactate dehydrogenase (LDH)	S		210–420 U/L
Lead	Whole blood	<40 mcg/dL Toxic: ≥100 mcg/dL	<1.93 mcmol/L Toxic: ≥4.83 mcmol/L
Lipase	S		Adult: 10–150 U/L
Magnesium	S	1.3–2.1 mEq/L	0.65–1.05 mmol/L
Osmolality	S		275–295 milli-osmoles/kg
Phosphorous, inorganic	S	2.7–4.5 mg/dL Greater than 60 years old: M: 2.3–3.7 mg/dL F: 2.8–4.1 mg/dL	0.87–1.45 nmol/L M: 0.74–1.2 nmol/L F: 0.90–1.3 nmol/L
Potassium	S	3.5–5.1 mEq/L	3.5–5.1 mmol/L
	P	3.5–4.5 mEq/L	3.5–4.5 mmol/L
Protein	S	6.4–8.3 g/dL	64–83 g/L
Sodium	S or P	136–146 mEq/L	136–146 mmol/L
Testosterone	S	mean ± 1 std error M: 572 ± 135 ng/dL F: 37 ± 10 ng/dL	mean ± 1 std error M: 19.8 ± 4.7 nmol/L F: 1.3 ± 0.3 nmol/L
Thyroxine, total	S	5–12 mcg/dL	65–155 nmol/L

Table continued on following page

APPENDIX 1. Continued

Test	Specimen	Reference Range (conventional units)	Reference Range (international units)
Triglycerides	S, after ≥12 hour fast	Greater than 60 years old: M: 5.0–10.0 mcg/dL F: 5.5–10.5 mcg/dL mg/dL	M: 65–129 nmol/L F: 71–135 nmol/L mmol/L
		20 to 29 years old M: 44–185 F: 40–128	M: 0.50–2.09 F: 0.45–1.45
		30 to 39 years old M: 49–284 F: 38–160	M: 0.55–3.21 F: 0.43–1.81

Test	Specimen	Conventional	SI Units
Tri-iodothyronine (total)	S	40 to 49 years old M: 56–298 F: 44–186 Greater than 50 years old M: 62–288 F: 55–247 120–195 ng/dL Greater than 60 years old: M: 105–175 ng/dL F: 108–205 ng/dL	M: 0.63–3.37 nmol/L F: 0.50–2.10 M: 0.70–3.25 F: 0.62–2.79 1.85–3.00 nmol/L M: 1.62–2.69 nmol/L F: 1.66–3.16 nmol/L
Urea nitrogen, blood (BUN)	S or P	7–18 mg/dL	2.5–6.4 mmol/L
Uric acid	S	M: 3.5–7.2 mg/dL F: 2.6–6.0 mg/dL	M: 0.20–0.42 mmol/L F: 0.15–0.35 mmol/L

Note that some laboratories may have reference ranges different from those listed above.
ABBREVIATIONS: M = male; F = female; S = serum; P = plasma; g = gram; mg = milligram; mcg = microgram; ng = nanogram; L = liter; dL = deciliter; mL = milliliter; mmol = millimole; mcmol = micromole; nmol = nanomole; mEq = milliequivalent.

INDEX

Note: Page numbers in *italics* refer to illustrations; page numbers followed by "t" refer to tables.

AAH (atypical adenomatous hyperplasia), 423–424
Abdominal pain, 279–288. See also *Pain, abdominal.*
Abetalipoproteinemia, and malabsorption, 309t
  biopsy for evaluation of, 320
ABG. See *Arterial blood gases.*
Absorptiometry, for measurement of bone density, 456
Accelerated idioventricular rhythm (AIVR), and ventricular
     arrhythmias, *103*
Achalasia, and risk of esophageal cancer, 304t
Achilles tendinitis, 680
  clinical features of, 707
Acid-base disorders, 48–56. See also *Acidosis; Alkalosis.*
  changes due to, 49t, 50t
  map of, *50*
  metabolic, anion patterns in, 55t
  mixed, 53–54
Acidemia, with chronic bronchitis, 561–562
Acidosis, 49
  and hypercapnia, 167
  and osteomalacia, 458
  and protein binding of calcium, 490
  causes of, 51, 51t
  hyperkalemia and, 45
  hypokalemia and, 44
  in asthma, 188
  loss of anions in, 51–52
  respiratory, 53–54, 54t
  with ethylene glycol toxicity, 244
Acquired immunodeficiency syndrome (AIDS), 374, 639–651. See also
     Human immunodeficiency virus (HIV).
  algorithm for diagnosis of, 648t–649t
  and malignant lymphomas, 391
  definition of, by CDC, 639
  diagnostic approach to, 642
  diarrhea-causing infections in, 21t
  epidemiology of, 640
  evaluation of HIV-positive patient and, 641–642
  incubation period for, 640
  indicator diseases for, 640t
  sinusitis associated with, 557
Acropachy, thyroid, in Graves' disease, 469
ACTH. See *Adrenocorticotropic hormone (ACTH).*
Actin-myosin crossbridge, cycling during systole, 79
Acute bronchitis, etiology of, 560
Acute lymphocytic leukemia (ALL), diagnosis of, 381
  treatment of, and long-term survival, 381
Acute myeloid leukemia (AML), survival rates and times in, 381
Acute myocardial infarction (AMI). See *Myocardial infarction (MI).*

Acute renal failure (ARF), 236–244
  differential diagnosis of, 236–239
  intrarenal, 238–239
    causes of, 238t
    clinical features of, 240
  laboratory findings in, 242t
  postrenal, 237–238, 237t
    clinical features of, 239–240
  prerenal, 236–237, 237t
    clinical features of, 239
  types of, diagnostic features of, 237t
  urinalysis in diagnosis of, 240, 241t
Acute tubular necrosis (ATN), 236, 237t, 239
  clinical features of, 240
  urinalysis results in, 241t
Acute venous thrombosis, 198–203. See also *Thrombosis.*
Addison's disease, and hyperkalemia, 46
  and watery diarrhea, 24
  definition of, 479
  delirium caused by, 773t
Addisonian crisis, 480
Adenocarcinoma, axillary lymph nodes in, 429
  esophageal, in Barrett's disease, 298
Adenomas, adrenal, and Cushing's syndrome, 474
    and hypertension, 34
  and risk of colorectal cancer, 330
  pituitary, and Cushing's syndrome, 473
  toxic, 469
    and thyrotoxicosis, 467
    epidemiology of, 468
    thyroid function tests for, 471
Adenomatous hyperplasia, atypical, 423–424
Adenopathy, and resection of solitary pulmonary nodules (SPNs), 176
  bilateral symmetrical hilar, in sarcoidosis, 220
Adrenal gland diseases, 473–483
  carcinomatous, DHEA-S levels in, 440, 441
Adrenal insufficiency, acute, in glucocorticoid deficiency, 480
  chronic, in glucocorticoid deficiency, 480–481
  hypercalcemia with, 493
Adrenocortical carcinoma, 441
Adrenocortical insufficiency, algorithm for diagnosis of, *483*
  diagnostic approach to, *483*
  manifestations of, 480t
Adrenocorticotropic hormone (ACTH), deficiency of, 479
  in stimulation test for evaluation of glucocorticoid deficiency, 481–482
  measurement of, for evaluation of Cushing's syndrome, 477, 479
  overproduction of, in Cushing's syndrome, 473
Adult respiratory distress syndrome (ARDS), 204–207
  diagnositic criteria for, 205t
  differential diagnosis of, 206t
Aeromonas hydrophila, as cause of infectious diarrhea, 619t
Affective changes, in multiple sclerosis, 800
AG. See *Anion gap (AG).*
Age, and atherosclerotic vascular disease, 33
  and cancer of unknown primary site (CUPS), 429
  and death rate in pneumonia, 562
  and etiology of bacterial meningitis, 630t
  and etiology of jaundice, 823
  and fatigue, 9
  and hepatic signs in infectious mononucleosis, 670
  and hyperkalemia, 46
  and hypertension, 32

Age (*continued*)
  and incidence of ankylosing spondylitis, 710
  and incidence of Wegener's granulomatosis, 215
  and ischemic colitis, 324
  and likelihood of multiple myeloma, 396
  and malignancy associated with lymphomas, 392
  and malignancy of solitary pulmonary nodules (SPNs), 173
  and mesangiocapillary GN, 261
  and nephrotic syndrome, 252
  and onset of Crohn's disease and ulcerative colitis, 324
  and onset of hereditary colorectal cancers, 331t
  and osteoporosis, 453
  and pretest likelihood of coronary artery disease, 73t
  and prevalence of diabetes mellitus type II, 502
  and prevalence of prostate carcinoma, 420
  and risk for activation of tuberculosis, 574
  and risk for acute bronchitis, 560
  and risk for autoimmune hepatitis, 853
  and risk for breast cancer, 412
  and risk for chronic hepatitis carrier state, 837
  and risk for colorectal cancer, 330
  and risk for CPPD, 706
  and risk for delirium, 770
  and risk for dementia, 776
  and risk for diabetes mellitus, by type, 498–499
  and risk for Goodpasture's syndrome, 208
  and risk for gout, 701
  and risk for idiopathic pulmonary fibrosis, 213
  and risk for malignant thyroid nodules, 470t
  and risk for migraine, 784
  and risk for myocardial infarction (MI), 117
  and risk for osteoarthritis, 697
  and risk for polyarthritides, 691t
  and risk for pulmonary embolism, 194t
  and risk for sarcoidosis, 217
  and risk for septic arthritis, 622
  and risk for stroke, 792
  and symptoms of hypothyroidism, 466
  and symptoms of meningitis, 629
  and terminal hair growth on face, 438
  and type of leukemia, 382
  and urinary incontinence, 28
  and use of alcohol, 813
  as contraindication to thrombolytic therapy, 120
  asthma severity and incidence patterns by, 184
  bimodal incidence curve for Hodgkin's disease by, 391
  on onset of inherited myopathies, 810t
AIDS. See *Acquired immunodeficiency syndrome (AIDS)*.
AIDS dementia complex, fever in, 646
Airflow obstruction, diseases associated with, 189
  in asthma, 184–185
  in chronic obstructive pulmonary disease (COPD), 190
AIVR (accelerated idioventricular rhythm), *103*
Alanine aminotransferase (ALT), for evaluation of chronic hepatitis,
    854–855
  for evaluation of hepatomegaly, 831
Albumin, measurement of, for evaluation of hepatomegaly, 831
  serum, for evaluation of chronic hepatitis, 855
Alcohol, acute hepatitis associated with, 839
  and acute pancreatitis, 338
  and anemia, 348–349
  and pain syndrome in lymphomas, 392
  as cause of cluster headache, 787

Alcohol (*continued*)
   blood, for evaluation of coma, 757
   ketoacidosis and, 52
   polyneuropathies associated with, 805–806
Alcoholism, 812–816
   and activation of tuberculosis, 574
   and dementia, 780
   clinical manifestations of, 813–815, 813t
   diagnostic approach to, 816, 816t
   epidemiology of, 813
   factors raising suspicion of, 816t
   hepatomegaly associated with, 829
   laboratory studies for evaluation of, 815–816
   working definition of, 812
Aldolase, for evaluation of myopathy, 807, 809
   levels of, in PM/DM, 730–731
Aldosterone, and hyperkalemia, 46
   and hypokalemia, 44
   functions of, 34
   plasma levels of, for evaluation of glucocorticoid deficiency, 482
Aldosteronism, and potassium levels, 38
   evaluation of, 37
   hypernatremia in, 43
   primary, 34
Alkaline phosphatase level, in cholestasis, 824
   in hepatitis, 840–841
Alkalosis, and protein binding of calcium, 490
   hypokalemia and, 44
   in asthma, 188
   metabolic, 52–53, 53t
   respiratory, causes of, 55t
ALL (acute lymphocytic leukemia), 381
Allergies. See also *Hypersensitivity.*
   and asthma, 185
   and rhinosinusitis, 557
Alpha-fetoprotein (αFP), and extragonadal germ cell tumors, 429
17-Alpha-hydroxylase, amenorrhea caused by deficiency of, 444t
Alport's syndrome, hematuria in, 231t
ALT. See *Alanine aminotransferase (ALT).*
Aluminum toxicity, 781
   and osteomalacia, 457–458
Aluminum toxicity dementia, 249
   chronic renal failure (CRF) in, 247
Alveolar proteinosis, pulmonary, 214–215
Alveolar-capillary membrane, damage to, in adult respiratory distress syndrome (ARDS), 204
Alveolitis, extrinsic allergic (hypersensitivity pneumonitis), 210
Alzheimer's dementia (DAT), 776–778
   delirium in, 778
Amenorrhea, 443–451
   algorithm for diagnosis of, 449
   clinical findings in, 445–448
   definition of, 443
   diagnostic approach to, 448–451
   differential diagnosis of, 443–445, 444t–445t
Amenorrhea/galactorrhea syndrome, hirsutism with, 437
American Cancer Society, 418t
American Psychiatric Association, definition of alcoholism by, 812
American Society for Gastrointestinal Endoscopy, 302
American Thoracic Society, 184
American Urologic Society, 421t
AMI. See *Myocardial infarction (MI).*
AML (acute myeloid leukemia), 381

Amylase, levels of, in pleural effusions, 166
  serum, associated with gallstones, 859
    in acute pancreatitis, 342
Amyloidosis, accompanying ankylosing spondylitis, 711
  differentiation of, from scleroderma, 736
  hepatomegaly associated with, 830
  malabsorption in, 311t
  polyneuropathies associated with, 806
  with multiple myeloma, 397
ANA. See *Antinuclear antibody (ANA)*.
ANCA. See *Antineutrophil cytoplasmic antibodies (ANCA)*.
Androgens, effects of, on women, 438t
  hirsutism caused by, 435
Anemia, 347–354
  acute leukemia and, 384
  acute renal failure and, 169
  and high-output heart failure, 78
  aplastic or sideroblastic, as risk factor for leukemia, 383
  autoimmune hemolytic, 350
    associated with leukemia, 385
  chronic renal failure and, 247
  definition of, 347
  differential diagnosis of, 347–349, 347t
  evaluation for, in chronic renal failure (CRF), 249
  Fanconi's, 365t. See also *Fanconi's syndrome*.
  folate deficiency and, 351–352
  hemolytic, 348t
    autoimmune, 350
      associated with leukemia, 385
    diagnosis of, 352
    in systemic lupus erythematosus (SLE), 721t
  diagnostic approach to, 353–354
  hypoproliferative, 721t
  in chronic disease, 351
  in Goodpasture's syndrome, 209
  in IIBD, 327
  in systemic lupus erythematosus (SLE), 721t, 725
  in Wegener's granulomatosis, 215
  iron deficiency, 351
  myelophthisic, 353
  pernicious. See *Pernicious anemia*.
  with multiple myeloma, 397, 400
Aneurysms, abdominal aortic, 62t
    diagnosis of, 284
  aortic, and gastrointestinal bleeding, 293
  and gastrointestinal bleeding, 291
  berry, clinical evaluation of, 795–796
Angina, intestinal, diagnosis of, 284
Angina pectoris, 59–76, 64t
Angiocardiography, for evaluation of chest pain, 74
Angiodysplasia, as cause of gastrointestinal bleeding, 291
Angiography, cerebral, for evaluation of dementia, 781
    for evaluation of headache, 790, 790t
  coronary, with ergot stimulation, 74
  for evaluation of Takayasu's arteritis, 738
  for evaluation of coma, 760
  for evaluation of gastrointestinal bleeding, 293–294
  for evaluation of mediastinal masses, 182
  pulmonary, for evaluation of pulmonary embolism (PE), 197
  renal, for evaluation of hematuria, 234
Angioimmunoblastic lymphadenopathy, 374
Angioma, as cause of gastrointestinal bleeding, 289
Animals, contact with, and infectious diarrhea, 615

Anion gap (AG), 51–52
in metabolic acid-base disorders, 55t
in multiple myeloma, 400
Ankylosing spondylitis (AS), 710–711
chronic interstitial pneumonitis in, 209t, 213
differential diagnosis of, 711
epidemiology of, 691t
laboratory features of, 694t
physical signs of, 693t
polyarthritis in, 690
symptoms of, 692t
Anorectal infections, associated with gonorrhea, 595
Anorexia, caused by tuberculosis, 575
in *Legionella pneumophila* infection, 569
in systemic lupus erythematosus (SLE), 719t
Anorexia nervosa, amenorrhea associated with, 448
Anoscopy, for evaluation of gastrointestinal bleeding, 294, 295
Anterior horn cell disease, myopathy associated with, 807
Anthrax, pneumonia associated with, 571t
Antibiotic therapy, *Clostridium difficile* infection following, 616
Antibodies, anticardiolipin, in systemic lupus erythematosus (SLE),
    725
anticentromere, for evaluation of scleroderma, 736
anti-GBM, in Goodpasture's syndrome, 209, 210
antineutrophil. See *Antineutrophil cytoplasmic antibodies (ANCA).*
antinuclear. See *Antinuclear antibody (ANA).*
antiphospholipid, in systemic lupus erythematosus (SLE), 725
IgM, in HBV infection, 843
    in Lyme disease, 667
in systemic lupus erythematosus (SLE), 721t, 725–726
precipitating, in hypersensitivity pneumonitis, 212
to double-stranded DNA, in SLE, 695, 725
to gangliosides, 806
to myelin-associated globulin, 806
Anti–double strand DNA, in systemic lupus erythematosus (SLE),
    695, 725
Antidromic reciprocating tachycardia (ART), 107–108
Antigens, HLA-B27, in ankylosing spondylitis, 711
    in spondyloarthropathies, 709
    in spondylitis with IBD, 715
HLA-Bw38, in psoriatic arthritis, 713
p24, as predictor for AIDS, 641
sources of, in hypersensitivity pneumonitis, 211t
Antineutrophil cytoplasmic antibodies (ANCA), for evaluation of
vasculitis, 740t
in Wegener's granulomatosis, 215, 741
Antinuclear antibody (ANA), and connective tissue disease, 735
for evaluation of polyarthritis, 695
for evaluation of scleroderma, 736
in PM/DM, 731
in systemic lupus erythematosus (SLE), 722, 724t
Antiphospholipid antibody syndrome, accompanying SLE, 721
Anti-ribonucleoprotein, in scleroderma, 736
Antistreptolysin O (ASO) titer, for evaluation of nephritic syndrome,
    260
Anti-topoisomerase, for evaluation of scleroderma, 736
Antitrypsin deficiency, in chronic hepatitis, 853
Anxiety, chest pain caused by, 60t
Aortic coarctation, and hypertension, 33, 36
Aortic dissection, abnormal hemodynamics with, 62t
chest pain caused by, 66t
Aortic regurgitation (AR), acute, 137–138
and valvular heart disease, 135–138
auscultation of, 147t

Aortic regurgitation (AR) *(continued)*
  chest pain caused by, 65t
  in ankylosing spondylitis, 710
  in systemic lupus erythematosus (SLE), 720
Aortic stenosis (AS), and valvular heart disease, 134–135
  auscultation of, 147t
  chest pain caused by, 65t
Aortic vascular graft, as indication for emergent evaluation, 295
Aorto-enteric fistula, as cause of gastrointestinal bleeding, 291, 292
Aortography, for evaluation of mediastinal masses, 182–183
APBs (atrial premature beats), in SVT, *94,* 94
Aphasia, aluminum toxicity dementia and, 249
Appendicitis, diagnosis of, 279, 282
Appetite, in malabsorption syndrome, 306
AR. See *Aortic regurgitation (AR).*
Arachnoiditis, chronic, in ankylosing spondylitis, 710–711
Arboviruses, encephalitis caused by, 635–637
  tropical, incubation period for, 657t
  types of, causing encephalitis, 636t
ARDS. See *Adult respiratory distress syndrome (ARDS).*
ARF. See *Acute renal failure (ARF).*
Arrhythmias, 85–115
  anatomic location of, 86
  and respiratory failure, 170
  atrioventricular block and, *108,* 108–111
  intraventricular conduction defects (IVCD) and, 112–115
  mechanism of, 86
  nonparoxysmal supraventricular, 99–102
  preexcitation syndromes and, 107–108
  supraventricular, 94–102
ART (antidromic reciprocating tachycardia), 107–108
Arterial blood gases, for evaluation of asthma, 187–188
  for evaluation of coma, 757
  for evaluation of dyspnea, 157
  for evaluation of PCP, 650
  for evaluation of respiratory failure, 169
  for evaluation of scleroderma, 737
  in ARDS, 207
Arterial occlusion, mesenteric, diagnosis of, 284
Arteriography, renal, 37
Arteritis, temporal (giant cell), 739–740, 790
  with PMR, 679
Arthralgias, 675–688
  conditions associated with, 736
  disorders characterized by, 676t–677t
  in sarcoidosis, 220
  in systemic lupus erythematosus (SLE), 718
Arthritis, and nephrotic syndrome, 254
  associated with IBD, 326, 715
  associated with Lyme disease, 666
  degenerative. See *Osteoarthritis (OA).*
  in Reiter's syndrome, 712
  in systemic lupus erythematosus (SLE), 718, 723t
  juvenile, and Lyme disease, 662
  peripheral, in ankylosing spondylitis, 710
    in spondyloarthropathies, 709
  pseudo-rheumatoid, clinical features of, 706
  psoriatic, 713–714
    epidemiology of, 691t
    laboratory features of, 694t
    physical signs of, 693t
    polyarthritis in, 690
    symptoms of, 692t
  reactive, 712

Arthritis (*continued*)
  rheumatoid (RA), and risk of septic arthritis, 622
    characteristics of arthrocentesis fluid in, 626t
    chronic interstitial pneumonitis in, 212
    epidemiology of, 691t
    laboratory features of, 694t
    physical signs of, 693t
    pleural effusions in, 165t
    polyarthritis in, 690
    symptoms of, 692t
    versus systemic lupus erythematosus (SLE), 722
  septic. See *Septic arthritis.*
Arthritis mutilans, 714
Arthrocentesis, for evaluation of polyarthritis, 695
Arthrography, for evaluation of musculoskeletal pain, 688
AS. See *Ankylosing spondylitis (AS); Aortic stenosis (AS).*
Asbestos, diseases associated with occupational exposure to, 869–872
  solitary pulmonary nodules (SPNs) from exposure to, 173
Asbestosis, 871
Ascites, cancer of unknown primary site (CUPS) and, 429
Asherman's syndrome, 445–446
  amenorrhea caused by, 444t
ASO (antistreptolysin O) titer, for evaluation of nephritic syndrome, 260
Aspartate aminotransferase (AST), for evaluation of chronic hepatitis, 854–855
  for evaluation of hepatomegaly, 831
  levels of, in alcoholism, 815, 816t
  serum concentration of, following MI, 130
Aspartate transaminase (AST), in hepatitis, 840
Aspergillosis, allergic bronchopulmonary, 186
Aspiration, fine needle, for diagnosis of adenopathy, 377–378
Aspirin, platelet dysfunction caused by, 365
AST. See *Aspartate aminotransferase (AST); Aspartate transaminase (AST).*
Asthma, 184–188
  and hypertension treatment, 35
  differential diagnosis of, 185
  extrinsic, definition of, 185
  occupational, 873–874, 873t
  severity scores for, 187, 187t
Ataxia-telangiectasia, 391
  and risk of leukemia, 383
Atherosclerosis, in end-stage renal disease, 248
  in nephrotic syndrome, 254
  in systemic lupus erythematosus (SLE), 720
Atherosclerotic plaques, thrombosis at sites of, 369
Atherosclerotic vascular disease, and hypertension, 33
ATN. See *Acute tubular necrosis (ATN).*
Atrial fibrillation, and supraventricular tachycardias (SVT), 99, 99
  and ventricular arrhythmias, 108
  evaluation of, with QRS complexes, 87
  in mitral regurgitation, 140
  in preexcitation syndromes, 107
Atrial flutter, and supraventricular tachycardias (SVT), 98, 98–99
  tachycardia and, 87
Atrial myxoma, 745
Atrial premature beats (APBs), in supraventricular tachycardias (SVT), 94, 94
Atrioventricular (AV) block, and arrhythmias, 108, 108–111
  first degree, 108, 108
  Mobitz type, 109–111, 111
  second-degree, 109, 109–110
  third-degree, 111, 111

Atrioventricular (AV) nodal reciprocating tachycardia (AVNRT), in supraventricular tachycardias (SVT), 94–95, *95*
Atrioventricular (AV) node, arrhythmias involving, 86
Atypical adenomatous hyperplasia (AAH), 423–424
Auer rods, in acute myeloid leukemia, 381
Auras, and seizures, 762
  in migraine, 786
Autoantibodies, in chronic hepatitis, 855
Autoimmune disorders, and adrenalitis, 479
  and chronic liver disease, 852–854
  and hemolytic anemia, 352
  and hypocalcemia, 496
  and multiple sclerosis, 799
  and primary idiopathic hypothyroidism, 466
  urinalysis indicating, 240
Autoimmune processes, mediastinal masses associated with, 181t
  pleural effusions caused by, 166
AV. See *Atrioventricular (AV)* entries.
AVNRT, 94–95, *95*
Axillary lymph nodes, in breast carcinoma, 429
Azotemia, in glomerulonephritis, 257
  in glucocorticoid deficiency, 481
  in Goodpasture's syndrome, 209, 210
  in membranoproliferative GN, 261

Babesiosis, identification of, 658
Babinski's signs, and evaluation of coma, 755
  with spinal cord compression, 407, 408
Bacilli, gram-negative, meningitis caused by, 632
Bacillus cereus, as cause of infectious diarrhea, 617t
Back pain, in cancer patients, 405
  in osteoporosis, 455
Bacteria, gram-negative, septic arthritis associated with, 623–624
  overgrowth of, in malabsorption, 308t, 318, 320
Bacterial dysentery, 19
Bacterial infections, and chronic diarrhea, 21t
Bacteriuria, 613
  asymptomatic, definition of, 610
BAL. See *Bronchoalveolar lavage (BAL)*.
Balanitis, in Reiter's syndrome, 712–713
Barium studies, for evaluation of chronic GI bleeding, 293, 296
  for evaluation of colorectal cancer, 333, 335
  for evaluation of esophageal diseases, 297–298
  for evaluation of IIBD, 327–328
  UGI, 300
Barrett's disease, and incidence of adenocarcinoma, 304t
  diagnosis of, 298
Bartter's syndrome, gout associated with, 705
  hypokalemia and, 44
Basal energy expenditure (BEE), definition of, 519–520
Basophilic stippling, in lead poisoning, 350
Bayes' theorem, for evaluation of malignancy of SPNs, 177
Becker's dystrophy, 810t
BEE (basal energy expenditure), definition of, 519–520
Behçet's disease, vasculitis associated with, 743
Bence-Jones protein, test for, in multiple myeloma, 400–401
Bence-Jones proteinuria, 399t
Benign prostate hypertrophy (BPH), versus prostate carcinoma, 420
Benzene, toxicity of, 875
Berger's disease, 231t
Bernard-Soulier syndrome, 366t
  platelet aggregation studies for evaluation of, 362

Bernstein test, for diagnosis of esophagitis, 298
Beta-hemolytic streptococci, septic arthritis associated with, 623
Beta-human chorionic gonadotropin (βHCG), and extragonadal germ
    cell tumors, 429
Biases, in evaluation of diagnostic tests, 7
Bifascicular block, intraventricular conduction defects (IVCD) and,
    115
Bile acid, in breath test for evaluation of malabsorption, 318
Bile salt, defective absorption of, and malabsorption, 309t
  intraluminal deficiency of, and malabsorption, 308t
Biliary tract disease, colic in, 858
  hepatitis in, 840
  hepatomegaly associated with, 830
Bilirubin, conjugated, 821–822
  jaundice caused by accumulation of, 821–825
  levels of, and scleral icterus, 854
    for evaluation of jaundice, 824
    in hepatitis, 840
  serum, for evaluation of abdominal pain, 287
  steps in metabolism of, 822t
  unconjugated, 821–822
Binswanger's disease, 778
Biopsy, bone, for assessment of renal osteodystrophy, 249
    for evaluation of osteomyelitis, 627
  bone marrow, for evaluation of hemostasis, 362
    for evaluation of leukemia, 384, 386
    in multiple myeloma, 401
  colorectal, for diagnosis of collagenous colitis, 325
    for evaluation of IIBD, 328
  diagnostic yield of, in cases of sarcoidosis, 223–224, 223t
    in fever of unknown origin (FUO), 538t
  for diagnosis of lymphomas, 393–394
  for diagnosis of Wegener's granulomatosis, 215
  for evaluation of breast cancer, 415–416
  for evaluation of Churg-Strauss vasculitis, 741
  for evaluation of dementia, 781, 783
  for evaluation of fever in immunocompromised host, 549
  for evaluation of fever of unknown origin (FUO), 540
  for evaluation of headache, 790
  for evaluation of hematuria, 235
  for evaluation of lymphomas, 392
  for evaluation of mediastinal masses, 183
  for evaluation of PAN, 741
  for evaluation of prostate carcinoma, 422, 423–424
  for evaluation of skin infections, 593
  for evaluation of solitary thyroid nodule, 471
  liver, for evaluation of chronic hepatitis, 855
    for evaluation of hepatitis, 850
    for evaluation of hepatomegaly, 832
    for evaluation of jaundice, 824
  lung, for assessment of pneumonia, 566
    for evaluation of PCP, 651
    for evaluation of Wegener's granulomatosis, 741
  lymph node, for evaluation of lymphadenopathy, 378
    for evaluation of lymphomas, 389
  muscle, for evaluation of mitochondrial myopathies, 809
    for evaluation of myopathy, 807, 809, 811
    for evaluation of PM/DM, 731–732
  nerve, for evaluation of polyneuropathies, 805
  open lung, for diagnosis of idiopathic pulmonary fibrosis, 214
  open pleural, for evaluation of asbestosis, 872
  reasons for, in gastric and duodenal disease, 302
  rectal, for evaluation of IIBD, 328

Biopsy (*continued*)
    renal, for evaluation of membranoproliferative GN, 261
      for evaluation of nephrotic syndrome, 252, 255
      for evaluation of RPGN, 262–263
    sensitivity of, for evaluation of colorectal cancer, 334
    skin, for evaluation of hypersensitivity vasculitis, 743
    small intestinal, for evaluation of malabsorption, 320
    temporal artery, 739
      for evaluation of polymyalgia rheumatica, 679
    transbronchial (TBL), for diagnosis of idiopathic pulmonary fibrosis,
      214
      for diagnosis of sarcoidosis, 221–222, 223
      in pulmonary alveolar proteinosis, 215
Bird fancier's lung, 211t
Bladder washout, for evaluation of urinary tract infections, 614
Bleeding, gastrointestinal, 289–296
    character of, 291–292
Bleeding disorders, 361–373
Bleeding time (BT), for screening platelet function, 362
Blood. See also *Hemato-* entries; *Hemo-* entries; *Hematuria.*
    evaluation of, in chronic diarrhea, 19
    in stool, in chronic diarrhea, 22
    loss of, and anemia, 348t
Blood counts, for evaluation of pleural effusions, 164–165
Blood cultures, for evaluation of infective endocarditis, 586–587
    for evaluation of vasculitis, 740t
Blood gases, arterial. See *Arterial blood gases.*
Blood pressure, postural changes and, 41
    systolic, in aortic regurgitation (AR), 136
Blood protein deficiencies, associated with thrombosis, 372
Blood studies, for evaluation of gastrointestinal bleeding, 293
    for evaluation of leukemia, 386–387
    preparation for, in malaria detection, 659t
Blood transfusion, and risk for hepatitis B and C, 852
Blood-urea nitrogen (BUN), and evaluation of congestive heart
      failure, 83
    and hyponatremia, 41
    for evaluation of prostate carcinoma metastasis, 422
    in acute renal failure, 236, 243
    in alcoholism, 816t
    in Goodpasture's syndrome, 209
    in nephritic syndrome, 258
    in systemic lupus erythematosus (SLE), 725
    in test for hypernatremia diagnosis, 43
Bloom syndrome, and risk of leukemia, 383
Blue rubber-bleb nevus syndrome, gastrointestinal bleeding associated
      with, 293
Boils, clinical features of, 592
    definition of, 590
Bone. See also *Osteo-* entries.
    involvement of, in sarcoidosis, 219t
    metabolic diseases of, 453–460
    scans of, for evaluation of prostate carcinoma metastasis, 423
    techniques for measuring density of, 456
Bone marrow disorders, and anemia, 348t
    and proliferation of cells, in leukemia, 381
    diagnosis of, 353
    nucleated red blood cells as indicators of, 350
Bone marrow transplantation, for chronic myelocytic leukemia, 385
Bone pain, in multiple myeloma, 397
    with chronic leukemia, 385
    with osteomalacia, 458–459
Borrelia burgdorferi, Lyme disease caused by, 662–667

Borrelia recurrentis, identification of, 658
Botulism, myopathy in, 808
Bowel disease. See also *Inflammatory bowel disease (IBD).*
   idiopathic inflammatory (IIBD), 323–328
     differential diagnosis of, 324t, 324–325
     epidemiology of, 324
   obstructive, diagnosis of, 283
BPH (benign prostate hypertrophy), versus prostate carcinoma, 420
Bradycardia, defined, 87
   in acute respiratory failure, 168
   mechanisms of, 86
   severe, 63t
Bradycardia-tachycardia syndrome, 93
Breast, benign disease of, and cancer, 412
   nodules in, and cancer, 411–418
Breast cancer, algorithm for diagnosis of, *417*
   and screening for colorectal cancer, 335
   diagnostic approach to, 416–417
   differential diagnosis of, 412–413
   epidemiology of, 412
   hypercalcemia with, 493
   medical history and physical examination in, 414t
   screening for, 415
     American Cancer Society, 418t
Breathing, difficulty in. See *Dyspnea.*
Bronchial fibrosis, in hypersensitivity pneumonitis, 212
Bronchial provocation tests, for evaluation of asthma, 188
Bronchiectasis, hemoptysis caused by, 159t, 160
Bronchitis, acute, 560–562
   chronic, 189
     and COPD, 190–191
     definition of, 560
   diagnostic approach to, 562
   differential diagnosis of, 560–562, 560t
   epidemiology of, 560
   hemoptysis caused by, 158, 160
   industrial, 874
Bronchoalveolar lavage (BAL), for diagnosis of sarcoidosis, 221
   for evaluation of PCP, 651
Bronchoscopy, for evaluation of hemoptysis, 160
   for evaluation of mediastinal masses, 182
   sensitivity of, in diagnosis of malignancy, 176
Bronchospasm, in asthma, 184
   stimuli precipitating, 185–186
Brucellosis, pneumonia associated with, 571t
BT (bleeding time), for screening platelet function, 362
Budd-Chiari syndrome, hepatomegaly associated with, 829
Buerger's disease, 739t
BUN. See *Blood-urea nitrogen (BUN).*
BUN/CREAT ratio, in acute renal failure, 242t, 243
   in hyponatremia, 41
Bundle of His, arrhythmias and, 86
Burkitt's lymphoma, 391
Bursal fluid, in evaluation of septic bursitis, 625, 627
Bursitis, 679–680
   and gout, 702
   clinical features of, 681t
   diagnostic approach to, 627
   septic, 623, 624

CAH. See *Chronic active hepatitis (CAH); Congenital adrenal
   hyperplasia (CAH).*

Calcification, evaluation of, in solitary pulmonary nodules (SPNs), 174
Calcium. See also *Hypercalcemia; Hypercalciuria.*
  levels of, in osteomalacia, 459
  serum, disorders of, 490–497
    in sarcoidosis, 220
  urinary, in sarcoidosis, 220, 223
Calcium pyrophosphate dihydrate deposition disease (CPDD), 704
  classification of, 706t
  diagnostic approach to, 708
  epidemiology of, 706
  versus osteoarthritis, 707t
Campylobacter fetus, 618t
  diarrhea caused by, in HIV-positive patients, 643–644
  foodborne disease caused by, 616t
Cancer. See also *Malignancy; Tumors.*
  breast nodules and, 411–418
  colon, and chronic diarrhea, 22
  gallbladder, 858
    associated with gallstones, 858
  head and neck, and risk of GI malignancy, 304t
  in IIBD, 324
  lung, 192. See also *Lung cancer.*
Cancer of unknown primary site (CUPS), 426–430
  adenocarcinoma as, 429
  algorithm for diagnosis of, *309*
  effective therapy for, 427t
  poorly differentiated carcinoma as, 429
Carbon dioxide, partial pressure of, and acute respiratory failure
      (ARF), 167
  in blood, 48–49
Carboxyhemoglobin test, for evaluation of coma, 757
Carcinoembryonic antigen (CEA), in colorectal cancer, 333
Carcinoid, bronchial, and Cushing's syndrome, 474
  immunocytochemistry for evaluation of, 428
  watery diarrhea associated with, 24
Carcinoma, adrenal, dehydroepiandrosterone sulfate levels in, 440
  adrenocortical, and Cushing's syndrome, 474
  colonic, and constipation, 15, 17
  hemoptysis caused by, 159t
  prostate, 420–425
  renal cell, with hematuria, 230
  risk for, in HBV carriers, 838
  thyroid, 462t, 463t
  transitional cell, with hematuria, 230
Cardiac arrhythmias, 85–115
Cardiac enzymes, in myocardial infarction (MI), 128–130
Cardiac tamponade, 63t
  during dialysis, 248
Cardiomyopathy, compensatory mechanisms in, 79
  in scleroderma, 734
Cardiovascular disorders, chest pain caused by, 60t
  hypertension as risk factor for, 32
Carotene, levels of, and fatty diarrhea, 24
Catecholamines, for evaluation of pheochromocytoma, 487
Catheterization, cardiac, for evaluation of infectious endocarditis, 588
      for evaluation of syncope, 766
Cauda equina syndrome, in ankylosing spondylitis, 710–711
  with spinal cord compression, 407
CBC. See *Complete blood count (CBC).*
CCU, utilization of, in myocardial infarction, 133
CDC staging system, for HIV-associated illness, 639
CEA, in colorectal cancer, 333
Celiac disease, and malabsorption, 310t
  and malignancy, 304t

Celiac disease (*continued*)
  biopsy for evaluation of, 320
  chronic diarrhea in, 21–22
Cellulitis, associated with septic bursitis, 624
  clinical features of, 591
  definition of, 590
  orbital, 557–558
Central nervous system (CNS), vasculitis involving, 741–743
Central nervous system (CNS) studies, in systemic lupus
      erythematosus (SLE), 726
Cerebrovascular disease, 792–798
  diagnostic approach to, 797–798
  differential diagnosis of, 792–793
  epidemiology of, 792
Ceruloplasmin, for evaluation of chronic hepatitis, 855
  synthesis of, in Wilson's disease, 853
Cervical adenitis, frequency of infections in, 375t
Cervical lymph nodes, and survival time in cancer of unknown primary
      site (CUPS), 428
Cervicitis, diagnostic approach to, 607–608
  in Reiter's syndrome, 712
  mucopurulent (endocervicitis), 599
CF. See *Cystic fibrosis (CF)*.
Chancroid, 604–605
  clinical features of genital ulcers in, 602t
Charcot's arthropathy, and secondary osteoarthritis, 698t
Chest pain, and angina, 59–76
  causes of, 60t
  diagnostic clues to causes of, 64t–69t
  in myocardial infarction (MI), 118
  in pneumonia, 562
  in pulmonary embolism, 194
CHF. See *Congestive heart failure (CHF)*.
Chlamydia, 595, 597
  and diarrhea, in the HIV-positive patient, 644
Cholangiography, for evaluation of gallbladder diseases, 860
Cholangitis, associated with choledocholithiasis, 859
Cholecystitis, 858
  chest pain caused by, 68t
  gallbladder diseases associated with, 859
  tests for, 860
Choledocholithiasis, pancreatitis associated with, 858
Cholelithiasis, 338, 857, 858
Cholera, as cause of infectious diarrhea, 617t
Cholescintigraphy, 824
  for evaluation of gallbladder diseases, 860
Cholestasis, delta bilirubin in, 822
  differential diagnosis of, 823t
Cholestatic jaundice, 821
Cholesterol, in gallstones, 859
  levels of, in hyperlipidemia, 512
  low and high density lipoprotein and, 515
Cholesterol emboli, 745
Chondrocalcinosis, 704
Chromosomes, in germ cell tumors, 428
  karyotype for evaluation of amenorrhea, 450
  locus for familial adenomatous polyposis, 331t
  Philadelphia, 382
  X, and familial hypophosphatemic rickets, 458
    and muscular dystrophies, 810t
Chronic active hepatitis (CAH), 838, 852
Chronic fatigue syndrome, 9
  working definition of, 10t

Chronic lymphocytic leukemia, diagnosis of, 382
  differentiation from other lymphoid malignancies, 384
Chronic myelocytic leukemia (CML), diagnosis of, 382
Chronic obstructive pulmonary disease (COPD), 189–192
  acute bronchitis associated with, 560
  differentiation of, from hypersensitivity pneumonitis,
    210
Chronic renal failure (CRF), 245–249
Chrug-Strauss vasculitis, 740t, 741
Chvostek's sign, in hypocalcemia, 494
  in malabsorption, 315–316
Cinefluoroscopy, for evaluation of esophageal diseases, 299
Cirrhosis, risk for, in hepatitis virus carriers, 838
CK. See *Creatine kinase (CK)*.
Clinical trials, hypertension treatment evaluations, 32
Clostridium botulinum, foodborne disease caused by, 616t
Clostridium difficile, diarrhea caused by, 619t
    in HIV-positive patients, 643
Clostridium perfringens, as cause of infectious diarrhea, 617t
  foodborne disease caused by, 616t
Clot stability test, for evaluation of secondary hemostasis, 364
Clubbing, chronic obstructive pulmonary disease (COPD) and, 191
CML (chronic myelocytic leukemia), diagnosis of, 382
CMV. See *Cytomegalovirus (CMV)*.
CNS. See *Central nervous system (CNS)* entries.
Coagulation, acquired disorders of, 367, 369
  and risk of DVT, 199t
  and risk of pulmonary embolism, 194t
  consumptive disorders of, 369
  disorders of, in chronic renal failure (CRF), 247
    with hematuria, 230
  in evaluation of secondary hemostasis, 364
  screening tests for disorders of, 363
Coccidioidomycosis, pneumonia associated with, 571t
Cogan's disease, vasculitis associated with, 743
Colic, body posture in, 286
Colitis, acute self-limited (ASLC), 22
  collagenous, 325
  following radiation therapy, 325
  infectious, 324
  pseudomembranous, 324
  segmental. See *Crohn's disease*.
  ulcerative, 323, 325t, 326, 334
Collagen-vascular disease, chronic renal failure (CRF) in, 246
  fever of unknown origin (FUO) accompanying, 535t
College of American Pathology, 413
Colonoscopy, for evaluation of colorectal cancer, 334
  for evaluation of gastrointestinal bleeding, 294
  for evaluation of IIBD, 328
  for evaluation of lower GI bleeding, 295
Colorectal cancer, 330–335
  prognosis of, 331t
Coma, 749–760
  anatomic localization of neurologic signs in, 753t
  and mortality, in diabetes mellitus, 503
  causes of, 750t
  clinical features of, 751–757
  diagnostic approach to, 760
  differential diagnosis of, 749–751
  laboratory studies in, 757–760
  typical signs of, 756t
Complement levels, for evaluation of systemic lupus erythematosus
    (SLE), 726

Complement levels (*continued*)
    for evaluation of vasculitis, 740t
    in nephritic syndrome, 259, 260, 261
Complete blood count (CBC), for evaluation of colorectal cancer, 332
    for evaluation of dyspnea, 157
    for evaluation of fever of unknown origin (FUO), 537
    for evaluation of lymphadenopathy, 377
    for evaluation of malaria, 658
    for evaluation of mediastinal masses, 180
    for evaluation of prostate carcinoma metastasis, 422
    for evaluation of urolithiasis, 273
Computed tomography (CT), abdominal, for evaluation of colorectal
       cancer, 333
      for evaluation of IIBD, 328
    chest, for evaluation of solitary pulmonary nodules (SPNs), 176
    for diagnosis of sarcoidosis, 221
    for evaluation of Alzheimer's disease, 778
    for evaluation of amenorrhea, 450
    for evaluation of cancer of unknown primary site (CUPS), 429
    for evaluation of coma, 758
    for evaluation of delirium, 775
    for evaluation of gastrointestinal bleeding, 295
    for evaluation of headache, 790, 790t
    for evaluation of hepatomegaly, 831–832
    for evaluation of HIV-associated fever, 646
    for evaluation of Huntington's disease, 779
    for evaluation of hydrocephalus, 780
    for evaluation of mediastinal masses, 181
    for evaluation of multi-infarct dementia (MID), 778
    for evaluation of otitis, 553
    for evaluation of pancreatitis, 343
    for evaluation of pheochromocytoma, 488
    for evaluation of prostate carcinoma, 423
    for evaluation of septic arthritis, 625, 627
    for evaluation of spinal cord compression, 408
    for evaluation of urolithiasis, 273–274
    quantitative, for measurement of bone density, 456
    versus magnetic resonance imaging (MRI), for evaluation of
       headache, 791
Computer protocol, for evaluation of myocardial infarction (MI), *132*
Conduction, aberrant, nonspecific, 115
    disturbances of, in MI, 124, 128
      simulating MI, 121t
Conduction block, P waves and QRS complexes in, 87
Condylomata acuminata, 603
Congenital adrenal hyperplasia (CAH), 439
    and hirsutism, 437
Congenital disorders, of coagulation factors, 365–367
Congenital hypothyroidism, 465
Congenital metabolic defects, hepatomegaly associated with, 830
Congestive heart failure (CHF), 77–84
    development of, with aortic regurgitation (AR), 136
    diagnostic approach to, *83*
    differentiation of, from ARDS, 205
    etiology of, 79t
    functional classification of, 80t
    symptoms of, 81t
Conjunctivitis, in Reiter's syndrome, 712
Conn's disease, 34
Connective tissue disease (CTD). See also *Sarcoidosis.*
    arthralgias or myalgias in, 676t
    chronic interstitial pneumonitis caused by, 212–213
    hematuria associated with, 230

Consciousness, and evaluation of coma, 753
  transient loss of, 762t
Constipation, 14–18
Contact dermatitis, caused by occupational exposure, 869
Contraceptives, hormonal, and amenorrhea, 448
Contractility, assessment of, in congestive heart failure, 79
COPD. See *Chronic obstructive pulmonary disease (COPD)*.
Cor pulmonale, in chronic obstructive pulmonary disease (COPD), 192
Coronary artery disease, risk factors for, 71t
Coronary care unit (CCU), utilization of, in myocardial infarction (MI), 133
Corticosteroids, and hypernatremia, 43
Cortisol, production of, by adrenal adenomas, 474
  urinary, for evaluation of Cushing's syndrome, 476
Cough, 25–27
  acute, causes of, 26t
  chronic, 26t, 27
  differential diagnosis of, 561t
  evaluation of, in HIV-positive patients, 647
  in pneumonia, 562
  with asthma, 186
  with pleural effusions, 163
Coxiella burnetti, Q fever caused by, 838–839
Coxsackie virus, hepatitis associated with infection by, 838
CPDD. See *Calcium pyrophosphate dihydrate deposition disease (CPDD)*; *Pyrophosphate dihydrate deposition disease (CPDD)*.
CPK. See *Creatine phosphokinase (CPK)*.
Crab louse, 605
Creatine kinase (CK), for evaluation of myopathy, 807, 809
  levels of, in myocardial infarction (MI), 128
  MB, in cardiac and noncardiac conditions, 131t
    in myocardial infarction (MI), 128
Creatine phosphokinase (CPK), levels of, in PM/DM, 730
  serum concentration of, following MI, *130*
Creatine phosphokinase isoenzyme (CK-BB), for evaluation of coma, 758
Creatinine, and diagnosis of hematuria, 233
  in acute renal failure, 236, 243
  in evaluation of prostate carcinoma metastasis, 422
  in Goodpasture's syndrome, 209
  in nephritic syndrome, 258, 259
  in systemic lupus erythematosus (SLE), 725
  in test of hypernatremia diagnosis, 43
  levels of, and hyponatremia, 41
Crepitus, in osteoarthritis, 699
  in scleroderma, 734
Crescentic glomerulonephritis, 262
CREST syndrome, 735
  anticentromere antibodies in, 736
  definition of, 733
Cretinism (congenital hypothyroidism), 465
Creutzfeldt-Jakob disease, dementia in, 781
CRF (chronic renal failure), 245–249
Crigler-Najjar syndromes, glucuronyl transferase deficiency in, 822
Crohn's disease, 315
  as cause of gastrointestinal bleeding, 291
  complications in, 326, 326t
  definition of, 323
  versus ulcerative colitis, 325t
Cryoglobulinemia, essential mixed, 744
Cryoglobulins, for evaluation of vasculitis, 740t
Cryptococcosis, extrapulmonary, as AIDS indicator, 640t
  fever accompanying, and HIV infection, 646

Cryptococcus neoformans, and respiratory symptoms in HIV-positive patients, 647
Cryptosporidia, diarrhea caused by, in HIV-positive patients, 643–644
Cryptosporidiosis, chronic symptomatic, as AIDS indicator, 640t
CSF analysis, for evaluation of multiple sclerosis, 801, 803
CT. See *Computed tomography (CT).*
CTD. See *Connective tissue disease (CTD).*
Cultures, blood, for evaluation of infectious diarrhea, 620
    for evaluation of septic arthritis, 627
  for evaluation of skin infections, 593
  urine, for evaluation of urinary tract infections, 613
CUPS. See *Cancer of unknown primary site (CUPS).*
Cushing's disease, definition of, 473
  hirsutism in, 437
  mediastinal masses associated with, 181t
Cushing's syndrome, 34, 473–479
  algorithm for diagnosis of, *478*
  anatomic localization tests in, 477t
  and hirsutism, 439
  arthralgias or myalgias in, 677t
  clinical features of, 475
  delirium caused by, 773t
  diagnostic approach to, 477–479
  differential diagnosis of, 473–474
  hypernatremia in, 43
  screening for, 38
Cutaneous symptoms, in Graves' disease, 469
  in systemic lupus erythematosus (SLE), 718–719
Cystic fibrosis (CF), and malabsorption, 307t
  bacterial sinusitis associated with, 557
  pneumonia associated with, 572t
Cystic liver diseases, hepatomegaly associated with, 830
Cystinuria, urolithiasis associated with, 271t
Cystitis, acute uncomplicated, 610, 612
  diagnostic approach to, 614
  hematuria in, 613
Cysts, breast, 412
Cytogenetics, in acute myeloid leukemia, 381
  in evaluation of cancer of unknown primary site (CUPS), 428
Cytokines, and asthma symptoms, 185
Cytology, for evaluation of pleural effusions, 166
Cytomegalovirus (CMV), and respiratory symptoms in HIV-positive patients, 647
  diarrhea caused by, in HIV-positive patients, 643–644
  differentiation of, from infectious mononucleosis, 669
  disseminated infection by, as AIDS indicator, 640t
  hepatitis associated with, 838, 844
  infectious mononucleosis caused by, 669t
  ulcerations and gastrointestinal bleeding associated with, in AIDS, 292

DAT. See *Alzheimer's dementia (DAT).*
de Quervain's thyroiditis, 467–468, 680
Decision analysis, to evaluate management of SPNs, 177
Deep venous thrombosis (DVT), 193, 198, 200
  and pulmonary embolism, 195
  diagnostic algorithm for evaluation of, 202–203, *202*
  differential diagnosis of, 199
  risk factors for, 199t
  symptoms of, 201t
Degenerative joint disease (DJD). See *Osteoarthritis (OA).*
Dehydroepiandrosterone, levels of, and adrenal cancer, 477

Dehydroepiandrosterone sulfate (DHEA-S), for evaluation of
    hirsutism, 440
Delirium, 769–775
  causes of, 772t–773t
  clinical features of, 771
  diagnostic approach to, 769, 771, 774–775
  differential diagnosis of, 770–771
    confusional state in, 774t
  epidemiology of, 770
  in Alzheimer's disease, 778
  pathogenesis of, 770
  versus dementia, 770–771
Delta wave, in preexcitation syndromes, 107
Dementia, 776–783
  causes of, 777t
  clinical definition of, 776
  diagnostic approach to, 781–783
  differential diagnosis of, 776–777
  lacunar, 778
  multi-infarct, 776–778, 779t
  Parkinsonism and, 778
  tests for (dementia batteries), 782
  treatable forms of, 779–781
  vascular, 778
  versus pseudodementia, 780t
Deoxynucleotidyl transferase (TDT), in acute lymphocytic leukemia,
    381–382
Depolarization, atrioventricular (AV) node, and arrhythmias, 86
  in preexcitation syndromes, 107
Depression, and fatigue, 11
  and hypertension, treatment of, 35
  in Alzheimer's disease, 778
  pseudodementia as cause of, 779
Dermatomyositis (DM), 809
  definition of, 728
  diagnostic approach to, 732
  differential diagnosis of, 729t–730t
  versus systemic lupus erythematosus (SLE), 722
Dermopathy, in Graves' disease, 469
Desquamative interstitial pneumonia (DIP), chest x-ray findings in, 214
Dexamethasone suppression tests, for assessment of Cushing's
    syndrome, 476–477
  for evaluation of adrenal carcinoma, 441
DHEA-S, for evaluation of hirsutism, 440
Diabetes insipidus, hypernatremia in, 42–43
Diabetes mellitus (DM), 498–511. See also *Insulin.*
  algorithm for classification of, *510*
  and nephrotic syndrome, 252, 254
  and risk of myocardial infarction (MI), 117
  clinical presentation of, in type I disease, 502–504
  criteria for screening tests in, 505t
  definition of, 498–499
  diagnosis of, 504–505, 506t–507t, 511
  differentiation of type I and type II, 509–511
  epidemiology of, 499–502
  gestational diabetes mellitus as a risk factor for, 499
  hyperkalemia and, 46
  impaired glucose tolerance (IGT) versus, 508–509
  malabsorption with, 314t
  osteoporosis accompanying, 454
  polyneuropathies in, 805
  types of, 500t–501t
  with chronic renal failure (CRF), 248

Diabetic ketoacidosis (DKA), 52
  clinical and laboratory presentations in, *503*
  rhinocerebral mucormycosis associated with, 557
Diagnostic testing, 3–8
Diaphoresis, in myocardial infarction (MI), 118
Diarrhea, and hypovolemic hypernatremia, 42
  associated with gastrointestinal bleeding, 292
  bloody, evaluation of, 23
  chronic, 19–24
    causes of, 20t
  diagnostic approach to, in HIV-positive patient, 644
  fatty, evaluation of, 24
  functional, 19
  infectious, 615–621, 617t–619t
  in HIV-positive patient, 643–644
  in IIBD, 325t
  metabolic acidosis caused by, 51
  secretory, and hypokalemia, 45
  watery, 22, 23, 24
Diastolic blood pressure (DBP), measurements of, for defining
    hypertension, 32
Diastolic murmurs, differential diagnosis of, 150–151
DIC. See *Disseminated intravascular coagulation (DIC)*.
Diet, and constipation, 14
  gluten-free, for diagnosis of celiac sprue, 21–22
  high-fiber, for treatment of constipation, 18
  purines in, and urolithiasis, 269t
Digital rectal examination (DRE), for evaluation of prostate carcinoma,
    421–422
Digitalis, and premature beats (palpitations), 85
DIP See *Desquamative interstitial pneumonia (DIP)*.
Diphtheria, as complication of pharyngitis, 554, 555
Disaccharidase deficiency, and malabsorption, 309t
Discoid rash, in systemic lupus erythematosus (SLE), 723t
Disorientation, and delirium, 770
Disseminated intravascular coagulation (DIC), 352–353, 368t
  associated with leukemia, 385
Diverticula, bleeding from, 291
  diseases of, and constipation, 15
Diverticulitis, diagnosis of, 283–284
DJD (degenerative joint disease). See *Osteoarthritis (OA)*.
DKA. See *Diabetic ketoacidosis (DKA)*.
DM. See *Dermatomyositis (DM); Diabetes mellitus (DM)*.
Donovanosis, 601
  clinical features of genital ulcers in, 602t
Doppler echocardiography, for evaluation of aortic regurgitation (AR),
    137, 138
  for evaluation of aortic stenosis (AS), 135
  for evaluation of mitral regurgitation, 140–141
  for evaluation of mitral stenosis (MS), 139
  for evaluation of mitral valve prolapse (MVP), 143
  for evaluation of pulmonic stenosis (PS), 149
  for evaluation of tricuspid regurgitation (TR), 144
  for evaluation of tricuspid stenosis (TS), 143
Doppler ultrasound, for evaluation of acute venous thrombosis, 201
Doubling time, of solitary pulmonary nodules (SPNs), 174
Dowager's hump, and osteoporosis, 455
Down's syndrome, and risk of leukemia, 383
  gout associated with, 705t
Downy cell lymphocytes, in infectious mononucleosis, 670t
DRE. See *Digital rectal examination (DRE)*.
Drugs. See also *Intravenous drug use*.
  acute renal failure caused by, 236–237
  acute tubular necrosis caused by, 240

Drugs (*continued*)
  amenorrhea caused by, 451t
  and abdominal pain, 286
  and nephrogenic diabetes insipidus, 43
  and urinary incontinence, 29
  anemia caused by, 348
  associated with abnormal glucose tolerance or diabetes mellitus, 508t
  associated with headache, in HIV treatment, 646
  associated with leukemia, 383
  associated with urolithiasis, 266
  associated with vasculitis syndrome, 744t
  asthma caused by, 186
  chronic diarrhea and, 21t
  coma caused by, 750–751
  constipation-causing, 15t
  fever associated with, 543
  gastrointestinal bleeding caused by, 292
  hematuria caused by, 231t
    false, 229
  hepatitis caused by, 839, 852
  hirsutism caused by, 436t
  hypercalcemia caused by, 493
  hyperkalemia and, 45–46
  hypersensitivity vasculitis caused by, 743
  hypocalcemia caused by, 496–497
  hypokalemia caused by, 44
  hyponatremia caused by, 40
  hypothyroidism caused by, 462t
  interactions with nutrients, 523, 524t–526t
  intrarenal acute renal failure caused by, 238t
  levels of, for evaluation of coma, 757
  lymphadenopathy caused by, 374
  myopathy induced by, 729t
  nephrotic syndrome caused by, 253t
  osteomalacia caused by, 457, 458
  pancreatitis caused by, 340
  scleroderma caused by, 733–734
  systemic lupus erythematosus (SLE) caused by, 721
Dual testing strategy, 7
Duchenne dystrophy, 810t
Ductal carcinoma in situ (DCIS), 411
Duodenal disease, 300–302
  chest pain caused by, 68t
  differential diagnosis of, 301t
Duroziz's sign, 136
DVT. See *Deep venous thrombosis (DVT)*.
D-xylose test, for evaluation of malabsorption, 317
Dysbetalipoproteinemia, familial, 513t
Dyspepsia, definition of, 300
Dysphagia, in dermatomyositis (DM)/polymyositis (PM), 730
Dysphasia, in aluminum toxicity dementia, 249
  in Alzheimer's disease, 778
  with migraine, 786
Dysplasia, fibromuscular, hypertension and, 33
Dyspnea, 155–157
  as symptom of CREST syndrome, 735
  evaluation of, in HIV-positive patients, 647
  in aortic stenosis (AS), 134
  in asthma, 186
  in emphysema, 189, 191
  in mitral stenosis (MS), 138
  in myocardial infarction (MI), 118
  in pulmonary alveolar proteinosis, 214

Dyspnea (*continued*)
  in pulmonary embolism (PE), 194
  in respiratory failure, 168
  with pleural effusions, 163
Dystrophy, myotonic, 808

EB. See *Epstein-Barr (EB) virus.*
Ebstein's anomaly, 107
ECG. See *Electrocardiography (ECG).*
Echocardiography, for evaluation of aortic regurgitation (AR), 137,
    138
  for evaluation of aortic stenosis (AS), 135
  for evaluation of chest pain, 72, 74
  for evaluation of congestive heart failure, 82
  for evaluation of infectious endocarditis, 587
  for evaluation of mitral regurgitation, 140–141, 141–142
  for evaluation of mitral stenosis (MS), 139
  for evaluation of mitral valve prolapse (MVP), 142–143
  for evaluation of pulmonic regurgitation (PR), 149
  for evaluation of pulmonic stenosis (PS), 149
  for evaluation of syncope, 766
  for evaluation of tricuspid regurgitation (TR), 144
  for evaluation of tricuspid stenosis (TS), 143
Ectopic ACTH production, Cushing's syndrome with, 474
Ectopic pregnancy, and PID, 597
  diagnosis of, 285
  evaluation for, in abdominal pain, 287
Ectopic thyroid tissue, thyroid scan for identification of, 472
Edema, hydrostatic pulmonary, versus ARDS, 205
  in adult respiratory distress syndrome (ARDS), 207
  in nephritic syndrome, 258
  in nephrotic syndrome, 253
Edrophonium injections, for evaluation of esophageal diseases, 299
  for evaluation of myasthenia gravis, 808, 810
EEG. See *Electroencephalogram (EEG).*
EGD. See *Esophagogastroduodenoscopy (EGD).*
Ehlers-Danlos syndrome, and secondary osteoarthritis, 698t
  aortic regurgitation (AR) in, 135–136
  gastrointestinal bleeding associated with, 293
  mitral valve prolapse (MVP) in, 142
EKG. See *Electrocardiography (ECG).*
Electrocardiography (ECG). See also *P waves; QRS complex; ST
    segment; T waves.*
  esophageal, for P wave identification, 87–88
  evolution of changes in MI on, 124, *125–129*
  exercise, for evaluation of chest pain, 74
  for evaluation of acute aortic regurgitation (AR), 138
  for evaluation of ankylosing spondylitis, 711
  for evaluation of aortic regurgitation (AR), 137, 138
  for evaluation of aortic stenosis (AS), 135
  for evaluation of chest pain, 72, 74
  for evaluation of coma, 757
  for evaluation of congestive heart failure, 82
  for evaluation of dyspnea, 157
  for evaluation of infectious endocarditis, 587–588
  for evaluation of mitral regurgitation, 140, 141
  for evaluation of mitral stenosis (MS), 139
  for evaluation of pulmonary embolism, 195
  for evaluation of pulmonic regurgitation (PR), 149
  for evaluation of pulmonic stenosis (PS), 149
  for evaluation of respiratory failure, 170
  for evaluation of scleroderma, 736
  for evaluation of syncope, 765

Electrocardiography (ECG) (*continued*)
    for evaluation of tricuspid regurgitation (TR), 144
    for evaluation of tricuspid stenosis (TS), 143
    hyperkalemia evaluation and, 45
    in myocardial infarction, 121t, 121–128
    in transmural versus subendocardial infarction, 116
    left ventricular infarction on, *126*
    markers for location of infarct on, 129t
    posterior infarction on, *128*
    reciprocal changes in MI on, 124
    signal averaged, for evaluation of syncope, 766
Electrodiagnostic tests, for evaluation of myopathy, 809
Electroencephalogram (EEG), for evaluation of coma, 759
    for evaluation of headache, 790, 790t
Electrolyte disorders, 39–47
Electrolyte levels, in coma, 757
Electromyography (EMG), for evaluation of myopathy, 807
    for evaluation of PM/DM, 731
Electrophysiologic testing, for evaluation of syncope, 766
ELISA. See *Enzyme-linked immunosorbent assay (ELISA)*.
EM. See *Erythema migrans (EM)*.
Emboli, cholesterol, 745
Embolism, pulmonary (PE), 193–197
    renal damage caused by, 230
Emery-Dreifuss dystrophy, 810t
EMG. See *Electromyography (EMG)*.
Emphysema, 189–190
    and chronic obstructive pulmonary disease (COPD), 191
    associated with antitrypsin deficiency and hepatomegaly, 830
    in hypersensitivity pneumonitis, 212
Empyema, laboratory findings in, 165t
Encephalitis, 635–638
    differential diagnosis of, 635t
    HIV, 646
    in infectious mononucleosis, 670
    viral, 635–638
Encephalopathy, hepatic, in carnitine deficiency, 809
    in chronic hepatitis, 854
    HIV, 646
    subacute arteriosclerotic, 778
    with mitochondrial myopathies, 809
Endocarditis, bacterial, with nephritic syndrome, 259
    CSF parameters in, 631t
    culture-negative, causes of, 586t
    early prosthetic valve, etiology of, *582*
    fungal, 584
    infective, 579–588
        associated with prosthetic valves, 579–580
        classification of, 580–584
        culture-negative, 584
        diagnostic approach to, 588
        differential diagnosis of, 584–586, 584t
        epidemiology of, 579–584
        gram-negative, 584
        intravenous drug use-associated, 579
        mediators of immune response in, 587t
        native valve involvement with, 579
        physical findings in, 585t
        symptoms of, 585t
        types of, 579–584
    IVDU-associated, 579, *581*
    late prosthetic valve, etiology of, *582*
    native valve, etiology of, *580*
    organisms causing, 537t

Endocarditis (*continued*)
    subacute bacterial, laboratory evaluation of, 740t
    versus bacteremia, in *Staphylococcus aureus* infection, 584t
Endocervicitis, 599
Endocrine disorders, amenorrhea caused by, 443
    and constipation, 15t, 17
    arthralgias or myalgias in, 677t
    malabsorption associated with, 314t
    mediastinal masses associated with, 181t
    myopathy associated with, 809
    polyneuropathies associated with, 806
Endoscopic retrograde cholangiopancreatography (ERCP), for
            evaluation of pancreatitis, 343
    hyperamylasemia following, 340
Endoscopy, for evaluation of colorectal cancer, 334
    for evaluation of esophageal diseases, 298
    for evaluation of gastrointestinal bleeding, 294
    for evaluation of varices, 295
    small bowel, for evaluation of chronic GI bleeding, 296
Energy expenditure factors, 521t
Entamoeba histolytica, diarrhea caused by, in HIV-positive patients,
            643
Enteritis, radiation, and malabsorption, 312t
    regional. See *Crohn's disease.*
Enteroclysis, for evaluation of GI bleeding, 296
Enterococci, and endocarditis, 583
Enteropathy, AIDS-associated, diarrhea caused by, 643–644
Enterotoxins, and infectious diarrhea, 615
Enteroviruses, meningitis caused by, 632–633
Enthesopathy, in ankylosing spondylitis, 710
Environmental factors, in asthma, 186
    in breast cancer, 412
    in IIBD, 324
    in lymphadenopathy, 375
Enzyme analysis, cardiac, 72
    for evaluation of AIDS, 641
Enzyme-linked immunosorbent assay (ELISA), for evaluation of
            Lyme disease, 667
Eosinophils, urinary, with hematuria, 233
Epicondylitis, lateral and medial (tennis and golfer's elbow), 680
Epidural disease, identification of, in spinal cord compression, 408
Epidural metastases, sites of, 406t
Epiglottitis, as a complication of pharyngitis, 555
Epilepsy, accompanying multiple sclerosis, 800
Epistaxis, and apparent gastrointestinal bleeding, 293
EPO. See *Erythropoietin (EPO).*
Epstein-Barr virus, and lymphomas, 391
    antibodies to, in infectious mononucleosis, 671
    hepatitis associated with, 838
    infectious mononucleosis caused by, 668–671, 669t
    pharyngitis with infection by, 555
ERCP. See *Endoscopic retrograde cholangiopancreatography
            (ERCP).*
Ergotism, 746
Erysipelas, clinical features of, 591
Erysipeloid, clinical features of, 592
Erythema, in gout, 702
Erythema migrans (EM), in Lyme disease, 666
Erythema nodosum, sarcoidosis associated with, 220
Erythrasma, clinical features of, 592
Erythrocyte sedimentation rate (ESR), in idiopathic pulmonary
            fibrosis, 214
    in IIBD, 327
    in multiple myeloma, 400

Erythrocyte sedimentation rate (ESR) (*continued*)
  in polyarthritis, 690
  in polymyalgia rheumatica, 679
  in vasculitis, 739
Erythrocytosis, 355–360
  classification of, 356t
Erythroid colony-forming units (CFU-E), for diagnosis of
     polycythemia vera, 359
Erythropoietin (EPO), levels of, 355
  in polycythemia vera, 359
Escape beats, in nonparoxysmal supraventricular arrhythmias, 100
Escape rhythm, 86
Escherichia coli, diarrhea caused by, 617t, 618t
  foodborne disease caused by, 616t
  meningitis caused by, 630t
Esophageal diseases, 297–299
  differential diagnosis of, 297–298, 298t
Esophageal lye stricture, and risk of malignancy, 304t
Esophagitis, Bernstein test for evaluation of, 298
  chest pain caused by, 67t
Esophagogastroduodenoscopy (EGD), for evaluation of esophageal
     diseases, 298
  for evaluation of gastric and duodenal disease, 301–302
  for evaluation of gastrointestinal bleeding, 294
  for evaluation of UGI disorders, 303t
Esophagoscopy, for evaluation of mediastinal masses, 182
Esophagram, for evaluation of mediastinal masses, 182, 183
ESR. See *Erythrocyte sedimentation rate (ESR)*.
Estrogens, and pulmonary embolism, 194t
  exposure to, and breast cancer, 412
Ethical considerations, and patient's values, 4
  and treatment decisions, 4
Ethmoiditis, clinical features of, 557
Ethylene glycol, ingestion of, and acid formation, 52
  toxicity of, 875
Euthyroid syndrome, tests for, 464t
  versus hypothyroidism, 465
Evoked potential studies, for evaluation of multiple sclerosis, 801, 802,
    803
Exercise, hematuria caused by, 230, 232
Extragonadal germ cell tumors, and alpha-fetoprotein (αFP), 429
  and beta-human chorionic gonadotropin (βHCG), 429
Extrinsic asthma, definition of, 185
Exudates, 162–163, *163*, 165t
  in pleural effusions, 162
Eyes, involvement of, in Lyme disease, 665t
  in sarcoidosis, 219t

Fabry's disease, 253t
  prolonged fever accompanying, 537t
Facial migraine, 786
False-negative rate, of Tuttle test, 299
False-positive rate, of triolein breath test for fat malabsorption, 318
  of Tuttle test, 299
Familial disorders. See also *Congenital* entries; *Inherited disorders*.
Familial hyperlipidemia, 513, 513t
Familial hyphosphatemic rickets, osteomalacia caused by, 458
Familial hypogonadotropic hypogonadism, amenorrhea caused by,
    444t
Fanconi's syndrome, 246, 365t
  and risk of leukemia, 383
  osteomalacia associated with, 458

Farmer's lung, 210, 211t
Fasciitis, following skin infections, 593
Fatigue, 9–13
  and symptoms of multiple sclerosis, 800
  associated with hepatitis, 836
  clinical features of, 11–12
  differential diagnosis of, 11t
  in infectious mononucleosis, 669
  in Lyme disease, 665t
  in systemic lupus erythematosus (SLE), 719t
  of ventilatory muscles, in COPD, 190
Fecal fat measurement, for evaluation of malabsorption, 316–317
Fecal occult blood test (FOBT), for evaluation of colorectal cancer,
    333, 335
Feminization, testicular, amenorrhea caused by, 444t
FEV. See *Forced expiratory volume (FEV)*.
Fever, causes of, 537t
  evaluation of, in patients from the tropics, 655–657
  HIV-associated, 644, 647
  in acute sinusitis, 558
  in immunocompromised host, 542–551
  in infectious mononucleosis, 670t
  in pneumonia, 562–563
  in systemic lupus erythematosus (SLE), 719t
  infections as source of, in immunocompromised host, 542
  patterns of, in malaria, 656
Fever of unknown origin (FUO), 533–540
  caused by tuberculosis, 575
  clinical features of, 536
  definition of, 533
  diagnostic approach to, 538t, 540
  differential diagnosis of, 533–536
  percentage of cases of, by diagnosis, 534t–535t
  work-up of patient with, 539t
Fiberoptic bronchoscopy, for sarcoidosis diagnosis, 223
Fibrin degradation, and secondary hemostasis, 364
Fibrinogen, in secondary hemostasis, 364
  inherited deficiency of, 366
  levels of, in nephrotic syndrome, 255
Fibroadenomas, 412
Fibrobullous apical disease, accompanying ankylosing spondylitis,
    711
Fibrocystic disease, versus breast cancer, 413
Fibromuscular dysplasia, hypertension and, 33
Fibromyalgia, diagnostic features of, 675, 678
  differential diagnosis of, 678
  tender point locations for, *678*
Fine needle aspiration (FNA), for evaluation of breast cancer, 415
  for evaluation of prostate carcinoma, 424
Fitz-Hugh-Curtis syndrome, upper abdominal pain in, 858
Fluids, daily requirements for, 521
Fluorescent antibody techniques, for evaluation of malaria, 660
FNA. See *Fine needle aspiration (FNA)*.
FOBT. See *Fecal occult blood test (FOBT)*.
Folate deficiency, and anemia, 351–352
Folliculitis, clinical features of, 592
  definition of, 590
Follow-up, as diagnostic procedure, 7–8
  for fatigue, 11
  JNC recommendations for, in hypertension, 33t
Foodborne infections, 615
  organisms causing, 616t
Forced expiratory volume (FEV), for asthma evaluation, 187
  for evaluation of COPD, 191

Forssman antibody, 671
αFP. See *Alpha-fetoprotein (αFP)*.
Framingham study, 32
FRC. See *Functional residual capacity (FRC)*.
Free thyroid index (FT$_4$I), 461
Friedreich's ataxia, simulating MI, on ECG, 121t
FT$_4$I. See *Free thyroid index (FT$_4$I)*.
Functional residual capacity (FRC), for evaluation of COPD, 191
Fungal disease, acute hypersensitivity pneumonitis caused by, 210
   glucocorticoid deficiency associated with, 479
   septic arthritis associated with, 624
FUO. See *Fever of unknown origin (FUO)*.
Furuncles, clinical features of, 592
   definition of, 590

G6PD. See *Glucose-6-phosphate dehydrogenase (G6PD)*.
Galactorrhea, and hirsutism, 439
Galactorrhea-amenorrhea syndromes, 444t
Gallbladder diseases, 857–861
   clinical features of, 858–859
   diagnostic approach to, 860–861
   differential diagnosis of, 858
   epidemiology of, 857–858
   laboratory studies for evaluation of, 858–859
Gallium-67 scan, for diagnosis of sarcoidosis, 221
   for evaluation of PCP, 650
Gallstones, 338, 857, 858
Gammaglutamyl transferase (GGT), levels of, in alcoholism, 816, 816t
Gardner's syndrome, 331t
Gastrectomy, malabsorption following, 312t
Gastric acidity, as risk factor for infectious diarrhea, 615
Gastric disease, 300–302
Gastric emptying, drugs affecting, 302
Gastric fluid, for evaluation of tuberculosis, 577
Gastric lavage, for evaluation of gastrointestinal bleeding, 294, 295
Gastric outlet obstruction, 301
Gastric resection, and risk of malignancy, 304t
Gastric ulcer, radiographic imaging for evaluation of, 300
Gastritis, chronic atrophic, and risk of malignancy, 304t
   diagnosis of, 300–301, 301t
Gastroenteritis, eosinophilic, and malabsorption, 311t
Gastroenterocolic fistulas, radiographic imaging for diagnosis of, 301
Gastrointestinal disorders, bleeding in, 62t, 289–296
   differential diagnosis of, 289–291, 289t
   chest pain caused by, 60t, 74–75
   in scleroderma, 734
   upper, 297–304
Gastrointestinal (GI) tract, blood from, in hemoptysis, 158
   diseases of, and constipation, 16t
Gastroparesis, radiographic imaging for diagnosis of, 301
Gaucher's disease, 374
   arthralgias or myalgias in, 677t
   hepatomegaly associated with, 830
GDM. See *Gestational diabetes mellitus (GDM)*.
Gender, and atherosclerotic vascular disease, 33
   and chronic lymphocytic leukemia, 382
   and chronic obstructive pulmonary disease (COPD), 190
   and creatinine excretion, 259
   and DVT incidence, 198
   and liver damage from alcoholism, 815
   and mitral stenosis (MS), 138

Gender (*continued*)
    and nephrotic syndrome, 252
    and osteoporosis, 455t
    and pretest likelihood of coronary artery disease, 73t
    and prevalence of fibromyalgia, 675
    and risk for ankylosing spondylitis, 710
    and risk for autoimmune hepatitis, 852
    and risk for gallstones, 857
    and risk for Goodpasture's syndrome, 208
    and risk for gout, 701
    and risk for malignant thyroid nodules, 470t
    and risk for myocardial infarction (MI), 117
    and risk for pituitary Cushing's syndrome, 473
    and risk for polyarthritides, 691t
    and risk for polymyalgia rheumatica, 679
    and risk for polymyositis (PM), 728
    and risk for pseudohypoparathyroidism, 496
    and risk for Reiter's syndrome, 712
    and risk for sarcoidosis, 217
    and risk for scleroderma, 733
    and risk for spondyloarthropathies, 709
    and risk for systemic lupus erythematosus (SLE), 718
    and risk for Takayasu's arteritis, 738
    and risk for urinary tract infections, 612
    and urinary incontinence, 28
    and urolithiasis, 265
Genetic factors. See also *Hereditary disorders.*
    in breast cancer, 412
    in migraine, 784
    in multiple sclerosis, 800
Genitourinary system, involvement in Lyme disease, 665t
Gestational diabetes mellitus (GDM), 499
    and perinatal morbidity, 504
    diagnostic criteria for, 506t–507t
GGT. See *Gammaglutamyl transferase (GGT).*
Ghon complex, 576
GI. See *Gastrointestinal (GI) tract.*
Giardia lamblia, diarrhea caused by, 617t
    in HIV-positive patients, 643–644
Gilbert's syndrome, 287
    jaundice in, 840
    unconjugated hyperbilirubinemia caused by, 822
Glanzmann's thrombasthenia, 366t
    platelet aggregation studies for evaluation of, 362
Glomerulitis, in Wegener's granulomatosis, 215
Glomerulonephritis (GN), 257–263. See also *Renal failure.*
    as cause of chronic renal failure (CRF), 245–246
    as complication of pharyngitis, 554
    crescentic, 262
    drugs causing, 231t
    following skin infections, 593
    in Goodpasture's syndrome, 208, 209
    in systemic lupus erythematosus (SLE), 719–720
    in Wegener's granulomatosis, 215
    PAN associated with, 741
    postinfectious, with intrarenal ARF, 240
    rapidly progressive (RPGN), 262
    urinalysis in, 241t
Glomerulopathy, definition of, 257
Glucocorticoid deficiency, 479–483
    clinical features of, 480–481
    differential diagnosis of, 479
Glucocorticoid excess. See also *Cushing's syndrome.*
    in osteoporosis, 453

Glucose, and pleural effusions, 166
  plasma, for diagnosis of diabetes mellitus, 505
    normal values for, 504t
Glucose intolerance. See also *Impaired glucose tolerance (IGT)*.
  in chronic pancreatitis, 340
  types of, 500t–501t
  with chronic renal failure (CRF), 248
Glucose tolerance test, oral, 509t
Glucose-6-phosphatase deficiency, gout associated with, 705t
Glucose-6-phosphate dehydrogenase (G6PD), level of, and treatment
    for malaria, 658
Glucuronyl transferase, deficiency of, in Gilbert's disease, 822
  role of, in bilirubin metabolism, 822t
Glutamic oxalacetic transferase, serum concentration of, following
    MI, *130*
Gluten-sensitive enteropathy, and malabsorption, 310t
Glycosuria, in nephrotic syndrome, 255
GN. See *Glomerulonephritis (GN)*.
Goiter, 463t
  definition of, 461
  hypothyroidism caused by, 462t
  toxic multinodular (MNG), 469, 470–471
    epidemiology of, 468
    hyperthyroidism with, 467
Gonadal dysgenesis, and primary amenorrhea, 443
Gonadal failure, idiopathic adrenal failure as risk factor for, 479
Gonadal resistance, amenorrhea caused by, 443
Gonadotropin, for evaluation of amenorrhea, 450–451
Gonococci, infection by, and risk of septic arthritis, 623
  sampling sites for culture of, 596t
Gonorrhea, 594–595
Goodpasture's syndrome, 159t, 208–209, 231t
  with nephritic syndrome, 262
Gottron's papules, in dermatomyositis (DM), 730
Gout, 690, 701–704
  and hypertension treatment, 35
  arthralgias or myalgias in, 676t
  diagnostic approach to, 703–704, 704t
  differential diagnosis of, 703
  disorders and physiological states in, 705t
  epidemiology of, 691t
  laboratory features of, 694t
  mechanisms underlying, 704
  physical signs of, 693t
  radiographic findings in, 703t
  stages of, 701–702
  symptoms of, 692t
  versus osteoarthritis, 699
Graft versus host disease (GVHD), fever associated with,
    543
Granulocytopenia, associated with leukemia, 384
Granuloma inguinale, 601
Granulomas, noncaseating, 217, 218t
Granulomatosis, allergic, with nephritic syndrome, 261
Granulomatous disorders, and FUO, 535t
  hepatomegaly associated with, 830
  ileocolitis with. See *Crohn's disease*.
Graves' disease, 462t, 463t, 467
  clinical features of, 468–469
  diagnosis of, with TSH, 465
  epidemiology of, 468
Gray platelet syndrome, 366t
Guillain-Barré syndrome, and respiratory failure, 168t
  in infectious mononucleosis, 670

Guillain-Barré syndrome (*continued*)
    nerve biopsy for evaluation of, 805
    polyneuropathies in, 806
GVHD. See *Graft versus host disease (GVHD)*.

HACEK organisms, 587
    and endocarditis, 583
Haemophilus influenzae, clinical features of skin infection by, 591
    meningitis caused by, 629, 630, 630t, 632
    pneumonia caused by, 566–567
Hair. See also *Hirsutism*.
    growth patterns of, in normal women, 438t
    types of, 436t
Hamartomas, gastrointestinal bleeding associated with, 293
Hamman-Rich syndrome, 213
Hampton's sign, for evaluation of gastric ulcers, 300
Handedness, as risk factor for osteoarthritis, 697
Harris-Benedict equation, for calculation of daily calorie
    requirement, 519–520
Hashimoto's thyroiditis, 462t, 463t, 466–467
    antibodies present in, 467
βHCG. See *Beta-human chorionic gonadotropin (βHCG)*.
HD. See *Hodgkin's disease (HD)*.
Headache, 784–791
    acute, algorithm for evaluation of, *788*
    chronic, algorithm for evaluation of, *789*
    classification of, 785t
    cluster, 787
    cold stimulus and, *788*
    diagnostic approach to, 789–791
    evaluation of, by imaging, 791t
      in HIV–positive patient, 645–647
    frequency of abnormal findings in, 790t
    in MPS, 686
    temporal classification of, 786t
    temporal patterns of, *785*
    tension-type, 787
Heart. See also *Atrial* entries; *Cardiac* entries; *Congestive heart
      failure; Endocarditis; Mitral valve; Murmur; Myocardial
      infarction (MI); Ventricular* entries.
    hemolysis caused by prosthetic valves in, 352
    Lyme disease involving, 665t, 666
    sarcoidosis involving, 219t
    valvular disease of, 134–151
Heart block, 86
Heart tones, in aortic regurgitation (AR), 136, 138
    in aortic stenosis (AS), 135
    in mitral regurgitation (MR), 140, 141
    in mitral stenosis (MS), 139
    in mitral valve prolapse (MVP), 142
    in pulmonic regurgitation (PR), 149
    in pulmonic stenosis (PS), 149
    in tricuspid regurgitation (TR), 144
    in tricuspid stenosis (TS), 143
Heberden's nodules, 698
Hematochezia, 295
Hematocrit, in pancreatitis, 342
    increased, algorithm for evaluation of, *359*
      laboratory findings associated with, 357t
Hematologic disorders, in systemic lupus erythematosus (SLE), 720,
    724t
Hematomas, chronic subdural, and dementia, 781
    fever caused by, 543

Hematuria, 229–235
  algorithm for evaluation of, *234*
  causes of, frequency of, 232t
  differential diagnosis of, 231t
  in glomerulonephritis, 257
  in nephritic syndrome, 257–258
  in Wegener's granulomatosis, 215
Hemicrania, chronic paroxysmal, 787
Hemiplegic migraine, 786
Hemochromatosis, and risk for chronic hepatitis, 853
  hepatomegaly associated with, 830
Hemodynamics, and chest pain, 59–61, 62t–63t
Hemoglobin, bilirubin from, 821
Hemoglobinopathy, hematuria and, 231t
Hemolysis, caused by prosthetic heart valves, 352
  mechanical, schistocytes as indicator of, 350
Hemolytic anemia. See *Anemia, hemolytic.*
Hemophilias, 365–366
Hemoptysis, 158–160
  causes of, 159t
  in DVT, 201t
  in Goodpasture's syndrome, 208
  massive, assessment of, 160
    causes of, 159t
  with mediastinal masses, 183
Hemorrhage, associated with erythrocytosis, 356
Hemorrhoids, as cause of gastrointestinal bleeding, 291
Hemostasis, 361–373
  common disorders of, laboratory findings in, 368t
  primary, algorithm for evaluation of, *370*
    differential diagnosis of, 364–365
    laboratory findings in, 362–363
  secondary, algorithm for evaluation of, *371*
    differential diagnosis of, 365–367, 369
    laboratory evaluation of, 363–364
Henderson-Hasselbalch equation, 48
Henoch-Schönlein purpura, 743–744
  IgA level in, 740t
  with nephritic syndrome, 259, 261–262
Hepatitis, alcoholic, 829, 852
  chronic, 829, 837–838, 852–856
  diagnosis of, 847t
  lupoid, 852–853
  non-A, non-B, 833
  toxic, 839–840
  viral, 833–851
    as cause of jaundice, 823–824
    chronic, 837–838
    clinical features of, 836–838
    diagnostic approach to, 844, 846–850
    differential diagnosis of, 838–840
    epidemiology of, 834–836
    laboratory tests for evaluation of, 840–844
    organisms causing, 833
    simplified diagnosis of, 848t
    symptoms in, 837t
Hepatitis viruses, epidemiology of, 834–835, 836
  laboratory tests for, 841, *841, 843,* 844, 844t–845t
    interpretation of, 848t–849t
  serologic course of, *842, 846*
Hepatomas, associated with hemochromatosis, 853
Hepatomegaly, 827–832
  associated with hemochromatosis, 854
  causes of, 828t–829t

Hepatomegaly (*continued*)
  clinical manifestations of, 830–831
  diagnostic approach to, 832
  differential diagnosis of, 827–830
  in infectious mononucleosis, 670
  in Q fever, 838–839
  laboratory studies for evaluation of, 831–832
Hereditary disorders. See also *Congenital* entries; *Familial* entries.
  anemia associated with, 349
  colorectal cancer associated with, 331t
  gastrointestinal bleeding associated with, 292
  nephrotic syndrome in, 253t
  of bilirubin metabolism, 822
  polyneuropathies associated with, 806
Hermaphroditism, amenorrhea caused by, 444t
Herpes genitalis, 603–604
Herpes simplex infection, clinical features of genital ulcers in, 602t
  diarrhea caused by, in HIV-positive patients, 643–644
  hepatic necrosis in infection by, 838
  pulmonary/esophageal, as AIDS indicator, 640t
Herpes simplex virus type 1 (HSV-1), encephalitis caused by,
      637–638
Herpes simplex virus type 2 (HSV-2), meningitis caused by,
      633–634
Herpes zoster, 71
  chest pain caused by, 60t
Heterophil agglutination test, reaction to, in infectious
      mononucleosis, 670
Heterophil antibodies, detection of, in infectious mononucleosis, 671
Hiatal hernia, as cause of gastrointestinal bleeding, 290
  chest pain caused by, 68t
Hirschsprung's disease, and constipation, 17
Hirsutism, 435–442
  algorithm for diagnosis of, *441*
  associated with amenorrhea, 447
  causes of, 436t
  diagnostic approach to, 440–442
  epidemiology of, 435
  idiopathic, 435, 437, 439t
  with adrenocortical carcinoma, 474
Histoplasma capsulatum, and respiratory symptoms in HIV-positive
      patients, 647
Histoplasmosis, pneumonia associated with, 571t
HIV. See *Human immunodeficiency virus (HIV).*
Hodgkin's disease (HD), 389
  immunostaining for evaluation of, 428
  risk of AML following treatment for, 383
Homans' sign, 201t
Homosexuality, and risk for hepatitis B and C, 852
  and risk for infectious diarrhea, 616
Hormones, abnormal levels of, in adrenocortical carcinoma, 474
  and prostate carcinoma, 420
  hirsutism caused by, 437
  levels of, and pituitary tumors, with amenorrhea, 447
Horner's syndrome, 179
Horton's histamine headache, 787
HPO. See *Hypothalamic-pituitary-ovarian (HPO) axis.*
HPT. See *Hyperparathyroidism (HPT).*
HSV-1. See *Herpes simplex virus type 1 (HSV-1).*
HSV-2. See *Herpes simplex virus type 2 (HSV-2).*
HTLV. See *Human T-cell leukemia virus (HTLV).*
HTLV-1. See *Human T-cell lymphotrophic virus, type 1 (HTLV-1).*
Human immunodeficiency virus (HIV). See also *Acquired
      immunodeficiency syndrome (AIDS).*

Human immunodeficiency virus (HIV) (*continued*)
  and lymphadenopathy, 392
  antibody test for, in evaluation of dementia, 783
  arthritis and skin disease in, 714
  CDC staging system for illness associated with, 639
  dementia associated with infection by, 781
  ELISA and Western blot analysis for identification of, 641
  infectious diarrhea associated with, 616
  pneumonia associated with, 572t
  prolonged fever in infections with, 533
  related conditions associated with gastrointestinal bleeding and,
      292
  tuberculosis associated with, 575
  vasculitis associated with, 745
Human T-cell leukemia virus (HTLV), 383
  lymphomas associated with, 391
Human T-cell lymphotrophic virus, type 1 (HLTV-1), myelopathy
      associated with, 799
Huntington's disease, 778–779
Hybridization probes, for evaluation of pneumonia, 566
Hydatid cyst, solitary pulmonary nodules (SPNs) caused by,
      172t
Hydrocephalus, dementia in, 779–780
17-Hydroxyprogesterone (17-OHP), levels of, and evaluation of
      hirsutism, 440
Hyperamylasemia, causes of, 338t
  following endoscopic retrograde cholangiopancreatography
      (ERCP), 340
  in trauma-induced pancreatitis, 339
Hyperbilirubinemia. See also *Jaundice*.
  in viral hepatitis, 833
Hypercalcemia, 490–494
  associated with urolithiasis, 266
  definition of, 490
  diagnostic approach to, 493–494
  differential diagnosis of, 491–493, 491t
  hypertonic hyponatremia in, 40
  in multiple myeloma, 397, 400
  intrarenal acute renal failure caused by, 238t
  pancreatitis associated with, 340
Hypercalciuria, and urolithiasis, 267t–269t
Hypercapnia, causes of, 168t
  in acute respiratory failure, 167, 168
  in ARDS, 206
  in chronic obstructive pulmonary disease (COPD), 190
Hypercortisolism, manifestations of, 475t
Hypergammaglobulinemia, associated with CLL, 385
  polyclonal, in systemic lupus erythematosus (SLE), 726
Hyperglycemia, hypernatremia in, 42
  in pancreatitis, 342
Hypergonadotropism, amenorrhea caused by, 443
Hyperkalemia, 45–46
  in acute renal failure, 238t, 244
  in glucocorticoid deficiency, 481
  in periodic paralysis (PP), 808
  intrarenal acute renal failure caused by, 238t
  simulating MI, on ECG, 121t
Hyperlipidemia, 512–515
  definition of, 512
  diagnostic approach to, 515
  etiology of, 512–513, 513t
  genetic classification of, 513t
  hyponatremia with, 39
  in nephrotic syndrome, 255

Hyperlipidemia (*continued*)
  with chronic renal failure (CRF), 248
  xanthomas mimicking tendinitis in, 680
Hypernatremia, 42–44
  blood-urea nitrogen (BUN) test for, 43
Hyperoxaluria, and urolithiasis, 269t–270t
Hyperparathyroidism (HPT), and urolithiasis, 267t
  hypercalcemia caused by, 491–492, 491t
  osteoporosis caused by, 453
  secondary, in renal osteodystrophy, 249
Hyperphosphatemia, in renal osteodystrophy, 249
Hypersensitivity, 218. See also *Allergies*.
  carotid sinus, and syncope, 766–767
  chronic interstitial pneumonitis caused by, 208–213
Hypersensitivity vasculitis, 743–744
Hypersplenism, anemia associated with, 349
Hypertension, 32–38
  as contraindication to thrombolytic therapy, 120t
  frequency of, in general population, 34t
  hypokalemia and, 44
  in acute respiratory failure, 168
  in nephritic syndrome, 258
  portal, as cause of gastrointestinal bleeding, 289
  secondary, 36–38
  with pheochromocytoma, 485
Hyperthyroidism, and dementia, 780
  and watery diarrhea, 24
  congenital, prevalence of, 466
  osteoporosis caused by, 453
  tests for, 464t
Hypertrichosis, causes of, 436t
  definition of, 435
Hypertriglyceridemia, familial, 513t
  pancreatitis associated with, 340, 342
Hyperuricemia, and gout, 702
  disorders and physiological states with, 705t
Hyperventilation, clinical features of, 793t
Hypervolemia, hypernatremia in, 43
  hyponatremia in, 41, 42
Hypoadrenalism, hyponatremia and, 40
Hypoalbuminemia, hypocalcemia associated with, 495
  in nephrotic syndrome, 255
Hypocalcemia, 494–497
  diagnostic approach to, 497
  differential diagnosis of, 495–497, 495t
  in nephrotic syndrome, 255
  in pancreatitis, 342
  in renal osteodystrophy, 249
  postsurgical, 496
  symptoms of, 494–495
Hypoglycemia, and HIV, 645
  in glucocorticoid deficiency, 481
Hypokalemia, 44–45
  in chronic renal failure (CRF), 246
  in IIBD, 327
  in periodic paralysis (PP), 808
Hypomagnesemia, hypocalcemia associated with, 496
Hyponatremia, 39–42
  and congestive heart failure, 83
  in glucocorticoid deficiency, 481
  in multiple myeloma, 400
Hypoparathyroidism, adrenal failure as risk factor for, 479
  idiopathic, hypocalcemia associated with, 495–496

Hypoperfusion, cerebral, and syncope, 761
Hypophosphatemia, and urolithiasis, 268t
  osteomalacia caused by, 458
Hypotension, in acute respiratory failure, 168
  transaminase levels in, 840
Hypothalamic-pituitary-ovarian (HPO) axis, hirsutism as
      perturbation of, 435
Hypothalamus, disorders of, and amenorrhea, 445t, 448
Hypothetico-deductive method, 3
Hypothyroidism, 465–467
  and dementia, 780
  classification of, 463t
  definition of, 465
  diagnostic approach to, 471
  following treatment for Graves' disease, 466
  goitrous, 463t
  hyponatremia and, 40
  idiopathic adrenal failure as risk factor for, 479
  tests for, 464t
Hypovolemia, as cause of acute renal failure, 236
  hypernatremia in, 42
  hyponatremia and, 40
  hypotonic hyponatremia and, 41
Hypoxanthine-guanine phosphoribosyl transferase, gout associated
      with, 705t
Hypoxemia, chronic, 191
    in adult respiratory distress syndrome (ARDS), 204, 206
    in chronic obstructive pulmonary disease (COPD), 190
    in pancreatitis, 342
    physiologic causes of, 167
    with chronic bronchitis, 561–562
Hypoxia, causes of, 169t
  in pneumonia, 563
  in respiratory failure, 169
  symptoms of, associated with respiratory failure, 168
Hysterectomy, 444t

IBD. See *Inflammatory bowel disease (IBD)*.
Ideal body weight (IBW), and basal energy expenditure (BEE),
      519–520
  for adults, 520t
Idiopathic adrenal failure, 479
Idiopathic hirsutism (IH), 439t
  defined, 435, 437
Idiopathic panhypopituitarism, amenorrhea caused by, 444t, 448
IE. See *Endocarditis, infective*.
IFA. See *Indirect fluorescent antibody (IFA) test*.
IGT. See *Impaired glucose tolerance (IGT)*.
IH. See *Idiopathic hirsutism (IH)*.
IM. See *Infectious mononucleosis (IM)*.
Imaging techniques. See also *Computed tomography (CT); Magnetic
      resonance imaging (MRI); Ultrasound; X-ray*.
  for evaluation of Cushing's syndrome, 477, 477t
  for evaluation of hepatomegaly, 831–832
  for evaluation of jaundice, 824
  for evaluation of osteomalacia, 460
  for musculoskeletal pain, 687–688
Immunocompromised host, definition of, 542
  fever in, 542–551
    diagnostic approach to, 550–551
    laboratory studies for evaluation of, 548–550
  infections in, 544t–545t
    frequency of, by type, 546t–547t

Immunocompromised host (*continued*)
    pneumonia in, 572t
        caused by *Staphylococcus aureus*, 569
        microbiologic diagnosis of, 566
    symptom absence in, 543, 548
    symptoms of meningitis in, 629
Immunocytochemistry, for evaluation of cancer of unknown primary
    site (CUPS), 427–428
Immunodeficiency, biopsy for evaluation of, 320
    malabsorption with, 313t
Immunoelectrophoresis, for evaluation of multiple myeloma, 401
Immunofluorescence screening assay, for evaluation of systemic
    lupus erythematosus (SLE), 725
Immunofluorescent staining, Goodpasture's syndrome diagnosis
    with, 209
Immunoglobulins, in MGUS, and subsequent malignant disease, 396
    in multiple myeloma, 396
    markers in chronic lymphocytic leukemia, 382
Immunologic disorders, in PM/DM, 731
    in systemic lupus erythematosus (SLE), 724t
Immunologic reactions, as cause of chronic pulmonary infiltrates,
    209t
    chronic interstitial pneumonitis caused by, 208–213
    in idiopathic inflammatory bowel disease, 324
    in nephritic syndrome, 261
    in sarcoidosis, 218
Immunoregulation disorders, associated with lymphomas, 391
Immunosuppression. See also *Immunocompromised host*.
    and activation of tuberculosis, 574
    and risk of infectious diarrhea, 616, 624
    drug-induced, and risk of malignant lymphomas, 391
    sinusitis associated with, 557
Impaired glucose tolerance (IGT), 499. See also *Glucose
    intolerance*.
    diagnostic criteria for, 506t–507t
    versus diabetes mellitus, 508–509
Impedance plethysmography (IPG), for evaluation of acute venous
    thrombosis, 201
Impetigo, clinical features of, 591–592
    definition of, 590
Impotence, in prostate carcinoma, 421
Impulse formation and conduction (heart), 86
Incontinence. See *Urinary incontinence*.
Indirect fluorescent antibody (IFA) test, for evaluation of Lyme
    disease, 667
Indium-111 scans, white cell, for evaluation of osteomyelitis, 627
Infections, dementia associated with, 780–781
    polyneuropathies associated with, 806
    solitary pulmonary nodules (SPNs) caused by, 172t
    susceptibility to, in nephrotic syndrome, 254
    vasculitis associated with, 744–745
Infectious mononucleosis (IM), 668–671
    diagnostic approach to, 671
    differential diagnosis of, 668–669
    epidemiology of, 668
    hepatitis associated with, 844
    heterophil-negative, 669, 669t
    symptoms of, 670t
Infective endocarditis (IE), 579–588
Inflammatory bowel disease (IBD), 22
    and risk of colorectal cancer, 330
    arthritis associated with, 715
    fatty liver associated with, 829–830

Influenza, pneumonia caused by, 570
Inherited disorders. See also *Congenital* entries; *Familial* entries; *Genetic factors; Hereditary disorders.*
   and risk for alcoholism, 813
Injury, and risk of DVT, 199t
Insulin. See also *Diabetes mellitus.*
   deficiency of, and hyperkalemia, 45
      and ketoacidosis, 52
   hypokalemia associated with, 44
Insulin-resistance syndromes, and hirsutism, 437
International Headache Society, 785t
Interstitial pneumonitis, chronic, 208–215
   lymphocytic (LIP), 214
Intraductal fibroadenomas, 412
Intravenous drug use, and risk of hepatitis B and C, 852
   and risk of septic arthritis, 623
   endocarditis associated with, 579, *581*
   osteomyelitis associated with, 624
   pneumonia associated with, 572t
Intravenous drug users, skin infections in, 591
Intravenous pyelogram (IVP), for evaluation of hematuria, 233
   for evaluation of urolithiasis, 273, 274–275
Intraventricular conduction defects (IVCD), 112–115, *112–115*
Intrinsic asthma, definition of, 185
Iodine-131 thyroid scan, for evaluation of mediastinal masses, 182
   for evaluation of thyroid disease, 465
IPG. See *Impedance plethysmography (IPG).*
Iron, serum levels of, and ferritin levels, in chronic hepatitis, 855
Iron deficiency, anemia due to, 351
   for evaluation of colorectal cancer, 332
Iron storage disorders. See also *Hemochromatosis.*
   hepatomegaly associated with, 830
Irritable bowel syndrome, 19, 284–285, 306
   and constipation, 15
Ischemic heart disease, evaluation of, as cause of chest pain, 75–76
Isochromosome, in germ cell tumors, 428
Isospora belli, diarrhea caused by, in HIV-positive patients, 643
IVCD. See *Intraventricular conduction defects (IVCD).*
IVDU. See *Intravenous drug use.*
IVP. See *Intravenous pyelogram (IVP).*

Janeway's lesions, in infectious endocarditis, 585, 585t
Jaundice, 821–825
   benign postoperative, 840
   biochemical classifications of, 821
   cholestatic, 821
   diagnostic approach to, 825, 825t
   differential diagnosis of, 823t
   hepatic, 821
   in acute cholecystitis, 859
   laboratory studies for evaluation of, 824
   obstructive. See *Cholestasis.*
   pathophysiology of, 821–822
   prehepatic, 821
Jodbasedow phenomenon, 462t
Joint aspiration, characteristics of fluid from, 626t
Joints, deformities of, in arthritis, 690, 697
   inflammatory disease of. See *Arthritis.*
   involvement of, in sarcoidosis, 219t
Junctional premature beat (JPB), and nonparoxysmal supraventricular arrhythmias, 100, *100*

Junctional rhythm (junctional escape), and nonparoxysmal
    supraventricular arrhythmias, 100–101, *101*

Kaposi's sarcoma, 292
    as AIDS indicator, 640t
    diarrhea caused by, in HIV-positive patients, 643–644
    in Class IV HIV-associated illness, 639
Karyotype. See also *Chromosomes.*
    in Turner's syndrome, 446
Kayser-Fleischer rings, in Wilson's disease, 854
Keratoderma blennorrhagicum, in Reiter's syndrome, 712
Ketoacidosis, 52
Kidneys. See also *Nephritic syndrome; Nephritis; Nephropathy;
    Nephrotic syndrome; Pyelonephritis; Renal failure.*
    in Lyme disease, 665t
    in sarcoidosis, 219t
    stones in, 264–275
Killip classification, for myocardial infarction (MI), 119t
Korsakoff's syndrome, 780
Kveim-Siltzbach skin test, for diagnosis of sarcoidosis, 217, 220–221

Lactase deficiency, and appetite, 306
    and malabsorption, 309t
Lactate dehydrogenase (LDH), concentration of, in pleural fluid,
    162
    levels of, in myocardial infarction (MI), 128, 130, *130*
        in PCP, 650
        in PM/DM, 731
        in pulmonary alveolar proteinosis, 214–215
Lactic acid, acidosis and, 52
Lactic acidosis, in asthma, 169, 188
Lactose intolerance, and watery diarrhea, 24
LAFB. See *Left anterior fascicular block (LAFB).*
Lambert-Eaton myasthenic syndrome, myopathy in, 808
LAP. See *Leukocyte alkaline phosphatase (LAP).*
Laparotomy, for evaluation of gastrointestinal bleeding, 295, 296
Latex agglutination tests, for evaluation of meningitis, 629
LCIS. See *Lobular carcinoma in situ (LCIS).*
LCM. See *Lymphocytic choriomeningitis (LCM) virus.*
LDH. See *Lactate dehydrogenase (LDH).*
Lead poisoning, basophilic stippling in, 350
Left anterior fascicular block (LAFB), *114*, 114
    QRS complex in, 114
Left posterior fascicular block (LPPB), 114–115, *115*
Left ventricular failure, and hemoptysis, 159
    in scleroderma, 734–735
Left ventricular output, in aortic stenosis, 134
Left-bundle-branch block (LBBB), *113*, 113–114
Legionella pneumophila, diagnostic tests for, 570t
    pneumonia caused by, 569
Legionnaires' disease, 571t
Leptospirosis, hepatitis associated with, 838
    pneumonia associated with, 571t
Leukemia, 381–387
    acute, symptoms of, 384–385
    chronic, 382, 385
    differential diagnosis of, 383–384
    differentiation from other hematologic disorders, 384
    epidemiology of, 382–383
    hepatomegaly associated with, 830
    Rai staging system for evaluation of, 386t
    suggested diagnostic approach to, 387

Leukocyte alkaline phosphatase (LAP), in chronic myelocytic
 leukemia, 382
Leukocytes, fecal, and chronic diarrhea, 19
 in peripheral blood smear, 350
Leukocytosis, in *Legionella pneumophila* infection, 569
 in leukemia, 382
 in pneumonitis, 210
 in Wegener's granulomatosis, 215
Leukoencephalopathy, progressive multifocal, as AIDS indicator,
 640t
Leukopenia, in systemic lupus erythematosus (SLE), 721t, 725
Levine's sign, 119
LGV. See *Lymphogranuloma venereum (LGV)*.
Lhermitte's sign, 407
Libman-Sacks endocarditis, in systemic lupus erythematosus (SLE),
 720
 stroke associated with, 794t–795t
LIP. See *Lymphocytic interstitial pneumonitis (LIP)*.
Lipase, serum, in acute pancreatitis, 342
Lipemia retinalis, hyperlipidemia associated with, 514
Listeria monocytogenes, foodborne disease caused by, 616t
 meningitis caused by, 630t, 632
Liver. See also *Hepatitis; Hepatomegaly; Jaundice, hepatic.*
 abscess of, 839
 damage to, associated with solvent exposure, 875
 enzymes of, in evaluation of coma, 757
 failure of, and hyperkalemia, 46
 fatty, 829
 hemostatic disorders accompanying disorders of, 368t
 insufficiency of, and malabsorption, 308t
 in Lyme disease, 665t
 in sarcoidosis, 219t
 urobilinogen levels in diseases of, 822
Liver disease, and gastrointestinal bleeding, 292, 293
Liver function tests, for evaluation of prostate carcinoma
 metastasis, 422
Liver-spleen scan, for evaluation of hepatomegaly, 832
Lobular carcinoma in situ (LCIS), 411
Locked-in syndrome, definition of, 749
Lofgren's syndrome, 220
Looser's zones, 460
LP. See *Lumbar puncture (LP)*.
Lumbago, in MPS, 686
Lumbar puncture (LP), for evaluation of coma, 758–759
 for evaluation of delirium, 775
 for evaluation of dementia, 781, 783
 for evaluation of headache, 790
 for evaluation of malaria, 658
 for evaluation of meningitis, 634–635
Lung cancer, 192
 and ectopic Cushing's syndrome, 474
 asbestos exposure and, 872
 identification of SPNs as, 171
 oat cell, 40
 squamous cell, hypercalcemia with, 493
Lungs. See also *Pulmonary entries; Pneumonia; Pneumonitis;
 Pneumothorax; Respiratory system.*
 biopsy of, in hypersensitivity pneumonitis, 212
 compliance of, in adult respiratory distress syndrome (ARDS),
 207
 fibrosis of, 204
 function of, and congestive heart failure, 81
 hemoptysis caused by abscess of, 159t
 involvement of, in sarcoidosis, 219t

Lungs (*continued*)
  occupational disorders of, 870t
  scan of, for evaluation of syncope, 766
Lupoid hepatitis, 852–853
Lupus anticoagulant, 725
Lupus erythematosus. See *Systemic lupus erythematosus (SLE)*.
Lyme disease, 662–667
  diagnostic approach to, 667
  differential diagnosis of, 663
  geographic distribution and epidemiology of, 662, *663*
  manifestations of, by stage, 664t–665t
  stages of, 663–666
Lymph nodes, axillary, in breast carcinoma, 429
  involvement of, in sarcoidosis, 219t
Lymphadenopathy, 374–379, 391. See also *Lymphomas*.
  differentiation of, from leukemia, 384
  in Class III HIV-associated illness, 639
  in infectious mononucleosis, 669, 670t
  in systemic lupus erythematosus (SLE), 719t, 720
  neoplastic, 375, 377t
  suggested diagnostic approach to, 378–379
Lymphangiectasia, intestinal, and malabsorption, 310t
Lymphangiography, for evaluation of prostate carcinoma, 423
Lymphatic obstruction, and malabsorption, 310t
Lymphatic system, in Lyme disease, 664t
Lymphocytes, Downy cell, in infectious mononucleosis, 670t
Lymphocytic choriomeningitis (LCM) virus, 633
Lymphocytic interstitial pneumonitis (LIP), 214
Lymphocytosis, in infectious mononucleosis, 670t
Lymphogranuloma venereum (LGV), clinical features of genital
      ulcers in, 601, 602t, 603
Lymphomas, 292, 389–394. See also *Lymphadenopathy*.
  and malabsorption, 310t
  brain, in Class IV HIV-associated illness, 639
  CNS, and HIV, 645
  diagnostic approach to, 393–394
  diarrhea caused by, in HIV-positive patients, 643
  differential diagnosis of, 392
  epidemiology of, 390
  identification of poorly differentiated, 428
  malignant, associated with lymphomatoid granulomatosis, 741
  small bowel, and watery diarrhea, 22
  staging evaluation for, 394, 394t
Lymphomatoid granulomatosis, 741
Lymphopenia, in sarcoidosis, 218

M mode echocardiography, for evaluation of aortic regurgitation
      (AR), 137
  for evaluation of aortic stenosis (AS), 135
  for evaluation of mitral regurgitation, 140, 141
  for evaluation of mitral stenosis (MS), 139
  for evaluation of mitral valve prolapse (MVP), 142
  for evaluation of pulmonic stenosis (PS), 149
  for evaluation of tricuspid regurgitation (TR), 144
  for evaluation of tricuspid stenosis (TS), 143
Macroglobulinemia, in lymphocytic interstitial pneumonitis, 214
Magnetic resonance imaging (MRI), for evaluation of Alzheimer's
      disease, 778
  for evaluation of headache, 790
  for evaluation of hepatomegaly, 832
  for evaluation of HIV-associated fever, 646
  for evaluation of hydrocephalus, 780

Magnetic resonance imaging (MRI) (*continued*)
　for evaluation of mediastinal masses, 181–182
　for evaluation of multi-infarct dementia (MID), 778
　for evaluation of multiple sclerosis, 801, 802
　for evaluation of pheochromocytoma, 488
　for evaluation of prostate carcinoma, 423
　for evaluation of spinal cord compression, 409
　versus computed tomography (CT), for evaluation of headache,
　　791
Malabsorption, 306–321
　algorithm for diagnosis of, *321*
　and hypocalcemia, 496
　classification and clinical findings in, 307t–314t
　in vitamin D-deficient osteomalacia, 457
　signs suggestive of underlying causes, 316
Malaise, associated with hepatitis, 836
　in infectious mononucleosis, 669, 670t
Malar rash, in systemic lupus erythematosus (SLE), 723t
Malaria, 653–660
　and nephrotic syndrome, 254
　CDC advice on, telephone number for, 669
　diagnostic approach to, 660
　differential diagnosis of, 657–658
　epidemiology of, 653–654
　hepatomegaly in, 839
　risk factors for, 656
　symptoms of, 656–657, 657t
Malignancy. See also *Cancer; Neoplasms; Tumors.*
　evaluation of hemoptysis for, 160
　gastrointestinal, screening for, 304t
　hematuria caused by, 230
　hypercalcemia associated with, 492–493
　lung, evaluation of, 176
　nonpulmonary, associated with solitary pulmonary nodules
　　(SPNs), 173
　of gastric ulcers, evaluation of, 300
　of solitary pulmonary nodules (SPNs), 171, 174
　pleural effusions caused by, 165t, 166
　risk of, in mediastinal masses, 178
　solitary pulmonary nodules (SPNs) caused by, 172t
　vasculitis associated with, 744
Malignant gammopathy, tests for confirmation of, 401
Mallory-Weiss tears, as a cause of gastrointestinal bleeding, 289, 292
Malnutrition, in nephrotic syndrome, 254
Maltase deficiency, and malabsorption, 309t
Mammography, for evaluation of breast cancer, 415
Management decisions, and diagnostic test outcomes, 5–7
Marasmus, 254
Marfan's syndrome, 71
　and aortic dissection, 62t
　and mitral valve prolapse (MVP), 142
　and secondary osteoarthritis, 698t
　aortic regurgitation (AR) caused by, 135
Marrow disorders. See *Bone marrow disorders.*
MAST. See *Michigan Alcohol Screening Test (MAST).*
Mast cells, pulmonary, activation of, in asthma, 184–185
MAT. See *Multifocal atrial tachycardia (MAT).*
May-Hegglin anomaly, 365t
MBP. See *Myelin basic protein (MBP).*
MCTD. See *Mixed connective tissue disease (MCTD).*
Mean corpuscular volume (MCV), for evaluation of anemia, 349–350
　in alcoholism, 815, 816t

Meckel's diverticula, evaluation of, 296
 with technetium-99m studies, 293
Mediastinal masses, 178–183, 180t, 181t
Mediastinoscopy, for evaluation of mediastinal masses, 182
Mediastinotomy, anterior, for evaluation of mediastinal masses, 182
Mediastinum, definition of, 178
 subdivision and contents of, 179t
Medications. See *Drugs.*
Medullary carcinoma, of breast, 411
Meigs' syndrome, 163t
Melanoma, stage II, 429
Melioidosis, pneumonia associated with, 571t
MEN (multiple endocrine neoplasia), 487t
Meningitis, 629–635
 and HIV, 645
 aseptic, 632–634
  causes of, 633t
  in infectious mononucleosis, 670
 bacterial, 629, 634
  CSF parameters in, 631t
 carcinomatous, CSF parameters in, 631t
 diagnostic approach to, 634–635
 etiologies of, suggested by historical and physical exams, 634t
 fungal, CSF parameters in, 631t
 viral, CSF parameters in, 631t
  pathogens causing, 632–634
  WBC count in, 632
Mental status disturbances, in hypocalcemia, 494
Mental status examination, Folstein, 782t
 for evaluation of delirium, 774
Mesangiocapillary glomerulonephritis, accompanying nephritic
  syndrome, 261
Mesothelioma, malignant, associated with asbestos exposure,
  871–872
Metabolic disorders, acid-base, anion patterns in, 55t
 and constipation, 15t, 17
 pancreatitis associated with, 340
Metabolic myopathies, 808–809
Metabolic studies. See also *Nutrition.*
 for evaluation of coma, 758
 for evaluation of urolithiasis, 274–275
Metal poisoning, nephrotic syndrome in, 253t
Metanephrines, urinary, for evaluation of pheochromocytoma,
  487–488
Metastases, epidural sites of, 406t
 in prostate carcinoma, 420
 solitary lung, 171
 spinal cord compression caused by, 405
Methacholine challenge test, for evaluation of bronchial
  hyperresponsiveness, 874
Methanol, ingestion of, and formic acid, 52
Metyrapone test, for evaluation of glucocorticoid deficiency, 482
MGUS. See *Monoclonal gammopathy of unknown significance
  (MGUS).*
MI. See *Myocardial infarction (MI).*
Michigan Alcohol Screening Test (MAST), 814, 815t
β_2-Microglobulins, level of, associated with AIDS, 641
Microhematuria, 235
 definition of, 229
MID. See *Multi-infarct dementia (MID).*
Migraine, 784, 786
 and hypertension treatment, 35
 clinical features of, 793t
 facial, 786

Migrainous neuralgia, 787
Milk-alkali syndrome, hypercalcemia with, 493
Milkman fractures, 460
Mites, infection by, 605
Mitochondrial myopathies, 809
Mitral regurgitation (MR), acute, 141–142
    and valvular heart disease, 140–142
    auscultation of, 146t
    chronic, 140–141
    in systemic lupus erythematosus (SLE), 720
Mitral stenosis (MS), 138–139
    and hemoptysis, 159
    auscultation of, 146t
Mitral valve prolapse (MVP), 71, 142–143
    auscultation of, 146t
    chest pain caused by, 64t
Mixed connective tissue disease (MCTD), 733
    and ANA, 695
    versus SLE, 722
MM. See *Multiple myeloma (MM)*.
Mobitz type I AV block, *109,* 109–110
Mobitz type II AV block, *110,* 110–111
Molluscum contagiosum, 603
Monoclonal gammopathy, clinical features of, 398t–399t
Monoclonal gammopathy of unknown significance (MGUS), 396
Mortality, associated with hospitalization for gastrointestinal
        bleeding, 289
    cumulative, in congestive heart failure, 77
    for pneumonia, 562
    from bleeding varices, 295
    from colorectal cancer, 330
    from postsurgical pancreatitis, 340
    in adult respiratory distress syndrome (ARDS), 206
    in CUPS, 426
    in esophagoastroduodenoscopy (EGD), 301–302
    in fatty liver of pregnancy, 829
    in Goodpasture's syndrome, 209
    in idiopathic pulmonary fibrosis, 213
    of nonoliguric and oliguric ARF, 239
    of surgery patients with erythrocytosis, 356
    risk of, intravenous pyelograms and, 233
Morton's neuroma, in entrapment neuropathy, 684
Motor response, and evaluation of coma, 744, 754
Mouth ulcers, in IIBD, 327
MPS. See *Myofascial pain syndromes (MPS)*.
MR. See *Mitral regurgitation (MR)*.
MRI. See *Magnetic resonance imaging (MRI)*.
MS. See *Mitral stenosis (MS); Multiple sclerosis (MS)*.
Mucosal lesions, in Reiter's syndrome, 713
Mucus plugging, in asthma, 184
Multifocal atrial tachycardia (MAT), *97,* 97–98
Multi-infarct dementia (MID), 776–778, 779t
Multiple endocrine neoplasia (MEN), 487t
Multiple myeloma (MM), 396–402
    and hyponatremia, 39, 41
    and nephrotic syndrome, 254
    diagnostic approach to, 402
    differential diagnosis of, 396–397
    osteoporosis accompanying, 454
    risk of AML following treatment for, 383
    symptoms of, 397, 400
Multiple sclerosis (MS), clinical features of, 800–801
    diagnostic approach to, 801–803
    differential diagnosis of, 802

Multiple sclerosis (MS) (*continued*)
  epidemiology of, 799–800
  versus systemic lupus erythematosus (SLE), 722
Murmur, in acute mitral regurgitation, 141
  in aortic regurgitation (AR), 136, 138
  in aortic stenosis (AS), 135
  in mitral regurgitation, 140, 141
  in mitral stenosis (MS), 139
  in mitral valve prolapse (MVP), 142
  in pulmonic regurgitation (PR), 149
  in pulmonic stenosis (PS), 149
  in tricuspid regurgitation (TR), 144
  in tricuspid stenosis (TS), 143
Muscular dystrophies, 810t
Musculoskeletal disorders. See also specific disorders, e.g.,
    Osteoarthritis.
  chest pain in, 60t, 71
  in systemic lupus erythematosus (SLE), 718
  pain in, diagnostic approach to, 686–688
  symptoms of, in scleroderma, 734
Musculoskeletal system, in Lyme disease, 664t, 666
Musset's sign, 136
MVP. See *Mitral valve prolapse (MVP).*
Myalgias, 675–688
  disorders characterized by, 676t–677t
  in dermatomyositis (DM)/polymyositis (PM), 728
  in infectious mononucleosis, 669
  in systemic lupus erythematosus (SLE), 718
Myasthenia gravis, myopathy in, 808
Mycobacterial infections, and respiratory symptoms, in
    HIV-positive patients, 647
  septic arthritis associated with, 624
Mycobacterium avium-intracellulare, diarrhea caused by, in
    HIV-positive patients, 643
  infection with, as AIDS indicator, 640t
  similarity of, to tuberculosis, 575
Mycobacterium kansasii infection, similarity of, to tuberculosis, 575
Mycobacterium tuberculosis, 574–578
Mycoplasma pneumoniae, diagnostic tests for, 568t
  pneumonia caused by, 567–568
  symptoms of, 568t
Myelin basic protein (MBP), in CSF, for evaluation of multiple
    sclerosis, 801
Myelitis, transverse, in infectious mononucleosis, 670
Myelography, for evaluation of spinal cord compression, 408
Myeloproliferative syndromes, and risk of leukemia, 383
Myelotoxicity, associated with benzene exposure, 875
Myocardial disease, primary, simulating MI on ECG, 121t
Myocardial infarction (MI), 62t, 116–133
  acute inferior diaphragmatic left ventricular, *127*
  and respiratory failure, 170
  cardiac enzymes in, 128–130
  chest pain in, 59, 64t, 70, 118
  clinical evaluation of, *132,* 132–133
  differential diagnosis of, 117, 117t
  echocardiography for diagnosis of, 130–131
  Killip classification for, 119t
  non–Q-wave, ECG evaluation of, 122
  Q-wave versus non–Q-wave, 117t
  silent (atypical presentation), 118–119, 118t
Myocardial ischemia, 59
Myocardial workload and contractility, and congestive heart failure,
    79t
Myofascial pain syndromes (MPS), 676t, 686

Myoglobinuria, in carnitine palmitoyl transferase deficiency, 809
  positive urine dipstick tests in, 229
Myonecrosis, following skin infections, 593
Myopathy, 807–811
  diagnostic approach to, 809–810
  differential diagnosis of, 807–809
  inherited, 810t
Myositis, connective tissue diseases associated with, 729t
  in systemic lupus erythematosus (SLE), 718
Myotonic disorders, 808
Myringotomy, for diagnosis of otitis, 553
Myxedema, with hypothyroidism, 465
Müllerian dysgenesis, 446
  amenorrhea caused by, 443, 444t

Narcotics, and chronic pancreatitis, 340
National Cholesterol Education Program (NCEP), 512
National Committee on Detection, Evaluation and Treatment of
        High Blood Pressure (JNC), 32, 33t
National Council on Alcoholism, definition of alcoholism by, 812
National Polycythemia Vera Study Group, 359
NCEP. See National Cholesterol Education Program (NCEP).
NCVs. See Nerve conduction velocities (NCVs).
Negative predictive value (NPV), 4–6
Neisseria gonorrhoeae, diarrhea caused by, in HIV-positive
        patients, 643–644
  infection by, 594–595
  septic arthritis associated with, 623
Neisseria meningitidis, infection by, 629, 630, 630t
Neoplasms, arthralgias or myalgias in, 677t
  as cause of gastrointestinal bleeding, 290, 291
  fever associated with, 542
  fever of unknown origin (FUO) accompanying, 534t–535t
  intrathoracic, chest pain caused by, 60t
  lymphadenopathy associated with, 374, 376t
  solitary pulmonary nodules caused by, 172t
Nephritic syndrome, 257–263
  diagnostic features of, 258–259, 259t
  diseases associated with, 260t
Nephritis, hereditary (Alport's syndrome), 231t
  urinalysis results in, 241t
Nephrocalcinosis, versus urolithiasis, 264
Nephrolithiasis, 264–275
  and chronic gout, 702
  and hypercalcemia, 492
Nephropathy, heroin, 252
  IgA, and chronic renal failure (CRF), 246
     hematuria caused by, 230
  IgG-IgA (Berger's disease), 262
Nephrotic syndrome, 251–255
  associated with nephritic syndrome, 261
  differential diagnosis of, 252–253
  epidemiology of, 252
  prevalence of primary glomerular disease in, 252t
  proteinuria in, 251
  secondary, causes of, 253t
  with multiple myeloma, 400
Nephrotoxicity, associated with solvent exposure, 875
Nerve conduction velocities (NCVs), for evaluation of myopathy, 807
  for evaluation of polyneuropathies, 805
  in evaluation of entrapment neuropathy, 682
Nervous system, involvement of, in sarcoidosis, 219t

Neuritis, optic, in multiple sclerosis, 800
Neurodegenerative disease, differentiation of, from multiple
    sclerosis, 802
Neurologic disorders, and constipation, 16t, 17
    in hypocalcemia, 494
    in systemic lupus erythematosus (SLE), 723t–724t
Neurologic symptoms, in spinal cord compression, 407–408, 409
    in systemic lupus erythematosus (SLE), 720
Neurologic system, involvement of, in Lyme disease, 664t, 666
Neuromuscular disorders, and constipation, 17, 18
Neuropathy, arthralgias or myalgias in, 676t–677t
    entrapment, 682–684
    peripheral, in renal failure, 247, 249
Neuropsychologic testing, 781–782
Neurotoxicity. See also *Toxicity; Toxins.*
    of organic solvents, 874–875
NGU. See *Nongonococcal urethritis (NGU).*
NHL. See *Non-Hodgkin's lymphoma (NHL).*
Niemann-Pick disease, 374
Nipple discharge, breast cancer and, 413, 415
Nitrite test, for evaluation of urinary tract infections, 613–614
Nitrogen balance, calculation of, 530
Nodules, 463t
    pulmonary, solitary, 171–177
    thyroid, 470, 472
        and risk for malignancy, 470t, 471
Nongonococcal urethritis (NGU), 598–599
Non–Hodgkin's lymphoma (NHL), 389–390
    classification of, 390t
    extranodal disease in, 392
    in Class IV HIV-associated illness, 639
Nonparoxysmal supraventricular arrhythmias, 99–102, *100, 101*
Nosocomial infections, of urinary tract, 612
NPV. See *Negative predictive value (NPV).*
Nursing home patients, pneumonia among, 572t
Nutrients, absorption sites of, 523t
    deficiencies of, clinical signs of, 528t–529t
Nutrition. See also *Diet; Vitamin deficiencies.*
    and activation of tuberculosis, 574
    and anemia, 348t
    and folate deficiency, 351–352
    and osteomalacia, 456–457
    and polyneuropathies, 806
    assessment of, 519–530
    defects of carbohydrate metabolism and, 808–809
    defects of lipid metabolism and, 809

OA. See *Osteoarthritis (OA).*
Obesity, as risk factor for diabetes mellitus type II, 502
    as risk factor for myocardial infarction, 117
    as risk factor for osteoarthritis, 697
    in idiopathic hirsutism, 439
OCBs. See *Oligoclonal bands (OCBs).*
Occupational disorders, 866t
    associated with solvent exposure, 874–875
Occupational medicine, 865–875
    diagnostic approach to, 868–869
    principles of, 865–869
Occupational risks, environmental, for pneumonia, 571t
    for alcoholism, 813
    for extrinsic allergic alveolitis, 210
    for hypersensitivity pneumonitis, 211t
    for osteoarthritis, 697

Occupational risks (*continued*)
  for solitary pulmonary nodules (SPNs), 173
  for urologic cancer, 230
Oculocephalic reflex, for evaluation of coma, 754
Oculovestibular reflex, for evaluation of coma, 754
OGTT. See *Oral glucose tolerance test (OGTT)*.
17-OHP. See *17-Hydroxyprogesterone (17-OHP)*.
Oligoarticular arthritis, with psoriatic arthritis, 714
Oligoclonal bands (OCBs), in CSF, for evaluation of multiple
    sclerosis, 801
Oliguria, in nephritic syndrome, 258
Ophthalmopathy, in Graves' disease, 469
Ophthalmoplegic migraine, 786
Oral glucose tolerance test (OGTT), 505, 509t
Oral ulcers, in systemic lupus erythematosus (SLE), 723t
Orbital cellulitis, 557–558
Orthodromic reciprocating tachycardia (ORT), 107
Osler's maneuver, for evaluation of pseudohypertension, 33
Osler's nodules, in infectious endocarditis, 585–586
Osmolal gap, 52
Osmolality, serum, and hyponatremia, 41
  urinary, in acute renal failure, 242t, 243
Osteoarthritis (OA), arthralgias or myalgias in, 676t
  associated with Wilson's disease, 854
  diagnostic approach to, 700
  differential diagnosis of, 699–700
  epidemiology of, 697–698
  secondary, 698t
  versus CPDD, 707t
  versus rheumatoid arthritis, 699–700
Osteodystrophy, renal, 247, 249, 457
Osteomalacia, 456–460
  classification of, 457t
  diagnostic approach to, 460
  differential diagnosis of, 456–458
  in nephrotic syndrome, 254
  oncogenic, 458
  phosphate-related, 457t, 458
Osteomyelitis, anaerobic, 625
  clinical features of, 624–625
  contiguous focus of infection in, 624–625
  diagnostic approach to, 628
  epidemiology of, 623
  hematogenous infection in, 624
  vascular insufficiency associated with, 625
Osteonecrosis, arthralgias or myalgias in, 677t
  magnetic resonance imaging (MRI) for evaluation of, 688
Osteopenia, 455–456, 456t
  vertebral, 455–456, 456t
  with hypercortisolism, 475, 475t
Osteoporosis, 453–456
  arthralgias or myalgias in, 677t
  classification of, 454t
  differential diagnosis of, 453–454, 454t, 456–458, 456t
  risk factors for, 455t
Osteosclerosis, 458
Otitis, 552–554
  diagnostic approach to, 553–554
  epidemiology of, 552
  etiology and clinical manifestations of, 552–553
Outflow tract abnormalities, amenorrhea caused by, 443
Outpatient setting, chest pain/angina in, 59
  diagnosis in, 7–8
  prevalence of fatigue seen in, 9

Ovaries, cancer of, and screening for colorectal cancer, 335
    clinical findings in amenorrhea and, 446–447
    cysts of, diagnosis of, 285
    polycystic. See *Polycystic ovary (PCO) syndrome.*
    premature failure of, and amenorrhea, 447
    tumors of, 445t
        testosterone-secreting, 437
Overlap syndrome, 733
Oxygen demand, and dyspnea, 155
Oxygenation, tissue, and acidosis, 52

P waves, for evaluation of arrhythmias, 87–88
    in atrial premature beats, 94
    in AV nodal reciprocating tachycardia (AVNRT), 94
    in ectopic atrial tachycardia (EAT), 96, 97
    in idioventricular rhythm (IVR), 103
    in junctional premature beat (JPB), 100
    in Mobitz type II AV block, 110–111
    in multifocal atrial tachycardia, 97–98
    in sinus arrest, 93
    in torsades de pointes, 106
    in ventricular fibrillation (VF), 105
    in ventricular premature beat (VPB), 102–103
    in ventricular tachycardia, 104–105
    in wandering atrial pacemaker, 95–96
    retrograde, in junctional rhythm, *101,* 101
Pacemaker, wandering atrial, 95–96, *96*
Paget's disease, and secondary osteoarthritis, 698t
    arthralgias or myalgias in, 677t
    low back pain in, 406t
    with breast cancer, 411
Pain. See also *Chest pain.*
    abdominal, 279–288
        and differential diagnosis of pancreatitis, 337
        causes of, 279t–282t
        differential diagnosis of, 279–285
        in chronic pancreatitis, 340
        in colorectal cancer, 332
    and breast cancer, 413
    back, in cancer patients, 405
        in osteoporosis, 455
    bone, in multiple myeloma, 397
        with chronic leukemia, 385
        with osteomalacia, 458–459
    central back, in multiple myeloma, 407
    chest. See *Chest pain.*
    gastrointestinal bleeding and, 292
    head, in sphenoid sinusitis, 557
    in acute pancreatitis, 340
    in multiple sclerosis, 801
    in osteomyelitis, 624
    in peptic ulcer disease, 300
    in tendinitis, 680
    in urolithiasis, 266
    low back, causes of, 406t
    referred, 286
    relief of, and diagnosis, 70
    with pleural effusions, 163
Palpitations, 85
Palsy, progressive supranuclear, in Parkinsonism, 778
PAN. See *Polyarteritis nodosa (PAN).*

Pancreas, evaluation of exocrine function of, 320
  insufficiency of, and chronic diarrhea, 21
    and malabsorption, 307t
    effects of, on appetite, 306
Pancreatic islet, carcinoma of, 474
Pancreatitis, 337–344
  abdominal pain with, 287
  acute, diagnostic approach to, 343–344
    hypocalcemia associated with, 496
  and fatty diarrhea, 24
  as cause of acute renal failure, 236
  associated with choledocholithiasis, 858, 859
  body posture in, 286
  chest pain caused by, 68t
  chronic, diagnostic approach to, 344
  clinical findings in, 341t
  conditions associated with, 339t
  differential diagnosis of, 337–340
  epidemiology of, 337
  in systemic lupus erythematosus (SLE), 720
  pleural effusions in, 165t
  postsurgical, 339–440
Pannus-producing arthropathies, 703t
PAP. See Prostatic acid phosphatase (PAP).
Papillary carcinoma, 411
Paraganglioma, immunocytochemistry for evaluation of, 428
Parallel testing strategy, 7
Parapneumonic exudate, 165t
Paraproteins, identification of, in multiple myeloma, 401
Parasites, chronic diarrhea caused by, 21t
  malabsorption due to, 313t
Parathyroid hormone (PTH), and hypercalcemia, 492
  serum levels of, in osteomalacia, 459
Parkinsonism, 778–779
Paroxysmal atrial tachycardia (PAT), 96
Paroxysmal attacks, in pheochromocytoma, 485, 486t
Paroxysmal nocturnal dyspnea (PND), and congestive heart failure, 81t
Partial thromboplastin time (PTT), in secondary hemostasis, 363
PAS. See Periodic acid–Schiff (PAS) reaction.
PAT. See Paroxysmal atrial tachycardia (PAT).
Pathogens, pneumonia-causing, 566
Pathophysiology, of asthma, 184–185
  of congestive heart failure, 78–79
PCO. See Polycystic ovary (PCO) syndrome.
PCP. See Pneumocystis carinii pneumonia (PCP).
PCWP. See Pulmonary capillary wedge pressure (PCWP).
PE. See Pulmonary embolism (PE).
Peak expiratory flow rate (PEFR), for asthma evaluation, 187
Pediculosis pubis, 605
PEEP. See Positive end-expiratory pressure (PEEP).
Pelvic inflammatory disease (PID), 597
  and ectopic pregnancy, 285
  diagnostic approach to, 608
  pain accompanying, 285
Peptic ulcer disease, as cause of gastrointestinal bleeding, 289
  as contraindication to thrombolytic therapy, 120t
  associated with erythrocytosis, 356
  diagnosis of, 283
  endoscopic predictors of further bleeding from, 294t
  pain of, 300
Percutaneous transthoracic needle biopsy, for evaluation of
    mediastinal masses, 182

Perfusion scan, for chest pain evaluation, 74
  for evaluation of acute venous thrombosis, 202
Pericarditis, as complication of uremia, 248
  chest pain caused by, 65t
  in scleroderma, 734
  in systemic lupus erythematosus (SLE), 720
  simulating MI on ECG, 121t
Perinatal morbidity, and gestational diabetes mellitus, 504
Periodic acid–Schiff (PAS) reaction, in pulmonary alveolar
        proteinosis, 215
Periodic paralysis (PP), 808
Peritoneal pain, differentiation of, from urolithiasis, 272t
Peritonitis, body posture in, 286
Peritonsillar abscess, 555
Pernicious anemia, and risk of malignancy, 304t
  diagnosis of, 318
  idiopathic adrenal failure as risk factor for, 479
  Schilling test for diagnosis of, 352
Peroxidase activity test, for diagnosis of hematuria, 229
PET. See Positron emission tomography (PET).
Peutz-Jeghers syndrome, 293
Peyer's patches, associated with lymphomas, 391
PFTs. See Pulmonary function tests (PFTs).
PGL. See Progressive generalized lymphadenopathy
        (PGL).
pH, alkaline, and evaluation of urolithiasis, 273
  and causes of pleural effusions, 166
  in buffer systems, physiological, 48
  monitoring of, for evaluation of esophageal diseases, 299
  stool, 23
  urinary, in hematuria, 229
    in struvite lithiasis, 270–271t
Phalen's sign, 683
Pharyngeal infections, associated with gonorrhea, 595
Pharyngitis, 554–556
  differential diagnosis of, 555–556
  epidemiology of, 555
  in infectious mononucleosis, 668, 669, 670, 670t
Pharyngotonsillitis, 669
Pheochromocytoma, 485–489
  algorithm for diagnosis of, 489
  and Cushing's syndrome, 474
  and high-output heart failure, 78
  and hypertension, 34–35
  clinical features of, 486t
  definition of, 485
  diagnostic approach to, 488–489, 488t
  differential diagnosis of, 486–487, 487t
  epidemiology of, 485
  immunocytochemistry for evaluation of, 428
  screening for, 38
    indications for, 487t
Philadelphia chromosome, in chronic myelocytic leukemia, 382
Phosphate, levels of, in osteomalacia, 459
5-Phosphoribosyl-1-pyrophosphate synthetase, gout associated with,
        705t
Photophobia, in migraine, 786
Photosensitivity, in systemic lupus erythematosus (SLE), 723t
Physical examination, for evaluation of solitary pulmonary nodules
        (SPNs), 174
Pick's disease, 778
PID. See Pelvic inflammatory disease (PID).
Pigeon fancier's disease, 210
PIN. See Prostatic intraepithelial neoplasia (PIN).

Pituitary, adrenocorticotropic hormone (ACTH) suppression in, 479
  amenorrhea caused by disease of, 445t, 447–448
  CT scan for evaluation of, in amenorrhea, 450
  disorders of, associated with malabsorption, 315
  involvement of, in Cushing's syndrome, 473
  tumors of, and amenorrhea, 444t
Plague, pneumonia associated with, 571t
Plasmodia, identification of, and malaria diagnosis, 658–659
  incubation period for, 657t
  life cycle of, *654*, 654–655
  malaria-causing, 653
Plasmodium falciparum, incubation period for, 657t
  chloroquine-resistant, 656
Platelet(s), disorders of, 366t
    in chronic renal failure (CRF), 247, 249
  dysfunctions of, 365
Platelet count, and aggregation studies, 362–363
  in thrombocytopenia, 364
Pleural effusions, 162–166, 165t
  causes of, 163t
Pleurisy, chest pain caused by, 66t
  in systemic lupus erythematosus (SLE), 720
Pleuroscopy, for evaluation of pleural effusions, 166
Plummer-Vinson syndrome, and risk of malignancy, 304t
PM. See *Polymyositis (PM).*
PMF. See *Progressive massive fibrosis (PMF).*
PMR. See *Polymyalgia rheumatica (PMR).*
PND. See *Paroxysmal nocturnal dyspnea (PND).*
Pneumocystis carinii pneumonia (PCP), and respiratory symptoms
      in HIV-positive patients, 647
  as AIDS indicator, 640t
Pneumomediastinum, chest pain caused by, 67t
Pneumonia, 562–573
  alcoholism associated with, 572t
  chest pain caused by, 67t
  community-acquired, 563t, 572t
  diagnostic approach to, 570–573
  environmental factors in, 571t
  epidemiologic categories of, 572t
  etiology of, 562, 562t
    based on presentation, 573t
  hemoptysis caused by, 160
  invasive diagnostic tests for evaluation of, 566t
  Pneumocystis carinii, 640t, 647
  postinfluenzal, 572t
  types of, and epidemiology, 562
  viral, as cause of ARDS, 205
Pneumonitis, chronic interstitial, 208–215
  desquamative interstitial (DIP), 214
  hypersensitivity (extrinsic allergic alveolitis), 210
  in systemic lupus erythematosus (SLE), 720
  lymphocytic interstitial, as AIDS indicator, 640t
  usual interstitial (UIP), 214
Pneumothorax, as complication of bronchoscopy, 176
  as complication of TTNA, 177
  as risk of thoracentesis, 164
  chest pain caused by, 66t
  tension as cause of, 62t
Polyarteritis nodosa (PAN), diagnostic evaluation of, 741
  laboratory evaluation of, 740–741, 740t
  with nephritic syndrome, 261
Polyarthritis, 689–696
  causes of, 691t
  diagnostic approach to, 695–696

Polyarthritis (*continued*)
  epidemiologic characteristics of, 691t
  in systemic lupus erythematosus (SLE), 718
  laboratory features of, 694t
  physical signs of, 693t
  symptoms of, 692t
  with psoriatic arthritis, 714
  with scleroderma, 734
Polyclonal gammopathy, in idiopathic pulmonary fibrosis, 214
Polycystic ovary (PCO) syndrome, 439t
  amenorrhea caused by, 445, 445t, 450
  clinical findings in, with amenorrhea, 447
  hirsutism in, 435, 437
Polycythemia, 355–360
  definition of, 355
  relative, laboratory features of, 357–358
  secondary, 360
Polycythemia vera, 356, 358–359
  diagnostic criteria in, 358t
  risk of AML following treatment for, 383
  symptoms of, 357t
Polymyalgia rheumatica (PMR), 678–679
  associated with temporal arteritis, 739
Polymyositis (PM), 809
  definition of, 728
  differentiation of, from scleroderma, 736
  epidemiology of, 728
Polymyositis-dermatomyositis, as cause of chronic interstitial
      pneumonitis, 213
Polyneuropathies, 804–807
  and myopathy, 808
  clinical features of, 804–805
  diagnostic approach to, 806–807
  differential diagnosis of, 805–806
  motor, 805
  sensory, 805
Polyposis, familial, and colorectal cancer, 331t, 334
      and risk of malignancy, 304t
Polyps, gastric, and risk of malignancy, 304t
Porphyria, polyneuropathies associated with, 806
Porphyrin, bilirubin from, 821
Positive end-expiratory pressure (PEEP), improvement of ARDS
      with application of, 206
Positive predictive value (PPV), 4–6
  of Bernstein test for esophagitis, 298
Positron emission tomography (PET), for evaluation of Alzheimer's
      disease, 778
  for evaluation of Huntington's disease, 779
Posttest likelihoods, 4–6, 6t. See also *Negative predictive value
      (NPV); Probability.*
Potassium. See *Hyperkalemia; Hypokalemia.*
Potassium hydroxide preparation, for evaluation of skin infections, 593
Pott's disease. See *Tuberculous osteomyelitis (Pott's disease).*
PP. See *Periodic paralysis (PP).*
PPD. See *Tuberculin (PPD) test.*
PPV. See *Positive predictive value (PPV).*
PR. See *Pulmonic regurgitation (PR).*
PR interval, in preexcitation syndromes, 107
Predictive values, of diagnostic procedures for jaundice, 825t
  of Monospot test, 671
Preexcitation syndromes, 107–108
Pregnancy, and high-output heart failure, 78
  diabetes mellitus during, 499
  fatty liver of, 829

Premature beats, palpitations caused by, 85

Presyncope, clinical features of, 793t

Pretest likelihood, of coronary artery disease in symptomatic
    patients, 73t

Primaquine, for treatment of malaria, 658

Prinzmetal's angina, 70

Probability, of abnormal test results in a panel, 6–7
  pretest, and diagnostic test results, 6t
    and interpretation of test results, 5–6, 6t

Probability thresholds, of diagnoses, 4

Proctitis, diarrhea associated with, 616
  infectious, in homosexual men, 608–609

Proctocolitis, and diarrhea, in HIV-positive patient, 644

Progestational challenge, for evaluation of amenorrhea, 450

Progressive generalized lymphadenopathy (PGL), and AIDS, 375

Progressive massive fibrosis (PMF), associated with silica exposure,
    872

Prolactin, serum levels of, and amenorrhea, 447, 450
    and hirsutism, 440, 441
    and related abnormal conditions, 451t

Prolactinoma, hirsutism with, 437, 440

Prostate carcinoma, diagnostic approach to, 425, 425t
  localized, 420–425
  pathology of, 424t
  staging of, 421t

Prostatic acid phosphatase (PAP), in prostate carcinoma, 421,
    422

Prostatic intraepithelial neoplasia (PIN), 423–424

Prostatic specific antigen (PSA), in prostate carcinoma, 421

Prostatitis, hematuria caused by, 230
  in Reiter's syndrome, 712

Prosthetic devices, and risk of septic arthritis, 623
  osteoarthritis associated with, 625

Proteases, emphysema related to, 189–190

Protein, concentration of, in exudates, 162
  requirements for, 520

Protein/creatinine ratio. See also *BUN/CREAT ratio*.
  in nephrotic syndrome, 254–255

Proteins, visceral, and nutrition status, 527t

Proteinuria, in glomerulonephritis, 257
  in nephritic syndrome, 258
  in nephrotic syndrome, 251, 254

Prothrombin time (PT), for evaluation of chronic hepatitis, 840,
    855
  for evaluation of hepatomegaly, 831
  in secondary hemostasis, 363

PS. See *Pulmonary stenosis (PS)*.

PSA. See *Prostatic specific antigen (PSA)*.

Pseudocysts, and chronic pancreatitis, 339
  and pancreatitis, 341, 341t
  differentiation of, from pancreatitis, 343

Pseudodementia, caused by depression, 779
  versus dementia, 780t

Pseudofractures, in osteomalacia, 460

Pseudogout, 704–708
  arthralgias or myalgias in, 676t
  as form of CPDD, 704
  characteristics of arthrocentesis fluid in, 626t
  clinical features of, 706
  diagnostic approach to, 708
  differential diagnosis of, 708
  versus osteoarthritis, 699

Pseudohermaphroditism, 443, 446
  amenorrhea caused by, 444t

Pseudohyperkalemia, 45
Pseudohypertension, 32–33
Pseudohypoparathyroidism, hypocalcemia associated with, 496
Pseudomonas aeruginosa, osteoarthritis associated with, 625
Pseudo-osteoarthritis, clinical features of, 706–707
Pseudo-rheumatoid arthritis, clinical features of, 706
Pseudoxanthoma elasticum, gastrointestinal bleeding associated
    with, 293
Psittacosis, pneumonia associated with, 571t
Psoriasis, arthritis associated with. See *Arthritis, psoriatic*.
Psychiatric illnesses, fatigue associated with, 9
Psychosocial concerns, and fatigue, 11
PT. See *Prothrombin time (PT)*.
PTH. See *Parathyroid hormone (PTH)*.
PTT. See *Partial thromboplastin time (PTT)*.
Pulmonary alveolar proteinosis, 214–215
Pulmonary artery pressure, in adult respiratory distress syndrome
    (ARDS), 207
Pulmonary capillary wedge pressure (PCWP), for evaluation of
    CHF, 78
Pulmonary disease, chest pain caused by, 60t
  chronic obstructive, 189–192
    prognosis in, 192
  in scleroderma, 735
  versus congestive heart failure, 77–78
Pulmonary embolism (PE), 63t, 193–197, 370
  chest pain caused by, 67t
  fever associated with, 543
  laboratory findings in, 165t
  physical signs of, 195t
  simulating MI, on ECG, 121t
  symptoms of, 194t
Pulmonary fibrosis, idiopathic, 213–214
Pulmonary function, in hypersensitivity pneumonitis, 212
  in systemic lupus erythematosus (SLE), 720
Pulmonary function tests (PFTs), for diagnosis of sarcoidosis, 223
  for evaluation of asbestosis, 871
  for evaluation of COPD, 191
  for evaluation of sarcoidosis, 221
  for evaluation of scleroderma, 737
Pulmonary hemorrhage, PAN associated with, 741
Pulmonary hypertension, and pulmonic regurgitation (PR), 149
  chest pain caused by, 67t
  in scleroderma, 735
  in systemic lupus erythematosus (SLE), 720
  in systemic sclerosis, 213
  tricuspid regurgitation (TR) associated with, 144
Pulmonary infarction, 194
Pulmonary nodules, solitary, 171–177
  causes of, 172t–173t
  diagnostic approach to, *175*, 175–177
Pulmonary regurgitation (PR), and valvular heart disease, 149
  auscultation of, 148t
Pulmonary stenosis (PS), and valvular heart disease, 145, 149
  auscultation of, 148t
Pupillary response, for evaluation of coma, 753
Purified protein derivative test. See *Tuberculin skin test*.
Purkinje network, arrhythmias and, 86
Pyelography, retrograde, for evaluation of hematuria, 233–234
Pyelonephritis, acute, clinical features of, 612
  diagnostic approach to, 614
  hematuria in, 613
  urinalysis results in, 241t
  white blood cell casts in, 613

Pyogenic bacteria, and respiratory symptoms, in HIV-positive
    patients, 647
Pyrophosphate dihydrate deposition disease (CPDD), gout
    accompanied by, 701
Pyuria, laboratory evaluation of, 613

Q fever, hepatitis associated with, 838
    pneumonia associated with, 571t
Q wave changes, in MI, 123–124, *123*
QRS complex, for evaluation of arrhythmias, 87
    in antidromic reciprocating tachycardia, 108
    in idioventricular rhythm (IVR), 103
    in LAFB, 114
    in LBBB, 113–114
    in LPFB, 115
    in Mobitz type II AV block, 110–111
    in preexcitation syndromes, 107
    in RBBB, 113
    in sinus arrest, 93
    in third-degree atrioventricular block, 111
    in torsades de pointes, 106
    in ventricular fibrillation (VF), 105
    in ventricular premature beat (VPB), 102–103
    in ventricular tachycardia, 105
Quincke's sign, 136
Quinsy, 554, 555

Race/culture, and hypertension, 32
    and incidence of diabetes mellitus, 502
    and osteoporosis, 454, 455t
    and prevalence of IIBD, 324
    and prevalence of prostate carcinoma, 420
    and prevalence of systemic lupus erythematosus (SLE), 718
    and risk for alcoholism, 813
    and risk for ankylosing spondylitis, 710
    and risk for gallstones, 858
    and risk for Gaucher's disease, 830
    and risk for multiple sclerosis, 799
    and risk for polyarthritides, 691t
    and risk for polymyalgia rheumatica, 679
    and risk for sarcoidosis, 217
    and risk for temporal arteritis, 739
    and type of leukemia, 382
Radiation, as leukemogenic agent, 383
Radiation therapy, colitis following, 325
Radiculopathy, clinical features of, 685t
Radiographic studies. See also *Radionuclide imaging; X-ray.*
    for evaluation of ankylosing spondylitis, 711
    for evaluation of colorectal cancer, 333
    for evaluation of congestive heart failure, 82
    for evaluation of gastric disease, 300–301
    for evaluation of gout, 702, 703t
    for evaluation of psoriatic arthritis, 714
    for evaluation of scleroderma, 736
    for evaluation of solitary pulmonary nodules (SPNs), 174
    for evaluation of urolithiasis, 273–274
    to distinguish osteoarthritis from CPDD, 707t
Radioimmunoassay, for evaluation of renal osteodystrophy, 249
Radiologic imaging, for evaluation of spinal cord compression,
    408–409
Radiologic procedures, for evaluation of pneumonia, 566

Radionuclide imaging, chromium-51 labeling, for diagnosis of
     erythrocytosis, 355
  cobalt-labeled cobalamin, 318
  for evaluation of acute renal failure, 244
  for evaluation of fever of unknown origin (FUO), 539–540
  for evaluation of gastric and duodenal disease, 302
  for evaluation of gastrointestinal bleeding, 293
  for evaluation of IIBD, 328
  for evaluation of polyarthritis, 695
  for evaluation of prostate carcinoma, 423
  for evaluation of spinal cord compression, 408
  for myocardial infarction (MI) diagnosis, 131
  gallium-67, for diagnosis of sarcoidosis, 221
    for evaluation of PCP, 650
  iodine-131, for assessment of thyrotoxicosis, 472
    for evaluation of mediastinal masses, 182
  technetium-99m, for evaluation of gallbladder diseases, 860
    for evaluation of RSD, 684
  venographic, 202
Radionuclide ventriculography, 131
Rapidly progressive glomerulonephritis (RPGN), 262
Raynaud's phenomenon, clinical features of, 734
  conditions associated with, 735
  dermatomyositis (DM)/polymyositis (PM) associated with, 730
  in systemic lupus erythematosus (SLE), 719t
RBCs. See *Red blood cells (RBCs)*.
Reciprocating tachycardia, in preexcitation syndromes, 107
Red blood cells (RBCs), abnormalities in, and causes of anemia, 350
  dysmorphic, in hematuria, 232
  in infection by *P. falciparum,* 655
  in nephritic syndrome, 258
  scan of tagged, for evaluation of lower GI bleeding, 293, 295, 296
Reed-Sternberg cells, in Hodgkin's disease, 389
Reflex sympathetic dystrophy (RSD), 684, 686
Reflux disease, diagnosis of, 299
Refsum disease, polyneuropathies associated with, 806
Reiter's syndrome, 711–712
  clinical features of, 712–713
  diagnostic approach to, 713
  epidemiology of, 691t, 712
  incomplete, definition of, 712
  laboratory features of, 694t, 713
  physical signs of, 693t
  polyarthritis in, 690
  symptoms of, 692t
Renal blood flow, cardiac and hepatic causes of diminution of, 236
Renal calculi, 264–275
  composition of, 265t, 274
  frequency of, 265t
  pathogens associated with, 611
  symptoms of, by urinary tract location, 272t
Renal disorders, associated with nephritic syndrome, 259–260, *260,*
    260t
  end-stage, factors accelerating, 246
    in patients with nephritic syndrome, 261
  hypokalemia in, 44
  in systemic lupus erythematosus (SLE), 719–720, 719t, 723t
  risk factors for infection in, 611t
  with scleroderma, 735
Renal failure, acute (ARF), 236–244
  chronic (CRF), 245–249
  hypocalcemia associated with, 496
  osteomalacia associated with, 457–458
  with multiple myeloma, 397, 400

Renal function, and congestive heart failure, 83
    and hypertension, 36
    in hypernatremia and nephrogenic diabetes insipidus, 43
    in systemic lupus erythematosus (SLE), 725
Renal insufficiency, 258
Renal osteodystrophy, 247, 249, 457
Renal tubular acidosis (RTA), and urolithiasis, 268t–269t
Renal vascular disease, and hypertension, 33–34
Renin, levels of, and hyperkalemia, 46
        and hypokalemia, 44
    measurement of, for evaluation of hypertension, 37–38
Renin-angiotensin-aldosterone system, hyperkalemia and, 46
Repolarization, and ST changes in MI, 122, 122–123
Respiratory failure, acute (ARF), 167–170
    in chronic obstructive pulmonary disease (COPD), 191–192
    prognostic clinical indicators in, 169
    symptoms of, in asthma, 186, 188
Respiratory infections, asthma in response to, 186
Respiratory system, evaluation of HIV-associated dysfunction of,
        647–651
    involvement of, in Lyme disease, 665t
Reticulocytes, in evaluation of anemia, 350
    in infection by *P. vivax* and *P. ovale*, 655
Reticuloendothelial system, formation of bilirubin in, 821
Reye's syndrome, CK-MB isoenzyme level in, 131t
Rhabdomyolysis, in acute renal failure, 238t
    in acute tubular necrosis, 240
Rheumatic diseases, and aortic stenosis, 134
    mitral stenosis (MS) caused by, 138
    vasculitis associated with, 743
Rheumatic fever, 554
Rheumatoid arthritis. See *Arthritis, rheumatoid.*
Rheumatoid factor, 695
Rhythms, automatic, 86
    ectopic atrial, 87
    supraventricular, 88–115
Ribonucleoprotein (RPN) titer, in MCTD, 733
Rickets, familial hypophosphatemic, osteomalacia caused by,
        458
Right-bundle-branch block (RBBB), 112, 112–113
Risk factors, contraindicating rectal examination, 349
    for acquired immunodeficiency syndrome (AIDS), 640
    for adult respiratory distress syndrome (ARDS), 205, 205t
    for breast cancer, 412
    for chronic renal failure (CRF), 248
    for colorectal cancer, 330, 335
    for coronary heart disease, 514t
    for HIV, evaluation of, in gastrointestinal bleeding, 292
    for ischemic heart disease, 70
    for myocardial infarction (MI), 116–117
    for pancreatitis, 340–342, 339–342
    for thromboembolism, 193
    for urologic cancer, 230
    for venous thromboembolism, 194t
    in contrast venography, 201
    in management of solitary pulmonary nodules (SPNs), 177
RNP. See *Anti-ribonucleoprotein.*
Roth's spots, in infectious endocarditis, 586
RPGN. See *Rapidly progressive glomerulonephritis
        (RPGN).*
RPN. See *Ribonucleoprotein (RPN) titer.*
RSD. See *Reflex sympathetic dystrophy (RSD).*
RTA. See *Renal tubular acidosis (RTA).*
Rubella, 669

SA. See *Sinoatrial (SA) block*; *Sinoatrial (SA) node.*
Sacroiliitis, and IBD, 715
  in spondyloarthropathies, 709
Salicylate intoxication, alkalosis and, 52
Salivary glands, involvement of, in sarcoidosis, 219t
Salmonella, as cause of diarrhea, 618t
    in HIV-positive patients, 643
  foodborne disease caused by, 616t
  osteomyelitis associated with, 624
Sarcoidosis, 217–224, 374
  algorithm for diagnosis of, 224
  arthralgias or myalgias in, 676t
  clinical features of, 219, 219t
  differential diagnosis of, 218–220, 222t
  history of related disorders in, 220
  hypercalcemia with, 493
  radiographic stages in, 222t
Scabies, 605
Scapuloperoneal dystrophy, 810t
Scarlet fever, as complication of pharyngitis, 554, 555
Schilling test, for chronic pancreatitis, 343
  for evaluation of anemia, 352
  for evaluation of vitamin B_{12} malabsorption, 318
  four-stage, 318t
Schistosomiasis, 839
  hematuria caused by, 230
Scintigraphy, bone, for evaluation of musculoskeletal pain, 688
Scleroderma, 733–737
  and risk of malignancy, 304t
  diagnosis of, 735, 737
  differential diagnosis of, 735–736
  urinalysis results in, 241t
Scleromyxedema, differentiation of, from scleroderma, 736
Sclerosis, systemic, 733–737. See also *Scleroderma.*
    versus systemic lupus erythematosus (SLE), 722
Secretin test, for evaluation of malabsorption, 320
  in chronic pancreatitis, 343
  intravenous, in screening for Zollinger-Ellison syndrome, 302
Seizures, absence, 762
  accompanying multiple sclerosis, 801
  differentiation of, from syncope, 761–762
  evaluation of, in HIV-positive patient, 645–647
  partial, clinical features of, 793t
Sensitivity, of diagnostic procedures, 4–6, 4t, 6t
Sepsis, following skin infections, 593
Septic arthritis, characteristics of arthrocentesis fluid in, 626t
  clinical features of, 623–624
  diagnostic approach to, 627
  epidemiology of, 622–623
  fungal infections associated with, 624
  joint aspiration for evaluation of, 625
Septicemia, 745–746
Serial testing strategy, 7
Serology, for evaluation of arboviral encephalitis, 637
  for evaluation of chronic hepatitis, 855
  for evaluation of dementia, 783
  for evaluation of fever of unknown origin (FUO), 538
  for evaluation of hepatitis, 849, 855
  for evaluation of hepatomegaly, 831
  for evaluation of infectious diarrhea, 620
  for evaluation of infectious mononucleosis, 670–671
  for evaluation of jaundice, 824
  for evaluation of Lyme disease, 667
  for evaluation of lymphadenopathy, 377

Serology (*continued*)
  for evaluation of pneumonia, 564
  interpretation of, for hepatitis B, 848t–849t
Serositis, in systemic lupus erythematosus (SLE), 723t
Serum amylase, associated with gallstones, 859
  for evaluation of abdominal pain, 287
Serum gastrin, for screening for Zollinger-Ellison syndrome, 302
  indications for measuring, 303t
Serum glutamic oxaloacetic transaminase (SGOT), 130
  in hepatitis, 840
Serum glutamic pyruvate transaminase (SGPT) in hepatitis, 840
Serum protein electrophoresis (SPE), for assessment of vasculitis, 740t
  for evaluation of multiple myeloma, 401
Sexual activity, headache associated with, 788
Sexual dysfunction, and hypertension treatment, 35
Sexually transmitted diseases (STDs), 594–609
  algorithm for evaluation and treatment of, in homosexual men, *608*
  classification of, 595t
  diagnostic approach to, 606–609
SGOT. See *Serum glutamic oxaloacetic transaminase (SGOT)*.
SGPT. See *Serum glutamic pyruvate transaminase (SGPT)*.
Sheehan's syndrome, amenorrhea caused by, 445t
  hypothyroidism associated with, 462t
Shigella, as cause of diarrhea, 618t
  in HIV-positive patients, 643–644
  foodborne disease caused by, 616t
Shock, cardiogenic, 63t
SIADH. See *Syndrome of inappropriate antidiuretic hormone (SIADH) secretion*.
Sick sinus syndrome (bradycardia-tachycardia syndrome), 93
Sickle cell anemia, osteomyelitis associated with, 624
Sigmoidoscopy, for diagnosis of IIBD, 327
  for evaluation of colorectal cancer, 334
  for evaluation of gastrointestinal bleeding, 294
  for evaluation of IIBD, 328
  for evaluation of infectious diarrhea, 620
  for evaluation of lower GI bleeding, 295
Silicosis, associated with occupational exposure, 872
Sinoatrial (SA) block, first degree, 90–91, *91*
  second degree, 91–92, *91*
  third degree, 92–93, *92*
Sinoatrial (SA) node, arrhythmias involving, 86
Sinus rhythms, *89*, 89–93, *90*, *93*
Sinus Wenckebach, 91
Sinusitis, 556–558
  diagnostic approach to, 558
  epidemiology of, 557
  frontal, clinical features of, 557
  maxillary, clinical features of, 557
  sphenoid, 557
  types of, and potential complications, 556
Sjögren's syndrome, accompanying systemic lupus erythematosus (SLE), 721
  and ANA, 695
  and interstitial pneumonitis, 209t, 213, 214
  laboratory evaluation of, 740t
  versus systemic lupus erythematosus (SLE), 722
Skin, abnormalities of, in hypocalcemia, 494
  in scleroderma, 734
  in chronic hepatitis, 854
  in Lyme disease, 664t
  in Reiter's syndrome, 712–713

Skin (*continued*)
  in sarcoidosis, 219t
  occupational disorders of, 869
  pigmentation of, in chronic adrenal insufficiency, 481
  rashes on, in infectious mononucleosis, 670
Skin infections, 590–593
  clinical features of, 591–592
  diagnostic approach to, 592–593
  epidemiology of, 590–591
  fungal, clinical features of, 592
  ulceronodular, clinical features of, 592
SLE. See *Systemic lupus erythematosus (SLE)*.
Sleep disturbance, in neuropathy, 687
Small-cell carcinoma, and Cushing's syndrome, 474
  immunocytochemistry for evaluation of, 428
Smoking, and chronic bronchitis, 189
  and chronic cough, 25
  and risk of lung cancer, 192
  and risk of myocardial infarction (MI), 117
  and solitary pulmonary nodules (SPNs), 173
Sodium. See also *Hypernatremia; Hyponatremia*.
  levels of, in nephritic syndrome, 258
  urinary, in acute renal failure, 242t, 243–244
Solitary pulmonary nodules (SPNs). See *Pulmonary nodules, solitary*.
Spastic colon, 19
Specificity, of diagnostic procedures, 4–6, 6t
  of multiple independent tests, 7
SPEP. See *Serum protein electrophoresis (SPE)*.
Spherocytosis, congenital, 350
Spinal cord compression, 405–409
  causes of, by site of primary tumor, 406t
  diagnostic approach to, 409
  differential diagnosis of, 405–408
  in ankylosing spondylitis, 710
Spirometry, for evaluation of asthma, 188
  for evaluation of dyspnea, 156–157
Spleen, involvement of, in sarcoidosis, 219t
Splenic infarcts, fever associated with, 543
Splenomegaly, and anemia, 349
  in chronic myelocytic leukemia, 382
  in infectious mononucleosis, 670t
  in systemic lupus erythematosus (SLE), 719t, 720
SPNs. See *Pulmonary nodules, solitary*.
Spondylitis, in spondyloarthropathies, 709
Spondyloarthropathies, 709–717
  arthralgias or myalgias in, 676t
  diagnostic approach to, 716–717
Sprue, and malabsorption, 311t. See also *Celiac disease*.
Sputum, character of, in pneumonia, 564
  evaluation of, in chronic cough, 25–26
  examination of, for evaluation of hemoptysis, 160
  for evaluation of tuberculosis, 577
ST segment, changes in, in MI, *122–123*
  elevation of, in MI, 124
Staphylococcus, and endocarditis, 583
  coagulase-negative, meningitis caused by, 632
  foodborne disease caused by, 616t
Staphylococcus aureus, as cause of infectious diarrhea, 617t
  meningitis caused by, 630t
  osteomyelitis associated with, 624, 625
  pneumonia caused by, 569
  septic arthritis associated with, 623
Staphylococcus epidermidis, osteomyelitis associated with, 625

Stasis, and risk of DVT, 199t
  and risk of pulmonary embolism, 194t
Status migrainosus, 787
Steatorrhea, 19
  and chronic diarrhea, 21
  and chronic pancreatitis, 340
  with malabsorption, 316–317
Stein-Leventhal syndrome, 435, 437
Stiffness, and musculoskeletal pain, 686–687
Still's disease, arthralgias or myalgias in, 676t
  prolonged fever accompanying, 537t
Stool, blood in, and colorectal cancer, 332
    and IIBD evaluation, 327, 328
  character and frequency of, in malabsorption, 315
  examination and culture of, in HIV-positive patient, 644
    in infectious diarrhea, 620
  fat levels in, in pancreatitis, 343
Storage disease, and lymphadenopathy, 374
Storage pool deficiency, platelet aggregation studies for evaluation
    of, 362
Strain gauge plethysmography (SGP), for evaluation of acute venous
    thrombosis, 201
Streptococci, osteomyelitis associated with, 624
  penicillin-sensitive, and endocarditis, 582–583
Streptococcus pneumoniae, diagnostic tests for, 567t
  meningitis caused by, 629, 630, 630t
  pneumonia caused by, 566
Stress, and angina, 71
  and glucocorticoid deficiency, 481
  metabolic, and risk of urolithiasis, 264–265
  urinary incontinence related to, 30t
Stress testing, for evaluation of syncope, 766
Stroke, as complication in MI, 120
  classification of, 794t
  clinical features of, 796t
  differentiation of, from multiple sclerosis, 802
  evolving or completed, 793
    clinical features of, 795
    diagnostic approach to, 797–798
    laboratory studies of, 797
Subendocardial infarction, 123, 116, 123
Sucrase deficiency, and malabsorption, 309t
Supraventricular arrhythmias, accompanying preexcitation, 107
Supraventricular rhythms, 88–115
Supraventricular tachycardias (SVT), 94–98, 94–99
Surface marker test, for evaluation of leukemia, 386
SVT. See Supraventricular tachycardias (SVT).
Syncope, 761–768
  causes of, 763t–764t
  diagnostic approach to, 767–768
  differential diagnosis of, 761–764
  laboratory evaluation of, 765
Syndrome of inappropriate antidiuretic hormone (SIADH) secretion,
    hyponatremia in, 40, 41–42
Synovial fluid analysis, for assessment of gout, 702
  for evaluation of CPDD, 707
Syphilis, 597–598
  and diarrhea, in HIV-positive patient, 644
  clinical features of genital ulcers in, 602t
  false positive test for, in SLE, 725
  in HIV-seropositive population, 642
  liver function in, 838
Systemic disorders, associated with nephritic syndrome, 259, 260t
  polyneuropathies associated with, 806

Systemic lupus erythematosus (SLE), 231t, 374, 718–727
    antinuclear antibody (ANA) test for, 695
    as cause of chronic interstitial pneumonitis, 212
    classification of, 723t–724t
    clinical features of, frequency of, 719t
    diagnostic approach to, 726–727
    differential diagnosis of, 721–722
    epidemiology of, 691t
    laboratory features of, 694t, 721t, 725–726
    physical signs of, 693t
    polyarthritis in, 690
    symptoms of, 692t
    with nephritic syndrome, 259
Systemic sclerosis, 733–737. See also *Scleroderma.*
    as cause of chronic interstitial pneumonitis, 212–213
Systolic murmurs, differential diagnosis of, 150
Sézary syndrome, 390

T waves, changes in, in MI, 123, *123, 124*
Tachycardia, antidromic reciprocating (ART), 107–108
    defined, 87
    in acute aortic regurgitation (AR), 137
    in acute respiratory failure, 168
    orthodromic reciprocating (ORT), 107
    reciprocating, 107
    reentrant (reciprocating), 86
    supraventricular, 94–99
    ventricular, 87, 103–105, *105*
    versus nonparoxysmal supraventricular arrhythmias, 99–100
    wide complex, etiology of, 88t
Tachypnea, with pulmonary embolism, 195t
Takayasu's arteritis, 33, 738
TBBX. See *Transthoracic bronchoscopic biopsy (TBBX).*
TBG. See *Thyroxine-binding globulin (TBG).*
TBL. See *Transbronchial lung (TBL) biopsy.*
T-cell analysis, for evaluation of acquired immunodeficiency
        syndrome (AIDS), 641
    for evaluation of HIV-positive patient, 642
T-cell subsets, for evaluation of fever in HIV-positive patient, 645
TDT. See *Deoxynucleotidyl transferase (TDT).*
Technetium-99m scan, 131
    for evaluation of gallbladder diseases, 861
    for evaluation of gastric and duodenal disease, 302
    for evaluation of gastrointestinal bleeding, 293
    for evaluation of hepatomegaly, 832
    for evaluation of osteomyelitis, 627
Telangiectasia, as a cause of gastrointestinal bleeding, 289
    hereditary hemorrhagic, 292
Tendinitis, 680, 682
Tensilon test (edrophonium IV injection), for evaluation of
        esophageal diseases, 299
    for evaluation of myasthenia gravis, 808, 810
Tensynovitis, volar flexor, 680
Teratomas, benign cystic, and amenorrhea, 447
Testosterone, deficiency of, and osteoporosis, 454
    ovarian neoplasms as source of, 437
    serum levels of, and hirsutism, 440
Tetany, in hypocalcemia, 494
TG. See *Triglycerides (TG).*
Thalassemia, diagnosis of, 353
Thallium-201 imaging, 131
    for chest pain evaluation, 74

Thermography, for evaluation of breast cancer, 416
Thiazide provocation test, for evaluation of hypercalcemia, 492
Thoracentesis, for evaluation of pleural effusions, 164
Thoracic CT, for evaluation of mediastinal masses, 181
Thoracotomy, for evaluation of mediastinal masses, 182
    for small-cell and non–small-cell carcinomas, 171
Thrombin time (TT), in secondary hemostasis, 364
Thromboangiitis obliterans, 745
Thrombocytopenia, 364, 365t
    and causes of hemostasis, 362
    associated with leukemia, 384
    immune, associated with CLL, 385
    in systemic lupus erythematosus (SLE), 721t, 725
Thromboembolism, risk factors for, 193, 194t
Thrombolytic therapy, for myocardial infarction (MI), 120, 120t
Thrombophlebitis, in systemic lupus erythematosus (SLE), 720
    superficial, 200
Thrombosis, 369–373
    acquired conditions with increased risk for, 372t
    acute venous, 198–203
        differential diagnosis of, 200t
        untreated, 199t
    associated with erythrocytosis, 356
    cavernous sinus, complications of, 558
    congenital conditions predisposing to, 370–372
    deep venous. See *Deep venous thrombosis (DVT)*.
    lupus anticoagulant associated with, 369
    renal vein, in systemic lupus erythematosus (SLE), 720
        nephrotic syndrome as cause of, 254
    venous sinus, clinical evaluation of, 796
Thrombotic thrombocytopenic purpura (TTP), 352
Thymoma, and Cushing's syndrome, 474
Thyroid. See also *Graves' disease*; *Goiter*; *Hashimoto's thyroiditis*;
        Hyperthyroidism; *Hypothyroidism*.
    diseases of, 461–472
    function of, and amenorrhea, 447
        in nephrotic syndrome, 255
    medullary cancer of, and Cushing's syndrome, 474
Thyroid disease, diagnostic approach to, 471–472
    epidemiology of, 465–466
Thyroid function tests, 461, 464t
    for evaluation of hypothyroidism, 467
    for evaluation of mediastinal masses, 183
Thyroid stimulating hormone (TSH), for evaluation of thyroid
        disease, 471–472
Thyroid storm, 468
Thyroiditis, 462t
    clinical features of, 469–470
    subacute, 463t, 467–468
    thyroid function tests for, 471
Thyroid-stimulating hormone (TSH), 461, 463
Thyrotoxicosis, 467–471
    and high-output heart failure, 78
    classification of, 462t
    diagnostic approach to, 471
    differential diagnosis of, with iodine-131, 465
    epidemiology of, 468
    hypercalcemia with, 493
    hypokalemia associated with, 44
    laboratory features of, 470
Thyrotropin-releasing hormone (TRH), levels of, in thyroid disease,
        463, 465
    use of, in stimulation test for diagnosis of thyroid disease,
        471–472

Thyroxine (T$_4$), in thyroid disease, 461

Thyroxine-binding globulin (TBG), 461

TIAs. See *Transient ischemic attacks (TIAs)*.

Ticks, transmission of Lyme disease by, 662

Tietze's syndrome, 71
  and chest pain, 69t

Tinel's sign, in entrapment neuropathy, 683

TLC. See *Total lung capacity (TLC)*.

Todd's paralysis, 762

Torsades de pointes, 87
  ventricular arrhythmias in, 105–106, *106*

Total lung capacity (TLC), for evaluation of COPD, 191

Toxic materials, acute renal failure caused by, 238

Toxic reactions, to aluminum, 247

Toxicity, and dosage, in occupational exposure, 865

Toxin assay, for evaluation of infectious diarrhea, 620

Toxins, as cause of dementia, 781
  as cause of tubular necrosis, 240
  environmental, and development of MS, 799
  gastrointestinal bleeding caused by, 292
  myopathy caused by, 809
  nephrotic syndrome caused by, 253t
  organic solvents as, 874
  reversible polyneuropathies associated with, 806

Toxoplasmosis, and HIV, 645–646
  CNS, as AIDS indicator, 640t
  differentiation of, from infectious mononucleosis, 669

TR. See *Tricuspid regurgitation (TR)*.

Tracheobronchial tree, hyperresponsiveness of, 184

Transaminases, elevation of, in hepatitis, *845*
  for evaluation of chronic hepatitis, 854
  levels of, in acute hepatitis, 824
    in alcoholic hepatitis, 852

Transbronchial lung (TBL) biopsy, for evaluation of sarcoidosis, 221–222

Transfer-RNA synthetases, antibodies against, in polymyositis (PM), 731

Transfusions, fever caused by, 543

Transient ischemic attacks (TIAs), clinical features of, 793, 793t, 795
  diagnostic approach to, 797
  in carotid or vertebrobasilar territories, 792, 795t
  laboratory studies of, 796–797

Transmural infarction, 116

Transrectal ultrasound (TRUS), for evaluation of prostate carcinoma, 423, 424t

Transthoracic bronchoscopic biopsy (TBBX), 176

Transthoracic needle aspiration (TTNA), 176–177

Transudates, differential diagnosis of, 162–163, *163*
  pleural effusions defined as, 162

Transurethral resection of prostate (TURP), 421

Trauma, abdominal, and acute pancreatitis, 338–339
  and pulmonary embolism, 194t
  headache associated with, 788

Treponema pallidum. See *Syphilis*.

TRH. See *Thyrotropin-releasing hormone (TRH)*.

Tricuspid regurgitation (TR), 144
  auscultation of, 148t

Tricuspid stenosis (TS), 143
  auscultation of, 147t

Trifascicular block, 115

Triglycerides (TG), levels of, in hyperlipidemia, 512

Triiodothyronine (T$_3$), in thyroid disease, 461

Triolein breath test, for fat malabsorption, 317–318

Trisomy 21 (Down's syndrome), and risk of leukemia, 383
   gout associated with, 705t
Tropical infectious disease, incubation periods for, 657t
Trousseau's sign, in hypocalcemia, 494
   in malabsorption, 315–316
TRUS. See *Transrectal ultrasound (TRUS)*.
Trypanosomiasis, identification of, 658
TS. See *Tricuspid stenosis (TS)*.
TSH. See *Thyroid-stimulating hormone (TSH)*.
T-suppressor lymphocytes, in hypersensitivity pneumonitis, 212
TT. See *Thrombin time (TT)*.
TTNA. See *Transthoracic needle aspiration (TTNA)*.
TTP. See *Thrombotic thrombocytopenic purpura (TTP)*.
Tuberculin (PPD) skin test, 574
   and type of tuberculosis, 575–576
   cross-reactivity with nontuberculous mycobacteria in, 577
   for evaluation of fever of unknown origin (FUO), 537
   for evaluation of HIV-positive patient, 642
Tuberculosis, 574–578
   abdominal, 575–576
   adrenocortical insufficiency caused by, 479
   bone and joint, 576
   diagnostic approach to, 578
   epidemiology of, 575
   genitourinary, 576
   laryngeal, 576
   lymph node, 576
   massive hemoptysis caused by, 159t
   meningeal, 575
   miliary, 576
   pericardial, 576
   pleural effusions in, 165t
   tests for, in evaluation of hemoptysis, 160
Tuberculous meningitis, CSF parameters in, 631t
Tuberculous osteomyelitis (Pott's disease), 624
Tubular disease, chronic renal failure (CRF) in, 246
Tularemia, pneumonia associated with, 571t
Tumor fever, 542
Tumor lysis syndrome, 241t
Tumors, hepatic, hepatomegaly associated with, 830
   pancreatic, and watery diarrhea, 24
   polyneuropathies associated with, 806
   resectable, as cause of dementia, 781
   virilizing, and hirsutism, 439
Turner's syndrome, 446
   amenorrhea caused by, 443, 444t
TURP (transurethral resection of prostate), 421
Tuttle test, for short-term pH monitoring, 299
Twin studies, of diabetes mellitus type I, 499
   of diabetes mellitus type II, 502
   of IIBD, 324
   of leukemia, 383
   of multiple sclerosis, 800
Tylosis, and risk of malignancy, 304t
Tympanometry, for diagnosis of otitis, 553
Typhoid fever, jaundice in, 838

UIP (usual interstitial pneumonitis), 214
Ulcerative colitis, and screening for colorectal cancer, 334
   complications in, 326
   definition of, 323
   versus Crohn's disease, 325t

Ulcerative proctitis, 323
Ulcerative skin lesions, definition of, 590
Ulcers, genital, clinical features of, 602t, 606–607, *607*
    mucosal, and infectious diarrhea, 615
Ultrasonic duplex scan, for evaluation of acute venous thrombosis,
        200–201
Ultrasound, abdominal, for evaluation of colorectal cancer, 333
    Doppler, 201
    for evaluation of acute renal failure, 244
    for evaluation of breast cancer, 415
    for evaluation of chronic renal failure (CRF), 249
    for evaluation of gallbladder diseases, 859
    for evaluation of hepatomegaly, 831
    for evaluation of pancreatitis, 343
    for evaluation of pleural effusions, 164
    for evaluation of prostate carcinoma, 423
    for evaluation of Takayasu's arteritis, 738
    for evaluation of urolithiasis, 273–274
    renal, for evaluation of hematuria, 233
UPEP. See *Urine protein electrophoresis (UPEP)*.
Urethritis, in males, 598t, 606, *606*
    in Reiter's syndrome, 712
    nongonococcal (NGU), 598–599
    urinary tract infections associated with, 612
Uric acid, urolithiasis associated with, 270t
Urinalysis, for evaluation of acute renal failure (ARF), 241t
Urinary incontinence, 28–31
    acute versus chronic, 28
    chronic, mechanisms of, 30t
    complications of, 29t
Urinary tract infections, 610–614
    complicated, risk factors for, 611t
    epidemiology of, 612
    hematuria in, 230
    intrinsic, chronic renal failure (CRF) in, 246
    laboratory features of, 613–614
Urine, for evaluation of tuberculosis, 577
Urine output, and diagnosis of hypernatremia, 43–44
Urine protein electrophoresis (UPEP), for evaluation of multiple
        myeloma, 401
Urolithiasis, 264–275
    and renal tubular acidosis (RTA), 268t–269t
    differential diagnosis of, 265
    differentiation of, from peritoneal pain, 272t
    epidemiology of, 265
    stone type and metabolic abnormalities in, 267t–271t
    struvite, 270–271t
    with hematuria, 230
Usual interstitial pneumonitis (UIP), 214
Uterine cancer, and screening for colorectal cancer, 335
Uveitis, acute anterior, in ankylosing spondylitis, 710
    in Reiter's syndrome, 712

V̇A/Q scan. See *Ventilation-perfusion (V̇A/Q) scan*.
Vaginitis, 599–601
    diagnostic approach to, 607
    in Reiter's syndrome, 712
    symptoms and laboratory features of, 600t
    urinary tract infections associated with, 612
Valvular heart disease, 134–151
    auscultation of, 146t–148t
Vanillylmandelic acid (VMA), urinary, for evaluation of
        pheochromocytoma, 487–488

Varices, endoscopy for evaluation of, 295
Vascular congestion, hepatomegaly associated with, 827, 828
Vascular diseases, diagnosis of, 284
   renal, 246
Vascular ectasia, as a cause of gastrointestinal bleeding, 289, 290
Vasculitic syndromes, 738–745
Vasculitis, 738–746
   blood cultures for evaluation of, 740t
   central nervous system involvement in, 741–743
   dementia syndrome associated with, 781
   diagnostic approach to, 746
   diffuse granulomatous, in Wegener's granulomatosis, 215
   drugs associated with, 744t
   HIV-associated, 739t
   hypersensitivity, 743–744
   hypocomplementemic, 744
   in systemic lupus erythematosus (SLE), 720
   laboratory evaluation of, 740t
   topological classification of, 739t
   urinalysis results in, 241t
Vasoactive intestinal peptide (VIP), level of, and watery diagnosis, 24
Vasoconstriction, peripheral, in acute respiratory failure, 168
Vegetative state, definition of, 749
Venography, contrast, for evaluation of DVT, 201
Ventilation-perfusion (Va/Q) scan, for evaluation of pulmonary embolism, 196, 196t
Ventricular arrhythmias, 87, *102*, 102–106, *103, 105, 106*, 108
Ventricular fibrillation (VF), and ventricular arrhythmias, *105*, 105, *106*
Ventricular hypertrophy, simulation of MI on an ECG, 121t
Ventricular premature beat (VPB), and ventricular arrhythmias, *102*, 102–103
Ventricular tachycardia (VT), and ventricular arrhythmias, *103*, 103–105
Vertigo, episodic or positional, clinical features of, 793t
VF. See *Ventricular fibrillation (VF).*
Vibrio parahemolyticus, as cause of infectious diarrhea, 619t
   foodborne disease caused by, 616t
Villous adenoma, 45
Vincent's angina, 669
VIP. See *Vasoactive intestinal peptide (VIP).*
Viral hepatitis, 833–851
Virchow's triad, 193, 198
Virilization, and hirsutism due to elevated androgen levels, 438
   associated with amenorrhea, 447
Virus infections, multiple sclerosis as, 799
Vitamin B$_{12}$, hypokalemia and, 44
Vitamin deficiencies, and chronic, 780
   and hemostatic disorders, 368t
   arthralgias or myalgias in, 677t
   associated with malabsorption, 315
   in anemia, 350–351, 352
   in Crohn's disease, 327
   in osteomalacia, 456–458, 456t
   Schilling test for, 318
Vitamin intoxication, hypercalcemia with, 493
VMA. See *Vanillylmandelic acid (VMA).*
von Willebrand's disease, 365–366, 366t
   acquired, 247t
   tests for, 363
VPB. See *Ventricular premature beat (VPB).*
VT. See *Ventricular tachycardia (VT).*

Waldenström's macroglobulinemia (WM), 396
hyponatremia in, 39
Waldeyer's ring, associated with lymphomas, 391
Water, infectious diarrhea caused by microorganisms in, 615
Watermelon stomach, 290
Weakness, in myopathy, 807
Wegener's granulomatosis, 159t, 215, 231t, 246, 739t, 741–742
chronic interstitial pneumonitis caused by, 209t
laboratory evaluation of, 740t
solitary pulmonary nodules (SPNs) caused by, 172t
with nephritic syndrome, 261
Weight loss, with malabsorption, 306
Weil's syndrome, 838
Wenckebach AV block, 109–110, 109
Wernicke's encephalopathy, 780
Westermark's sign, 196
Western blot analysis, for evaluation of HIV infection, 641
Whipple's disease, biopsy for evaluation of, 320
malabsorption in, 311t
prolonged fever accompanying, 537t
White blood cells (WBC) count, for evaluation of pneumonia, 562.
    See also *Leukemia; Leukocytes; Leukocytosis.*
White matter symptoms, in multiple sclerosis, 800
Wilson's disease, and Fanconi's syndrome, 458
and secondary osteoarthritis, 698t
delirium caused by, 772t
hepatitis associated with, 853
Kayser-Fleischer rings in, 854
neurologic symptoms of, 854
Wiskott-Aldrich syndrome, 365t, 391
WM. See *Waldenström's macroglobulinemia (WM).*
Wolff-Parkinson-White syndrome, 107
simulating MI, on ECG, 121t
Wood's light examination, for evaluation of skin infections, 593
Workplace, criteria for relating environment to disease in, 868–869
types of hazardous exposures in, 867t

Xanthelasma, in hyperlipidemia, 514
Xanthomas, with hyperlipidemia, 514
X-ray, abdominal, for evaluation of abdominal pain, 288
    for evaluation of pancreatitis, 343
chest, in ARDS, 207
    for diagnosis of ARDS, 204
    for diagnosis of lymphomas, 393
    for diagnosis of sarcoidosis, 221
    for evaluation of aortic regurgitation (AR), 137, 138
    for evaluation of aortic stenosis (AS), 135
    for evaluation of asthma, 188
    for evaluation of COPD, 191
    for evaluation of dyspnea, 156
    for evaluation of hemoptysis, 160
    for evaluation of lymphadenopathy, 377
    for evaluation of mediastinal masses, 178, 182
    for evaluation of mitral regurgitation (MR), 140, 141
    for evaluation of mitral stenosis (MS), 139
    for evaluation of pleural effusions, 164
    for evaluation of prostate carcinoma metastasis, 423
    for evaluation of pulmonary embolism, 195–196
    for evaluation of pulmonic regurgitation (PR), 149
    for evaluation of pulmonic stenosis (PS), 149
    for evaluation of respiratory failure, 169

X-ray (*continued*)
    for evaluation of silicosis, 872
    for evaluation of solitary pulmonary nodules (SPNs), 175
    for evaluation of tricuspid regurgitation (TR), 144
    for evaluation of tricuspid stenosis (TS), 143
    for evaluation of tuberculosis, 576–577
    for hypersensitivity pneumonitis, 210
    in Goodpasture's syndrome, 209
    in idiopathic pulmonary fibrosis, 213–214
    in pulmonary alveolar proteinosis, 214
    in Wegener's granulomatosis, 215
    exposure to, as risk factor in leukemia, 383
    for diagnosis of hematuria, 233
    for evaluation of osteoarthritis, 699
    for evaluation of otitis, 553
    for evaluation of septic arthritis, 625
    joint, for evaluation of polyarthritis, 695
    lateral neck, for evaluation of pharyngitis, 556
    skull, for evaluation of headache, 790, 790t
    small bowel, for evaluation of Crohn's disease, 328
        for evaluation of malabsorption, 320

Yellow fever, jaundice in, 838
Yersinia enterocolitica, as cause of infectious diarrhea, 619t
    foodborne disease caused by, 616t

Zollinger-Ellison (ZE) syndrome, 22
    and peptic ulcer disease, 300
    and watery diarrhea, 24
    appearance of, on UGI series, 301
    malabsorption in, 312t
    peptic ulcer disease in, 300
    screening for serum gastrin in, 302